World Headquarters
Jones and Bartlett Publishers
40 Tall Pine Drive
Sudbury, MA 01776
978-443-5000
info@jbpub.com
www.jbpub.com

Jones and Bartlett Publishers Canada
6339 Ormindale Way
Mississauga, Ontario L5V 1J2
CANADA

Jones and Bartlett Publishers International
Barb House, Barb Mews
London W6 7PA
UK

Jones and Bartlett's books and products are available through most bookstores and online booksellers. To contact Jones and Bartlett Publishers directly, call 800-832-0034, fax 978-443-8000, or visit our website, www.jbpub.com.

Substantial discounts on bulk quantities of Jones and Bartlett's publications are available to corporations, professional associations, and other qualified organizations. For details and specific discount information, contact the special sales department at Jones and Bartlett via the above contact information or send an email to specialsales@jbpub.com.

Production Credits
Executive Editor: Kevin Sullivan
Associate Editor: Amy Sibley
Production Director: Amy Rose
Production Editor: Tracey Chapman
Senior Marketing Manager: Emily Ekle
Manufacturing and Inventory Coordinator: Amy Bacus
Composition: Auburn Associates, Inc.
Cover Design: Kate Ternullo
Cover Image: © emin kulyev/Shutterstock, Inc.
Printing and Binding: Courier Westford
Cover Printing: Courier Westford

Library of Congress Cataloging-in-Publication Data
Nursing care of the pediatric surgical patient / [edited by] Nancy Tkacz
  Browne ... [et al.]. — 2nd ed.
    p. ; cm.
  Rev. ed. of: Nursing care of the general pediatric surgical patient /
  edited by Barbara V. Wise ... [et al.]. 2000.
  Includes bibliographical references and index.
  ISBN-13: 978-0-7637-4052-8 (casebound)
  ISBN-10: 0-7637-4052-7 (casebound)
  1. Children—Surgery—Nursing.   I. Browne, Nancy Tkacz.
  II. Nursing care of the general pediatric surgical patient.
  [DNLM: 1. Pediatric Nursing.   2. Perioperative Nursing.   3. Child.
  4. Infant.   WY 161 N97416 2007]
  RD137.N87 2007
  610.73′677—dc22
                            2006025212
6048

Printed in the United States of America
10 09 08 07 06   10 9 8 7 6 5 4 3 2 1

Nursing Care of the Pediatric Surgical Patient

Second Edition

Editors

Nancy Tkacz Browne, MS, RN, CPNP
Division of Pediatric Surgery
University of Illinois at Chicago
Chicago, IL

Laura M. Flanigan, MSN, RN, PNP
Pediatric Nurse Practitioner
Division of Pediatric Surgery
Morgan Stanley Children's Hospital of New York
New York, NY

Carmel A. McComiskey, MS, APRN-BC, CPNP-AC
Pediatric Nurse Practitioner
Division of Pediatric Surgery
University of Maryland Hospital for Children
Baltimore, MD

Pam Pieper, MSN, RN, ARNP, BC
Pediatric Surgery NP/CNS
Division of Pediatric Surgery
University of Florida Health Science Center—
  Jacksonville and Clinical Associate Professor
University of Florida College of Nursing
  Jacksonville, FL

Associate Editors

Jeannette Diana-Zerpa, MSN, RN, ARNP
Miami Children's Hospital
Department of Pediatric Surgery
Miami, FL

Lynne D. Farber, MSN, RN, CPNP
Clinical Instructor Pediatric Surgery
School of Medicine
University of North Carolina, Chapel Hill
Chapel Hill, NC

Frances T. Gill, MSN, RN, CPNP
Coordinator of Advanced Practice
Pediatric General Surgery
Alfred I. DuPont Hospital for Children
Wilmington, DE

Betty R. Kasson, MS, RN, CNS, PNP
Carmel Valley, CA

JONES AND BARTLETT PUBLISHERS
Sudbury, Massachusetts
BOSTON   TORONTO   LONDON   SINGAPORE

Editor Dedications

Laura Flanigan

I would like to express my gratitude to the late Robert E. Gross. While a nursing student at Children's Hospital in Boston, I read his text *The Surgery of Infancy and Childhood* and was spellbound. I knew then where I hoped I would be able to direct my professional life. I will be forever grateful to Dr. Judson Randolph for giving me the opportunity to live my dream and continuing to be an inspiration. Thanks to Dr. R. Peter Altman and Dr. Charles Stolar for giving me the opportunity to practice and always being there when I need them. And, of course, thanks to my husband Dan, who has never begrudged the time and energy that I have devoted to my nursing practice.

Carmel McComiskey

To Jim, Kate, and Molly: I am so blessed to call you my family. To my nursing colleagues at the bedside at the University of Maryland, who work tirelessly every day to heal people's children as if they were their own. Mary Ellen and Rita, my partners, for their faith in my expertise that challenges me to continue to learn. To Katrina, who taught me there is nothing a mother won't learn to do for her children. To the surgeons at the University of Maryland, who pay me to do what I love. To all my APSNA colleagues, whose quest for excellence has changed Pediatric Surgical Nursing.

Pam Pieper

To my parents for teaching me to believe in myself; to Dr. Joe Tepas, my mentor, friend, and partner in pediatric surgery for over 20 years and without whom my career surely would have taken another trajectory; and to my husband, Bob McMichael, for his love and tolerance of my professional escapades; may he understand how much I truly love him.

Nancy Tkacz Browne

To my parents, Marjorie & Albin Tkacz, who instilled in me a sense that if I worked hard enough, I could do anything. To my sister, Betsy, and my nieces, Anna & Laura…for their love, laughter, and the incredible joy that they bring to my life. To Donna, Mary, Deb, & Dave who represent the truest meaning of friendship & loyalty. To Mark & Ai-Xuan for believing and taking a chance. To Albert W. Dibbins who believes that I can be taught anything. . . . Al is my hero, my mentor, and my friend. And to Allen, my husband and partner, whose love defines unconditional support.

Betty Kasson

To Jim, whose emotional and technical support make all things possible. To Dakin and Nancy, Chris and Gina, who make the world a better place. And to Maya, whose small star burns so brightly. I would also like to acknowledge the contributions of my APSNA colleagues who improve the surgical care of children and their families every day.

Jeannette Diana-Zerpa

For my mother who cares for me always, and for my husband, Carlos, and our children who light my life.

Lynne Farber

I would like to acknowledge and thank the outstanding Pediatric Surgery group at UNC: Tim Weiner, J. Duncan Phillips, and Patricia Lange for their insight and numerous edits (and re-edits) of the "tubology" chapter. My sincere appreciation and thanks to Amy Lamm, Bill Adamson, and Dan von Allmen for their support and guidance. Most of all, I would like to acknowledge my wonderful husband, Mark Farber, for his endless patience, surgical expertise, and technical support.

Frances Gill

To my surgical "family" at the Alfred I. DuPont Hospital for Children who consistently demonstrate the art and science of caring for children as if they were their own. Most especially, to Philip J. Wolfson, MD who has been my mentor, my colleague, my editor, and my dearest friend. He has taught me everything I know in Pediatric Surgery with unyielding support and patience. He is my hero. To Christopher Giaquinto, PA-C, who has shown unbelievable fortitude in helping with clinical photography and computer skills extraordinaire! To my APSNA partners who strive to improve the surgical care of children entrusted to us. Lastly, to my beautiful daughter Jill who fills the world with her giving spirit, her wit, and her smile each day. She has given me unconditional love and support throughout this project. She is my angel.

Contributors

Cynthia A. Bishop, RN, MSN, CPNP
Nurse Manager, Surgery MSA
Ambulatory Care Department
J. W. Riley Hospital for Children
Indianapolis, IN

Suzanne Borkowski, MS, PNP, ETN
Formerly, Pediatric Nurse Practitioner at
    Pediatric Surgery and Nursing
Women and Children's Hospital of Buffalo
Buffalo, NY

Caroline Braas, RN, BSN, CCTC
Renal Transplant Coordinator
St. Christopher's Hospital for Children
Philadelphia, PA

Nancy Tkacz Browne, MS, RN, CPNP
Division of Pediatric Surgery
University of Illinois at Chicago
Chicago, IL

Leona Lee Burnham, RN, MSN
Clinical Nurse Specialist Pediatric Surgery
Southern Illinois University School of Medicine
Springfield, IL

Mary Ellen Carter, MSN, RN
Clinical Nurse Specialist, Pediatric Surgery
Division of Pediatric Surgery
J.W. Riley Hospital for Children
Indianapolis, IN

Teri Coha, RN, MSN, APN, CWOCN
Clinical Nurse Specialist
Pediatric Surgery
Children's Memorial Hospital
Chicago, IL

Mary Ellen Connolly, MSN, CPNP
Pediatric Nurse Practitioner
Division of Pediatric Surgery
University of Maryland Medical Center
Baltimore, MD

Jeannette Diana-Zerpa, MSN, RN, ARNP
Department of Pediatric Surgery
Miami Children's Hospital
Miami, FL

Neil Ead, RN, MSN, CPNP
Nurse Practitioner
Division of Pediatric Surgery
Hasbro Children's Hospital
Providence, RI

Lynn E. Fagerman, MSN, APRN-BC, PNP
Pediatric Nurse Practitioner
Developmental Medicine
DeVos Children's Hospital
Grand Rapids, MI

Kathleen Falkenstein, PhD, PNP
Assistant Professor Drexel University
Nurse Practitioner, GI and Transplant
Department of Nursing
St. Christopher's Hospital and Drexel University
Philadelphia, PA

Lynne D. Farber, MSN, RN, CPNP
Clinical Instructor, Pediatric Surgery
School of Medicine
University of North Carolina, Chapel Hill
Chapel Hill, NC

Laura M. Flanigan, MSN, RN, PNP
Pediatric Nurse Practitioner
Division of Pediatric Surgery
Morgan Stanley Children's Hospital of New York
New York, NY

M. Elizabeth Foster, RN, MS, CWOCN
Dallas, TX

Kurt Freer, RN, MSN, CRNP
Nurse Practitioner, Liver Transplant Coordinator
Division of Pediatric Gastroenterology, Hepatology &
    Liver Transplant
St. Christopher's Hospital for Children
Philadelphia, PA

Frances T. Gill, MSN, RN, CPNP
Coordinator of Advanced Practice
Pediatric General Surgery
Alfred I. DuPont Hospital for Children
Wilmington, DE

Kathleen O'Connor Guardino, RN, MSN
Clinical Nurse Specialist
Pediatric Surgery
Schneider Children's Hospital
New Hyde Park, NY

Linda J. Haga, RN, CPN
Nurse Clinician Pediatric Surgery
Children's National Medical Center
Washington, DC

Beverly Bynum Haynes, RN, BSN, CPN
Nurse Clinician Pediatric Surgery
The Children's Hospital of Alabama
Birmingham, AL

Lori J. Howell, RN, MS
Executive Director, The Center for Fetal Diagnosis and
    Treatment
Clinical Associate, University of Pennsylvania School
    of Nursing
Division of General, Thoracic, and Fetal Surgery
The Children's Hospital of Philadelphia
Philadelphia, PA

Betty R. Kasson, MS, RN, CNS, PNP
Carmel Valley, CA

Melanie A. Kenney, RN, MA, CPNP
Research Assistant
Division of Pediatric Cardiology
Children's Hospital of Iowa
University of Iowa Healthcare
Iowa City, IA

Michael J. Kinney, RN, BSN
Renal Nurse Clinician
Department of Nephrology
St. Christopher's Hospital for Children
Philadelphia, PA

Melinda Klar, RN
Clinical Trials Coordinator
Department of Surgery
University of Tennessee Graduate School of Medicine
Knoxville, TN

Kim Knoerlein, ARNP, MS
Advanced Registered Nurse Practitioner
Pediatrics/Neonatology
Dartmouth-Hitchcock Medical Center
Lebanon, NH

Amy W. Lamm, MSN, RN, CPNP
Clinical Instructor Pediatric Surgery Division
University of North Carolina
Chapel Hill, NC

Kathleen M. Leack, RN, BSN
Surgical Nurse Clinician
Children's Hospital of Wisconsin
Milwaukee, WI

Wendy Lord Mackey, APRN, MSN, CORNL
Nurse Practitioner
Pediatric Otolaryngology
Yale University
New Haven, CT

Renee C. B. Manworren, RN, MS, CNS
Pediatric Clinical Nurse Specialist and Clinical
    Manager
Pain Management Team
Children's Medical Center Dallas
Dallas, TX

Carmel A. McComiskey, MS, APRN-BC, CPNP-AC
Pediatric Nurse Practitioner
Division of Pediatric Surgery
University of Maryland Hospital for Children
Baltimore, MD

Kimberly Haus McIltrot, MS, RN, CPNP
Nurse Practitioner, Pediatric Surgery
Division of Pediatric Surgery
Johns Hopkins Hospital
Baltimore, MD

Wendy M. McKenney, MS, ARNP
Neonatal Nurse Practitioner
Intensive Care Nursery
Dartmouth-Hitchcock Medical Center
Lebanon, NH

Lisa Meadows, RN, MSN, APRN, BC
Pediatric Nurse Practitioner
Child Health Advocacy and Outreach
St. Louis Children's Hospital
St. Louis, MO

Susan R. Miesnik, RNC, MSN, CRNP
Perinatal Nurse Practitioner
Division of General, Thoracic, and Fetal Surgery
The Center for Fetal Diagnosis and Treatment
The Children's Hospital of Philadelphia
Philadelphia, PA

Robin Moushey, MSN, RN
Health Education Nurse Specialist
Family Resource Center
St. Louis Children's Hospital
St. Louis, MO

Dorothy M. Mullaney, ARNP, MHSc
Neonatal Nurse Practitioner
Neonatology
Dartmouth-Hitchcock Medical Center
Lebanon, NH

Danuta E. Nowicki, RN, MN, CPNP
Nurse Practitioner, Pediatric Surgery
Division of Pediatric Surgery
Children's Hospital Los Angeles
Los Angeles, CA

Kimberly O'Dowd, RN, MS, CPNP
Pediatric Nurse Practitioner
Division of Pediatric Surgery, University of Illinois
    at Chicago
University of Illinois Medical Center
Chicago, IL

Mary E. Otten, RN, MSN, CPNP
Pediatric Nurse Practitioner
Cincinnati Children's Hospital Medical Center
Cincinnati, OH

Pam Pieper, MSN, RN, ARNP, BC
Pediatric Surgery NP/CNS
Division of Pediatric Surgery
University of Florida Health Science Center—
    Jacksonville and Clinical Associate Professor
University of Florida College of Nursing
Jacksonville, FL

Frances N. Price, RN, MS, CPNP
Nurse Practitioner Pediatric Surgery
Department of Pediatric Surgery
The Children's Hospital
Denver, CO

Susan M. Quinn, RNC, MS, ARNP
Neonatal Nurse Practitioner
Neonatology
Dartmouth-Hitchcock Medical Center
Lebanon, NH

Valerie E. Rogers, MS, RN, CPNP, CWOCN
Doctoral Student
School of Nursing
University of Maryland, Baltimore
Baltimore, MD

Laura E. San Miguel, RNCS, MSN, PNP
Pediatric Nurse Practitioner
Madison, NJ

Jennifer Seigel, RN, CPNP
Pediatric Nurse Practitioner
St. Louis Children's Hospital
St. Louis, MO

Tina Shapiro-Stolar, MSN, ARNP
Formerly, Nurse Practitioner for
    Division of Pediatric Surgery
Miami Children's Hospital
Miami, FL

Judith J. Stellar, MSN, CRNP
Surgery Clinical Nurse Specialist
Department of Nursing
The Children's Hospital of Philadelphia
Philadelphia, PA

Marilyn Miller Stoops, RN, MSN, CNP
Pediatric Nurse Practitioner
Department of Pediatric, General, and Thoracic
    Surgery
Cincinnati Children's Hospital Medical Center
Cincinnati, OH

Kerin L. Worley, RD, LDN, CSP
Pediatric Dietician
Nutrition and Food Services
North Carolina Children's Hospital
Chapel Hill, NC

Kelli B. Young, RN, MSN, CRNP
Surgical Advanced Practice Nurse
Division of General, Thoracic, and Fetal Surgery
The Children's Hospital of Philadelphia
Philadelphia, PA

Beth T. Zimmermann, RN, MS, APRN, CCNS
Advanced Practice Nurse/Clinical Nurse Specialist
Division of Pediatric Surgery
University of Chicago Comer Children's Hospital
Chicago, IL

Preface

We are pleased to present the second edition of *Nursing Care of the General Pediatric Surgical Patient*. Our mission as editors is to provide updated information about current best nursing practice regarding common pediatric surgical conditions. This textbook is designed to both educate and assist the pediatric surgical nurse in providing expert nursing care for children undergoing surgery. By compiling current teaching into one easy reference, we hope to develop the standard by which all pediatric surgical nursing care can be measured.

In this second edition, the editors added information about thoracic problems, bariatric surgery, tube care, and current resources. Authors updated basic knowledge about classic pediatric surgical diagnoses with current strategies shown to improve patient outcomes.

Diagnosis-related teaching tools developed by the authors are now available in English and Spanish. These teaching sheets can be downloaded at www.apsna.org and www.jbpub.com. We permit—in fact, encourage—you to reproduce these teaching sheets for your families. We include two samples of these family teaching sheets on the following pages. All of the teaching sheets follow the same format. We hope these tools will help parents understand their child's illness and prove to be an invaluable resource in your practice.

Teaching Sheets

■ Gastrostomy

What is a gastrostomy?

A gastrostomy is the creation of a new opening into the stomach. A small incision(stoma or opening) is made in the skin and stomach wall. A feeding or gastrostomy tube (G-tube) is inserted into the stomach. This tube delivers the medicine or food necessary for your child to grow or feel better.

Who gets a gastrostomy tube?

Children need gastrostomy tubes if they are born with any medical condition that prevents a child from eating enough and swallowing safely. A child who is premature, who has an abnormal esophagus, chronic lung disease, failure to thrive, short bowel syndrome, or heart disease with poor feeding and growth may need another way to get food and medicine. Children with pseudo-obstruction or other problems moving food from the stomach into the intestines might require a gastrostomy for emptying food or air from the stomach.

How is the decision made that surgery is needed?

Your physician will discuss reasons for the operation with you and will help you decide if your child will benefit from a gastrostomy tube.

What can I expect from surgery?

Children usually gain weight and feel better when they receive needed food and medicine. These improvements may also help them fight off germs and prevent infections.

Tips for the day of surgery—what to bring, what to leave home.

Bring your child's favorite doll or toy to the hospital. Caretakers should wear comfortable clothes and are welcome to stay with their child during the hospital stay.

When will my child be able to go home?

Your child will go home when s/he is comfortable and able to take food and fluids. Before discharge, your nurse will teach you how to care for your child's gastrostomy tube, give feedings, medications, and troubleshoot common problems.

How much time should I plan off work?

Many parents take off approximately two weeks for their child's surgery and recovery at home. We can write a letter to your employer explaining the need for you to be with your child during this time.

What care is needed at home after surgery?

Care of the incision: Wash your hands with antimicrobial soap before touching the gastrostomy area. You may use warm soap and water to gently clean around the gastrostomy site twice a day or as needed. Make sure that you remove all the crusted areas on the skin around the tube. You may use diluted hydrogen peroxide (1/2 peroxide, 1/2 water) and Q-tips to clean the site for the first two weeks. After cleaning, rinse with water and pat dry.

Activity limitations: Your child may participate in all normal activities including lying on his/her stomach as long as the tube is secure so that it will not accidentally be pulled out. Make certain the G-tube is carefully secured under his/her clothing.

Diet: Children will be provided with a nutritional plan before leaving the hospital. Fluids that can be given through the gastrostomy tube are milk, formula and water. Liquid medications or well-crushed pills diluted with liquid may also be given. Always flush the G-tube with water before and after each feeding or medication.

Bathing: For one week following the surgery, your child should avoid swimming or soaking in a bathtub.

Medication: Your physician or nurse practitioner will provide a prescription for pain medication prior to discharge from the hospital. If your child's pain is not controlled on this medication, please call the surgeon.

When should I call the surgery team?

Call with temperature greater than 101F., redness around the G-tube site, an increase in gastrostomy drainage, accidental tube dislodgement, nausea, vomiting, diarrhea, pain uncontrolled by medications prescribed, or any questions or concerns. The postoperative appointment should be scheduled prior to your child's discharge from the hospital.

What should I tell my child's teacher?

When your physician allows your child to return to school, tell your child's teacher and school nurse about your child's gastrostomy. You will want to tell them what to do and whom to call in an emergency. A spare gastrostomy tube or "to go kit" should always accompany your child to school.

What are the long-term consequences?

A gastrostomy will provide the extra nutrition and medicine necessary for your child to reach his or her very best potential in life.

Will this affect growth and development?

Children who are G-tube fed have the same development as other children. They will grow better with the optimum amount of calories the G-tube can deliver.

Is there anything else I need to know to care for my child?

Simply, keeping the gastrostomy site clean and dry, and tension off the site will prevent the majority of complications with a gastrostomy tube. ALWAYS keep a spare tube available, and replace **immediately** if the tube accidentally is pulled out. You are not alone, and only a phone call away if there are new questions or concerns after discharge from the hospital.

Please reproduce and distribute this sheet to your surgery families. This teaching sheet can also be downloaded at www.APSNA.org.

■ Appendectomy

What is appendicitis?

The appendix is a very small, narrow pouch attached to the intestine. Its purpose is not known. Food and stool can get trapped within this "pouch" and cause it to swell and become inflamed or infected. Occasionally other substances can obstruct this pouch and cause the same result. The appendix must be removed before it bursts or "perforates" and spreads the infection within the abdomen.

Who gets appendicitis?

Appendicitis can occur at any age but is most common in children between the ages of 4 and 15 years.

How is appendicitis diagnosed?

Children with appendicitis usually first complain of pain around their umbilicus (belly button) and do not want to eat. The pain gradually moves to the right lower part of the abdomen. There may be nausea, vomiting and a small amount of diarrhea. Some children have a fever but not always.

Your child's doctor will begin by examining your child for other problems that can "look like" appendicitis. They will gently push on your child's abdomen to find the spot that is the most tender. They may ask your child to move around or jump up and down. In some cases, it is necessary to do a rectal exam (put a gloved finger in the rectum).

After the exam, your doctor will have blood drawn to look for an increase in the number of white blood cells which may indicate an infection. It is often also helpful to get an ultrasound or CT scan to help make the diagnosis.

How is the decision made that surgery is needed?

If the physical exam, blood tests and scans all point to an infection in the appendix, your doctor will usually recommend an operation to remove the appendix. In some cases, if the appendix has already "burst" it may be better to put a thin drain tube into the abdomen to remove the infected fluid and give your child antibiotics to treat the infection before we remove the remaining appendix.

What can I expect from surgery?

Your child's surgery will take about an hour. After surgery s/he will have intravenous (IV) fluids and medicines until s/he can take fluids by mouth. S/he may have a thin, clear tube draining fluid from the abdomen. In most cases s/he will have three very small incisions but there may be just one slightly longer incision.

Tips for the day of surgery—what to bring, what to leave home.

Bring your child's favorite comfort things; blankets, stuffed animal, small toys etc. Do not bring food, clothes, or large, heavy toys.

When will my child be able to go home?

Your child will be able to go home when they do not have a temperature over 101 F, are eating their regular diet and can take pain medicines by mouth. This is usually 1-2 days unless your child's appendix perforated in which case s/he will be in the hospital slightly longer.

What care is needed at home after surgery?

Bathing: Your child can take a shower 3-5 days after surgery and a bath in 7 days.

Activity: They should be out of bed and walking around but not riding a bike, playing sports or other contact activities.

Diet: Your child can eat any foods that are appropriate for age.

Medication: Most children need some pain medicine for a few days after coming home. Often acetaminophen (Tylenol®) or ibuprofen (Motrin®) is enough to control the pain and soreness.

When should I call the surgery team?

You should call the surgeon if your child has a temperature over 101 F, vomiting, diarrhea, increased or different abdominal pain or is not eating. You should also call if your child has an incision that looks redder, swollen, or begins to drain fluid.

What should I call my pediatrician for, and when should we see him/her?

You should call your child's pediatrician if s/he has a sore throat, runny nose, earache, cough or rash. If you are not sure whom to call, begin with your pediatrician. S/he may suggest you call the surgeon.

When can my child return to school or daycare? Will I need a note to excuse him/her from PE?

Children can usually return to school one week after going home. They should not participate in sports or physical education for 4 weeks. They should not lift anything over 10 pounds (including backpacks) for 4 weeks. Ask the surgery team for an excuse note for school.

What are the long term consequences?

There are no long term effects of having your appendix removed.

Will this affect growth and development?

Your child may lose a small amount of weight before s/he feels like eating her/his usual diet and amounts. S/he should return to her/his previous weight soon and have no other effects.

Foreword

Florence Nightingale published *Notes on Nursing* in 1859. That first publication elucidated for the individual who wished to become a nurse (there were no schools of nursing in those times) the need to be mindful of the patient in all manner of ways. Nightingale was concerned about fresh air, light, warmth, cleanliness, and the proper selection and administration of diet. Nightingale was the first to collect data in order to provide evidence-based care to her patients. As you read this textbook, you will note that the use of evidence in the provision of nursing care is the basis for care provided to pediatric surgical patients.

Today we have "holistic" nursing care, "evidence-based" nursing care, premier schools of nursing, and well educated, discerning men and women in every nursing arena. Nurses continue to follow Nightingale's credo "in all things place the patient in the center of concern." Specialized, family-focused care of the child is the central theme.

The more experienced nurses among us remember a time when surgical patients remained on bed rest without food or drink for long periods of time. Chest tubes were connected to a three glass bottle system and children were fully restrained while receiving intravenous fluid therapy. Large abdominal wounds were the norm, and colostomy closure was rarely considered.

Nursing and surgical care have changed. Society and technology have driven advances in all levels of nursing care. Bedside nurses are exhorted to take charge of their patients, managing numerous types of complicated equipment, ever-changing products, increasing amounts of documentation, and incredibly ill patients. Advanced practice nurses (APNs) have developed expanded roles where they manage groups of patients and care teams while providing education for families, nurses, and residents. APNs must weave the role of researcher, administrator, mentor, and program coordinator into their practice. Evidence-based support for each of these endeavors is found within these pages.

The first edition of *Nursing Care of the General Pediatric Surgical Patient* was published in 2000. It has become a guide for those who provide care to pediatric surgical patients and their families as well as for nursing educators. The new edition, highly endorsed by the American Pediatric Surgical Nurses Association (APSNA), takes *Nursing Care of the General Pediatric Surgical Patient* to the level of required reading and ownership. This book provides the bedside nurse with disease process information, multiple references, instruction guides, and tools to be used with patients and families. Advanced practice nurses will glean information to enrich and guide clinical practice as they incorporate increasing responsibility into their roles. Finally, you are welcome to download the diagnosis-related teaching sheets in English and in Spanish from www.apsna.org and www.jbpub.com for use with your patients and families.

This text is thoughtfully prepared and beautifully presented to promote excellence in pediatric surgical nursing. We hope that all individuals who share high ideals of practice will find this book a valuable resource. APSNA encourages you to read, learn, utilize, share, and enjoy!

Beth T. Zimmermann, RN, MS, APN, CCNS
President, APSNA 2005–2006

Linda J. Haga, RN, CPN
President, APSNA 2006–2007

Frances T. Gill, MS, CRNP
President-Elect, APSNA 2006–2007

Special Acknowledgments

When we, as editors, were convinced to take on the task of revising the first edition of *Nursing Care of the General Pediatric Surgical Patient,* we felt that our commitment was contingent upon the assistance of four additional colleagues. We were able to persuade Jeannette Diana-Zerpa, Lynne Farber, Fran Gill, and Betty Kasson to join us in this project. Though at that point we had nothing professionally to offer them except placing their names in the Acknowledgement section, all agreed without hesitation to help without thought of professional recognition. Their selfless dedication to children, families, colleagues, and education is the truest example of the total professional.

We divided our group into four teams. Each editor had a "buddy" who shared the responsibility of coordinating approximately eight chapters per team. Over the months, it became apparent that the contribution of our "buddies" needed to be recognized formally. We are appreciative of Jones and Bartlett for agreeing to name Jeannette A. Diana-Zerpa, Lynne D. Farber, Frances T. Gill, and Betty R. Kasson as Associate Editors of *Nursing Care of the Pediatric Surgical Patient.*

Our journey began in May of 2005 with a timetable of 18 months until publication. The efforts of Jeannette, Lynne, Fran, and Betty have enabled us to bring this project to completion on schedule. This has involved enormous effort on the part of many. But without our "buddies," we could never have achieved the quality and timely completion of this textbook.

Laura M. Flanigan
Carmel A. McComiskey
Pam Pieper
Nancy Tkacz Browne

Acknowledgments

The creation of the Second Edition of *Nursing Care of the Pediatric Surgical Patient* is a true collaboration of many professionals committed to the care of surgical children. The Editors and Associate Editors would like to extend our appreciation to all who contributed to the reality of this work.

First and foremost, we thank the 55 contributing authors who gave considerable time and effort in the creation of this edition. All authors have a "day job" which often consumes much more than a traditional 40-hour work week. Additionally, all have other roles and responsibilities which needed their attention these past months. All found the time to review, research, write, and edit their parts of this project. Several had personal crises during the writing phase of this edition. Yet, despite offers to place their book responsibilities elsewhere, all authors insisted on completing their commitment both to the editors and to the children we care for in our practices. We salute the chapter authors who are the heart and soul of this edition.

We also extend our sincere gratitude to the American Pediatric Surgical Nurses Association (APSNA). All Editors and Associate Editors are longstanding APSNA members and all have had the privilege of serving on the APSNA Board of Directors. We acknowledge the APSNA Board of Directors for 2005–2006 and 2006–2007 for their leadership in supporting this second edition. The organization has again made education a top priority in its quest to champion the highest quality of care possible for infants and children undergoing surgery. In particular, the Editors would like to recognize Linda J. Haga, ASPNA President 2006–2007, for finding a publisher for the second edition and skillfully convincing us as Editors of the wonderful opportunity of textbook editing.

We salute the members of ASPNA who were not directly involved in the creation of this textbook. These members assumed other organizational responsibilities when a significant percentage of our membership became involved with this revision. APSNA has many other projects that are just as deserving, and the membership rose to the occasion. We thank them for that and for their consistent commitment to the care of the pediatric surgical patients in their practices.

We would like to thank our pediatric surgical colleagues. The partnership between the pediatric surgeon and the pediatric surgical nurse is a true model for delivery of quality patient care for children. Nationally, the American Pediatric Surgical Association (APSA) has recognized the contribution that APSNA and pediatric surgical nurses everywhere make to improve the care of their patients. At the practice level, you will find that many of these chapters have acknowledgments of individual pediatric surgeons who have supported this textbook in many ways. Examples include contributions of pictures, discussion, and editing. Collaboration is the truest word to use.

We would also be remiss if we did not thank our pediatric surgical colleagues outside of nursing and medicine. These are the men and women who ensure that the pediatric surgery practices run smoothly. Each practice has a different model, but all have been aware of the Editor's and Authors' project responsibilities. And all have helped in their individual ways. We thank them.

We would like to thank all the people who took the time to review these chapters. In particular, we would like to thank Kathy Iurlano, Trupti Parik, and Kerri Keller for taking the time to give their thoughts and constructive criticisms. They represent a large group of colleagues who cheerfully gave of their time without asking for recognition. Thank you to all.

We would like to thank Jones and Bartlett Publishers who agreed to produce the second edition of this textbook. They have made this process achievable for a group of nurses who are very experienced at taking care of surgical children but novices at textbook editing. In particular, we would like to recognize Kevin Sullivan for quietly and efficiently guiding our textbook through the Jones and Bartlett system. Also, our thanks to Amy Sibley whose quiet, patient personality efficiently kept us on task. Amy was always immediately accessible for questions or needs. She answers her own phone, and we are not sure she has voice mail, a rare and appreciated trait as we often had limited time to contact her. We also wish to recognize Tracey Chapman who has patiently and skillfully guided us through the editing process.

The reader will see artwork throughout the textbook that illustrates pediatric surgical anatomy and procedures. Several pieces of the artwork have been produced by the daughters of chapter authors. We thank these young women for sharing their special talent with their mothers and with us. We also want to acknowledge the technical assistance of Christopher Giaquinto who spent hours of his time preparing pictures and figures for the text.

The Editors would like to thank two of the "unsung heroines" of this textbook. The first is Suzanne Borkowski who agreed to take on the task of updating the Resource section of the original textbook. Sue, a former APSNA president, took a fresh look at this section and expanded it beautifully. All the contact information is current as of publication date. But in anticipation that websites and contact information change, Sue made the suggestion that we place these resources on the APSNA Web site (www. apsna.org) to be updated regularly. APSNA is in the process of making this suggestion a reality.

The editors also thank Leona Burnham for taking on the task of creating a glossary of pediatric surgical nursing terminology. Leona took the original work and expanded it to a new level. Her section is a tutorial for any nurse new to the field of pediatric surgical nursing. And many of us experienced in this field learned a few new things also! Leona's contribution may be one of the most important in this textbook, and we are indebted to her dedication to this project.

APSNA has support from many arenas . . . one of these areas is Web site support. Gerry Daney has been the contact between our Web site and APSNA for several years. His ideas and technical expertise have contributed greatly to the organization's growth. Gerry is the person who makes the ideas happen. For example, his expertise will enable you, the reader, to go to www.apsna.org and download information from the Resource List or Teaching Sheets for your professional use. Thank you, Gerry.

As the world becomes smaller through technology, we recognize our responsibility to be sensitive to the cultural needs of our patients and families. Ideas abound on making our textbook international. Our first step is the addition of Teaching Sheets for pediatric surgical procedures written in Spanish. These correspond to the clinical chapters in the book and are available to download at www. apsna.org and www.jbpub.com. We are indebted to Nilda Nagle, Jeannette Diana-Zerpa, Carlos Zerpa, and Sofia Morales, MSN, RN, ARNP who translated each of the 41 Teaching Sheets from English to Spanish. Aware that there are differences within the Spanish language, we also collaborated with translation professionals to verify interpretation. Gracias, Nilda, Jeannette, Carlos, and Sofia!

Our professional future is found in our nursing students. We can think of no finer example than Hiwot Woldgeorgis. Hiwot attends the University of Missouri at Columbia and is currently a junior in their excellent undergraduate nursing program. During a research rotation in Chicago last summer, Hiwot watched as editor Nancy Browne struggled with some of the early organizational tasks of textbook editing. Hiwot offered to help and has done so in numerous ways. When an author needed help with literature searches, Hiwot efficiently found pertinent references and sent them to the author in a timely manner. She gave feedback about chapter selection and content. Remember her name as we suspect that she will be editing her own textbook at some point in her career. At present, she is dedicated to pursuing a career in perinatal nursing. We still hope to persuade her to join us in pediatric surgical nursing.

We owe a special debt of gratitude to the editors and authors of the First Edition of *Nursing Care of the General Pediatric Surgical Patient*. Barbara Wise, Chris McKenna, Gail Garvin, and Bethany Harmon edited the first edition that was published in 2000. They and their authors, most of whom came back for the Second Edition, produced from scratch the first (and to our knowledge only) textbook specifically devoted to the nursing care of the general pediatric surgical patient. The effect of their pioneering efforts are felt every day as the first edition is used as a resource in the care of children internationally. Their tireless initial work has made our task infinitely easier.

Finally, the Editors salute Clara Lindley. Prior to this textbook, Clara did not have a connection with pediatric surgical nursing. However, we can say unequivocally that the quality of this textbook owes a great debt to Clara's contribution. In the transition from our first publisher to the current company, the textbook's digital files were lost. This committed us as Editors and authors to work off a paper copy, to make changes on the paper copy and then convert these changes to a Word document. You can imagine the potential for error involved. Our only alternative seemed to be retyping the entire textbook. Time prohibited this choice. At this point, Clara was discovered by Editor Pam Pieper. Clara was aware of a technology that scanned our paper copies and turned them into an electronic document that we could edit. Clara literally scanned almost every chapter, table, and figure so that we were able to submit an entirely electronic copy to our publisher on time. Clara spent hours of her own time in this endeavor. We sincerely thank her and appreciate her efforts.

The production of this second edition was a labor of love from countless individuals. Each and every one of us has done so in the hopes that children everywhere will have a little easier path because of the knowledge imparted by these pages.

Laura Flanigan
Carmel McComiskey
Pam Pieper
Nancy Tkacz Browne

Introduction

Sitting Vigil
A Pediatric Surgical Nursing Tradition

The modern era of pediatric surgery in North America began in Boston shortly after World War I when Dr. William E. Ladd, a Harvard-trained general surgeon, made a decision to limit his practice to the surgical care of infants and children. Dr. Ladd was distressed by the quality of surgical care offered to these small patients and was determined to improve it. With meticulous attention to detail, he began to keep accurate medical records which included signs and symptoms, the surgical procedure, and outcomes. He developed policies and uniform methods of care for each surgical disease. Dr. Ladd spent countless hours in the pathology department studying both microscopic and gross specimens. Using all the information that he gleaned, he constantly evolved new procedures and methods of care.

In 1927, Dr. Ladd became the Surgeon-in-Chief of the Children's Hospital in Boston. He was a great teacher and established the first pediatric surgical training program. In 1941, the first modern American pediatric surgical textbook titled *Abdominal Surgery of Infancy and Childhood* was published, coauthored by Dr. Ladd and his trainee, Dr. Robert E. Gross.

Dr. Gross went on to succeed Dr. Ladd as Surgeon-in-Chief in 1947. Dr. Gross had incredible drive, initiative, imagination, and attention to detail. His department at the Children's Hospital in Boston was renowned throughout the world. In 1953, Dr. Gross's now-classic text *The Surgery of Infancy and Childhood* was published. It became the gospel of pediatric surgery. Many of the procedures described in his text are still done today.

The growth of pediatric surgery in this country was documented in 1997 in *The Genealogy of North American Pediatric Surgery* by Drs. Philip Glick and Richard Azizkhan. They stated "There is a long golden cord that stretches from Dr. Ladd to the present, binding all of us together as in no other specialty." According to the genealogy, Dr. Gross trained 69 pediatric surgeons, with 15 of those going on to start their own training programs across the country. Dr. Judah Folkman, a pediatric surgeon and scientist who succeeded Dr. Gross, stated that "Dr. Gross introduced surgical techniques that saved the lives of countless thousands of babies and children throughout the world." It is impossible to accurately describe the awe and respect awarded Dr. Gross by not only his trainees but also by the generations of pediatric surgeons that have followed. He had established the "epicenter of the pediatric surgical revolution."

As Dr. Ladd and Dr. Gross were developing the specialty of pediatric surgery, there were nurses at the Children's Hospital in Boston who had to learn, grow, and develop nursing techniques to care for these patients.

Very little is documented about how nurses reacted to this revolution in surgery, but we know they were there. We suspect that many might have been skeptical at first, but as they saw patient outcomes change, we are sure they became supporters.

Nurse anesthetists were common in these early days, but not all were able to keep up with these new pediatric surgeons. One exception was Miss Betty Lank. "Bess" was recognized as a pioneer in this "new" specialty. Between 1935 and 1969, she labored in the operating rooms at the Children's Hospital in Boston, where she designed new equipment and developed new techniques to deal with the ever more complex procedures being done by Ladd and Gross.

The students at the Children's Hospital in Boston's School of Nursing often comprised a major part of staffing on all shifts. This school (and others like it) had very strong traditions and high standards. Diploma nursing schools had three year, year round programs which combined intensive classroom and practical experience. The hours were long and responsibility came quickly. These young women (there were no male nurses during the Ladd and Gross years) developed early expertise in pre- and postoperative care. They also spent at least three months in the operating room and were competent operating room nurses by the time this rotation was over. Many students stayed on at the hospital following graduation. Positions in the operating room and on the surgical floors were considered the premier jobs.

The staff nurses on the surgical infant, toddler and children's floors had to have stamina and skill. They were the ones who made the observations and documented what happened to patients as they recovered from these procedures, newly developed by Ladd and Gross. On the basis of what these nurses learned, the hospital developed a policy and procedure book that very specifically outlined the care to be given to patients after certain surgical procedures. The head nurse and supervisor ran their floors as absolute monarchies. Virtually all communication between the nurse and surgeon came via the head nurse. She was expected to be fully informed about every aspect of every patient under her care. Head nurses were appointed to their positions because of their clinical expertise.

Dr. Ladd and Dr. Gross worked in an era prior to the innovation of the neonatal or pediatric intensive care unit

> *"If you have knowledge, let others light their candles at it."*
> **Margaret Fuller**

and before the development of any of the modern technology we now take for granted. As patients began to come out of the operating room with surgical diagnoses that had previously been fatal, a new nursing role was conceived called the "constant care" nurse. Each surgical floor had a room set aside for the most critically ill infants and children. In that room would be several of the most skilled nurses who were assigned to care for these very ill patients. One pediatric surgeon of the time said, "Great technical, surgical skill would come to nothing without the dedication of the nurses charged with the care of those tiny fragile patients." Without ventilators, intravenous pumps, or monitors, these nurses sometimes seemed to bring these patients through the postoperative period with the sheer force of their will. Student nurses were sometimes assigned to work with these nurses to try to somehow pick up that intangible something that they seemed to possess that made them great pediatric surgical nurses.

In this new operating room arena created by Ladd and Gross, there were some other nurses performing some very special roles. Dr. C. Everett Koop, one of the early, new breed of pediatric surgeons said, "Nothing in surgery is as satisfying as working with a skilled operating room nurse who knows the way you think, as well as the way you operate. You're like dancing partners; no words need to be spoken in a synchronized duet."

Marie Dresser was a graduate of the Boston Children's Hospital School of Nursing who went to work in the operating room there after graduation. One day, after working with Marie on a number of occasions, Dr. Gross simply went to the supervisor of the OR and told her that he wished Marie to be assigned to all his cases. In time, she worked exclusively for Dr. Gross in the operating room, the clinical office, and, on occasion, made patient rounds with him. This was the role known as the "designated scrub nurse." Marie and Dr. Gross were the model for many a successful team. Marie was the epitome of a true perioperative nurse. She developed long-term relationships with patients and families. She was a teacher and counselor for the residents. She maintained constancy on the service when the boss was not present. She was the forerunner of the advanced practice nurse. Many a young pediatric surgeon, upon finishing his training with Dr. Gross, would ask a talented, young OR nurse to join him in practice as he went off to bring Dr. Gross's vision to yet another children's hospital.

Now there are opportunities for the modern, pediatric nurse to concentrate on pediatric surgery as a staff nurse, a clinical specialist, a pediatric nurse practitioner, a trauma coordinator, or a teacher. These are new times with new challenges and lots of work to be done.

As pediatric surgery grew across the country, pediatric surgical nurses in many institutions practiced in isolation from one another. Some of these nurses began to meet at the annual conference of the American Pediatric Surgical Association (APSA) that was founded in 1970. Over time, a group of pediatric surgical nurses who collaborated with pediatric surgeons came to exchange ideas and advice at these meetings.

By May 1991, these nurses realized the value of formalizing our professional subspecialty. Thirty-one pediatric surgical nurses met in Orlando, Florida at APSA for a breakfast session where they strategized to form their own association. By 1993, these nurses had formally created an organization complete with name, Board of Directors, bylaws, dues, policies, and an educational program. The American Pediatric Surgical Nurses Association (APSNA) was born. Pediatric surgical nurses who were "descendants" of Marie Dresser and Miss Betty Lank finally had a professional home.

Since 1993, APSNA has grown tremendously. The organization consists of nearly 300 members who practice in a multitude of roles that are related to caring for the pediatric surgical child. Initial educational conferences were 4 hours in length. Today, APSNA's Annual Educational Conference is three days long with poster sessions, research presentations, plenary sessions, and discussion groups. Collaboration with pediatric surgeons has continued, with many surgeons presenting at APSNA's conference.

Through APSNA, pediatric surgical nurses now communicate through an email listserv, website, and the organizational newsletter, *Sutureline*. Continuing education and scholarship have been a theme from the organization's birth and that tradition continues today. One of the nicest traditions of APSNA is that the organization created a way to recognize excellence in pediatric surgical nursing with the development of the Founder's Award. Finally, excellence in our professional subspecialty can be formally recognized and appreciated.

In 1998, APSNA addressed the fact that pediatric surgical nursing did not have a formal textbook. Much of our teaching was from our pediatric surgical mentors but so much of pediatric surgical nursing goes beyond an understanding of pathology and procedures. APSNA leadership set the goal of compiling and publishing a textbook devoted entirely to the nursing care of the general pediatric surgical patient. The editors and authors were all experts in pediatric surgical nursing. It was with great pride that this ground-breaking textbook was published in 2000.

As we publish the second edition of the APSNA textbook seven years later, we are gratified to see how far our profession has progressed over time. Equally as gratifying is to see the advances in pediatric surgical care and outcomes for thousands of infants and children. Pediatric surgical nurses are challenged to continue their professional growth and to pass along our history to our next generation of colleagues.

Pediatric surgical nursing has made significant advances since Dr. Ladd and the nursing team at Boston Children's Hospital began their pioneering work in 1927. However, there is a constant thread that binds all pediatric surgical nurses together. And that thread, of course, is the children and their families.

Pediatric surgical nurses across the decades have had the privilege of "sitting vigil" with countless families as they watch their children struggle to recover from their particular circumstances.

> "Knowledge increases in proportion to its use—that is, the more we teach, the more we learn."
>
> **H.P. Blavatsky**

Whether the surgery is life-threatening or routine, every parent faces the fear of leaving their child at the OR doors. More than once, a pediatric surgical nurse has accompanied a child into the OR and "watched" on behalf of a mother until she and her child were reunited postoperatively. Such trust is an enormous responsibility which has been borne by generations of pediatric surgical nurses.

Pediatric surgical nurses have a proud history and an exciting future. We owe a great debt to our predecessors and we bear the responsibility to continue their proud tradition. In times of exhaustion and seemingly insurmountable challenges, pediatric surgical nurses are often sustained by the privilege of our relationships with children and families. We are invited into their lives at their most vulnerable times, and we are entrusted with their most cherished possession. Families look to us for hope and comfort. While our skills must be excellent, our humanity is often what families remember.

Excellent pediatric surgical care improves the quality of thousands of lives each year. Most of these children go on to a whole life. However, there are those who fight valiantly but are not able to survive the obstacles placed in their path. We dedicate this textbook to the children represented by Jennifer, Steven, Antonio, Ashley, Roland,

Grant, Yolanda, Marcia, Stephanie, and Stefano. We all miss you and who you would have been. But your being was enough to fill our hearts with lessons learned and joyful times. And our thoughts, prayers, and tremendous respect are expressed through the parent names of Christina, Rafael, Kathy, Myra, Jennifer, Ginger, Lorraine, Sharon, Katrina, Dave, Mark, Teresa and Nick. These parents, and countless others, have allowed us to sit vigil with them as they shared their children with us. The tradition continues.

Laura M. Flanigan
Carmel A. McComiskey
Pam Pieper
Nancy Tkacz Browne

Jeannette A. Diana-Zerpa
Lynne D. Farber
Frances T. Gill
Betty R. Kasson

Special Considerations in the Care of the Pediatric Surgical Patient

1

Perioperative Preparation of the Child and Family

By Kathleen M. Leack

Those who care for the pediatric surgical population recognize that multiple factors make this population challenging and unique. Children and families need information and preparation before the surgical experience. Whether the child is having a minor outpatient surgery or an emergent life-saving procedure, it is an extraordinary stressor for the child and family (Wollin, Plummer, Owen, Hawkins, Materazzo, & Morrison, 2004). Assessment and guidance are necessary for a thorough preoperative plan. The nurse must possess an understanding of child development to care for the child and family.

Nursing teams have a unique role in the continuum of care of the child throughout the operative experience. Perioperative care of the pediatric surgical patient includes not only provision of preoperative information to the family but also physical preparation of the patient. A general knowledge of the proposed surgical procedure and care of a patient in the operating room suite is necessary and should also include a specific understanding of a child's airway and the physiologic response to surgery and anesthesia.

The purpose of this chapter is to provide general recommendations for preoperative preparation. The information provided is meant to inform health care team members about the psychological and physical needs of children who require surgery. These needs are addressed in the context of the family. This chapter also discusses the care of the pediatric surgical patient in the preoperative holding room, the operating room suite, and subsequent transfer to the postanesthesia care unit (PACU). For additional information about procedures or diagnoses, please refer to appropriate chapters in this text.

■ Child Development

The surgical experience is known to be stressful to the child and the family. How children see and grasp their experiences and surroundings is completely dependent on their cognitive and emotional developmental level. The statement, "children are not little adults" holds true when it comes to surgical preparation of the child. A young child is not able to comprehend the importance of lying still for a painful procedure (in order that the procedure can be completed more expeditiously). Conversely, a teenager does not require simple "baby talk" explanations before the procedure. Care providers can overestimate the skill and development of a younger child while underestimating those same skills in an adolescent (Wilson, Nagy, & Jessee, 2001). Each child must be approached at his/her appropriate level.

Child development theories developed by Piaget (1968) and Erikson (1985) describe cognitive and personality development that follows a predictable course. These stages of child development pertain to both cognitive and emotional development. The child's developmental level and coping strategies affect the way that the child will respond to surgery (Smith & Callery, 2004). The practitioner must understand these sequential stages in order to provide a supportive environment for the child. Using developmental framework methodology allows the provider to work with and provide information to the child in a calm, supportive, and honest manner. Table 1-1 provides an overview of developmental stages and supportive techniques discussed in this section.

One concept that crosses all developmental levels is that of attachment and concern about separation. Much has been written about strengthening a child/parent bond (as with premature hospitalized infants) and the negative effects that arise when this bond does not occur. There are natural times when separation of parent and child is necessary (parents leaving for work or vacation). A surgical procedure is an unnatural time of separation. The issue of separation is significant for both parent and child. Even though a surgical procedure may be minor and short in duration (to the health care team), much is expected of both the child and the parent in terms of trust in the care provider. Parents put trust in the surgical team to provide expert surgical care in addition to providing a safe, warm, and supportive experience for the child. Children trust that they will return to their parents.

Child Coping

Coping strategies vary from child to child, and each child can develop a greater repertoire of strategies with matu-

Table 1-1	**Developmental Stages and Influence on Preoperative Preparation**				
Age	**0–1 yr**	**1–3 yr**	**3–6 yr**	**6–12 yr**	**12–18 yr**
Cognitive	Dependent on senses; developing motor skills	Egocentric thought; language comprehension better than verbal skills	Very inquisitive; still egocentric	Logical thought; can consider other points of view; understands body functioning (age 9)	Mature reasoning; deductive and hypothetical thought; higher level of understanding about body function and effects of illness
Psychosocial	Developing trust; relies on consistent response to needs	Developing ability to control own body and emotions	More independent active imagination; mixes fantasy with reality	Achievement oriented; developing mastery and self-esteem	Development of identity and autonomy
Specific fears	Separation from primary caregivers; strangers	Separation; dark; abandonment; threat to body boundary	Separation; loss of control; bodily injury; imagined threats	Loss of control (body or emotional); bodily harm; separation from family and peers	Loss of self-control or autonomy; disfigurement; disability
Coping ability	Depends on parental presence	Depends on parental presence; decreases in unfamiliar environment	Depends on parental presence; some internal coping skills	Small repertoire of coping skills; can be taught skills; preparation useful	Greater number of coping skills
Interventions	Ensure parental presence; limit strangers; keep normal routine	Parental presence; opportunities to control own body; therapeutic play security objects	Parental presence; explain what will be experienced, participate in care	Parental, peer, or other adult support; preparation; teaching coping skills; privacy; participation in care	Parental and peer support; preparation; teach coping skills; ensure privacy; participate in care; complete discussion of surgery

Sources: From Busen (2001); Erikson (1985); Piaget (1968); Wilson et al. (2001).

rity. How the child defines the stress of the surgical experience is integral to facilitating adaptive coping (LaMontagne, 2000). When a combination of information and coping skills are provided to adolescents who have intense anxiety about their surgical procedure, their anxiety decreases (LaMontagne, Hepworth, Cohen, & Salisbury, 2003).

During the preoperative assessment, the care provider should explore the child's coping strategies. An individualized preoperative plan to facilitate coping should be developed (Kain, Caldwell-Andrews, & Wang, 2002). For younger children, separation from parents may be the greatest stressor. Other children fear the painful or unknown aspects of the experience. Preparation programs help the child develop a better understanding of the surgical experience. Programs that include parents in the operating room (OR) or provide preoperative sedation are advantageous to children who fear separation.

Strategies for Preparation

Many children report that they were nervous or worried about surgery (Wollin et al., 2004). Children's negative reactions result from their fears and misconceptions. Of great concern is the evidence of emotional distress and behavioral disturbance both before and after surgery and after hospitalization (Ferrari, 2002). Before surgery, agitation requiring physical restraint has been noted. After surgery, psychological upset, such as bedwetting, nightmares, and disturbances in eating and sleeping patterns, have been documented (Kain et al., 2002). Preoperative preparation programs reduce or eliminate children's fears and anxiety, which in turn decreases the incidence of preoperative emotional distress and behavioral disturbance. Regardless of the length of the operative procedure and hospital encounter, children should be prepared for their experience.

■ Providing Information

An increasing number of surgical procedures are being performed on an outpatient basis. This shift means that parents assume more responsibility for the psychological preparation of children before surgery. Regardless of where the surgery takes place, parents are instrumental in providing and reinforcing information for preparation of the child (O'Connor-Von, 2000). Parents who receive both written and verbal information state that once they review the written information, the verbal information alone seems insufficient (Spencer & Franck, 2005; Bellew, Atkinson, Dixon, & Yates, 2002).

Nursing staff should direct the parents to appropriate sources for information.

Examine the child and family's previous experience with and knowledge of surgery and hospitalization. A child's preoperative anxiety may be a reflection of the parent's anxiety (Kain et al., 2002; Zuwala & Barber, 2001). Children today are also exposed to health and medical information from television, computer games, and peers; this information can precipitate a child's misconception of the surgical experience. Ask the child what he or she believes will happen and correct any misunderstanding that the child might have (Smith & Callery, 2004). In addition to focusing on the surgical experience, the child needs specific information about why surgery is indicated. When children draw pictures of their internal organs, they often misplace them in the body, and when asked about function of that organ, they describe it incorrectly (Schmidt, 2001). It is therefore helpful to describe the organ and its function with an anatomically correct drawing in addition to describing the purpose of the surgical procedure.

Nursing staff should provide the child with concrete information. Use descriptive and simple comparisons, specifically detailing colors, sounds, feelings and sensations, size, and shapes. Tailor words to the developmental level of the child (Koopman, Baars, Chaplin, & Zwinderman, 2004). Avoid words that the child may not understand or define a word for the child when a suitable synonym does not exist. For example, "surgery" is another word for "operation." Avoid words that may have negative implications, such as "shot" or "put to sleep," as well as emotionally charged words; use "make an opening" rather than "cut you open." The language of the operating room can be easily misinterpreted by both children and their families. Try to use terms consistent with those the family uses to reinforce explanations.

The questions that a child may ask may be very different than what the health care provider may expect; it is important that the health care provider closely listens to questions that children pose (Koopman et al., 2004; Smith & Callery, 2004). For example, when discussing the role of anesthesia, many children share that they fear they will waken in the middle of surgery; questions asked then center on that theme. Explain that the child will be monitored closely and will not awaken until the operation is finished.

Provide children with both procedural and sensory information. Preoperative procedural information should detail the sequence of operative events. Sensory information focuses on the sights, sounds, smells, tastes, and sensations of the operative experience. Descriptions, pictures, and videotapes provide some information about the look of the operating room but lack the multisensory information children use to explore new experiences.

■ Active Participation

Provide the child with opportunities to practice his or her surgical role. Allow the child to be an active participant in the surgical process. For example, ask the child to help hold the mask over his or her mouth and nose, rather than just placing the mask on the child's face. Provide the child with a genuine choice if and when there is one. For example, "do you want to walk or ride in the wagon to surgery?" rather than "are you ready to go to surgery?" Suggest positive coping strategies during stressful times. For example, "you can squeeze my hand until it's over."

■ Preoperative Preparation Program

Preoperative preparation programs provide information, familiarize the family with the surgical process, encourage emotional expression, and teach coping strategies (Cote, Todres, Ryan, & Goudsouzian, 2001). Nurses and child life specialists facilitate these programs. Child life specialists strive to reduce the impact of stressful life events that affect the development, health, and well-being of children and families. The child life specialist focuses preparation efforts on the child's point of view. The nurse or child life specialist clarifies medical information and terminology for the child and family. In addition, each program should incorporate a multicultural approach to child preparation (O'Conner-Von, 2000).

Therapeutic Play

Children use play both to express their understanding of the world and to learn more about the world. They can master stressful situations through play. Structured play activities that are designed to facilitate self-expression, develop coping mechanisms, and promote psychological well-being of children undergoing medical procedures and hospitalization are termed *therapeutic play*. Use therapeutic play activities in preoperative preparation programs to facilitate children's understanding of surgery and to address fears and clarify misconceptions related to the surgical equipment being used and the procedures being performed. The tools of therapeutic play are similar to the tools of child's play, and may consist of stuffed animals, anatomically correct dolls, puppets, drawings, toy medical equipment, and real medical equipment (Kain et al., 2002).

■ Psychological Preparation: The Parents

In most cases, the presence of parents in the hospital is beneficial to the child and helps normalize the environment, provide support, and reduce stress. To decrease the stress and anxiety of parents whose children are having surgery, specific stressors and coping styles must be identified (LaMontagne, 2000). For the parent, the most stressful aspects of a child's hospitalization are related to the loss of the familiar parental role and uncertainty regarding both the outcome of the medical situation and the predictability of events. Encourage parents to perform their usual caregiving tasks. Support parents as they advocate for their child.

Interventions aimed at reducing parental stress during their child's surgery directly influence their child's coping and response to the surgical experience (Kain et al., 2002). Preoperative anxiety in parents directly influences the anxiety of their child. Parents desire comprehensive information on their child's condition; this can decrease their anxiety (Spencer & Franck, 2005).

■ Preoperative Consultation

Preoperative Consultation: Surgeon

A child may see the pediatric general surgeon electively or emergently. After examination and determination that a surgical procedure is indicated, the surgeon provides information about the child's diagnosis and proposed surgical procedure. The surgeon explains the surgical procedure, the risks and benefits of that procedure, the expectations for and length of recovery, the potential complications, the inpatient versus outpatient status, and the timing of the procedure.

Informed Consent

Informed consent has become a fundamental process in the practice of modern medicine (Nwomeh, Waller, Caniano, & Kelleher, 2005). Informed consent involves the surgeon providing information to the parents and caregivers in a detailed and understandable manner. The information should include a description of the underlying condition for which the surgery has been recommended, the details of the proposed surgical procedure; and the risks, benefits, and alternatives to that procedure. After this information is disclosed, adequate time should be allowed for discussion, including a question-and-answer period between the surgeon and the legal guardian.

After all questions have been answered, informed consent is obtained from the legal guardian (usually the parent). The documentation of this informed consent discussion consists of a parental signature on the surgical consent form and documentation from the surgeon in the child's medical record.

Although much of the informed consent discussion occurs between the surgeon and parent, the input of the patient must also be solicited. The procedure should be explained to the child in a manner that the child understands. For older children, assent (the agreement of someone who is not competent to give legally valid informed consent) should be sought (Nwomeh et al., 2005; Busen, 2001).

The role of the nurse in the informed consent process is to ask the parents whether they have spoken with the surgeon about the proposed procedure. If the parents report that the discussion has occurred, that they understand the information that was provided, and that their questions have been answered, the nurse may witness the signature of the parent on the surgical consent document. If the parents have questions that pertain to the nuances of the procedure or other aspects of surgical care, the surgeon should be notified. It is within the realm of nursing practice to provide information that clarifies the discussion between the surgeon and family (Phippen & Wells, 2000).

Preoperative Consultation: Anesthesiologist

A preoperative meeting with the anesthesia team is another important aspect of preparation. This meeting may occur several days before the proposed procedure or on the day of surgery. Many institutions have a preanesthetic clinic in which the patient can be seen before the procedure. The children best suited for this clinic, with exceptions, are those with complex medical histories or other anesthetic difficulties. Written information discussing the role of the anesthesiologist also helps parents understand the need for this additional preoperative evaluation (American Society of Anesthesiologists [ASA], 2005; Ferrari, 2004).

The anesthesiologist obtains a health history identifying potential anesthetic difficulties. The history includes a review of a patient's response to previous anesthetics and any family history of adverse anesthetic experiences. A physical examination is completed, with a focus on cardiopulmonary assessment, an airway examination (to assess for intubation difficulty), and assessment of other anatomic considerations that may make interventions, such as insertion of intravenous line or positioning, difficult. It is through this process that intraoperative and postoperative anesthetic risks are determined (Garcia-Miguel, Serrano-Aguillar, & Lopez-Bastida, 2003). The American Society of Anesthesiologists has developed a classification system to stratify the risk of anesthesia according to that patient's state of health (Table 1-2) (ASA, 2004).

In addition to reviewing anesthesia and its risks and benefits, the anesthesiologist discusses postoperative pain control strategies. Parents expect information on anesthesia, the operative experience, and postoperative pain management techniques. The child and the parent should be reassured that alleviating postoperative discomfort is the goal of all who care for the child. Many methods of postoperative pain management should be discussed with the parents (Cote et al., 2001) When parents are provided with written information, there is an increase in verbal communication with, and instruction from, care providers (Bellew et al., 2002). Parents report higher satisfaction when both verbal and written information is provided.

■ Preoperative Assessment: Nursing Assessment

Preoperative Medical History

The patient's nursing team should obtain a thorough history and perform a physical examination before any procedure. Essential elements of the exam include review of allergies, recent and chronic illnesses/conditions, illness exposure, current medications, immunization status, birth history, family medical history, review of body systems,

Table 1-2	Perioperative Management: American Society of Anesthesiologists (ASA) Classification
Class I	Healthy patients with localized pathologic processes
Class II	Patients with mild systemic diseases
Class III	Patients with severe systemic disease that limits activity but is not totally incapacitating
Class IV	Patients with an incapacitating disease that is a constant threat to life
Class V	Patients who are not expected to survive 24 hours with or without the surgical procedure
Class VI	Patients who have been declared brain dead but whose organs will be removed for donor purposes

Source: Fortunato (2000).

and complete physical examination (Black & Hawks, 2005). Table 1-3 provides a review of body systems and the implications for anesthesia.

Language and Culture

Health care providers work with families from various cultural, religious, and educational backgrounds. To be effective, these factors need to be incorporated into the plan of care. Before the family interview or the physical examination of the patient, the family should be asked which language they prefer.

Suboptimal communication occurs with families who have limited English proficiency when assisted only by family members or by health care professionals who have limited second-language skills (Burbano O'Leary, Frederico, & Hampers, 2003; Flores et al., 2003). The preferred method of communication with families who need language assistance is to use the skills of a dedicated interpreter who has passed a proficiency examination. If an interpreter is not available when assessment or communication with the family is needed, telephone interpretation systems are available (Advisory Board, 2005).

Some families may request advisement of a family member or a clan or church elder when they are considering the information provided by the surgical team. Although these situations can be challenging, the surgical team must include these individuals (Ells & Caniano, 2002). Some cultures practice alternative and complementary rituals in addition to traditional health care (Black & Hawks, 2005). Attending to these culturally based requests contributes to family-centered care.

History of Present Illness

The perioperative nurse, while conducting the preoperative assessment and patient history, must take into consideration the condition of the patient. Most assessments (discussed in this chapter) occur with the patient who has an electively scheduled surgery. However, these assessments also pertain to the child who is hospitalized and is requiring an urgent operation. Despite the urgency of surgery, the nurse must obtain an adequate history regarding the events and symptoms that occurred before presentation (Cote et al., 2001).

Allergies

Many medications and products may cause sensitivity or allergic reactions. Extra precautions must be taken for patients who report a history of allergy or sensitivity to anesthetics or other drugs (Fortunato, 2000). Many patients have a sensitivity to products applied to the skin, such as tape, surgical scrub, and skin preparation products. Avoid these products in the operative process (Fortunato).

Latex

There has been increased awareness of the risk of allergic reactions from latex-containing products. The reaction is triggered by the latex antigen, which is also present in the powder found on latex gloves (AORN, 2004). The reactions include contact urticaria, bronchial asthma, anaphylactic shock, and death (Fortunato, 2000). Latex products should be avoided or used cautiously in all patients with a history of spina bifida or urologic conditions requiring repeated surgeries. Children with an undiagnosed latex allergy may give a history of urticaria or swelling of the lips and face after contact with latex balloons or foods that share common antigenic properties to latex, such as papayas, bananas, kiwi, raw potatoes, chestnuts, and avocados (Holzman et al., 2005; Ferrari, 2002). In 1998, in response to this issue, the US Food and Drug Administration mandated that product packaging include documentation of latex content (AORN).

Document all of the child's allergies in the medical record. Place an allergy band on one of the child's extremities to identify an allergy. If the allergy (e.g., latex) has direct implications for the operating room personnel, notify the operating room staff (AORN, 2004).

Current Medications

Review with the parent that antipyretics, and any over-the-counter medications should be included in the patient's list of current medications (Black & Hawks, 2005). In addition, information about use of herbal substances, weight loss aids, and illicit drugs should be obtained (Busen, 2001; Ferrari, 2002). Review medications influencing electrolyte status, clotting, or cardiovascular function with the anesthesiologist before surgery. Certain medications (e.g., anticonvulsants, anticoagulants) may require preoperative laboratory evaluation. Plan for alternative routes for enteral medications if postoperative NPO status is expected.

Birth History

Obtain a prenatal and neonatal history. Conditions associated with prematurity, such as apnea, subglottic stenosis, bronchopulmonary dysplasia, patent ductus arteriosus, and intraventricular hemorrhage may affect the anesthetic plan (Cote et al., 2001). Inquire about the child's birth weight, length of hospital stay, and ventilatory support.

Table 1-3	Preoperative Assessment: Review of Body Systems and Physical Examination	
Review of Systems	**Conditions**	**Anesthetic/Surgical Implications**
Head, eyes, ears, nose, throat	1. Hearing or vision loss 2. Loose or broken teeth	1. Impairs communication. 2. Unintentional loss or injury or aspiration during intubation.
Respiratory	1. Airway disturbances (narrow airway, tracheostomy, home oxygen, home ventilation) 2. History of asthma, bronchopulmonary dysplasia, or cystic fibrosis 3. Smoking history	1. Difficult intubation (laryngomalacia, micrognathia); increased risk of sleep apnea. 2. Describe severity, symptoms, triggers, and last exacerbation; optimize medical management in anticipation of surgery. 3. Irritable airway or bronchospasm may occur; tobacco decreases hemoglobin which decreases oxygen delivery to healing wound; smokers may be more susceptible to thrombus.
Cardiovascular	1. Cardiac murmurs	1. Identify cardiac condition before surgery; may require subacute bacterial endocarditis prophylaxis.
Gastrointestinal	1. NPO status 2. History of vomiting or diarrhea 3. Constipation 4. Malnutrition 5. Metabolic disorders	1. Develop plan for usual oral medications. 2. Laboratory confirmation & fluid and electrolyte restoration. 3. Consider preoperative bowel cleansing. 4. Optimize nutrition in anticipation of surgery. 5. Dietary restrictions may need to be modified.
Neurologic	1. Intracranial hemorrhage risk 2. Seizures 3. Developmental delays	1. Anesthesia can alter intracranial and cerebral perfusion pressures. 2. Assess frequency, duration, and characteristics of seizures; anesthesia and preoperative anxiolytics may alter seizure threshold. 3. Anesthetic implications of degenerative neuromuscular disorders.
Endocrine	1. Diabetes 2. Adolescent females 3. Thyroid 4. Obesity	1. Schedule early in day; document normal insulin requirements & serum glucose range. 2. Determine menarche, menstrual cycle, & last menstrual period; rule out pregnancy (laboratory testing). 3. Maintain thyroid replacement; postoperative hypothyroidism can lead to hypotension and bradycardia. 4. Adipose tissue is less vascular—wounds prone to dehiscence.
Musculoskeletal	1. Contractures, plegias	1. Prevent intraoperative injury; careful intraoperative positioning.
Dermatologic	1. Alterations in skin integrity 2. Contagious skin conditions	1. Prevent further injury; prevent transmission of infections; higher risk for wound infections. 2. Isolation precautions.

(continues)

Table 1-3	*(continued)*	
Review of Systems	**Conditions**	**Anesthetic/Surgical Implications**
Hematologic/oncologic	1. Anemias/blood disorders 2. Receiving chemotherapy	1. Require further laboratory evaluation. 2. Chemotherapy can alter both cardiac and pulmonary functions.
Urologic	1. Home catheterization routine	1. May require indwelling catheter post-operatively.
Mental health	1. History of mental health treatment	1. Provide supportive environment; follow established treatment plan.

Adolescent Females

Most female patients who have achieved menarche require a urine pregnancy test before surgery. If the young woman is a mother, assess the details about her pregnancy and whether she is currently breastfeeding. If this is the case, a lactation specialist should be consulted to work with this patient after surgery so that she may maintain her milk supply.

Anesthetic History

Inquire about the child's previous anesthetic experiences. A significant past anesthetic history could include airway problems, previous tracheal intubation, or difficult or long-term venous access (Ferrari, 2002). Review the problems that can occur after anesthesia, including nausea, vomiting, and prolonged recovery. Ask about a family history of malignant hyperthermia.

Children with Multiple Health Issues

It is common to work with a child who has multiple health care needs. Ask whether the child has any special health care directives, such as a do-not-resuscitate (DNR) or altered code order. If this is the case, the anesthesia and surgical team should discuss this with the family (Oldham, Colombani, Foglia, & Skinner, 2005; ASA, 2001).

Any adaptive equipment that the child uses (e.g., wheelchair, braces) should be available after surgery. The nurse can work with the parents to develop a patient-specific plan of care.

Bleeding History or Anemia

A bleeding history should include assessment of frequent bruising, excessive or frequent nose bleeds, or slow-healing skin lesions. Depending on the nature of the child's hematologic issues, preoperative transfusion or clotting factor administration may be indicated.

Patients should also be assessed for any existing history of anemia or difficulty with clotting. Anemia may impair oxygen delivery during the operation, so a preoperative work-up may be necessary (Oldham et al., 2005).

Recent Illness/Illness Exposure and Infectious Disease and Isolation Practices

Preoperative history should include exposure to communicable diseases, presence of skin lesions, and signs of infection (e.g., fever, cough) (Black & Hawks, 2005). Children who have exposure to chickenpox or other childhood communicable diseases are prohibited from elective surgery to avoid cross-contamination between patients. Children with a recent history of bronchitis, respiratory syncytial virus (RSV), cough, or cold and those with asthma are at greater risk for irritable airway, laryngospasm, bronchospasm, postoperative hypoxemia, and atelectasis with anesthesia (Ferrari, 2002). However, recent opinion suggests that many of these children can be safely taken through the anesthetic experience (Tait & Malviya, 2005). Endotracheal intubation does continue to be a key contributing factor for exacerbation of respiratory symptoms (cough, bronchospasm) as well as oxygen desaturation (Cote et al., 2001). For children who have a known infectious disease (e.g., methicillin-resistant *Staphylococcus aureus* [MRSA], vancomycin-resistant *Enterococcus faecium* [VRE], etc.), document and institute isolation precautions.

For children requiring isolation, documentation includes an identification band placed on the child's extremity, notation on the preoperative documents, and identification on the child's chart. The operating room team should be notified so that isolation precautions can be maintained across the continuum of care.

Family Medical History

It is unnecessary to obtain a full family medical history. Instead, the examiner should focus on information that assists in the development of the anesthetic and surgical plan. Specifically, the examiner should address family reactions to anesthetic agents (e.g., prolonged paralysis) or a family history of neurodegenerative conditions, inherited blood disorders, or unexpected deaths (Cote et al., 2001; Ferrari, 2002). Signs and symptoms of pseudocholinesterase deficiency, malignant hyperthermia, and inherited blood disorders, such as sickle cell, should also be included in the family screening.

■ Preoperative Care: Physical Preparation

Laboratory Testing

Routine laboratory testing of pediatric surgical patients is no longer recommended. Laboratory testing should be determined by the medical condition of the child and the nature of the surgery to be performed. Tests should be restricted to those for whom the results will affect surgical management (Garcia-Miguel et al., 2003).

Bowel Preparation

In some instances, preoperative bowel cleansing may be needed. The goal of bowel cleansing is to prevent contamination of the abdominal cavity from fecal soiling during intestinal or abdominal surgery (Black & Hawks, 2005). There are multiple methods for mechanical emptying of intestinal contents. In addition, some procedures may warrant enteral antibiotic cleansing. Some preparations are completed in the home setting; it is important that the family understand the directions for the preparation. In other instances, a child may be admitted to the hospital on the day before surgery for this preparation.

Transfusion

The surgeon may request that the patient have blood typing and crossmatching completed with blood prepared and available for surgery. In some instances, preoperative transfusion is indicated. If a child needs a transfusion, packed red blood cells are the preferred product. In most instances, children do not need the volume that a unit of whole blood contains; all that is needed are the red cells to ensure adequate oxygen-carrying capacity (Cote et al., 2001).

Before a transfusion or the surgical procedure in which the transfusion may occur, the surgeon explains the indications, risks, and benefits of blood transfusion to the parents. After discussion and time allowed for answering of the families' questions, consent is obtained and the document is placed with the patient's medical records. If circumstances allow, directed blood donation by a family member or friend can be arranged. In instances when blood transfusion is likely and the parents have religious or cultural beliefs that preclude this intervention, the surgeon should discuss the use of alternative blood volume–expanding products (Benson, 1989; Ferrari, 2002). In some cases, the surgeon may need to obtain a court order to mandate that the child undergo transfusion. These issues need to be handled before surgery with care and sensitivity.

Preoperative Scrubs and Hair Removal

Preoperative showers and scrubs with antimicrobial soaps decrease microbial colony counts. However, they have not been definitively shown to decrease postoperative surgical wound infection (Mangram, Horan, Pearson, Silver, & Jarvis, 1999). However, the longer the time span between hair removal and the procedure, the higher the incidence of postoperative wound infection (Oldham et al., 2005; Phippen & Wells, 2000). Hair is not removed unless it interferes with the incision; the intraoperative team removes hair when indicated.

Dietary Restrictions

Once the timing of the procedure has been determined, review preoperative dietary restrictions with the patient and the family. Children have higher fluid requirements for size than adults, and prolonged preoperative fasting may cause dehydration, hypoglycemia, ketosis, and discomfort from hunger (Culpepper, 2000). Therefore, periods of fluid restriction must be minimized so that dehydration is avoided before anesthesia. Warner (1999) concluded that in healthy children, no increase in gastric volume or decrease in gastric pH occurred when the child was allowed apple juice 2 hours before surgery, as compared with children who fasted for longer periods of time. Therefore, abstinence from clear liquids longer than 2 hours before surgery is unnecessary. Current preoperative fasting recommendations for healthy children have been developed by the Society of Pediatric Anesthesiologists and incorporate these recommendations (Table 1-4).

Surgical Site Marking

The Joint Commission for the Accreditation of Healthcare Organizations (JCAHO) has developed guidelines to promote safe surgery. Practice requirements include marking sites where laterality occurs (e.g., with extremities).

Table 1-4	Preoperative Fasting Recommendations for Infants and Children	
Type of Meal	**Recommendation for Fasting Period**	
Clear liquids	2 hr before surgery	
Breast milk	4 hr before surgery	
Infant formula	6 hr before surgery	
Non-human milk	6 hr before surgery	
Light meal	6–8 hr before surgery	

Source: Summary of Fasting Recommendations to Reduce the Risk of Pulmonary Aspiration, Warner/American Society of Anesthesiologists, 1999.

JCAHO recommends that the patient and/or guardian mark the intended surgical site in the presence of the surgeon, who should then initial the intended site. Surgeries performed on the wrong site are completely preventable; site marking practices eliminate multiple factors that may lead to wrong site surgery (Joint Commission on Accreditation of Healthcare Organizations [JCAHO], 2004; JCAHO, 2003).

Preoperative Medication

Most clinicians selectively recommend pharmaceutical agents in addition to psychological preparation for surgery (Cote et al., 2001). The primary goal of preoperative sedation is the quiet induction of anesthesia. The effects of premedication decrease anxiety and an awareness of the environment in addition to providing analgesia (Fortunato, 2000).

Midazolam may be ordered as part of the preoperative sedation plan, because it reduces preoperative anxiety and provides amnesia and sedation (Gregory, 2002). Because anxiety reduction is the primary purpose of preoperative sedatives, the oral route is considered superior to the intravenous, intramuscular, or rectal route in children. Effective amnesia is achieved within about 10 minutes (Kain et al., 2000; Brosius & Bannister, 2003). A recent change in the oral formulation of midazolam makes it more palatable (Gregory). One investigator has found that the use of intravenous midazolam administered orally provides a more reliable sedation (Brosius & Bannister). Decreased postoperative negative behaviors (separation anxiety, nightmares) followed the use of preoperative midazolam when anxiety was decreased at the time of separation from a parent and at the induction of anesthesia (Kain, Mayes, Wang, & Hofstadter, 1999; Kain et al., 2000).

Final Preoperative Organization

As time nears for the surgical procedure, the nurse completes the final preoperative preparation. Parents and other family members should be ready to accompany the child. A child may choose to carry a favored toy or other comfort item to surgery (Gregory, 2002). Have the child and family ready for surgery at the prearranged time in order to maintain the flow of the operating room schedule. When preoperative delays occur, inform the surgeon and the operating room charge nurse. Table 1-5 provides a summary of the final preoperative details.

■ Preoperative: Holding Room

The holding room is the area immediately preceding entry into the operating room. The holding room nurse verifies patient identification, reviews the paperwork, and monitors the patient for adverse reactions to preoperative medication (Fortunato, 2000). A calm environment provides an easy transition into the operating room. Efforts are made to promote patient comfort and to minimize anxiety by using distraction techniques, such as toys and videos (Dunn, 1997).

In the holding room, the family meets again with the surgeon and anesthesiologist to review the plan and to address questions or concerns. The family also meets with the operating room nurse who will be caring for the child. The operating room nurse discusses his or her role and the manner in which the family will be updated during the surgical procedure. The child life specialist or chaplain may also be helpful to the family.

When parent-accompanied induction is planned, the parent, in appropriate attire, accompanies the child into the operating room suite (Table 1-6). If the parent(s) is not accompanying the child through induction, nursing staff should transfer or carry the child into the operating room and ask parents to wait in the assigned area. Explain when and where the parents will be able to see their child after the surgical procedure is completed. A parent paging system may be used for parent updates or to alert parents when the operation is nearing completion.

■ Postanesthesia Care Unit

Responsibilities of the PACU nurse include minimizing anxiety and controlling postoperative pain. Postoperative pain is managed with intermittent narcotics or initiation of patient/parent-controlled analgesia, epidural infusions, or other medications. For further information about postoperative pain management, refer to Chapter 5 in this text.

Table 1-5 **Final Preoperative Organization**

Patient Identification	Name Banding
Documentation	Completed preoperative checklist
Allergies	Allergy banding
Isolation requirements	Maintain isolation throughout operative experience; notification of OR team; isolation band; isolation "sticker" on chart
Laboratory testing	Urine HCG testing; verification of sickle cell testing; blood banding; results of pertinent labs on chart
NPO status	Review with parent last time child ate/drank
Jewelry/nail polish	Removal of nail polish & all jewelry (including body piercings)
Items to OR	Surgical consent; old medical records; radiographs
Personal items	Patient may choose preferred item to take to OR. Remove contact lenses; secure glasses or hearing aids; remove dental prosthesis; label personal items
Medication administration	Administration and documentation of ordered medication: midazolam, DDAVP, certain preoperative antibiotics, patient's daily meds (if any)
Procedures	Transfusion; enema administration
Language barrier(s)	Provision of interpreter

Sources: Phippen & Wells (2000); Fortunato (2000); Ferrari (2002).
DDAVP, vasopressin; HCG, human chorionic gonadotropin; OR, operating room.

Developmentally focused comfort activities aid in decreasing pain and anxiety. Allowing an infant to suckle on a pacifier, holding the inconsolable toddler, and using distraction techniques, such as toys, music, and videotapes for the preschooler helps settle the postoperative child. If older children and adolescents have questions about their surgical procedure and current status, these should be answered honestly.

Parental Presence

Many institutions have implemented programs in which the parents are allowed into the PACU. Parental presence during this early phase of a child's recovery can alleviate much of the child's excitement and stress (Gregory, 2002).

In the case of children with special health care needs, the parent can assist the child and can enhance the staff's ability to assess the child.

■ Other Considerations

Operative Care across the Continuum

Children receive surgical care electively, urgently, or emergently. Children's needs and assessments must be tailored to the timeline available. However short a preoperative time may be, the nurse must possess assessment and organizational skills to safely ready the child and family for surgery.

Table 1-6 **Parental Presence at Anesthesia Induction**

1. Parents must want to be present. No parent is forced to be with his or her child for anesthesia induction; however, a suitable substitute may be sought.
2. Patient safety is of the utmost importance. Children with airway problems and young children may be excluded from the program.
3. The parent is prepared preoperatively for the experience and supported emotionally after the experience by a familiar nurse.
4. The parent should be informed about the sequence of events, how the child will look during anesthesia induction, and how the child may react, as well as what the parents' role will be.
5. The parent may sit next to the child or comfort the child in the parent's lap as inhalation anesthesia commences.
6. Parents are encouraged to touch, sign, tell stories, and reassure their children during anesthesia induction.
7. The parent should be escorted from the induction area when the child is no longer aware of his surroundings.

Sources: Romino et al. (2005); Cote et al. (2001).

Same Day Surgery/Outpatient Surgery Center

As many as three million children undergo a surgical procedure each year. Sixty percent of the surgeries that are completed require a same-day stay surgery (Kain et al. 2002; Lauro & Berman, 2002). Those procedures occur either in a hospital or in a free-standing outpatient surgical center. If the procedure is performed in an outpatient surgical center, the child is generally in good health or has a systemic disease that is under good control (Gregory, 2002).

Hospitalized Patients

Some children require hospitalization after the surgical procedure. Sometimes, a child who is hospitalized may require surgery. In this instance, the inpatient nursing team prepare the child for surgery. Special inpatient considerations include "add-on" cases, in which the child is fit into the previously scheduled operative schedule. The inpatient nurse arranges or provides for preoperative preparation of the child and family and is the liaison who provides updates on the probable time of surgery.

Critically Ill Patients

Critically ill children may also require surgery. These children come to the operating room from the inpatient setting, from the emergency department, or from the trauma room. Treatment of shock and metabolic derangements before surgical intervention increase the success of the operative procedure (Clancy et al., 2001). The critical care nurse provides preoperative preparation for the family and usually receives the child back after surgery.

Out of the Operating Room Procedures

Procedures on Inpatient Wards and Procedures in Clinics/Physician Offices

Procedures ranging from chest tube insertion to removal of an ingrown toenail are performed outside of the operating room. Regardless of the procedure, the patient and family must be informed, the child must be medicated, and appropriate environmental precautions must be used.

Procedural Sedation

The concept and practice of procedural sedation are increasing. The patient's well-being and comfort as well as avoidance of undue stress must be ensured during procedures performed out of the operating room. The goal of procedural sedation is to provide pain management in addition to pharmacologically induced cooperation of a patient. Use preprocedure/conscious sedation protocols

to achieve this goal. Failure to complete a risk assessment before procedural sedation may increase adverse events during sedation (Hoffman, Nowakowski, Troshynski, Berens, & Weisman, 2002). Appropriate procedural sedation is safe, is adequate for the procedure, and provides comfort for the child. There are well-defined guidelines for monitoring and managing a patient during and after sedation. Any caregiver providing or assisting with procedural sedation must be knowledgeable about sedation guidelines (Committee on Drugs/American Academy of Pediatrics, 2002).

■ Conclusion

Preoperative preparation encompasses cognitive, psychological, and physical preparation of the child for surgery. Just as each child's physical presentation is unique, so are the psychological needs of each child. Preparation of the child and family for surgery must focus on their unique needs and must include a holistic approach to the physical and psychological preparation of the child. Parental presence facilitates a more positive coping response from the child, and parents must be included in the child's surgical experience. Attempts to individualize preoperative preparation are beneficial to the child's overall surgical experience.

■ Acknowledgment

We would like to recognize the contributions of Renee C.B. Manworren and Marti Fledderman to the perioperative chapter presented in the first edition of this textbook.

References

The Advisory Board Company. (2005, February 28). *Pediatric Interpretation Issues*. [Original Inquiry Brief]. Washington, D.C.

American Society of Anesthesiologists. (2001). *Ethical guidelines for the anesthesia care of patients with do-not-resuscitate orders*. Retrieved October 15, 2005, from American Society of Anesthesiologists Web site: http://www.asahq.org/publicationsAndServices/standards/09.html

American Society of Anesthesiologists. (2004). *Standards for basic anesthetic monitoring*. Retrieved October 15, 2005, from American Society of Anesthesiologists Web site: www.asahq.org/publicationsAndServices/standards/02.pdf

American Society of Anesthesiologists. (2005). *When your child needs anesthesia*. Retrieved October 15, 2005, from American Society of Anesthesiologists Web site: http://www.asahq.org/patientEducation/childanes.htm

AORN Latex Guideline. (2004). *AORN Journal, 79*, 653–672.

Bellew, M., Atkinson, K., Dixon, G., & Yates, A. (2002). The introduction of a paediatric anaesthesia information leaflet: An audit of its impact on parental anxiety and satisfaction [Electronic version]. *Pediatric Anesthesia, 12*, 124–130.

Benson, K. (1989). The Jehovah's Witness patient: Considerations for the anesthesiologist. *Anesthesia & Analgesia, 69*, 647–656.

Black, J., & Hawks, J. (2005). *Medical-surgical nursing: Clinical management for positive outcomes* (7th ed.). St. Louis, MO: Elsevier Saunders.

Brosius, K., & Bannister, C. (2003). Midazolam premedication in children: A comparison of two oral formulations on sedation score and plasma Midazolam levels. *Anesthesia & Analgesia, 96*, 392–395.

Burbano O'Leary, S., Federico, S., & Hampers, L. (2003). The truth about language barriers: One residency program's experience. *Pediatrics, 111*, 569–573.

Busen, N. (2001). Perioperative preparation of the adolescent surgical patient. *AORN Journal, 73*, 337–363.

Clancy, J., McVicar, A., & Boyd, S. (2001). The surgical neonate. *British Journal of Perioperative Nursing, 11*, 21–27.

Committee on Drugs/American Academy of Pediatrics. (2002). Guidelines for monitoring and management of pediatric patients during and after sedation for diagnostic and therapeutic procedures: Addendum [Electronic version]. *Pediatrics, 110*, 836–838.

Cote, C., Todres, I., Ryan, J., & Goudsouzian, N. (2001). *A practice of anesthesia for infants and children* (3rd ed.). Philadelphia: WB Saunders.

Culpepper, T. (2000). AANA journal course: Update for nurse anesthetists—intraoperative fluid management for the pediatric surgical patient. *AANA Journal, 68*, 531–538.

Dunn, D. (1997). Responsibilities of the preoperative holding area nurse. *AORN Journal, 66*, 820–838.

Ells, C., & Caniano, D. (2002). The impact of culture on the patient-surgeon relationship [Electronic version]. *Journal of the American College of Surgeons, 195*, 520–530.

Erikson, E. (1985). *Childhood and society, 35th anniversary edition.* New York: W.W. Norton & Company.

Ferrari, L. (2002). Do children need a preoperative assessment that is different from adults? *International Anesthesiology Clinics, 40*, 167–186.

Ferrari, L. (2004). Preoperative evaluation of pediatric surgical patients with multisystem considerations [Electronic version]. *Anesthesia & Analgesia, 99*, 1058–1069.

Flores, G., Laws, M., Mayo, S., Zuckerman, B., Medina, L., Abreu, M., et al. (2003). Errors in medial interpretation and their potential clinical consequences in pediatric encounters [Electronic version]. *Pediatrics, 111*, 6–15.

Fortunato, N. (2000). *Berry & Kohn's operating room technique* (9th ed.). St. Louis, MO: Mosby.

Garcia-Miguel, F., Serrano-Aguillar, P., & Lopez-Bastida, J. (2003). Preoperative assessment [Electronic version]. *The Lancet, 362*, 1749–1757.

Gregory, G. (2002). *Pediatric anesthesia* (4th ed.). New York: Churchill Livingstone.

Hoffman, G., Nowakowski, R., Troshynski, T., Berens, R., & Weisman, S. (2002). Risk reduction in pediatric procedural sedation by application of an American Academy of Pediatrics/American Society of Anesthesiologists process model [Electronic version]. *Pediatrics, 109*, 236–243.

Holzman, R., Brown, R., Hamid, R., Hirschman, C., Kinsella, S., Petrovich, C., et al. (2005). *Natural rubber latex allergy: Considerations for anesthesiologists.* Retrieved October 15, 2005, from American Society of Anesthesiologists Web site: http://www.asahq.org/publicationsAndServices/latexallergy.pdf

Joint Commission on Accreditation of Healthcare Organizations (JCAHO). (n.d.). *Help prevent errors in your care: For surgical patients* [patient brochure]. Retrieved October 12, 2005, from Joint Commission on Accreditation of Healthcare Organizations Web site: http://www.jcaho.org/general+public/gp+speak+up/wrong_site_brochure.pdf

Joint Commission on Accreditation of Healthcare Organizations (JCAHO). (2004). *Procedures requiring surgical site marking.* Retrieved October 12, 2005, from Joint Commission on Accreditation of Healthcare Organizations Web site: http://www.jcaho.org/accredited+organizations/hospitals/standards/hospital+faqs/provision+of+care/anesthesia+care/site_marking.htm

Joint Commission on Accreditation of Healthcare Organizations (JCAHO). (2003). *Universal protocol for preventing wrong site, wrong procedure, wrong person surgery.* Retrieved October 12, 2005, from Joint Commission on Accreditation of Healthcare Organizations Web site: http://www.jcaho.org/accredited+organizations/patient+safety/universal+protocol/universal_protocol.pdf

Kain, Z., Caldwell-Andrews, A., & Wang, S. (2002). Psychological preparation of the parent and pediatric surgical patient [Electronic version]. *Anesthesiology Clinics of North America, 1*, 29–44.

Kain, Z., Hofstadter, M., Mayes, L., Krivutza, D., Alexander, G., Wang, S., et al. (2000). Midazolam: Effects on amnesia and anxiety in children [Electronic version]. *Anesthesiology, 93*, 676–684.

Kain, Z., Mayes, L., Wang, S., & Hofstadter, M. (1999). Postoperative behavioral outcomes in children: Effects of sedative premedication [Electronic version]. *Anesthesiology, 90*, 758–765.

Koopman, H., Baars, R., Chaplin, J., & Zwinderman, K. (2004). Illness through the eyes of a child: The development of children's understanding of the causes of illness [Electronic version]. *Patient Education and Counseling, 55*, 363–370.

LaMontagne, L. (2000). Children's coping with surgery: A process-oriented perspective [Electronic version]. *Journal of Pediatric Nursing, 15*, 307–312.

LaMontagne, L., Hepworth, J., Cohen, F., & Salisbury, M. (2003). Cognitive-behavioral intervention effects on adolescents' anxiety and pain following spinal fusion surgery. *Nursing Research, 52*, 183–190.

Lauro, H., & Berman, L. (2002). Cutting-edge pediatric anesthesia for the outpatient. *Same Day Surgery Reports, BB#513*, 1–7.

Mangram, A., Horan, T., Pearson, M., Silver, L., & Jarvis, W. (1999). Guideline for prevention of surgical site infection. *Infection Control and Hospital Epidemiology, 20*, 247–278.

Nwomeh, B., Waller, A., Caniano, D., & Kelleher, K. (2005). Informed consent for emergency surgery in infants and children [Electronic version]. *Journal of Pediatric Surgery, 40*, 1320–1325.

O'Connor-Von, S. (2000). Preparing children for surgery—an integrative research review. *AORN Journal, 71*, 334–343.

Oldham, K., Colombani, P., Foglia, R., & Skinner, M. (Eds.). (2005). *Principles and practice of pediatric surgery.* Philadelphia: Lippincott Williams & Wilkins.

Phippen, M., & Wells, M. (2000). *Patient care during operative and invasive procedures* (2nd ed.). Philadelphia: W.B. Saunders Company.

Piaget, J. (1968). *Psychological studies.* D. Elkind (Ed) (A. Tenzer, Trans). New York: Random House.

Romino, S., Keatley, V., Secrest, J., & Good, K. (2005). Parental presence during anesthesia induction in children. *AORN Journal, 81*, 780–792.

Schmidt, C. (2001). Development of children's body knowledge, using knowledge of the lungs as an exemplar [Electronic version]. *Issues in Comprehensive Pediatric Nursing, 24*, 177–191.

Smith, L., & Callery, P. (2004). Children's accounts of their preoperative information needs. *Journal of Clinical Nursing, 14*, 230–238.

Spencer, C., & Franck, L. (2005). Giving parents written information about children's anesthesia: Are setting and timing important? [Electronic version]. *Pediatric Anesthesia, 15*, 547–553.

Tait, A., & Malviya, S. (2005). Anesthesia for the child with an upper respiratory tract infection: Still a dilemma? [Electronic version]. *Anesthesia & Analgesia, 100*, 59–65.

Warner, M. (1999). Practice guidelines for preoperative fasting and the use of pharmacologic agents to reduce the risk of pulmonary aspiration: Application to healthy patients undergoing elective procedures: A report by the American Society of Anesthesiologists Task Force on preoperative fasting [Electronic version]. *Anesthesiology, 90*, 896–905.

Wilson, H., Nagy, C., & Jessee, P. (2001). Children's understanding of illness: Students' assessments [Electronic version]. *Journal of Pediatric Nursing, 16*(6), 429–437.

Wollin, S., Plummer, J., Owen, H., Hawkins, R., Materazzo, F., & Morrison, V. (2004). Anxiety in children having elective surgery [Electronic version]. *Journal of Pediatric Nursing, 19*, 128–132.

Zuwala, R., & Barber, K. (2001). Reducing anxiety in parents before and during pediatric anesthesia induction. *AANA Journal, 69*, 21–25.

CHAPTER

2

Fluid and Electrolyte Management of the Pediatric Surgical Patient

By Neil Ead

Fluid management in the pediatric surgical patient is a critical element of pediatric care. Fluid and electrolyte management of pediatric patients must be extremely precise if these patients are to maintain homeostasis. This chapter reviews considerations in maintaining the fluid and electrolyte status in the pediatric surgical patient in the preoperative, intraoperative, and postoperative phases. It includes a review of deficits, maintenance, and replacement strategies used in the pediatric surgical patient.

■ Body Fluid Compartments and Composition

Three key factors influence fluid and electrolyte balance and are different in infants and small children than those of the adult: internal distribution of water, insensible water losses, and kidney function (Tuggle, 2003). The first major concern is how infants and small children distribute and regulate water. The newborn is made up of approximately 75% to 80% total body water (Merenstein & Gardner, 2003). This falls to about 60% by the time the child reaches 1 year of age (O'Neill, Grosfeld, Fonkalsrud, Coran, & Caldamone, 2003). Not only is there proportionately more water in the child's body but it is also dis-

tributed differently than that of the adult. Body fluids are distributed in two main functional compartments: intracellular fluid (ICF) and extracellular fluid (ECF). The primary intracellular cation is potassium, and the primary electrolyte in the ECF is sodium. In the neonate, most of the water is located in the extracellular space. Less body water is in the extracellular space in the adult. The ECF is located outside the cells and includes the intravascular and interstitial fluid. The extracellular space is located within the blood vessels, around the cells, and around the brain and spinal cord. The ICF is located within the cell. Approximately half of a child's ECF is exchanged every 24 hours (Bindler & Howry, 2005). This means that the infant has a greater daily fluid requirement with little fluid volume reserve. Thus, any increase in fluid loss rapidly leads to dehydration (Wheeler, 2002). Infants and small children also have a greater proportion of body surface area than that of adults; this places them at greater risk for fluid losses from evaporation (Binkley, Beckett, Casa, Kleiner, & Plummer, 2002). Changes in the ECF volume are the most frequent and important abnormalities encountered in the surgical patient (Sarti, DeGaudio, Messineo, Cuttini, & Ventura, 2001).

The next important factor contributing to the child's fluid status is that of insensible water loss, which is the invisible, continuous, passive loss of water from the skin (evaporation), lungs (respiration), and metabolism (Hand, 2001). One can estimate daily insensible water losses by multiplying 300 mL by the child's body surface area. In addition to insensible water losses being greater in children, they are often increased with illness or as a result of selected medical treatments (Wessel, 2001). Fever increases insensible water losses by about 10mL/kg for each degree centigrade above 37°C (van Wissen & Breton, 2004).

The final physiologic factor affecting a small child's fluid status is the maturity of the kidneys (Drukker & Guignard, 2002). During the first 2 years of life, the kidneys are functionally immature and unable to effectively concentrate or dilute urine. Therefore, low specific gravity may be falsely reassuring in the infant with dehydration. In addition, the mechanisms for sodium regulation are not yet mature. They are also inefficient at excreting the products of metabolism. Therefore, the infant or small child who receives excessive amounts of fluid may be unable to increase urine output to compensate, resulting in hypervolemia. In summary, fluid and electrolyte imbalances may progress quickly in small infants and children.

Normal Exchange of Fluid and Electrolytes

Osmosis is the movement of a fluid through a semipermeable membrane from a solution that has a lower solute concentration to one that has a higher solute concentration. Osmolality refers to the number of particles (proteins and electrolytes) per liter of water. A solution with the same osmolality as blood plasma is called isotonic (Cook, 2003). Normal serum osmolality ranges from approximately 272 to 300 mOsm/L. Acute changes in the serum osmolality produce free water shifts. Free water moves from an area of low osmolality to an area of higher osmolality (Allison, 2004). A decreased serum osmolality usually indicates low sodium concentration, whereas an increased serum osmolality usually indicates a high concentration of sodium (Behrman, Kliegman, & Jenson, 2004).

Preoperative Considerations

A critical part of assisting the pediatric surgical patient in maintaining fluid and electrolyte balance is preoperative assessment and identification of risk factors for imbalance. Preoperative laboratory analysis of electrolyte levels should be checked if indicated by the history and physical examination. Abnormalities should be corrected

before any surgical procedure is performed, unless surgery is needed to correct a life-threatening problem (Maharaj et al., 2005). Medical management of preexisting conditions can affect fluid and electrolyte balance (Holliday, Segar, & Friedman, 2003).

Preexisting conditions, such as diabetes mellitus, liver disease, and renal insufficiency, may be aggravated by surgical stress, thereby increasing a child's risk of fluid and electrolyte imbalances. Preoperative medications may affect the excretion of water and electrolytes. Preoperative surgical regimens, such as the administration of enemas or laxatives, may increase fluid loss from the gastrointestinal tract. Preoperative enteral fluid restrictions are used to reduce nausea, vomiting, and aspiration risk in the surgical patient. The neonate or young infant, who is often fed every 3 hours, may not tolerate prolonged periods without enteral feedings. Lengthy preoperative oral intake restriction may be unavoidable in the acutely ill child, but it can lead to significant dehydration without the administration of adequate intravenous fluids. In the healthy infant undergoing elective surgery, prolonged oral fluid restrictions may not be necessary. There are less fluids found in the stomach after 2 hours in patients who have consumed small amounts of clear liquid than in those who have fasted (Reiling & McKellar, 2004).

Typically, clear liquids are allowed up to 2 hours before surgery. To avoid this problem, small infants may be scheduled as the first elective surgical cases of the day.

In summary, whether the patient is scheduled electively or emergently, fluid administration is goal-directed (Gan et al., 2002). In some cases, ongoing fluid resuscitation may continue throughout the intraoperative and postoperative periods. In others, perioperative fluid restrictions are indicated (Joshi, 2005).

Calculating Fluid and Electrolyte Requirements

Fluid management should be approached by dividing water and electrolyte requirements into deficit, maintenance, and replacement therapy (Marko, Layon, Caruso, Moxingo, & Gabrielli, 2003). Fundamental to any system of fluid management is an accurate determination of the current volume and hydration status of the patient. Deficit therapy refers to the evaluation and management of the losses of fluid and electrolytes that occurred before the patient's presentation. There are three essential components to deficit therapy: (1) accurate estimation of the severity of dehydration, (2) determination of the type of deficit that has occurred, (3) development of an approach to replete the deficit. Infants and children are relatively sensitive to small degrees of dehydration. Regardless of the management approach adopted to guide therapy, clinicians should take into account the changing physiology of the pediatric surgical patient (Hughes, 2004).

The most common patient problems associated with fluid and electrolyte balance during surgery include fluid volume deficit, sodium and water imbalances, and potassium imbalances. Fluid volume deficit is an imbalance in isotonic body fluids related to either abnormal fluid loss or decreased oral intake. Children with acute surgical illnesses may have significant fluid and electrolyte deficits from poor oral intake, vomiting, diarrhea, peritonitis, sepsis, burns, or hemorrhage (Nager & Wang, 2002).

The effect of fluid loss on the surgical patient depends on the amount of fluid lost and the speed at which those losses occur. Excessive or rapid losses quickly progress to a state of shock (Wessel, 2001). The clinical signs and symptoms of classic dehydration are the result of ECF volume depletion: hypovolemia, decreased cardiac output, and decreased tissue perfusion. When approximately one third of ECF volume has been lost, profound physiologic disturbances become evident (Cote, Todres, Goudsouzian, & Ryan, 2001). Intravascular volume must be rapidly restored to maintain adequate tissue perfusion for normal organ function, particularly if the child is emergently transferred to the operating room (Merenstein & Gardner, 2003). Dehydration is often characterized as mild, moderate, or severe (Armon, Stephenson, MacFaul, Eccleston, & Werneke, 2001). The degree of severity of dehydration is estimated from the patient's history and physical condition at the time of presentation (Behrman et al., 2004). In children with mild dehydration (1%–5%), the findings are largely historical. Children with moderate dehydration (6%–10%) may present with symptoms of dehydration and electrolyte disturbance. Physical findings may include changes in skin turgor, weight loss, sunken eyes and fontanel, slight lethargy, and dry mucous membranes. With severe dehydration (11%–15%), the child may exhibit cardiovascular instability (AHA, 2001). Percent dehydration is calculated based on estimates of associated weight loss in kilograms. Once the loss of weight is determined, the percent of weight loss from baseline is used to extrapolate the percent hydration. No single piece of laboratory data can predict the severity of dehydration. Symptoms typically associated with mild, moderate, and severe dehydration are featured in Table 2-1.

The child's fluid deficit refers to the estimated measurement of fluids lost during the illness before therapy. This assessment is helpful for further approximation of fluid losses and estimation of replacement therapy. Replacement therapy is guided by estimated losses. For each estimated percent of body weight lost, 10 mL/kg of replacement fluid is usually indicated (Behrman et al., 2004). Extracellular fluid volume deficit is the most common fluid imbalance in the surgical patient. The most common causes include loss of gastrointestinal fluids from vomiting, nasogastric suction, diarrhea, ostomy, fistula, and tube drainage (Mythen, 2005).

The type of deficit that has occurred can be further estimated using electrolyte values. The type of dehydration is defined by the tonicity of the patient's serum (Ball & Bindler, 2006). On this basis, states of dehydration are commonly referred to as isotonic or isonatremic, hypotonic or hyponatremic, and hypertonic or hypernatremic. Isotonic dehydration is characterized by proportionate losses of sodium and water. Serum osmolality ranges between approximately 270 and 300 mOsm/L and serum sodium level between 130 and 150 mEq/L. Intake is inadequate to balance losses, and losses are primarily extracellular. Hypotonic dehydration results when sodium losses are proportionately greater than fluid loss. Serum osmolality is less than 270 mOsm/L, whereas serum sodium level is greater than 150 mEq/L. Fluid shifts from the extracellular to the intracellular compartment in an attempt to reach equilibrium. Hyponatremic dehydration is primarily extracellular. This occurs in severe prolonged vomiting and diarrhea, burns, and renal disease. Use of hypotonic solutions in the treatment of dehydration can also result in hypotonic/hyponatremic dehydration. Initial rehydration may be administered over a relatively rapid period of time (within 24 hours) in isotonic and hypotonic dehydration (Sweeney, 2005). Hypertonic dehydration is characterized by greater fluid loss in proportion to sodium. Serum osmolality is greater than 310 mOsm/L, and serum sodium level is greater than 150 mEq/L. Extracellular fluid volumes remain relatively normal at the expense of the cell. Therefore, signs and symptoms of dehydration may be initially absent.

Symptoms of dehydration are often dangerously late and occur simultaneously with symptoms of intracellular dehydration. It may occur in patients who receive hypertonic intravenous fluids or tube feedings as well as in conditions like diabetes insipidus. Patients with hypertonic dehydration must be given special attention because of serious complications. Plasma sodium levels are slowly corrected by no more than 10 mEq/L/day (Lain & Wong 2002). The period for correction of deficits is usually 48 hours or longer to avoid central nervous system changes from cerebral edema. There are many approaches to the correction of fluid volume deficits. Regardless of the ap-

Table 2-1	Severity of Clinical Hydration		
Clinical Assessment	Mild	Moderate	Severe
% body weight lost	Up to 5% (40–50 mL/kg)	6%–9% (60–90 mL/kg)	10% or more (1001 mL/kg)
Level of consciousness	Alert, restless, thirsty	Irritable or lethargic (infants and very young children); alert, thirsty, restless (older children and adolescents)	Lethargic to comatose (infants and young children); often conscious, apprehensive (older children and adolescents)
Blood pressure	Normal	Normal or low; postural hypotension (older children and adolescents)	Low to undetectable
Pulse	Normal	Rapid	Rapid, weak to nonpalpable
Skin turgor	Normal	Poor	Very poor
Mucous membranes	Moist	Dry	Parched
Urine	May appear normal	Decreased output (<1 mL/kg/hr); dark color; increased specific gravity	Very decreased or absent output
Thirst	Slightly increased	Moderately increased	Greatly increased unless lethargic
Fontanel	Normal	Sunken	Sunken
Extremities	Warm; normal capillary refill	Delayed capillary refill (>2 sec)	Cool, discolored; delayed capillary refill (.3–4 sec)
Respirations	Normal	Normal or rapid	Changing rate and pattern

Source: Reprinted with permission (Ball and Bindler, 2006).

proach, certain principles must be followed. The restoration of cardiovascular function and preservation of cerebral and renal perfusion are of primary concern. Therapy should be initiated with isotonic fluid. The solution of choice is usually physiologic and is within close proximity to serum osmolality. Lactated Ringer's solution or 0.9% sodium chloride is given as a bolus of 10 to 20 mL/kg (AHA, 2001). Total body correction of fluid deficits may require a considerable period of time.

The primary electrolytes lost with most fluid volume deficits are sodium and potassium. Sodium deficits are generally corrected with isotonic fluid administration. Potassium is an intracellular ion and is generally not replaced until adequate renal function is ensured. The primary site of potassium clearance is the kidney. Therefore, potassium should not be administered in the child with oliguria. A rising creatinine concentration, changes in the blood urea nitrogen to creatinine ratio, and hyperkalemia are indicators of renal failure (Kluckow & Evans, 2001). The maximum concentration of potassium in replacement fluid is 40 mEq/L (Tuggle, 2003). The adequacy of deficit therapy needs to be constantly re-evaluated by continuous monitoring of the clinical condition. Therefore,

it is essential that the surgical team assess the fluid needs of the patient throughout the entire period of surgical management. The preoperative phase may involve fluid resuscitation with significant deficits. Fluid and electrolytes are provided throughout the perioperative period. If significant deficits exist, correction continues during surgery and well into the postoperative phase.

Intraoperative Management

Intraoperative management is influenced by deficit replacement, increases in vascular capacitance, losses due to hemorrhage, and anticipated losses due to sequestration (Kaye & Grogono, 2000). The focus during the postoperative phase is directed toward correction of deficits, both cumulative and ongoing, and later adjustment for the return of sequestered fluid to the venous system (Lefever-Kee & Paulanka, 2000).

During the operative procedure, the fluid choice reflects the most dominant fluid loss. Simple elective procedures in a well-hydrated child may result in insignificant losses. Hypotonic fluids may be adequate to replace minimal free water and minimal electrolyte losses (Kudsk, 2003). In the child who presents with significant preoperative deficits or the child who undergoes procedures associated with significant sequestration (third spacing), the use of isotonic solutions is indicated (van Wissen & Breton, 2004). For procedures in which significant blood loss has occurred, blood products may be administered. Selected blood products may also be administered to correct hematologic deficits, as occur in the oncology patient.

■ Sequestration/Third-Spacing

As previously mentioned in this chapter, the ECF is composed of the intravascular fluid (plasma) and the interstitial fluid. Sequestration or "third spacing" is defined as the movement of water and solute from the intravascular space to the interstitium. Increased capillary permeability causes plasma proteins to diffuse from the intravascular fluid compartment into the interstitial space. Plasma proteins are colloidal. They create an osmotic pressure gradient that sequesters fluid from the vascular space into the interstitium (Metheny, 2000). This movement of fluids, electrolytes, and proteins benefits neither the cell nor the vascular space (Redden & Wotton, 2001). This occurs to some degree with any type of inflammatory process, but it may be profound and life threatening in major prolonged abdominal or thoracic procedures, trauma, burns, and sepsis. In these situations, intravascular depletion may be significant enough to progress to cardiovascular collapse. Common sites of sequestration in abdominal surgery are the bowel and the peritoneal space. Pulmonary effusions may occur in association with thoracic surgery. With the systemic inflammatory response seen in sepsis and its accompanying profound capillary leak, sequestration may be more generalized, resulting in severe peripheral edema. Sepsis accompanied by the sequestration associated with surgery further complicates resuscitation during the postoperative period (Carcillo & Fields, 2002).

Patients who have significant amounts of sequestered fluid from the vascular space show all the signs of fluid volume deficits previously discussed. Urinary output may become diminished and more concentrated over time, and perfusion parameters may be altered. Hemoglobin and hematocrit may be elevated initially due to hemoconcentration, but fluid resuscitation may have a dilutional effect on the serum to where hemoglobin and hematocrit may be normal or low. In addition, if fluid is shifted into the peritoneum and bowel, the abdomen may become distended. Peripheral edema may be noted around the eyes, hands, feet, and genitalia. If untreated, the symptoms may progress to hypotension and, eventually, complete cardiovascular collapse. The surgical nurse must be constantly alert for early signs of third-space shifting. Meticulous measurements and monitoring of intake and output, specific gravity, abdominal girth, weight, severity of peripheral edema, and vital signs are a priority. Third-space losses cannot be directly measured (Radhakrishnan et al., 2005), and their intravenous replacement must be approximated. Sequestered fluid is almost always isotonic, and its replacement may be given as an isotonic crystalloid balanced salt solution, such as lactated Ringer's solution. Occasionally, serial administration of albumin and diuretics may be administered in order to facilitate re-absorption and excretion of sequestered fluid. Colloid should be used with caution. With profound capillary leak, administered colloid may sequester, taking with it additional fluid.

As the causative inflammation, surgical trauma, or infection decreases, capillary permeability returns to normal, sequestered fluid begins to reabsorb, and observable sites of edema begin to resolve. This usually begins over the first 24 to 48 hours after surgery. If fluid therapy is not adjusted at this time, the potential for intravascular fluid overload is great. Isotonic solutions are usually discontinued, and infusion rates are lowered as fluid is mobilized and urine output increases and becomes more dilute.

■ Implications for Postanesthesia Care

The transition to postanesthesia care maintains the focus on maintenance, correction of deficits and changes in vascular capacitance, and accounts for anticipated losses. The effects of anesthesia may include significant and prolonged changes in vascular capacitance. Systemic vasodilatation may alter cardiac preload enough to require adjustments in fluid management during the postanesthesia recovery phase. The patient may transition to the postanesthesia care unit with ongoing deficits and ongoing losses, which further contribute to the development of cardiovascular collapse. This generally requires ongoing replacement and maintenance with isotonic solutions (Cook, 2003). Resuscitation efforts may be maintained. If a prolonged period of resuscitation is anticipated, admission to a critical care setting may be considered, which often results in eliminating a short stay in the postanesthesia care unit.

Daily Maintenance Fluid and Electrolyte Requirements

Intravenous maintenance solutions contain the proportions of fluid and solutes required for basal needs. They may be used to replace the normal physiologic losses associated with basal metabolism, insensible fluid loss from the skin (evaporation) and lungs (respiration), and urine losses (Puglise, 2003). The aim of maintenance therapy is to replace water and electrolytes that are lost under ordinary conditions. Maintenance fluids are designed to maintain water and electrolyte homeostasis with the use of minimal renal compensatory mechanisms. They may be used solely over short periods of time but are not recommended over a prolonged period without a source of nutrition, especially in the small infant. Prolonged starvation may result in increased postoperative complications. The addition of 5% to 10% glucose to the maintenance fluid for the usual brief period of parenteral therapy in the child who is not previously malnourished provides sufficient calories to suppress severe ketosis. However, when prolonged periods of postoperative caloric restriction are anticipated, parenteral nutrition may be indicated until adequate enteral intake is re-established (Nehra, 2002).

The calculation of a patient's specific maintenance fluid requirement can be based on weight or surface area. The most commonly applied formulas used to calculate maintenance requirements are based on body weight and assume a healthy basal metabolic rate (Table 2-2).

Conditions associated with substantial increases in metabolism include, but are not limited to, prematurity, fever, prolonged respiratory distress, severe pain, and sepsis. In situations where the metabolic rate is elevated, fluid needs are increased (Hill, 2000). Formulas for calculating fluid requirements are extremely useful, but clinicians must follow patient responses to therapy that may necessitate adjustments in those calculated volumes. Circulatory parameters are monitored, and serum electrolyte, hemoglobin, and hematocrit values may be monitored closely. Accurate accounting of intake and output is essential throughout the perioperative period. The total fluid intake includes all sources of fluid administered enterally and parenterally. Output totals consider all measurable losses, which often include urine output; drainage from tubes, stomas, or fistulae; and losses from the gastrointestinal tract. As mentioned earlier, it may be difficult to estimate losses due to sequestration or third spacing. Certain disease states may further necessitate adjustments in fluid maintenance strategies. Conditions associated with selected congenital cardiac anomalies, renal failure, or increased intracranial pressure may require restrictions that complicate fluid therapy. However, if calculated fluid requirements take into account patient responses, anticipated ongoing losses, and existing disease states, the accuracy of fluid and electrolyte therapy is more likely. Stable perfusion parameters, normal electrolytes, and intake and output totals that are relatively equal are usually good clinical indicators of effective management (Hughes, 2004).

Electrolyte maintenance requirements are based on the patient's weight or body surface area. Pediatric dosages for sodium and potassium are expressed as milliequivalents (mEq) and are calculated using body weight in kilograms (kg) per day (mEq/kg/day). The sodium requirement is approximately 3 mEq/kg/day. The potassium requirement is approximately 2 mEq/kg/day (Blonshine, 2000).

Replacement of Ongoing Losses

Replacement fluid therapy is designed to replace ongoing abnormal fluid and electrolyte losses that continue during therapy and are generally related to persistent vomiting, diarrhea, nasogastric tube drainage, stoma output, wound drainage, pleural fluid, and fistula losses. Isotonic solutions are most appropriate for all drains requiring irrigation. Other solutions may contribute to further electrolyte abnormalities. The loss of water and electrolytes in stool is usually negligible unless diarrhea is present (Larson, 2000). Those losses can be, but are not often, measured and are usually not accounted for in the calculation of deficit or maintenance requirements. Therefore, they must be added to fluid therapy. Moreover, output from these sources may result in losses that are not consistent with selected maintenance fluids. Acid-base balance and serum electrolyte levels may assist the clinician in choosing fluid replacement solutions. Acid-base balance may be dramatically affected by losses via gastrointestinal fistulae, ileostomy, or stool. Hence, it may be inaccurate to simply increase the volume of maintenance fluids in an attempt to compensate for those losses. Replacement solutions are given in addition to mainte-

Table 2-2	Scale: Daily Maintenance Fluid Needs
Weight	**Fluid Needs/24 hr**
0–10 kg (0–22 lb)	100 mL/kg
11–20 kg (24–44 lb)	1,000 mL plus 50 mL/kg>10 kg
>20 kg (>44 lb)	1,500 mL plus 20 mL/kg>20 kg

nance fluid therapy. Replacement fluid choices may vary, depending on the source of the output. For example, lactated Ringer's solution has a buffering effect and is preferable to replace ileostomy output when loss of bicarbonate is expected. Sodium chloride in a 0.45% solution with added potassium may be used to replace nasogastric output when sodium and, to a lesser extent, potassium losses are expected. Excessive losses of potassium are often seen in severe diarrhea. Table 2-3 represents the average loss of electrolytes from various sites.

The rapidity with which an abnormal loss is replaced varies and depends on the amount and the rate of loss and the size of the patient. Infants may have a relatively small amount of actual fluid lost, although proportionately, it represents a large percentage of their circulating volume. Losses may be replaced over 2- to 8-hour intervals, depending on the size of the child and the extent of the losses over time. In most cases, it is advisable to replace large ongoing fluid losses promptly (Suhayda & Walton, 2002).

■ Types of Intravenous Solutions

Intravenous fluid therapy is administered in order to correct electrolyte abnormalities, replete fluid deficits in one or more compartments (ICF, ECF, or both), and correct acid-base imbalance (Cook, 2003). Crystalloid solutions consist of various concentrations of glucose and solutes in a water solution (Table 2-4). There are three classifications based on osmolality of the fluid and its relationship to serum osmolality. Normal serum osmolality is 280 to 300 mOsm/kg. Osmosis occurs with a 10% difference of that range. Thus, isotonic solutions have a range of 250 to 330 mOsm/L. When these solutions are administered, there is no shift of fluid into the cell. Isotonic crystalloid is not a volume expander. Approximately one third of iso-

tonic crystalloid administered during fluid resuscitation remains within the vascular space. Common isotonic solutions include lactated Ringer's solution or 0.9% sodium chloride. These preparations are generally administered to the surgical patient with resuscitation during the preoperative, intraoperative, and immediate postoperative period. Within the first 24 to 48 hours after surgery, sequestered fluid begins to return to the vascular space largely via the lymphatics. This effect is enhanced when the patient mobilizes. Isotonic fluids are then discontinued, and fluids may be reduced to maintenance alone to avoid fluid overload. Urine output also increases as fluid begins to mobilize. Patients particularly at risk at this time are those with renal failure or cardiovascular compromise.

Hypotonic solutions have an osmolarity below 250 mOsm/L. When they are administered, they cause a shift of fluid into the cell. A hypotonic solution such as 0.45% sodium chloride is appropriate for patients who need cellular hydration, as seen in patients experiencing diabetic ketoacidosis or in patients who undergo prolonged diuretic therapy. Hypertonic solutions have an osmolality greater than 330 mOsm/L. A hypertonic solution draws fluids from the cell; an example of this would be solutions containing 3% to 5% sodium chloride. These are rarely used in the surgical patient except in cases of severe hyponatremia or water intoxication. Patients receiving these solutions should be closely monitored.

Colloids are solutions containing large particles of protein, sugars, starch, or complex carbohydrate molecules, such as albumin, dextran, hydroxyethyl starch, and gelatin derivatives. They exert high osmotic pressures, drawing fluid into the vascular space. Blood may also be considered a colloid and true volume expander. Blood products are most often ordered when surgical procedures represent real or potentially significant blood loss,

Table 2-3	Composition of Gastrointestinal Secretions			
Type	**Na (mEq/L)**	**K (mEq/L)**	**Cl (mEq/L)**	**HCO₃ (mEq/L)**
Salivary	10	25	130	30
Stomach	60	10	130	
Duodenum	140	5	80	
Ileum	140	5	104	30
Colon	60	30	40	
Pancreas	140	5	75	115
Bile	45	5	100	35

Source: Reprinted with permission (Siegler, M., Azizkhan, R., & Weber, T., 2003).

Table 2-4	Composition of Commonly Used IV Fluids						
Fluid	Dextrose Mg/mL	Na mEq/L	K mEq/L	Ca mEq/L	Mg mEq/L	Cl mEq/L	Other
Lactated Ringer's	0	130	4	3	0	109	28 lactate
0.9% Sodium chloride	0	154	0	0		154	
5% Dextrose	50	0	0	0	0	0	
5% Dextrose in 0.45% sodium chloride	50	77	0	0	0	77	
Plasmalyte	0	140	5	0	3	98	
Normosol	0	140	5	0	3	90	27 lactate

Source: Reprinted with permission (Holmes and Walley, 2003).

as occurs in trauma and in replacement strategies in the oncology patient.

Oral Rehydration Solutions

The ability to select from different types of fluids and customize the infusion prescription to the patient's needs is a large part of ensuring positive patient outcomes. Oral rehydration solutions are successfully used in treating many children with mild isotonic, hypotonic, or hypertonic dehydration. Vomiting is not a contraindication (Ozuah, Avner, & Stein, 2002). These solutions have traditionally played a role in the treatment of mild acute dehydration, particularly for the child with gastroenteritis (Larson, 2000). Frequent, small frequent doses of oral rehydration solutions may be administered in order to avoid emesis.

Intravenous fluids remain the treatment of choice for moderate-to-severe fluid volume deficit in the surgical patient. Oral hydration strategies are reserved for stable patients and patients with mild losses during the preoperative phase up to 2 hours before surgery. Generally, the acutely ill patient requiring surgery is not taking in adequate volume to correct deficits with oral rehydration solutions alone. In those cases, oral rehydration solutions may supplement intravenous fluid management. They may also be appropriate in the postoperative period once the surgical condition has been stabilized with intravenous therapy. They may also be started before the patient advances to a clear liquid diet after surgery if the patient is slow to return to normal gastrointestinal function.

Adequacy of Intravenous Fluid Therapy/Clinical Response to Fluid Replacement Therapy

Dynamic fluid and electrolyte management requires ongoing assessment and goal-directed fluid management strategies. It is essential to closely monitor and assess patient responses to volume restoration. Clinicians must be aware of the child's preoperative and intraoperative fluid management and must possess a working knowledge of hemodynamic monitoring, the effects of anesthesia, fluid and electrolyte balance, and acid-base balance in order to structure appropriate fluid and electrolyte therapy in a timely manner. This must be prevalent throughout the perioperative period.

Assessment and intervention priorities are initially focused on airway maintenance and assessment of respiratory and circulatory function (ABCs). Once concerns for airway and respiratory function have been addressed, perfusion parameters are serially assessed. Increased heart rate and vasoconstriction are the child's primary compensatory mechanisms in a decreased cardiac output state (AHA, 2002). Circulatory assessment priorities include monitoring of heart rate, mental status, skin color and temperature, pulse quality, capillary refill time, urine output, and daily weights. Early fluid volume deficits may be characterized by mild tachycardia and listlessness, urine output may be decreased, and skin turgor may be diminished and may appear mottled. Capillary refill time is also sluggish (> 2 seconds). Mucous membranes may be dry, and tears may be absent during crying in the infant beyond the newborn period. Fontanelles and eyes may be sunken. Later, extremities are cool or cold, and capillary refill time is markedly delayed. Tachycardia becomes more severe, and as the diastolic pressure drops, a widened pulse pressure may be noted. Hypotension is a late sign in children with hypovolemia and becomes evident as compensatory mechanisms fail and the patient progresses to cardiovascular collapse (AHA). At this stage, end-organ perfusion becomes compromised. The resulting anaerobic metabolism at a cellular level results in a build-up of pyruvic acid (Guyton, 2006). Serum electrolyte and blood gas analysis demonstrates a metabolic acidosis. Generally, this condition is corrected with the restoration of fluid and electrolytes, and rarely is the administration of sodium bicarbonate solutions necessary. If the patient experiences ongoing losses of bicarbonate, as in the case of high stoma or fistula output, buffering agents, such as sodium acetate, may be added to intravenous fluids. Once enteral feedings are instituted and losses of this nature are ongoing, buffering agents may be added to the patient's enteral regimen.

Conversely, excessive urine output may indicate fluid overload or an abnormal endocrine response to injury, as in the case of diabetes insipidus. Overhydration must be avoided just as aggressively as underhydration since overhydration may result in excessive free water and subsequent water intoxication. This can be a life-threatening complication of fluid therapy that requires early identification and intervention. Patients should be weighed daily, particularly infants and small children. Any abrupt weight gain should alert the clinician to the possibility of fluid overload. In these cases, chest radiographs show an increase in heart size and pulmonary effusion.

As deficits are corrected, perfusion parameters should normalize and all sources of output should begin to approximate total intake. Urine output is maintained at 1 to 2 mL/kg/hour. Urine specific gravity usually ranges from 1.005 in a well-hydrated patient to 1.020 as the urine becomes more concentrated. Serum electrolytes begin to normalize. These values are not only important to the safe administration of anesthesia, but they also continue to be important throughout the perioperative period to assess responses to fluid maintenance and replacement therapy. Serial physical examinations, initially driven by the ABCs, later become more focused.

Conclusion

Fluid and electrolyte management represents an important aspect of pediatric surgical nursing. An understanding of the physiology of fluid requirements and the response to anesthesia and surgery is essential for the care of these children. Standard formulas for fluid therapy are helpful, but they must be modified to account for the rapidly changing physiology of the child and his or her individual responses to prescribed interventions. Hemodynamic monitoring and assessment of laboratory values assist the clinician in determining the adequacy of therapy, but clinical assessment remains the mainstay in the evaluation of fluid and electrolyte management.

Acknowledgment

I would like to acknowledge the important contribution made by Nancy Rabin, who authored this chapter for the first edition of this textbook.

References

AHA. (2001). Fluid therapy and medications. In M. F. Hazinski, A. Zaritsky, V. Nadkarni, R. Hickey, S. Schesnayder, & R. Berg (Eds.), *Pediatric advanced life support: Provider manual*. Dallas, TX: AHA.

Allison, S. (2004). Fluid, electrolytes and nutrition. *Clinical Medicine*. 4(6), 573–378.

Armon, K., Stephenson, T., MacFaul, R., Eccleston, P., & Werneke, U. (2001). An evidence and consensus based guideline for acute diarrhea management. *Archives of Diseases in Children*, 85, 132–142.

Ball, J., & Bindler, R. (2006). Alterations in fluid and electrolyte balance, and acid-base balance. In J. Ball & R. Bindler (Eds.), *Child health nursing: Partnering with children & families*. Upper Saddle River, NJ: Pearson Prentice Hall.

Behrman, R., Kliegman, R., & Jenson, H. (2004). *Nelson textbook of pediatrics* (17th ed.). Philadelphia: Saunders.

Bindler, R., & Howry, L. (2005). *Pediatric drug guide*. Upper Saddle River, NJ: Prentice Hall.

Binkley, H., Beckett, J., Casa, D., Kleiner, D., & Plummer, P. (2002). National athletic trainers' association position statement: Exertional heat illness. *Journal of Athletic Training*, 37, 329–343.

Blonshine, S. (2000). Sodium, potassium, and ionized calcium. *AARC Times*, 24(4), 46–48.

Carcillo, J., & Fields, A. (2002). Clinical practice parameters for hemodynamic support of pediatric and neonatal patients in septic shock. *Critical Care Medicine*. 30(6), 1365–1377.

Cote, C., Todres, I., Goudsouzian, N., & Ryan, J. (2001). *Practice of anesthesia for infants and children* (3rd ed.). Philadelphia: Saunders.

Cook, L. (2003). I.V. fluid resuscitation. *Journal of Infusion Nursing*, 26(5), 296–303.

Drukker, A., & Guignard, J. (2002). Renal aspects of the term and preterm infant: A selective update. *Current Opinion in Pediatrics*, 14, 175–182.

Gan, T., Soppitt, A., Maroof, M., El Moalem, H., Roberston, K., Moretti, E., et al. (2002). Goal-directed intraoperative fluid administration reduces length of hospital stay after major surgery. *Anesthesiology*, 97(4), 820–826.

Guyton, A. (2006). *Textbook of medical physiology*. Philadelphia: Saunders.

Hand, H. (2001). The use of intravenous therapy. *Nursing Standard*, 15(43), 47–55.

Hill, A. (2000). Initiators and propagators of the metabolic response to injury. *World Journal of Surgery*, 24, 624–629.

Holliday, M., Segar, W., & Freidman, A. (2003). Reducing errors in fluid therapy management. *Pediatrics*, 111(2), 424–425.

Hughes, E. (2004). Principles of post-operative patient care. *Nursing Standard*, 19(5), 43–56.

Joshi, G. (2005). Intraoperative fluid restriction improves outcome after major elective gastrointestinal surgery. *Anesthesia & Analgesia*, 101(2), 601–605.

Kaye, A., & Grogono, A. (2000). Fluid and electrolyte physiology. In R. Miller (Ed.), *Anesthesia*. Philadelphia: Lippincott, Williams, & Wilkins.

Kluckow, M., & Evans, N. (2001). Low systemic blood flow in hyperkalemia in preterm infants. *Journal of Pediatrics*, 138(1), 227–232.

Kudsk, K. (2003). Evidence of conservative fluid administration following elective surgery. *Annals of Surgery*, 238, 649–650.

Lain, I., & Wong, C. (2002). Hypernatremia in the first few days: Is the incidence rising? *Archives of Disease in Childhood*, 87, 158–162.

Larson, C. (2000). Safety and efficacy of oral rehydration therapy for the treatment of diarrhea in gastroenteritis in pediatrics. *Pediatric Nursing, 26*, 177–179.

Lefever-Kee, J., & Paulanka, B. (2000). *Fluid and electrolytes with clinical application*. Albany, NY: Delmar Publishers.

Maharaj, C., Kallam, S., Malik, A., Hassett. P., Grady, D., & Laffey, J. (2005). Preoperative intravenous fluid therapy decreases postoperative nausea and pain in high risk patients. *Anesthesia and Analgesia, 100*, 675–682.

Marko, P., Layon, A., Caruso, L., Moxingo, D., & Gabrielli, A. (2003). Burn injuries. *Current Opinion in Anesthesiology, 16*, 183–191.

Merenstein, G., & Gardner, S. (2003). *Handbook of neonatal intensive care* (5th ed.). St. Louis, MO: Elsevier.

Metheny, N. (2000). *Fluid and electrolyte balance*. Philadelphia: Lippincott.

Mythen, M. (2005). Postoperative gastrointestinal tract dysfunction. *Anesthesia and Analgesia, 100*, 196–204.

Nager, A., & Wang, V. (2002). Comparison of nasogastric and intravenous methods of rehydration in pediatric patients with acute dehydration. *Pediatrics, 109*(3), 566–572.

Nehra, V. (2002). Fluid electrolyte and nutritional problems in the postoperative period. *Clinical Obstetrics and Gynecology, 45*(2), 537–544.

O'Neill, J., Grosfeld, J., Fonkalsrud, E., Coran, A., & Caldamone, A. (Eds.). (2003). Fluid and electrolyte management. In *Principles of pediatric surgery* (2nd ed.). St. Louis, MO: Mosby.

Ozuah, P., Avner, J., & Stein, R. (2002). Oral rehydration, emergency physicians, and practice parameters: A national survey. *Pediatrics, 109*(1), 259–261.

Puglise, K. (2003). Fluids and electrolytes. *Journal of Infusion Nursing, 26*(3), 127–128.

Radhakrishnan, R., Xue, H., Weisbrodt, N., Moore, F., Allen, S., Laine, G., et al. (2005). Resuscitation-induced intestinal edema decreases the stiffness and residual stress of the intestine. *Shock, 24*(2), 165–170.

Redden, M., & Wotton, K. (2001). Clinical decision making by nurses when faced with third-space fluid shift. *Gastroenterology Nursing, 24*(4), 182–191.

Reiling, R., & McKellar, D. (2004). Outpatient surgery. In *Elements of contemporary practice*. Publication of the American College of Surgeons, WebMD Professional Publishing: Danbury, CT.

Sarti, A., DeGaudio, R., Messineo, A., Cuttini, M., & Ventura, A. (2001). Glomerular permeability after surgical trauma in children: Relationship between microalbuminuria and surgical stress score. *Critical Care Medicine, 29*(8), 1626–1629.

Suhayda, R., & Walton, J. (2002). Preventing and managing dehydration. *Medsurg Nursing, 11*(6), 267–278.

Sweeney, J. (2005). What causes hyponatremia? *Nursing, 35*(6), 18.

Tuggle, D. (2003). Fluid and electrolyte management. In M. Ziegler, R. Azizkhan, & T. Weber (Eds.), *Operative pediatric surgery*. New York: McGraw-Hill.

van Wissen, K., & Breton, C. (2004). Perioperative influences on fluid distribution. *Medsurg Nursing, 13*(5), 304–311.

Wheeler, M. (2002). Anesthesia for neonatal surgical emergencies. In A. Schwartz (Ed.), *Publication of the American Society of Anesthesiologists*. Philadelphia: Lippincott Williams and Wilkins.

Wessel, D. (2001). Managing low cardiac output syndrome after congenital heart surgery. *Critical Care Medicine, 29*(Suppl.), s220–s230.

3

Nutrition in the Pediatric Surgical Patient

By Amy W. Lamm and Kerin L. Worley

Nutritional management of the pediatric surgical patient is both dynamic and "challenging" because it involves satisfying the increased nutritional and metabolic demands of surgical conditions in an individual who already bears the high-energy requirements for growth. Recent advances in medical nutrition therapy have not only improved survival and decreased morbidity but have also minimized the impact on the ultimate growth and development of children because of the ability to safely provide adequate nutrition.

■ Nutritional Assessment and Estimation of Nutritional Requirements

Nutritional assessment should be completed at the time of the initial visit, then continually during hospitalization, and also, when clinically indicated, in the outpatient setting. Adequate assessment is necessary to identify patients in need of nutritional therapy as well as those at risk for malnutrition who may benefit from nutrition support before or after surgery.

Growth and Growth History

Nutrient requirements in the pediatric population must consider the need for growth and development. The growth velocity during infancy is higher than in any other stage of development (Table 3-1).

Full-term infants double their birth weight by 4 to 6 months of age and triple their birth weight by 1 year of age (Chumlea, 2005; Davis & Stanko-Kline, 2003). By the end of the first year of life, body length increases by 50% (Chumlea; Teitelbaum & Coran, 2000). Infants and children should be measured using the metric system for weight (kg), height (cm), and head circumference (<2 years of age). These measurements should be obtained on admission to the hospital and at regular intervals throughout hospitalization. Children should be weighed with an accurate digital or beam balance scale with minimal clothing and without shoes. Infants should be weighed without a diaper. The recumbent length in children younger than 2 years of age should be measured supine on a flat length board. Height is measured with a stadiometer and moveable headboard in children 2 or 3 years of age who are able to stand independently. These measurements should be plotted on age-specific and sex-specific growth curves; weight-age, height-age, weight-for-height, head

Table 3-1	Growth Velocity of Normal Infants and Children		
Age	Weight (g/day)	Length (cm/month)	Head Circumference (cm/week)
Premature	15–30	0.5	0.1–0.6
< 3 mo	25–35	2.6–3.5	0.5
3–6 mo	15–21	1.6–2.5	0.5
6–12 mo	10–13	1.2–1.7	0.5
1–3 yr	4–10	0.7–1.1	
4–6 yr	5–8	0.5–0.8	
7–10 yr	5–12	0.4–0.6	

Source: From Body composition of reference children from birth to age 10 years, by S.J. Fomon, F. Haschke, E.E. Ziegler, & S.E. Nelson, 1982, *American Journal of Clinical Nutrition, 35,* p.1169. © 1982 by the American Society for Clinical Nutrition. Adapted with permission.

circumference-age, and body mass index (kg/m²)-age using the 2000 Centers for Disease Control and Prevention and National Center for Health Statistics growth curves (Olsen, Mascarenhas, & Stallings, 2003). When measurements of premature infants are plotted on the growth curve, corrections should be made for gestational age until 24 months of age (Davis & Stanko-Kline, 2003).

Growth charts are simple and effective tools for identifying patients who are at nutritional risk. Children who are less than the fifth percentile for weight-age, height-age, or weight-height are at nutritional risk and require more detailed nutritional assessment and rehabilitation. If previous measurements are available, growth progress and deviations in growth rates can be followed. Growth rates that have dropped off (downward crossing of two major percentiles on Centers for Disease Control and Prevention/National Center for Health Statistics curves) or sudden unexpected accelerations in growth should be investigated. Downward crossing of growth percentiles may be an indicator of failure to thrive as a result of medical, chromosomal, metabolic, nutritional, or environmental factors. Serial monitoring of arm anthropometrics (midarm circumference and triceps skinfold) is helpful either when a child is immobile for an extended time or for continued monitoring of fat and muscle deposition during nutritional rehabilitation (Corrales & Utter, 2005; Olsen et al., 2003).

Diet History

A detailed diet history documents the child's current feeding practices and intake. A diet history, including a 24-hour recall, should be used to determine the adequacy of intake and food preferences and to identify cultural or religious eating practices or food intolerances. Appetite, food allergies, gastrointestinal intolerance (diarrhea, constipation, vomiting, gastroesophageal reflux), and eating behaviors should be evaluated to help determine the child's nutri-

tional risk or previous intolerance. Estimation of dietary energy, protein, and micronutrient intake helps explain possible causes for failure to thrive, establishes the nutritional risks of a surgical patient, and determines the patient's needs in the postoperative setting.

Estimating Energy and Protein Requirements

Measured energy expenditure using indirect calorimetry is an accurate method of "estimating" energy needs. However, it is costly and time consuming and is not always available. Nutritionists estimate energy and protein requirements using equations predicting resting energy expenditure (Table 3-2) on the basis of weight, sex, and age (National Research Council, 1989). The recommended dietary allowance (RDA) can also be used as a guideline for determining initial requirements for energy and protein. Table 3-3 outlines the RDAs for energy and protein on the basis of age.

Caloric Needs Based on Stress Factors and Chronic Illness

The RDAs may need to be adjusted for children who are ill or for those with a chronic disease. For example, infants and children with chronic lung disease, short bowel syndrome, immunodeficiency, cystic fibrosis, or congenital heart disease require additional energy, protein, and micronutrients to thrive and grow.

The additional calories are indicated based on stress factors such as fever, minor surgery, major surgery, infection, and burns. Table 3-4 lists the recommended increases in energy on the basis of these stress factors. One should not consider the increases cumulatively; if a patient has more than one of the stressors, the largest percentage increase should be used to calculate caloric needs. For example, if a trauma patient with multiple fractures

Table 3-2	Predicting Resting Energy Expenditure from Body Weight (kg)		
	Males		**Females**
Age Range (yr)	**Equation to Derive Resting Energy Expenditure (kcal/day)**	**Age Range (yr)**	**Equation to Derive Resting Energy Expenditure (kcal/day)**
0–3	$(60.9 \times wt) - 54$	0–3	$(61.0 \times wt) - 51$
3–10	$(22.7 \times wt) + 495$	3–10	$(22.5 \times wt) + 499$
10–18	$(17.5 \times wt) + 651$	10–18	$(12.2 \times wt) + 746$
18–30	$(15.3 \times wt) + 679$	18–30	$(14.7 \times wt) + 496$

Note: From *Predicting resting energy expenditure from body weight (kg)* by WHO, 1985. Expert Consultation Technical Support Series. Reprinted by permission of the World Health Organization.

is septic, calories increase by 40% to 60% (moderate to severe infection).

Close nutritional monitoring and clinical assessment are necessary in the hospital setting, especially in the neonatal and pediatric intensive care units. The child's clinical course may change dramatically in a short period of time, and, therefore, energy and protein delivery need to be adjusted. Many factors influence nutritional assessment and monitoring in the intensive care setting. Fluid status is extremely variable, and weight and vis-

ceral proteins are directly influenced by third spacing of fluid and diuresis. Therefore, subjective clinical assessment of the pediatric patient must be used in congruence with objective data.

Catch-Up Growth

Catch-up growth requirements should be provided when nutritional status is suboptimal and the child has failed to thrive. Accelerated growth is achieved by providing calories and protein in excess of the RDA requirements (Davis & Stanko-Kline, 2003). In order for a child to experience catch-up growth, an additional 20% to 30% of the child's baseline energy requirement may be necessary. Guidelines for calculating catch-up growth requirements are detailed in Table 3-5. The calculation of catch-up growth should be considered an estimate of caloric and protein needs. However, a better indication of sufficient growth requirements is weight gain at or above the expected rate for age.

Table 3-3	Recommended Dietary Allowances for Energy and Protein	
	Energy (kcal/kg/day)	**Protein (gm/kg/day)**
Infants		
0–6 mo	108	2.2
6–12 mo	98	1.6
Children		
1–3 yr	102	1.2
4–6 yr	90	1.1
7–10 yr	70	1.0
Males		
11–14 yr	55	1.0
15–18 yr	45	0.9
19–24 yr	38	0.8
Females		
11–14 yr	47	1.0
15–18 yr	40	0.8
19–24 yr	38	0.8

Source: From *Recommended daily allowances* (10th ed.), by the National Academy of Sciences, 1989, Washington, DC: National Academies Press. © 1989 by the National Academy of Sciences. Reprinted with permission.

Table 3-4	Percentage Recommended Increase of Calorie Needs Based on Stress Factors
Fever—12% for every 1° > 37°C
Minor surgery—10%
Major surgery—20%–30%
Long bone fractures—15%–30%
Infection—20% mild; 40% moderate; 60% severe
Multiple trauma with patient on ventilator—50%–70%
Long-term growth failure—35%–50%
Burns—25%–115% (depending on percent total body surface area burn)

Source: From *The metabolic management of the critically ill* (p. 36), by D. Wilmore, 1977, New York: Plenum Medical Book Co. Copyright 1977 by Plenum Medical Book Co. Adapted with permission.

Table 3-5 Estimating Catch-Up Growth Requirements

1. Plot the child's height and weight on the National Center for Health Statistics growth chart.
2. Determine the child's recommended calories for age (RDA).
3. Determine the ideal weight (50th percentile) for the child's height.
4. Multiply the RDA calories by ideal body weight for height (kg).[a]
5. Divide this value by the child's actual weight.

Catch-up growth requirement:

$$\frac{\text{RDA calories for age}^b \times \text{ideal weight for height (kg)}}{\text{Actual weight}}$$

Protein requirements:

$$\frac{\text{RDA for protein for age} \times \text{ideal weight for height}}{\text{Actual weight}}$$

[a] Ideal weight for age can be used in this part of the equation.

[b] Catch-up growth equations for children with developmental delay may utilize RDA for height age. (Determine at what age present height would be at 50th percentile. Use RDA for that age.)

Source: From Growth failure (p. 400), by Corrales K.M. & Utter S.L. (2005). In P.Q Samour & K. King (Eds.), Handbook of Pediatric Nutrition (3rd ed.). Sudbury, MA: Jones and Bartlett Publishers. Copyright 2005 by Jones and Bartlett Publishers. Reprinted with permission.

Patients who are severely malnourished may initially require normal caloric intake for age for the first 7 to 10 days, followed by a gradual increase toward the goal for catch-up growth in order to avoid refeeding syndrome. It is recommended that a multivitamin be given in order to prevent micronutrient deficiencies. Catch-up growth requirements should continue until the child achieves previous or age-appropriate growth percentiles. Accelerations in length may occur several months after catch-up growth in weight (Corrales & Utter, 2005).

Developmental Disabilities

Children with special health care needs are at increased risk for malnutrition (Reilly, Skuse, & Poblete, 1996; Sullivan et al., 2002; Sullivan et al., 2000). Studies have shown that up to 90% of children with developmental disabilities have feeding problems requiring assistance, such as feeding tube placement. Nutritional assessment of children with developmental disabilities includes measurements of anthropometric characteristics, body composition, growth velocity, caloric intake, energy expenditure, biochemistry, feeding skills, and nutritional risk factors in the context of the child's medical history (Zemel & Stallings, 2003).

Children with Prader-Willi syndrome or spina bifida generally have decreased energy needs, in comparison to healthy children without disability, due to a lower basal metabolic rate, decreased muscle tone, and limited motor activity. Energy needs in children with these conditions should be calculated per centimeter of height, because they often have shorter stature and tend to become overweight (Table 3-6). Children with cerebral palsy (without limited mobility) may have increased energy needs due to an abnormal resting energy expenditure, and inadequate caloric intake. Caloric needs in children with these developmental disabilities should also be determined on the basis of height, while accounting for activity level and severity of condition (Table 3-6). However, energy needs must be modified according to growth (Cloud, 2005).

Growth, including weight and height, should be monitored on growth charts specific to the clinical condition in children with developmental disabilities. These anthropometric measurements are important in assessing nutrition status. Triceps skinfold thickness and mid-upper arm circumference measurements are useful for estimating total body fat and muscle mass. Weight-height

Table 3-6 Guidelines for Estimating Caloric Requirements Based on Height in Children with Developmental Disabilities

Condition	Caloric Recommendation (kcal/cm)
Prader-Willi syndrome	Maintain growth: 10–11
	Slow weight loss: 8.5
Cerebral palsy: Mild (5–11 years of age)	14
Cerebral palsy: Severe, limited mobility (5–11 years of age)	11
Down syndrome (5–11 years of age)	Girls: 14.3
	Boys: 16.1
Motor dysfunction: nonambulatory (5–12 years of age)	7–11
Motor dysfunction: ambulatory (5–12 years of age)	14
Spina bifida (> 8 years of age)	Maintain weight: 9–11
	Promote weight loss: 7

Source: From Nutrition and feeding of the developmentally disabled, by C. Rokusek & E. Heindicles, 1985, Brookings, SD: South Dakota University Affiliated Program, Interdisciplinary Center for Disabilities. Adapted with permission.

relationships, including body mass index, are particularly good indicators of being under- or overweight in developmentally delayed children (Cloud, 2005). Close nutritional monitoring with frequent assessments every 3 to 6 months can help prevent malnutrition and growth failure in this special population (Zemel & Stallings, 2003).

Noncaloric Nutrients

Vitamins and minerals are essential micronutrients that serve as enzyme cofactors and structural components of the body. The micronutrient requirements of infants are derived from the nutrient content and volume of human milk consumed by a typical, healthy infant. The preterm infant requires more calcium, phosphorus, and magnesium than the full-term infant. These needs are typically met with fortified breast milk or premature infant formula, thus minimizing the risk of osteopenia (Groh-Wargo, 2000). For children and adolescents, the micronutrient requirements are based on RDAs (National Research Council, 1989).

Laboratory Data

Various laboratory tests are available to assess nutritional status. Vitamin (vitamins A, D, and E) and mineral (calcium, magnesium, phosphorus, copper, and zinc) serum levels may be useful in specific circumstances in individuals who are at risk or who require supplementation to promote healing. Laboratory assessment of renal and hepatic function helps determine requirements and delivery of nutrition according to the clinical situation. Evaluation of visceral protein status is particularly important. Persistent protein losses postoperatively may result from wounds, fistulas, or burns, dramatically increasing the need for energy and protein provision to maintain adequate synthesis and promote healing. Albumin and total protein have long half-lives (20 days) because of their large extravascular volume distribution and also vary considerably depending on fluid status. Ongoing or acute protein evaluation can most effectively be assessed with pre-albumin, which is a rapid-turnover protein with a half-life of 2 days. Therefore, it is a good indicator of acute changes in nutritional status. It is a relatively inexpensive, reliable measurement of visceral protein status that is not affected by hydration. Pre-albumin levels transiently decrease during the acute postsurgical phase. Measurements should be obtained initially and biweekly in the early recuperative phase to evaluate the adequacy of nutritional support (Beck & Rosenthal, 2002; Frantz, 2003; Teitelbaum & Coran, 2000).

■ Metabolic Consequences of Injury and Nutritional Repletion

The body's initial response to injury (e.g., surgery, sepsis, trauma, burns, acute inflammatory conditions) is the release of cytokines, which mediate the metabolic and immune response to injury. Counterregulatory hormones (e.g., catecholamines, glucagon, and cortisol) rapidly rise in response to cytokines. These counterregulatory hormones counteract the synthetic effects of insulin and insulin-like growth factor-1 (IGF-l) and cause a sequence of metabolic events that includes the catabolism of endogenous stores of protein, carbohydrate, and fat to fuel the body's ongoing metabolic response to stress. The loss of endogenous tissue resulting from a hypermetabolic and hypercatabolic state can lead to a poor clinical outcome in the absence of appropriate nutritional and metabolic support (Hill & Hill, 1998; Ljungqvist, Nygren, Soop, & Thorell, 2005; Pierro, 2002). As the body's acute metabolic response to injury resolves, anabolic metabolism adapts to restore catabolic losses. In children, the body now resumes growth. The goal then in the critically ill child is to initiate nutritional resuscitation early to promote growth recovery. The catabolic state also contributes to early nitrogen losses caused by either injury or starvation. The visceral protein stores (pre-albumin, albumin, transferrin, and retinol-binding protein) are then depleted to provide energy for the body. Urinary nitrogen losses also increase as a result of protein and fat catabolism (gluconeogenesis in the liver and lipolysis). Not only are visceral proteins used for gluconeogenesis in the liver, but altered protein metabolism during acute metabolic stress also occurs. The liver preferentially synthesizes acute-phase proteins (i.e., C-reactive protein), which start a cascade of events signaling an immune response and repair of the body (Coss-Bu et al., 2001; Hill & Hill, 1998).

Nutritional Repletion During Metabolic Stress

In general, infants and children in the postoperative period have energy requirements similar to their basal metabolic rate (Falcao & Tannuri, 2002; Pierro, 2002). The underlying acute illness or pathophysiology may be more of a factor in determining energy needs than the operative trauma itself (Chwals, Letton, Jamie, & Charles, 1995; Pierro). Neonates, who have reduced body stores, have increased baseline energy demands in the presence of injury and prolonged stress, and both under- and overfeeding may be associated with negative outcomes (Garza et al., 2002). Appropriate nutrition must be provided for the maintenance of protein status, growth, and wound healing in the postoperative period. In newborn infants, there is a moderate and immediate postoperative increase in resting energy expenditure that peaks 4 hours after surgery. In addition, there is a rapid return of energy expenditure to baseline 12 to 24 hours after surgery. This rapid return is possibly due to higher circulating levels of endogenous opioids, which serve as a protective mechanism to blunt the stress response in the first 48 hours of life (Pierro). In the postoperative period, critically ill infants may require fewer calories to meet their basal metabolic needs as a result of their reduction in activity and insensible losses while sedated in a thermoneutral intensive care environment (Falcao & Tannuri; Garza et al.). Thus, overfeeding is a potential risk if caloric repletion during the acute phase of metabolic stress is based on predicted requirements for healthy infants (Chwals, 1994; Falcao & Tannuri). As the acute-phase response subsides and the body resumes anabolic metabolism (growth), caloric administration should be progressively increased (Chwals et al.).

Risks Associated with Overfeeding

Overfeeding the critically ill infant or child may lead to respiratory compromise or hepatic dysfunction. Overfeeding of carbohydrates, regardless of adequacy of energy, increases lipogenesis, which is an energy-requiring process characterized by an increase in carbon dioxide production (V_{CO_2}) relative to oxygen consumption (V_{O_2}). In infants, increased carbon dioxide production, resulting from excess carbohydrate administration, increases the respiratory rate that is necessary to remove excess CO_2. However, in the infant with chronic lung disease or acute pulmonary compromise, the body may be unable to compensate for the increased CO_2 production and, consequently, CO_2 retention may occur. Substituting lipid for some of the carbohydrate administered may lead to reduced CO_2 production and lipogenesis. Hepatic cellular injury may also result from excessive carbohydrate delivery because of increased insulin levels, which increase glucose oxidation and lipogenesis. Hepatic cellular injury may therefore result from steatosis (deposition of fat in the liver) or intrahepatic cholestasis. The postoperative patient is at risk of overfeeding if the substrate delivery is not limited and energy needs are overestimated (Garza et al., 2002; Shulman & Phillips, 2003). Measurement of energy expenditure by indirect calorimetry may be used in determining precise caloric delivery in order to avoid overfeeding the critically ill pediatric patient (Chwals, 1994; Turi et al., 2001).

Refeeding Syndrome

The pediatric surgical patient often presents for interventions because of chronic conditions associated with malnutrition. It is extremely important to avoid the potential complications associated with refeeding these children as appropriate nutrition is reestablished postoperatively. Refeeding syndrome is characterized by the metabolic and physiologic alterations that occur when severely malnourished patients are refed too rapidly. Refeeding disrupts the adaptive state of decreased metabolism induced by semistarvation in the malnourished child. It involves a rapid increase in the basal metabolic rate as well as significant fluid and electrolyte shifts. There is a sudden reduction in serum levels of potassium, magnesium, and phosphate, in addition to glucose and fluid intolerance (Penny, 2003). Clinical symptoms may include vomiting, diarrhea, and edema, ultimately leading to respiratory failure and circulatory collapse (Corrales & Utter, 2005). Thus, children who are malnourished and have anthropometric measurements less than the fifth percentile should be refed slowly in order to avoid these metabolic disturbances and clinical complications.

Refeeding syndrome may be observed with enteral and parenteral feeds. During refeeding, carbohydrates should be gradually increased while maintenance amounts of protein, lipids, and vitamins are given. Serum potassium, phosphorus, glucose, and magnesium levels should be monitored daily for approximately 1 week in patients at risk for refeeding syndrome. These electrolyes should be replenished as needed, either in parenteral feedings or through enteral supplementation. Potassium can be added to oral rehydration solutions if patients are also dehydrated. A multivitamin, including thiamin, should also be added as appropriate nutrition is reestablished. Throughout the refeeding process, it is essential to monitor the patient's oral and intravenous intake as well as urinary and stool output, weight gain, and vital signs, including body temperature and cardiac and respiratory function. Careful assessment and management of nutritional status and metabolic changes can prevent the potentially lethal complications associated with refeeding syndrome (Wessel & Samour, 2005).

■ Enteral Nutrition Support

Enteral nutrition (EN) is the preferred method for meeting nutritional requirements of infants or children who have a functioning or partially functioning gastrointestinal tract but are unable or unwilling to safely and adequately achieve oral intake (Fig. 3-1). EN is used in

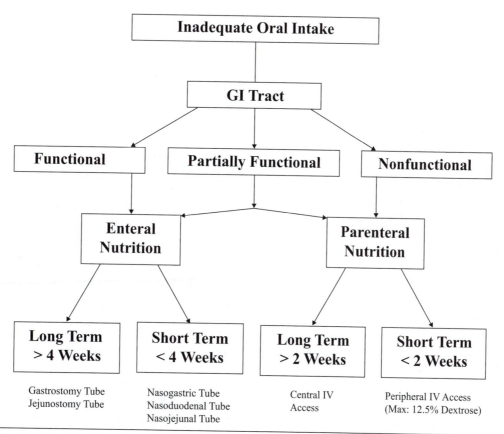

Figure 3-1 Algorithm for Enteral and Parenteral Nutrition

conjunction with an oral diet if intake is inadequate, and it may also be used to transition infants or children from parenteral nutrition to an oral diet. EN assists not only in nutrient delivery but it is also critical in maintaining gastrointestinal mucosal integrity and immunologic function (Shulman & Phillips, 2002). EN accelerates the time to full gut recovery, attenuates the hypermetabolic response to injury, is less costly than parenteral nutrition, and may improve the outcome for critically ill or traumatized patients (Frantz, 2003; Irving, Simone, Hicks, & Verger, 2000). EN support is a more efficient and physiologic use of nutrient substrates than is parenteral nutrition. In the critically ill surgical, trauma, or burn patient, enteral feedings may prevent the development of gastrointestinal bacterial translocation and prevent the development of sepsis. Finally, EN decreases the risk of hepatobiliary complications that occur with parenteral nutrition support (Frantz; Shulman & Phillips; Teitelbaum & Coran, 2000).

Enteral Access

The determination of enteral access should be based on the functional status of the gastrointestinal tract and the duration of nutritional support. Gastric feedings are the most physiologic route of delivery and are recommended when the risk of aspiration is minimal and tolerance is adequate (Shulman & Phillips, 2002). Generally, orogastric or nasogastric tubes are indicated for short-term enteral nutrition (4–6 weeks). Anticipated long-term nutrition requires a percutaneous or surgically placed feeding tube (DeChicco & Matarese, 2003). Duodenal/jejunal feedings are necessary when gastric feedings have failed because of delayed gastric emptying, frequent vomiting, severe gastroesophageal reflux, or aspiration (Nevin-Folino & Miller, 2005).

Formula Selection

A primary consideration in choosing the appropriate formula includes identifying patient-specific nutrient requirements, including energy, protein, and fluid needs. Clinical status, disease state, gastrointestinal function, and length of nutritional support are also important factors to consider. The choice of formula is also age dependent and sometimes disease or injury specific (e.g., cystic fibrosis, necrotizing enterocolitis, short bowel syndrome, immunodeficiency, burn, or head trauma).

Breast milk is recommended for use in children younger than 1 year of age; if breast milk is not available, commercial infant formulas should be used. Breast milk contains docosahexaenoic acid and arachidonic acid, which are long-chain fatty acids that enhance brain development and visual acuity (Chang & Kleinman, 2003). Infant formulas, such as Enfamil LIPIL and Similac Advance, now include docosahexaenoic acid and arachidonic acid in efforts to imitate breast milk, which is considered the "gold standard." Standard infant formulas are cow's milk based, fortified with iron, and provide 20 kcal/ounce. Soy formulas, such as ProSobee and Isomil, may be used in infants with cow's milk protein intolerance or suspected lactose intolerance. However, 20% to 50% of infants who are allergic to cow's milk protein are also allergic to soy protein and require a protein hydrolysate formula (e.g., Pregestimil, Alimentum, and Nutramigen) (Davis & Stanko-Kline, 2003). Amino-acid–based formulas, such as Neocate and EleCare, are used for infants with severe protein hypersensitivity or malabsorption (Akers & Groh-Wargo, 2005). Specific malabsorptive conditions (e.g., short bowel syndrome, intestinal resection, gastroschisis, intestinal atresia, and biliary atresia) may require hydrolyzed protein or amino acid formulas with medium chain triglyceride (MCT) oil to improve enteral absorption. Table 3-7 outlines the indications for use and the formula characteristics of the many specialized infant formulas currently available.

Infants with increased energy needs due to chronic illness or failure to thrive may require formulas with increased caloric density. Carbohydrate (Polycose, Moducal) or fat (MCT oil, Microlipid) additives should be used to concentrate formulas greater than 24 kcal/ounce, thus minimizing volume. Breast milk may also be fortified up to 30 kcal/ounce using modulars or standard infant formula powders. As caloric density is increased, the infant should be monitored for feeding intolerance, dehydration, and electrolyte abnormalities (Nevin-Folino & Miller, 2005).

Prepared formulas for children 1 to 10 years of age have a standard caloric density of 30 kcal/ounce and are often used for enteral tube feedings (Davis & Stanko-Kline, 2003). However, some pediatric populations that have high energy demands (e.g., patients with burns, severe lung disease, or failure to thrive) or are severely fluid restricted (e.g., patients with liver or heart failure or traumatic brain injuries) may benefit from a concentrated formula, such as Resource Just For Kids (1.5 kcal/mL). Fiber-supplemented formulas are now routinely used for long-term enteral support. Fiber may help to improve stool consistency and normalize bowel function (Slavin, 2003). Formula selection should once again be based on the child's clinical presentation (e.g., degree of malnutrition, presence of chronic disease, or traumatic injury).

Adult product formulations, such as Ensure and Jevity, are recommended for children over 10 years of age. These formulas are appropriate only in older children and adults because they have increased amounts of protein, sodium, potassium, chloride, and magnesium and decreased amounts of iron, zinc, calcium, phosphorus, and vitamin D (Davis & Stanko-Kline, 2003).

Types of Infusions

Intermittent (bolus) and continuous infusions, or a combination of both, are used for nutrient delivery. When enteral feeds are initiated, slow, continuous infusions are generally better tolerated than bolus feedings (Davis & Stanko-Kline, 2003). Intermittent gastric feedings may be administered over short periods of time (20–30 minutes), depending on tolerance. Intermittent or bolus feedings are practical for home enteral feedings because they allow ambulatory children to be more mobile between feedings. If continuous infusion is necessary because of poor nutrient absorption or feeding intolerance, portable feeding pumps are available. When patients are fed directly into the small bowel, continuous infusion is recommended. Nocturnal continuous infusion is beneficial if the patient is receiving supplemental enteral nutritional support because it allows the patient to eat by mouth during the day (Shulman & Phillips, 2002).

Initiation and Advancement

Initiation and advancement of enteral feedings should be based on the age and weight of the patient as well as the structure and function of the gastrointestinal tract (Table 3-8). A full-strength isotonic formula should generally be used when starting enteral feeds. However, postoperative patients with impaired gastrointestinal function may initially require an oral hydration solution (e.g., Pedialyte or Infalyte) or a dilute formula and slower feeding advancements than the standard recommended progression. Simultaneous advancements in feeding concentration and volume should be avoided (Nevin-Folino & Miller, 2005). Feeding intolerance, as evidenced by abdominal distention and pain, vomiting, and/or increased stool output, should be monitored for during feeding advancement. Gastric residuals should be checked before a bolus feeding or every 4 hours during advancement of continuous feedings if the patient develops signs of intolerance. Decrease the rate or bolus volume if the residual is more than double the hourly continuous infusion rate or is more than twice the bolus volume, and recheck the residual in 1 hour (Davis, 1998). If residuals remain excessive, feedings may need to be temporarily held and restarted at the previously tolerated concentration and volume (Nevin-Folino & Miller).

Table 3-7 Infant and Pediatric Formulas

Formula Classification	Indications	Infant Formulas (Birth–1year) (cal/ounce)	Toddler (>4–18 mo) & Pediatric Formulas (1–10 yr) (cal/ounce)	Adult (>10 years) (cal/ounce)
Standard cow's milk-based	Term infant with a normally functioning GI tract	Human milk (20 cal/ounce) Similac Advance with Iron[a] (20 cal/ounce) Enfamil LIPIL with Iron[b] (20 cal/ounce) Carnation Good Start Supreme DHA and ARA[d] (20 cal/ounce)	Similac 2 Advance[a] (20 cal/ounce) Enfamil Next Step[b] (20 cal/ounce) Good Start 2 Supreme[d] (20 cal/ounce)	
Preterm cow's milk-based	Low birth weight infants (hospital use only) < 34 wk gestation and/or weight < 2 kg	Similac Special Care Advance with Iron[a] (24 cal/ounce) Enfamil Premature LIPIL with Iron[b] (24 cal/ounce)		
Transitional	Premature infants after discharge from the hospital until 1 year of age	Similac NeoSure Advance[a] (22 cal/ounce) Enfamil EnfaCare LIPIL[b] (22 cal/ounce)		
Lactose free	Primary or secondary lactose intolerance	Similac Lactose Free[a] (20 cal/ounce) Enfamil LactoFree LIPIL[b] (20 cal/ounce) Good Start Supreme Soy[d] (20 cal/ounce)	PediaSure[a] (30 cal/ounce) Kindercal[b] (32 cal/ounce) Nutren Junior[d] (30 cal/ounce) Resource Just For Kids[c] (30 cal/ounce)	Ensure[a] (32 cal/ounce) Osmolite[a] (32 cal/ounce) Nutren 1.0[d] (30 cal/ounce)
Standard fiber containing (lactose free)			PediaSure w/ Fiber[a] (30 cal/ounce) Kindercal[b] w/ Fiber (32 cal/ounce) Nutren Junior[d] w/ Fiber (30 cal/ounce) Resource Just For Kids[c] w/ Fiber (30 cal/ounce) COMPLETE Pediatric[c] w/ Fiber (30 cal/ounce)	Ensure w/ Fiber[a] (32 cal/ounce) Jevity w/ Fiber[a] (32 cal/ounce)
Soy-based lactose free	Cow's milk protein sensitivity or lactose-intolerance	Similac Isomil Advance[a] (20 cal/ounce) Enfamil ProSobee LIPIL[b] (20 cal/ounce)	Similac Isomil 2 Advance[a] (20 cal/ounce) Enfamil Next Step ProSobee[b] (20 cal/ounce)	

(continues)

Table 3-7 (continued)

Formula Classification	Indications	Infant Formulas (Birth–1year) (cal/ounce)	Toddler (>4–18 mo) & Pediatric Formulas (1–10 yr) (cal/ounce)	Adult (>10 years) (cal/ounce)
		Good Start Supreme Soy[d] (20 cal/ounce)	Good Start 2 Essentials Soy[d] (20 cal/ounce)	
Semi-elemental (casein hydrolysates)	Allergies, malabsorption, and impaired GI function	Similac Alimentum[a] (20 cal/ounce), Nutramigen LIPIL[b] (20 cal/ounce), Pregestimil[b] (20 cal/ounce)	Peptamen Junior[d] (30 cal/ounce), Pepdite One+[e] (30 cal/ounce)	Peptamen[d] (30 cal/ounce), Perative[a] (39 cal/ounce)
Elemental	Allergies, impaired GI function, malabsorption	Neocate[e] (20 cal/ounce), EleCare[a] (20 cal/ounce)	Neocate 1+[e] (30 cal/ounce), Neocate Junior[e] (30 cal/ounce), Pediatric EO28[e] (30 cal/ounce), Vivonex Pediatric[c] (24 cal/ounce), EleCare[a] (30 cal/ounce) 1–3 year olds	Vivonex[c] (30 cal/ounce), Tolerex[c] (30 cal/ounce)
Disease specific	Low renal solute load and/or renal insufficiency	Similac PM 60/40[a] (20 cal/ounce)		
	Chylothorax, steatorrhea, and/or liver disease	Portagen[b]	Portagen[b]	Portagen[b], Lipisorb[c] (40 cal/ounce)
	Fluid restriction and/or increased metabolic needs		Resource Just for Kids 1.5[b] (45 cal/ounce)	Nepro[a] (60 cal/ounce), Nutren 1.5[d] (45 cal/ounce), Nutren 2.0[d] (60 cal/ounce), Ensure Plus[a] (45 cal/ounce), Pulmocare[a] (45 cal/ounce), TwoCal HN[a] (60 cal/ounce)

ARA, arachidonic acid; DHA, docosahexaenoic acid; GI, gastrointestinal.
[a]Ross Laboratories, Inc, Columbus, OH.
[b]Mead Johnson Nutritionals, Evansville, IN.
[c]Novartis, St. Louis Park, MN.
[d]Nestle Clinical Nutrition, Deerfield, IL.
[e]Scientific Hospital Supplies, Gaithersburg, MD.

Table 3-8	Suggestions for Initiation and Advancement of Continuous, Bolus, and Cyclic Tube Feeding		
Age	Initial Infusion	Advances	Goal
Continuous Feedings			
< 12 mo	1–2 mL/kg/hr	1–2 mL/kg every 2–8 hr	6 mL/kg/hr
1–6 yr	1 mL/kg/hr	1 mL/kg every 2–8 hr	4–5 mL/kg/hr
> 6 yr	25 mL/hr	25 mL/hr every 2–8 hr	100–150 mL/hr
Bolus Feeding			
< 12 mo	10–60 mL/2–3 hr	10–60 mL/feeding	90–180 mL/4–5 hr
1–6 yr	30–90 mL/2–3 hr	30–90 mL/feeding	150–300 mL/4–5 hr
> 6 yr	60–120 mL/2–3 hr	60–90 mL/feeding	240–480 mL/4–5 hr
Cyclic Feedings			
< 12 mo	1–2 mL/kg/hr	1–2 mL/kg/2 hr	60–90 mL/hr 12–18 hr/d
1–6 yr	1–2 mL/kg/hr	1–2 mL/kg/2 hr	75–125 mL/hr 8–16 hr/d
> 6 yr	25 mL/hr	25 mL/hr/2 hr	100–175 mL/hr 8–16 hr/d

Source: From *Contemporary nutrition support practice* (p. 358), by A. Davis in L.E. Matarese & M.M. Gottschlich (Eds.), Suggestions for Initiation and Advancement of Continuous, Bolus, and Cyclic Tube Feeding: Pediatrics, Philadelphia: Saunders. © 1998, with permission from Elsevier.

■ Parenteral Nutrition Support

Parenteral nutrition (PN) should be considered for infants and children in whom EN is either contraindicated or poorly tolerated. Parenteral energy needs are approximately 10% to 15% lower than enteral needs due to the lack of energy required for digestion and absorption (Cox & Melbardis, 2005). Congenital gastrointestinal malformations, necrotizing enterocolitis, hypermetabolic states (e.g., burns, severe trauma, severe chronic lung disease, and immunodeficiency), and organ failure are disease states in which PN support may be indicated. PN is often administered in conjunction with EN support, depending on the acuity and severity of the injury or disease state. PN delivery should be considered in patients who are unable to tolerate adequate EN delivery for a significant period of time (> 5 days) because of prolonged gastrointestinal dysfunction. The initiation of PN does not preclude the simultaneous administration of enteral feedings (Kerner, 2003).

Parenteral Access

Peripheral-vein parenteral nutrition (PPN) may be useful for 1 to 2 weeks of nutrition support, either to supplement enteral nutrition delivery or as the sole source of nutrition (Fig. 3-1). The use of lipid emulsions in addition to protein and carbohydrate solutions enables safe nutrient delivery using a solution less than 900 mOsm/L (dextrose concentrations should not exceed 12.5 g/dL). Highly concentrated dextrose solutions (>12.5 gm/dL) infused through a peripheral vein can quickly induce thrombophlebitis; these solutions should be infused only in central venous catheters. PPN is indicated for patients when short-term need is anticipated and for whom PPN can complement early initiation of enteral feedings. PPN rarely provides adequate protein and calories to meet nutritional goals. Central venous catheters are indicated in patients needing long-term (> 2–4 weeks) partial PN or when all requirements need to be met parenterally. Peripherally inserted central catheters may be placed for PN, because they provide an economical means of central venous access which is less invasive and have lower risks than surgically placed central venous catheters (e.g., Broviac and Hickman catheters). However, if peripherally inserted central catheter access is not feasible, a surgically placed central venous catheter may be necessary. The catheter tip is typically advanced to the junction of the superior vena cava and the right atrium to facilitate rapid dilution of the hyperosmolar solution with blood (Cox & Melbardis, 2005).

Parenteral Nutrient Delivery

The initiation and advancement of parenteral nutrition should be a gradual process with careful monitoring of fluid and glucose and tolerance (Cox & Melbardis, 2005). PN substrates should be advanced according to recommended guidelines for age and weight in order to reach appropriate nutritional goals safely (Table 3-9). Protein, calories, and fluid requirements may vary depending on the patient's surgical intervention, severity of injury, or the

Table 3-9 Initiation and Advancement of Parenteral Nutrition[a]

Initiation of Substrates

	Preterm Infants	Term Infants, Children, and Adolescents
Dextrose (glucose infusion rate [GIR] = mg/kg/min) $GIR = \dfrac{(mL/day\ TPN \times \%\ dextrose)}{Weight\ (kg) \times 144}$ (not to exceed a GIR = 5 mg/kg/min)	5%–10%	5%–10%
Amino acids	0.5–1 g/kg/day	1 g/kg/day
Lipids	0.5–1 g/kg/day	1 g/kg/day

Advancement of Substrates

	Preterm Infants	Term Infants, Children, and Adolescents
Dextrose	2.5% or (increase GIR by 1–2 mg/kg/min)	5% or (increase GIR by 1–2 mg/kg/min)
Amino acids	0.5–1 g/kg/day	1 g/kg/day
Lipids	0.5 g/kg/day	1 g/kg/day

Substrate Goals

	Recommended (% calories from substrate)	Preterm Infants	Term Infants	Children (1–11 years)	Adolescents
Dextrose (mg/kg/min)	60%	12–15	14 (Maximum)	14 (Maximum)	8 (Maximum)
Amino acids (g/kg/day)	10%–12%	2.5–4	2.5–3	1.5–2	1
Lipids (g/kg/day)	30% (60% of calories)	3	2–3	2–3	2–3
Kcal (kcal/kg/day)		100–120	80–100	60–80	40–60

From The University of North Carolina Hospitals Department of Pharmacy. Adapted with permission.

[a]The TPN Guidelines used at UNC Hospitals are provided for educational purposes only. The information presented in this document is not intended to and does not constitute medical or legal advice. UNC Hospitals is not liable for any use, including incorrect or improper use, of these guidelines. Individual institutional guidelines and local standards of care must be used when prescribing TPN.

presence of burns. General guidelines for caloric distribution are 40%–60% from carbohydrate (dextrose infusion), 10%–12% from protein (amino acids), and 25%–50% from fat (lipids). Unless otherwise specified, micronutrient (vitamin and trace mineral) supplements are generally added to pediatric PN as a standard according to the patient's weight. Electrolytes should be added to the PN solution to account for normal requirements as well as any additional losses, as evidenced by serum electrolyte levels (see Table 3-10 for normal electrolyte requirements).

Parenteral nutrition may be prepared in a 2-in-1 solution in which dextrose and amino acids are combined

Table 3-10 Normal Electrolyte Requirements for Parenteral Nutrition

	Infants & Toddlers	Children	Adolescents
Sodium (mEq/kg/day)	2–4	2–4	2–3
Potassium (mEq/kg/day)	1–3	1–3	1–2
Calcium (mEq/kg/day)	1–2	0.5–1	0.25–0.5
Magnesium (mEq/kg/day)	0.25–0.5	0.25–0.5	0.25–0.5
Phosphate (mmol/kg/day)	1–1.5	0.5–1	0.5–0.75

Source: From UNC Health Care Department of Pharmacy. Adapted with permission.

and connected to a separate lipid infusion using a Y-connector. A 3-in-1 PN solution containing lipids, amino acids, and dextrose in one container may be more convenient; however, these total nutrient admixtures are more influenced by increases in pH and temperature and may limit the amount of calcium and phosphorus that can be added without precipitation. L-cysteine may be added to PN to increase calcium and phosphorus solubility, and filters are recommended to prevent the delivery of precipitates (Cox & Melbardis, 2005).

In infants and children requiring long-term PN, cyclic delivery (over 12–16 hours per day) is safe and effective. This allows greater mobility and promotes a more normal routine for the child. The infusion rate should be tapered over the last 1 to 2 hours to slowly decrease the dextrose infusion and therefore prevent hypoglycemia when the infusion is stopped. The total volume of PN should be gradually decreased as infants and children are able to tolerate advancements in enteral feedings (Cox & Melbardis, 2005).

Monitoring of Adequacy and Tolerance of Parenteral Nutrition

Monitoring parenteral nutrition is important to avoid complications. Baseline laboratory parameters, such as electrolytes and chemistries (including calcium, phosphorus, and liver function tests), pre-albumin, and albumin should be obtained to evaluate renal function, glucose control, hydration, and baseline nutritional status when PN is initiated. Monitoring for primary micronutrient deficiencies is important in patients receiving long-term PN in the hospital or at home (Table 3-11).

Parenteral Nutrition Complications

Complications associated with PN may be infectious, mechanical, or metabolic. Infectious complications are typically due to catheter-related sepsis. Mechanical complications may be related to the initial placement of the catheter, thrombosis, or catheter occlusion. Metabolic complications include micro- or macronutrient abnormalities, overfeeding, and PN-associated cholestasis.

Infectious Complications

Infectious complications are a common cause of morbidity in patients receiving long-term PN (Szeszycki & Benjamin, 2005). In a patient receiving PN, the presence of fever is indicative of central venous catheter-related infection until all other sources have been ruled out. Catheter-related sepsis is typically confirmed when identical organisms are recovered from the central venous catheter and peripheral blood cultures (Fuhrman, 2003; Teitelbaum & Coran, 2000). Microorganisms can infect the catheter by entering the connection site, migrating along the subcutaneous tract, or traveling through the bloodstream from a distant septic site. It is also possible that the organism may be due to bacterial translocation from the gastrointestinal tract (Fuhrman; Teitelbaum & Coran; Vanderhoof & Young, 2002). The glucose content in PN is a good medium for bacterial growth. It is therefore recommended that PN be administered through a dedicated port of a central line (Szeszycki & Benjamin). A line infection is treated with the appropriate intravenous antibiotics via the catheter. An attempt to salvage the line should be made; however, in cases in which the pathogen is a fungus or a persistent bacterium, catheter removal is necessary. Manipulation of the central venous catheter has been identified as the most influential factor in developing line-related sepsis, and the most effective treatment of catheter-related sepsis is prevention. Therefore, strict adherence to catheter care protocols and practice of aseptic techniques are the most important factors in preventing catheter-related infections (Fuhrman).

Table 3-11	Recommended Labs for Monitoring Pediatric Parenteral Nutrition	
	Recommended Laboratory Tests	
Initial	Order weekly	Na, K, Cl, CO$_2$, BUN, creatinine, glucose, calcium, Mg, Phos, total protein, albumin [total bilirubin/direct bilirubin, AST, ALT, alkaline phosphatase, GGT (LFTs)], triglycerides
While advancing	Order daily	Na, K, Cl, CO$_2$, Ca, Mg, phosphorus
When stable	Order weekly	Na, K, Cl, CO$_2$, BUN, creatinine, glucose, calcium, Mg, phosphorus, total protein, albumin
	Order bimonthly	Total bilirubin/direct bilirubin, LFTs, triglycerides
Long term	Order bimonthly	Na, K, Cl, CO$_2$, BUN, creatinine, glucose, calcium, Mg, phosphorus
	Order monthly	Total protein, albumin, prealbumin, LFTs, triglycerides

Source: From UNC Health Care Department of Pharmacy. Adapted with permission.

BUN, blood urea nitrogen; AST, aspartate transaminase; ALT, alanine aminotransferase; LFT, liver function test; GGT, gamma-glutamyltransferase.

Mechanical Complications

Mechanical complications of PN can be related to catheter insertion or use. Catheter insertion complications include pneumothorax, air embolism, vessel injury, and malposition of the catheter tip. Most catheter insertion complications can be prevented with the use of appropriately trained and experienced personnel. Other PN-associated mechanical complications include venous thrombosis, catheter rupture, clotting, and occlusion. Hyperosmolar solutions increase the risk of vessel wall injury and thrombosis. The most common risk to a peripheral catheter is phlebitis due to infiltration. Peripheral venous infusate should be limited to an osmolarity of 700 to 900 mOsm/L; this type of preparation necessitates the use of lipids, which are isotonic, and a maximum dextrose solution of 12.5% (Fuhrman, 2003).

Another mechanical complication of both peripheral and central catheters is catheter occlusion, which can be caused by waxy lipid deposits, calcium phosphate, or other mineral precipitates. The appropriate catheter-clearing agent should be used according to the type of occlusion (Hoagland & Gahn, 2000).

Metabolic Complications

Metabolic complications related to PN encompass macronutrient and micronutrient abnormalities. Macronutrient complications are caused by an excess, deficiency, or imbalance of dextrose, protein, or lipids. Micronutrient-related complications are the result of excess or inadequate delivery of fluids, electrolytes, vitamins, minerals, and trace elements. Most metabolic complications can be minimized by closely monitoring PN and by following specific guidelines (Fuhrman, 2003; Szeszycki & Benjamin, 2005).

Long-term PN is associated with liver and biliary system complications. PN-associated cholestasis is the most common metabolic complication and is the leading cause of death in PN-dependent children who acquired short bowel syndrome in the prenatal or postnatal periods (Btaiche & Khalidi, 2002; Wessel, 2000). PN-associated cholestasis occurs in 30% to 60% of infants with short bowel syndrome (Wessel). Cholestasis refers to impaired canalicular secretion of bile or frank biliary obstruction (Fulford, Scolapio, & Aranda-Michel, 2004; Jeejeebhoy, 2005). The pathophysiology of cholestatic liver disease is still unclear, but it is likely that the etiology is multifactorial.

Risk factors for developing PN-associated cholestasis include prematurity, long duration of PN, and short bowel syndrome (Teitelbaum & Coran, 2000). Premature infants are at a greater risk for developing PN-associated cholestasis because of the physiologic immaturity of their hepatic excretory systems (Btaiche & Khalidi, 2002). A direct correlation has been shown between cholestatic jaundice and the duration of parenteral nutrition (Btaiche & Khalidi). Patients with the least amount of residual intestine are at the greatest risk for developing PN-related cholestasis (Fulford et al., 2004).

Possible causal mechanisms for PN-related cholestasis that have been explored include excessive or deficient components of the PN solution, overfeeding, inadequate gastrointestinal tract stimulation, and sepsis (Wessel, 2000; Btaiche & Khalidi, 2002). Almost every possible ingredient in the PN solution has been identified as the causative agent of cholestasis at some point (Teitelbaum, & Coran, 2000).

Excessive calories (overfeeding) from all or individual energy substrates (amino acids, dextrose, or lipids) or an imbalance of calories may contribute to liver dysfunction. Excessive dextrose infusion may result in increased delivery of free fatty acids to the liver, resulting in steatosis (fatty liver) but not cholestasis (Btaiche & Khalidi, 2002; Fulford et al., 2004). Administration of excess fat calories has been reported to cause abnormalities in liver enzymes; however, PN cholestasis was described in the literature long before lipids were included as part of the infusion (Fulford et al.). Phytosterols found in intravenous lipid compounds are suspected to play a role in the development of cholestasis (Teitelbaum & Coran, 2000). Excessive glycine, methionine, and degradation products of tryptophan may actually promote cholestasis (Btaiche & Khalidi; Jeejeebhoy, 2005). Taurine is required in the conjugation and subsequent excretion of bile salts; therefore, a taurine deficiency could play a role in the development of cholestasis (Teitelbaum & Coran). Since this discovery, taurine is now frequently added to neonatal amino acid mixtures; however, further studies will be required to determine its affect on cholestasis (Teitelbaum & Tracy, 2001). The trace elements copper and manganese can be hepatotoxic, and although the amounts of these elements in the PN solution are typically well below toxic levels, they are both excreted by the liver, and cholestasis reduces the excretion and increases the retention of these elements. It is recommended that copper be reduced and manganese be omitted from PN solutions provided to patients with cholestasis (Cox & Melbardis, 2005).

A lack of gastrointestinal stimulation results in a cascade of events that could each potentially cause or increase cholestasis. The initial effects of bowel rest include decreased intestinal motility and decreased secretion of cholecystokinin with an increase in intestinal permeability (Btaiche & Khalidi, 2002). Cholecystokinin is a peptide hormone that causes gallbladder contraction and induces intrahepatic bile flow. A lack of cholecystokinin would therefore lead to biliary sludge, cholelithiasis, and cholangitis (Fulford et al., 2004; Teitelbaum & Tracy, 2001). Synthetic cholecystokinin and ursodiol are sometimes given in an effort to improve bile flow. Ursodiol has been used with varying success. Early cholecystectomy may be recommended in some patients receiving long-term PN (Vanderhoof & Young, 2002). However, the most effective treatment for clearing cholestasis may be to increase the enteral feedings (Sigalet, 2001).

Another potential mechanism for PN-associated liver damage is bacterial overgrowth and translocation. These bacteria may form endotoxins that release cytokines, which are injurious to the liver. The use of enteral antimicrobials may be effective in reducing intraluminal bacteria and endotoxins, thereby decreasing bacterial translocation (Teitelbaum & Coran, 2000).

Potential measures that may be useful in the prevention and treatment of PN-associated cholestasis include early initiation and advancement of enteral feeds, avoidance of overfeeding, maintenance of adequate macronutrients, prevention of sepsis, cycling PN infusions, and pharmacologic interventions. Initiating even small amounts of enteral feedings may reduce intestinal stasis, diminish bacterial translocation, and improve bile flow (Btaiche & Khalidi, 2002). Strict aseptic protocols should be followed in order to minimize the occurrence of sepsis (Teitelbaum & Coran, 2000). It may also be beneficial to cycle the PN infusion to less than 16 hours per day. The potential benefits of cycling PN include prevention and treatment of cholestasis; however, this practice is still controversial. From a practical point of view, it is helpful to cycle PN to allow greater freedom of movement and daily activities (Fulford et al., 2004; Price, 2000). This may not be possible for premature infants because they are at increased risk for developing hypoglycemia because of their limited glycogen stores and the immaturity of their glucose regulatory mechanisms (Btaiche & Khalidi).

■ Special Conditions in Nutritional Support of the Pediatric Surgical Patient

Inflammatory Bowel Disease

Inflammatory bowel disease (IBD) refers to ulcerative colitis and Crohn's disease, which are chronic, inflammatory disorders of the gastrointestinal tract. Although the etiology of IBD is unknown, heredity, environment, and immunologic response appear to be contributing factors in its development (Young & Vanderhoof, 2000). Ulcerative colitis is primarily limited to the mucosa of the colon and rectum, with minimal involvement of the terminal ileum (Wessel & Samour, 2005). Crohn's disease involves transmural inflammation, which may occur in any portion of the gastrointestinal tract (Young & Vanderhoof). The two diseases often have similar clinical presentations, including abdominal pain, diarrhea, gastrointestinal blood and protein loss, weight loss, and growth failure (Wessel & Samour). Treatment for both conditions includes medical and/or surgical therapy. Various pharmacologic agents may produce clinical improvement and induce remission. Ulcerative colitis may be cured surgically with removal of the diseased colon and rectum. An endorectal ileal pull-through with creation of an ileal reservoir or pouch for fecal storage is commonly the surgical procedure of choice for ulcerative colitis. Crohn's disease is often managed surgically with resections of involved segments of bowel; however, surgery does not eliminate the risk of recurrence. Complications of Crohn's disease, including growth retardation, intestinal obstruction, perforation, enteric fistulas, abdominal abscesses, and perianal disease, often necessitate surgical intervention (Fonkalsrud, 2000).

Nutritional therapy also plays an important role in the management of IBD because malnutrition is the main cause of growth failure in patients with this disorder, occuring in approximately 30% of children with IBD. Permanent growth stunting is three times more likely in patients with Crohn's disease than in patients with ulcerative colitis (Hait, Bousvaros, & Grand, 2005; Heuschkel & Walker-Smith, 2003; Wessel & Samour, 2005). Inadequate intake, malabsorption, nutrient losses, drug-nutrient interactions, and increased nutrient requirements contribute to this growth retardation (Wessel & Samour). Nutrient deficits in IBD include protein, calcium, vitamin D, magnesium, folic acid, iron, and zinc, and are often associated with malabsorption due to mucosal inflammation and losses from diarrhea or fistula drainage. Oral micronutrient supplementation in children may be considered but is not generally required because of the variability of the disease remission periods. However, folic acid is often necessary for patients taking sulfasalazine because this medication significantly interferes with folate absorption (Heuschkel & Walker-Smith; Young & Vanderhoof, 2000). Vitamin B_{12} deficiencies may occur in patients with resections or disease in the terminal ileum (Wessel & Samour).

Nutritional rehabilitation in children with IBD involves oral dietary therapy, enteral nutrition with tube feedings, and/or PN. A well-balanced diet high in calories and protein should be encouraged. An intake of 140% to 150% of the RDA of energy and protein for age is often required to achieve catch-up growth in children with IBD (Hait et al., 2005; Wessel & Samour, 2005). Liquid nutrition supplemental formulas may be helpful in increasing caloric and protein intake. Restrictions of various foods, including fiber, refined sugars, and dairy products, should generally be based on individual patient tolerance rather than the risk of potential intolerance (Wessel & Samour). Lower fiber foods may be indicated in patients with active, severe disease because the traditional view holds that fecal residue may be irritating to the bowel (Young & Vanderhoof, 2000).

Enteral feedings have been shown to improve nutrition and growth, thus improving overall well-being. Exclusive enteral nutrition via continuous infusion may be effective in reducing inflammation and inducing remission in patients with active Crohn's disease (Wessel & Samour, 2005; Young & Vanderhoof, 2000). Children with treatment-resistant Crohn's disease may benefit from several weeks of exclusive enteral nutrition before surgery, resulting in a better postoperative course. In addition, early institution of enteral feeds after surgery reduces postoperative complications and results in better weight gain (Heuschkel & Walker-Smith, 2003). Short-term supplemental enteral therapy may involve placement of a nasogastric tube for nocturnal feedings, and longer therapies may involve the surgical or endoscopic placement of a gastrostomy tube. Elemental formulas or polymeric diets (Modulen IBD) have been shown to be effective in inducing remission in children with Crohn's disease and may be more useful in promoting linear growth than steroids (Hait et al., 2005; Heuschkel & Walker-Smith; Wessel & Samour).

PN should be used in selected children who have bowel obstructions, have short bowel syndrome due to resection, or are unable to tolerate adequate amounts of enteral nutrition because of active IBD (Wessel & Samour, 2005). Although PN is effective in the treatment of acute disease, it is associated with multiple complications, as discussed earlier.

Appropriate nutrition is essential for the optimal management of children with IBD. Early identification of growth failure and provision of nutritional therapy through enteral or parenteral routes is effective in decreasing bowel inflammation and promoting maximal growth potential.

Short Bowel Syndrome

Short bowel syndrome presents one of the most significant challenges in the nutritional management of the pediatric surgical patient. This complex disorder is defined as the spectrum of malabsorption that occurs after resection of a major portion of the small intestine for congenital or acquired lesions (Sigalet, 2001; Vanderhoof & Langnas, 1997; Wales et al., 2005). Malabsorption often involves micronutrients, such as vitamins and minerals; fluids; electrolytes; and macronutrients, including proteins, fats, and carbohydrates (Goulet, 1998; Vanderhoof & Young, 2002; Warner, Vanderhoof, & Reyes, 2000). Various factors affect the degree of malabsorption, including the age of the patient, the underlying condition necessitating bowel resection, and the length and segment of the remaining bowel (Sigalet).

Preterm infants with short bowel syndrome have a different prognosis than older children because of their capacity for additional longitudinal growth of the residual small bowel (Goulet, 1998; Wales et al., 2005). The length of the small intestine in a 27-week preterm infant is approximately 115 cm, whereas the term infant has a small intestine length of approximately 250 cm (Goulet; Vanderhoof & Langnas, 1997; Vanderhoof & Young, 2002). Short bowel syndrome is characterized by intestinal resections, leaving less than 30% of the normal small intestine length. In term infants, short bowel syndrome is generally defined as residual small intestine length less than 75 cm, which is often associated with some degree of malabsorption (Weseman & Gilroy, 2005).

The etiology of short bowel syndrome may be congenital or acquired. In the prenatal period, short bowel syndrome may be caused by isolated intestinal atresia, multiple atresias of the small intestine, meconium ileus or plug, gastroschisis, or extensive Hirschsprung's disease involving the small intestine. In the neonatal and postnatal period, short bowel syndrome is most commonly the result of necrotizing enterocolitis (Sigalet, 2001; Vanderhoof, 2003; Vanderhoof & Young, 2002). Necrotizing enterocolitis predominantly occurs in premature infants and often causes ischemic injury of the small intestine, leaving nonviable bowel requiring resection (see Chapter 13). Older children may develop a volvulus with intestinal ischemia or may have extensive Crohn's disease, tumors, radiation enteritis, or suffer abdominal trauma leading to small bowel resection and short bowel syndrome (Vanderhoof).

The anatomy of the remaining small intestine has a significant impact on the nutritional management and long-term outcome of patients with short bowel syndrome (Fig. 3-2). The site of greatest nutrient absorption occurs in the jejunum, while the reabsorption of water and electrolytes occurs predominantly in the ileum. Therefore, patients with an ileal resection may be more susceptible to fluid losses from osmotic diarrhea, which may increase

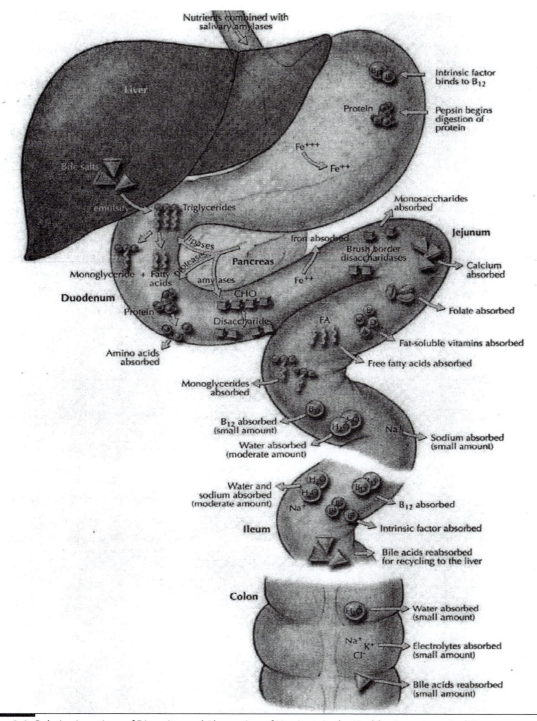

Figure 3-2 Relative Locations of Digestion and Absorption of Nutrients in the Healthy Gastrointestinal Tract

Source: From Short bowel syndrome: A nutritional and medical approach. Reprinted from *CMAJ* 14-May-02; 166(10), Pages 1297–1302 by permission of the publisher. © 2002 CMA Media Inc.

with feedings high in carbohydrates (Vanderhoof, 2003). In addition, absorption of vitamin B_{12}–intrinsic factor complex and bile salts may be significantly impaired after ileal resection. Fat-soluble vitamins, such as A, D, E, and K, and fats are also malabsorbed with loss of the ileum because of the lack of bile salts. Regulation of intestinal motility by nutrients and gastrointestinal hormones may

be impaired by ileal resection (Vanderhoof & Young, 2002). The ileocecal valve (ICV) controls the exit of fluid and nutrients from the small intestine into the colon and helps prevent the reflux of colonic bacteria into the small bowel. Thus, loss of the ICV may exacerbate nutrient malabsorption by decreasing transit time of nutrients from the small intestine into the colon and by contributing to bacterial overgrowth with intestinal mucosal inflammation (Vanderhoof). Preservation of the colon often improves the prognosis of the patient with short bowel syndrome. The colon is important in absorbing fluid, electrolytes, and short-chain fatty acids from malabsorbed carbohydrates, thus providing energy from additional calories (Sigalet, 2001; Vanderhoof; Vanderhoof & Young).

Over time, the residual small intestine adapts by increasing the transit time and thus nutrient contact time with the small bowel. The length and anatomy of the remaining small bowel affect its capacity to adapt. At the time of bowel resection, a minimal jejunoileal length of approximately 25 cm with an ICV or 40 cm of small intestine without an ICV is generally required for adequate adaptation to allow eventual independence from parenteral nutrition to occur (Vanderhoof, 2003). During the adaptation process, the intestinal musculature hypertrophies with an increase in bowel diameter and wall thickness and lengthens slightly, which increases the mucosal surface area for absorption. Hyperplasia of the mucosa also occurs with an increased number of enterocytes, as well as increased villus height and crypt depth for enhanced absorption (Goulet, 1998; Matarese et al., 2005; Sigalet, 2001; Vanderhoof).

During the adaptation process, the patient with short bowel syndrome progresses through three phases. The first phase after small bowel resection is characterized by limited absorption and diarrhea (Matarese et al., 2005). PN is the primary source of fluid and nutrition to promote normal growth during this time (Goulet, 1998; Matarese et al.; Vanderhoof & Young, 2002). PN replaces proteins, vitamins, minerals, and energy stores depleted as a result of the stress of surgery. During this period, fluid intake and output must be monitored closely. A separate replacement fluid solution is administered as needed for excess stool or ostomy output. Clinical and laboratory data, including electrolytes, liver function tests, and protein status, including albumin and pre-albumin levels, should be monitored to ensure sufficient nutritional restoration (Vanderhoof & Young).

After small bowel resection, enteral feedings should be initiated at a very slow rate via continuous gastric infusion after the postsurgical ileus resolves. Delivering even small amounts of diluted trophic feeds at 1 mL/hr may be beneficial to the newborn in stimulating intestinal adaptation, preventing the development of parenteral nutrition-associated cholestasis, and inhibiting bacterial translocation (Frantz, 2003; Teitelbaum & Coran, 2000; Vanderhoof & Young, 2002). EN may be the single most important factor in the successful management of short bowel syndrome because intestinal mucosal growth and function are largely dependent on the presence of food in the gut (Frantz; Vanderhoof & Young, 2001).

During the second phase of adaptation, fluid and electrolyte losses diminish and absorption is improved (Matarese et al., 2005; Vanderhoof & Young, 2002). Enteral nutrition is administered via continuous infusion and is advanced as tolerated. The concentration of the formula is initially advanced at low volumes to a goal of 0.67 kcal/mL or 20 kcal/ounce, followed by a gradual increase in the enteral feeding rate. In this way, transition from parenteral to enteral feedings may be accomplished while avoiding fluid overload (Vanderhoof & Young, 2002; Vanderhoof & Young, 2001). Small bolus oral feedings of 10 to 15 mL two to three times per day may be beneficial in promoting developmentally appropriate stages of feeding and preventing oral aversion (Warner et al., 2000). Breast milk, if available, or hypoallergenic semi-elemental formula containing predigested hydrolyzed protein may be used in infants with short bowel syndrome younger than 1 year of age. These formulas, including Nutramigen, Pregestimil, and Alimentum, are well tolerated by most infants with short bowel syndrome and reduce the risk of intestinal allergy caused by increased epithelial permeability to food antigens. Elemental amino acid formulas such as Neocate have an even lower allergenicity and may be used in very susceptible patients (Vanderhoof & Young, 2001; Warner et al.).

Because infants have a greater tolerance for fat than carbohydrates, a formula with a modest carbohydrate content is preferred. Carboyhdrates are digested rapidly, creating a high osmotic load in the gut that produces watery stools and contributes to fluid loss (Vanderhoof & Young, 2001; Warner et al., 2000). Most pediatric hydrolysate formulas have a higher percentage of calories from fat (between 40% and 50% of total calories). Pregestimil, Alimentum, and EleCare contain most of their fat calories in MCTs, which may be better absorbed because of their water solubility. However, these MCT formulas may create a higher osmotic load in the gut and impair intestinal adaptation (Vanderhoof & Young, 2001). Formulas that contain the vast majority of fat in the form of long-chain triglycerides include Nutramigen and Neocate. Long-chain triglycerides have a higher caloric density and are more effective in stimulating intestinal adaptation. As the gut is forced to work harder in digestion of nutrients, intestinal adaptation is enhanced. Therefore, a formula should be selected that contains either predominantly long-chain fats or a mixture of long- and medium-chain fats to promote absorption in the patient who has short bowel syndrome (Vanderhoof & Young, 2002; Vanderhoof & Young, 2001; Warner et al.).

Older children with short bowel syndrome can generally tolerate fiber-supplemented enteral formulas, which are higher in carbohydrates and lower in fat, with more complex protein sources. These formulas produce a firmer stool and allow fermentation of malabsorbed carbohydrate in the large bowel. These produce short-chain fatty acids, which increase intestinal adaptation and provide additional calories for colonic absorption (Vanderhoof, 2003). However, children with significant inflammation in their distal small bowel and colon from bacterial overgrowth may require a high-fat, low-carbohydrate formula, such as Pulmocare. The impact of formula choice on intestinal adaptation is important, regardless of age, and awareness of the residual intestinal anatomy assists in the selection of the optimal formula (Vanderhoof & Young, 2002; Vanderhoof & Young, 2001).

As adaptation progresses and absorption improves, enteral feeding rates are advanced and PN can be reduced (Vanderhoof & Young, 2001). During the second phase of adaptation, it is also important to continue to monitor the patient's nutritional status with daily weight and laboratory data (Teitelbaum & Coran, 2000). Tolerance of enteral feeding advancement is determined in a variety of ways. Stool volumes greater than 20 to 40 mL/kg/day indicate the need to slow the rate of feeding advancement or to hold feedings at the current rate for several days. Measuring stools for reducing substances also indicates carbohydrate malabsorption in small infants (Vanderhoof & Young, 2002; Vanderhoof & Young, 2001). In addition, a stool pH of less than 5.5 suggests carbohydrate malabsorption in patients with an intact colon (Vanderhoof & Young, 2002).

During the last phase, maximal adaptation is established and efforts are made to wean the patient from PN. This phase can last months to years and may take place at home, fostering a more normal environment for psychosocial development (Vanderhoof & Young, 2002; Teitelbaum & Coran, 2000). PN continues to be reduced proportionately to EN advancement (Vanderhoof & Young). The amount of time that PN is administered is decreased initially. Eventually, PN is either reduced to several nights per week or is completely discontinued (Matarese et al., 2005; Vanderhoof & Young).

Because the ultimate goal is to reach full enteral feedings, special efforts must be made to preserve normal oral motor development; feeding difficulties often occur if solid foods are withheld or delayed during normal developmental stages. Children with short bowel syndrome should follow the developmentally appropriate stages of eating throughout the adaptation process. Because of their decreased osmotic load, high-fat, high-protein solid foods such as meats should be introduced initially in children with short bowel syndrome (Vanderhoof & Young, 2002; Vanderhoof & Young, 2001; Warner et al., 2000). As new foods are introduced, enteral tolerance must continue to be monitored closely. Watery diarrhea may increase as enteral feedings are advanced, contributing to fluid and electrolyte losses. Urine output and specific gravity must be measured in order to assess hydration status. Frequent monitoring and correction of electrolyte losses, specifically sodium, in the serum and stool output help prevent dehydration (Vanderhoof & Young, 2002; Wessel & Samour, 2005). After ileal resection, it may be helpful to give cholestyramine in order to decrease secretory diarrhea by binding malabsorbed bile acids in the colon. However, this medication should not be given when bile acid deficiency already exists, because it could exacerbate nutrient malabsorption of fat-soluble vitamins by further depleting the supply of bile salts (Vanderhoof, 2003; Vanderhoof & Young, 2002). An antimotility agent, such as loperamide, may also be effective in slowing intestinal transit and decreasing the loss of fluid and nutrients (Vanderhoof). Monitoring for micronutrient deficiencies, such as calcium, magnesium, iron, and zinc, as well as vitamins A, D, E, and B_{12}, becomes essential as the child is weaned off PN and enteral tube feedings are replaced with oral nutrient intake (Vanderhoof & Young, 2002; Matarese et al., 2005). Appropriate supplementation of these nutrients may be necessary to avoid deficiency states (Vanderhoof & Young, 2001). Finally, long-term nutritional status and growth, including height, rate of weight gain, and weight-for-height ratio must be carefully monitored over time.

Most long-term complications associated with short bowel syndrome are a result of long-term PN and include central venous catheter complications, as discussed previously. Bacterial overgrowth in short bowel syndrome can exacerbate these catheter-related infections and can cause further nutrient malabsorption as a result of mucosal inflammation and competition with the host for other nutrients. Treatment for bacterial overgrowth involves administration of broad-spectrum antibiotics, often in a rotating schedule to prevent development of resistant organisms. PN-related liver disease is the major cause of death in children with short bowel syndrome. Although its etiology is poorly understood, several protective mechanisms reduce PN-associated liver disease. These include provision of at least 20% to 30% of total caloric needs through aggressive EN, prevention of small bowel bacterial overgrowth, and avoidance of catheter-related sepsis. Cholestasis also may occur in children on long-term PN, ultimately contributing to liver failure.

Long-term survival of children on PN is 80% to 85% (Vanderhoof & Young, 2002).

Various surgical options can be considered in the patient with bacterial overgrowth and severe malabsorption. The tapering enteroplasty is a procedure in which the antimesenteric bowel is resected longitudinally. This surgical procedure may help improve peristalsis, thus reducing bacterial overgrowth and increasing absorption in the excessively dilated bowel (Warner et al., 2000). Intestinal lengthening procedures such as the serial transverse enteroplasty and the Bianchi procedure may be performed on dilated small bowel, reducing the diameter of the intestine without loss of surface area. These bowel-lengthening procedures are also effective in reducing bacterial overgrowth and increasing intestinal absorption (Kim et al., 2003; Vanderhoof, 2003).

Intestinal failure may be defined as the inability to maintain nutritional and fluid status without the use of PN (Warner et al., 2000). In most patients with intestinal failure, complications of long-term PN may become life threatening (Weseman & Gilroy, 2005). In this subset of children with intestinal failure, small bowel transplantation may be considered. In patients with irreversible PN liver disease, combined liver/bowel transplantation is an option. Rejection and infection secondary to translocation of bacteria and fungi into the bloodstream are significant complications of intestinal transplantation. Determining the appropriate immunosuppression to control graft-versus-host disease while preventing posttransplantation lymphoproliferative syndrome remains a challenging problem. However, intestinal transplantation may offer a potential long-term alternative in patients with limited options (see Chapter 30). The nutritional management of infants and children with short bowel syndrome continues to present a significant challenge to the health care team and must be met with a comprehensive, multidisciplinary approach for successful outcomes (Vanderhoof, 2003).

■ Conclusion

Nutritional monitoring with support using EN and PN is a crucial component of the success of postsurgical pediatric patients. Both minor and major surgeries place pediatric patients at risk for poor dietary intake postoperatively, and recuperation and recovery may be inhibited if adequate provision of nutrients is not maintained. Close monitoring of intake, laboratory data, growth, and clinical status allows for improved identification of nutritional risk and timely introduction of nutritional support.

■ Acknowledgment

The authors would like to recognize the work of Annie McKenna and Jose M. Saavedra, authors of "Nutrition in the Pediatric Surgical Patient" in the first edition of this textbook.

References

Akers, S., & Groh-Wargo, S. (2005). Normal nutrition during infancy. In P. Q. Samour & K. King (Eds.), *Handbook of pediatric nutrition* (3rd ed., pp. 75–106). Sudbury, MA: Jones & Bartlett.

Beck, F. K., & Rosenthal, T. C. (2002). Pre-albumin: A marker for nutritional evaluation. *American Family Physician, 65,* 1575–1578.

Btaiche, I. F., & Khalidi, N. (2002). Parenteral nutrition-associated liver complications in children. *Pharmacotherapy, 22,* 188–211.

Chang, T. L., & Kleinman, R. E. (2003). Standard and specialized enteral formulas. In W. A. Walker, J. B. Watkins, & C. Duggan (Eds.), *Nutrition in pediatrics* (3rd ed., pp. 935–944). Hamilton, Ontario: Decker.

Chumlea, W. C. (2005). Physical growth and maturation. In P. Q. Samour & K. King (Eds.), *Handbook of pediatric nutrition* (3rd ed., pp. 1–10). Sudbury, MA: Jones & Bartlett.

Chwals, W. J. (1994). Overfeeding the critically ill child: Fact or fantasy? *New Horizons, 2,* 147–155.

Chwals, W. J., Letton, R.W., Jamie, A., & Charles, B. (1995). Stratification of injury severity using energy expenditure response in surgical infants. *Journal of Pediatric Surgery, 30,* 1161–1164.

Cloud, H. H. (2005). Developmental disabilities. In P. Q. Samour & K. King (Eds.), *Handbook of pediatric nutrition* (3rd ed., pp. 287–306). Sudbury, MA: Jones & Bartlett.

Corrales, K. M., & Utter, S. L. (2005). Growth failure. In P. Q. Samour & K. King (Eds.), *Handbook of pediatric nutrition* (3rd ed., pp. 391–406). Sudbury, MA: Jones & Bartlett.

Coss-Bu, J. A., Klish, W. J., Walding, D., Stein, F., O'Brian Smith, E., & Jefferson, L. S. (2001). Energy metabolism, nitrogen balance, and substrate utilization in critically ill children. *American Journal of Clinical Nutrition, 74,* 664–669.

Cox, J. H., & Melbardis, I. M. (2005). Parenteral nutrition. In P. Q. Samour & K. King (Eds.), *Handbook of pediatric nutrition* (3rd ed., pp. 525–557). Sudbury, MA: Jones & Bartlett.

Davis, A. M. (1998). Pediatrics. In L. E. Matarese & M. Gottschlich (Eds.), *Contemporary nutrition support practice* (pp. 347–364). Philadelphia: Saunders.

Davis, A. M., & Stanko-Kline, R. (2003). Pediatrics. In L. E. Matarese & M. Gottschlich (Eds.), *Contemporary nutrition support practice* (2nd ed., pp. 357–373). St. Louis, MO: Saunders.

DeChicco, R. S., & Matarese, L. E. (2003). Determining the nutrition support regimen. In L. E. Matarese & M. Gottschlich (Eds.), *Contemporary nutrition support practice* (2nd ed., pp. 181–187). St. Louis, MO: Saunders.

Falcao, M. C., & Tannuri, U. (2002). Nutrition for the pediatric surgical patients: Approach in the peri-operative period. *Revista do Hospital das Clinicas, 57*(6), 299–308.

Fonkalsrud, E. W. (2000). Inflammatory bowel disease and gastrointestinal neoplasms. In K. W. Ashcraft, J. P. Murphy, R. J. Sharp, D. L. Sigalet, & C. L. Snyder (Eds.), *Pediatric surgery* (3rd ed., pp. 545–570). Philadelphia: Saunders.

Frantz, F. W. (2003). Enteral nutrition. In P. Mattei (Ed.), *Surgical directives: Pediatric surgery* (pp. 25–33). Philadelphia: Lippincott Williams & Wilkins.

Fuhrman, M. P. (2003). Complication management in parenteral nutrition. In L. E. Matarese & M. Gottschlich (Eds.), *Contemporary nutrition support practice* (2nd ed., pp. 242–262). St. Louis, MO: Saunders.

Fulford, A., Scolapio, J. S., & Aranda-Michel, J. (2004). Parenteral nutrition-associated hepatotoxicity. *Nutrition in Clinical Practice, 19*, 274–283.

Garza, J. J., Shew, S. B., Keshen, T. H., Dzakovic, A., Jahoor, F., & Jaksic, T. (2002). Energy expenditure in ill premature neonates. *Journal of Pediatric Surgery, 37*, 289–293.

Goulet, O. (1998). Short bowel syndrome in pediatric patients. *Nutrition, 14*, 784–787.

Groh-Wargo, S. (2000). Recommended enteral nutrient intakes. In S. Groh-Wargo, M. Thompson, J. H. Cox, & J. V. Hartline (Eds.), *Nutritional care for high-risk newborns* (3rd ed., pp. 231–263). Chicago: Precept Press.

Hait, L., Bousvaros, A., & Grand, R. (2005). Pediatric inflammatory bowel disease: What children can teach adults. *Inflammatory Bowel Disease, 11*, 519–527.

Heuschkel, R., & Walker-Smith, J. A. (2003). Inflammatory bowel disease. In W. A. Walker, J. B. Watkins, & C. Duggan (Eds.), *Nutrition in pediatrics* (3rd ed., pp. 635–647). Hamilton, Ontario: Decker.

Hill, A. G., & Hill, G. L. (1998). Metabolic response to severe injury. *British Journal of Surgery, 85*, 884–890.

Hoagland, R. L., & Gahn, B. F. (2000). Parenteral nutrition: Nursing care for the infant receiving parenteral nutrition. In S. Groh-Wargo, M. Thompson, J. H. Cox, & J. V. Hartline (Eds.), *Nutritional care for high-risk newborns* (3rd ed., pp. 195–207). Chicago: Precept Press.

Irving, S. Y., Simone, S. D., Hicks, F. W., & Verger, J. T. (2000). Nutrition for the critically ill child: Enteral and parenteral support. *Advanced Practice in Acute Critical Care, 11*, 541–558.

Jeejeebhoy, K. N. (2005). Management of PN-induced cholestasis [Electronic version]. *Practical Gastroenterology, 24*, 62–68.

Kerner, J. A. (2003). Parenteral nutrition. In W. A. Walker, J. B. Watkins, & C. Duggan (Eds.), *Nutrition in pediatrics* (3rd ed., pp. 957–985). Hamilton, Ontario: Decker.

Kim, H. B., Fauza, D., Garza, J., Oh, J. T., Nurko, S., & Jaksic, T. (2003). Serial transverse enteroplasty (STEP): A novel bowel lengthening procedure. *Journal of Pediatric Surgery, 38*, 425–429.

Ljungqvist, O., Nygren, J., Soop, M., & Thorell, A. (2005). Metabolic perioperative management: Novel concepts. *Current Opinion in Critical Care, 11*, 295–299.

Matarese, L. E., O'Keefe, S. J., Kandil, H. M., Bond, G., Costa, G., & Abu-Elmagd, K. (2005). Short bowel syndrome: Clinical guidelines for nutrition management. *Nutrition in Clinical Practice, 20*, 493–502.

National Research Council. (1989). *Recommended dietary allowances* (10th ed.). Washington: National Academy Press.

Nevin-Folino, N., & Miller, M. (2005). Enteral nutrition. In P. Q. Samour & K. King (Eds.), *Handbook of pediatric nutrition* (3rd ed., pp. 499–524). Sudbury, MA: Jones & Bartlett.

Olsen, I. E., Mascarenhas, M. R., & Stallings, V. A. (2003). Clinical assessment of nutritional status. In W. A. Walker, J. B. Watkins, & C. Duggan (Eds.), *Nutrition in pediatrics* (3rd ed., pp. 6–16). Hamilton, Ontario: Decker.

Penny, M. E. (2003). Protein-energy malnutrition: Pathophysiology, clinical consequences, and treatment. In W. A. Walker, J. B. Watkins, & C. Duggan (Eds.), *Nutrition in pediatrics* (3rd ed., pp. 174–194). Hamilton, Ontario: Decker.

Pierro, A. (2002). Metabolism and nutritional support in the surgical neonate. *Journal of Pediatric Surgery, 37*, 811–822.

Price, P. T. (2000). Parenteral nutrition: Administration and monitoring. In S. Groh-Wargo, M. Thompson, J. H. Cox, & J. V. Hartline (Eds.), *Nutritional care for high-risk newborns* (3rd ed., pp. 91–107). Chicago: Precept Press.

Reilly, S., Skuse, D., & Poblete, X. (1996). Prevalence of feeding problems and oral motor dysfunction in children with cerebral palsy: A community survey. *Journal of Pediatrics, 129*, 877–882.

Shulman, R. J., & Phillips, S. (2002). Enteral and parenteral nutrition. In C. H. Lifschitz (Ed.), *Pediatric gastroenterology and nutrition in clinical practice* (pp. 417–448). New York: Marcel Dekker.

Shulman, R. J., & Phillips, S. (2003). Parenteral nutrition in infants and children. *Journal of Pediatric Gastroenterology and Nutrition, 36*, 587–607.

Sigalet, D. L. (2001). Short bowel syndrome in infants and children: An overview. *Seminars in Pediatric Surgery, 10*, 49–55.

Slavin, J. L. (2003). Dietary fiber. In L. E. Matarese & M. Gottschlich (Eds.), *Contemporary nutrition support practice* (2nd ed., pp. 173–180). St. Louis, MO: Saunders.

Sullivan, P. B., Juszczak, E., Lambert, B. R., Rose, M., Ford-Adams, M. E., & Johnson, A. (2002). Impact of feeding problems on nutritional intake and growth: Oxford feeding study II. *Developmental Medicine and Child Neurology, 44*, 461–467.

Sullivan, P. B., Lambert, B., Rose, M., Ford-Adams, M., Johnson, A., & Griffiths, P. (2000). Prevalence and severity of feeding and nutritional problems in children with neurological impairment: Oxford feeding study. *Developmental Medicine and Child Neurology, 42*, 674–680.

Szeszycki, E. E., & Benjamin, S. (2005). Complications of parenteral feeding. In G. Cresci (Ed.), *Nutrition support for the critically ill patient* (pp. 303–319). Boca Raton, FL: Taylor & Francis Group.

Teitelbaum, D. H., & Coran, A. G. (2000). Nutritional support of the pediatric surgical patient. In K. W. Ashcraft, J. P. Murphy, R. J. Sharp, D. L. Sigalet, & C. L. Snyder (Eds.), *Pediatric surgery* (3rd ed., pp. 17–37). Philadelphia: Saunders.

Teitelbaum, D. H., & Tracy, T. (2001). Parenteral nutrition-associated cholestasis. *Seminars in Pediatric Surgery, 10*, 72–80.

Turi, R. A., Petros, A. J., Eaton, S., Fasoli, L., Powis, M., Basu, R., et al. (2001). Energy metabolism of infants and children with systemic inflammatory response syndrome and sepsis. *Annals of Surgery, 233*, 581–587.

Vanderhoof, J. A. (2003). Short-bowel syndrome, including adaptation. In W. A. Walker, J. B. Watkins, & C. Duggan (Eds.), *Nutrition in pediatrics* (3rd ed., pp. 771–789). Hamilton, Ontario: Decker.

Vanderhoof, J. A., & Langnas, A. N. (1997). Short-bowel syndrome in children and adults. *Gastroenterology, 113*, 1767–1778.

Vanderhoof, J. A., & Young, R. J. (2002). Short bowel syndrome. In C. H. Lifschitz (Ed.), *Pediatric gastroenterology and nutrition in clinical practice* (pp. 701–721). New York: Marcel Dekker.

Vanderhoof, J. A., & Young, R. J. (2001). Enteral nutrition in short bowel syndrome. *Seminars in Pediatric Surgery, 10*, 65–71.

Wales, P. W., de Silva, N., Kim, J. H., Lecce, L., Sandhu, A., & Moore, A. M. (2005). Neonatal short bowel syndrome: A cohort study. *Journal of Pediatric Surgery, 40*, 755–762.

Warner, B. W., Vanderhoof, J. A., & Reyes, J. D. (2000). What's new in the management of short gut syndrome in children. *Journal of the American College of Surgeons, 190*, 725–736.

Weseman, R. A., & Gilroy, R. (2005). Nutrition management of small bowel transplant patients. *Nutrition in Clinical Practice, 20*, 509–516.

Wessel, J. J. (2000). Short bowel syndrome. In S. Groh-Wargo, M. Thompson, J. H. Cox, & J. V. Hartline (Eds.), *Nutritional care for high-risk newborns* (3rd ed., pp. 469–487). Chicago: Precept Press.

Wessel, J. J., & Samour, P. Q. (2005). Gastrointestinal disorders. In P. Q. Samour & K. King (Eds.), *Handbook of pediatric nutrition* (3rd ed., pp. 351–379). Sudbury, MA: Jones & Bartlett.

Young, R. J., & Vanderhoof, J. A. (2000). Nutrition in pediatric inflammatory bowel disease. *Nutrition, 16*, 78–80.

Zemel, B. S., & Stallings, V. A. (2003). Developmental disabilities. In W. A. Walker, J. B. Watkins, & C. Duggan (Eds.), *Nutrition in pediatrics* (3rd ed., pp. 580–590). Hamilton, Ontario: Decker.

CHAPTER

4

Vascular Access

By Melanie A. Kenney

Central venous catheters have advanced greatly during the past 30 years. Early animal studies demonstrated the safety and efficacy of administering hyperosmolar solutions through a central venous catheter (Dudrick, Wilmore, Vars, & Rhoads, 1968). The animals demonstrated adequate growth and development and a decreased incidence of thrombosis when the catheter tip was threaded into the superior vena cava. In a case study, Wilmore and Dudrick (1968) provided an infant with fluids and nutrition by means of a central venous catheter. After 44 days of intravenous nutrition, the infant's growth was appropriate for a 2-month-old child. Today, central venous catheters are used to provide parenteral nutrition solutions; to provide access for blood sampling, medications, and fluids; or to monitor a patient's hemodynamic stability. This chapter describes the various types of vascular access devices available, the care and maintenance of these devices, and the complications associated with their use.

■ Catheter Types

Two general types of central venous catheters exist: long term (partially implanted and totally implanted) and short term. Each catheter type has different features consistent with the anticipated duration of pediatric venous access required. Long-term central venous catheters provide vascular access for prolonged or lifelong therapies (e.g., chemotherapy, hemophilia therapy, parenteral nutrition, or other extended intravenous therapies). Short-term catheters function similarly to long-term catheters, but the duration of therapy is expected to be more limited.

Long-Term Partially Implanted Tunneled Devices (Hickman, Broviac, Groshong, Cook)

The first category, partially implanted venous access devices, consists of those commonly referred to by the name of the manufacturer or inventor, Hickman, Broviac, Groshong, and Cook. These are single-lumen or multiple-lumen catheters that are surgically placed in subcutaneous tunnels. The distal portion of the catheter exits the skin at what is referred to as the "exit site."

These catheters also feature a Dacron cuff that remains in the subcutaneous tunnel and promotes adherence of the surrounding tissue to the cuff, an anchoring process requiring several days to weeks. Theoretically, the cuff prevents the inadvertent removal or dislodgment of the catheter. The cuff also provides a mechanical barrier that inhibits the migration of organisms from the subcutaneous tunnel

(Fig. 4-1). These features, the subcutaneous tunnel and the Dacron cuff, have been theorized as the reasons for the lower infection rates of these catheters compared with those of short-term catheters (Baranowski, 1993; Gabriel et al., 2005). In addition, some catheters have two cuffs: one is the Dacron cuff and the other is an antimicrobial cuff that is located closer to the exit site to discourage bacterial migration in the initial postplacement period.

The Groshong catheter, developed in 1978, has an additional unique feature in its design: the catheter tip is closed and has a pressure-sensitive valve inside it. The process of introducing infusions or medications creates positive pressure and opens the valve outward. When negative pressure or suction is applied, the valve opens inward and allows blood sampling from the catheter. When the catheter is not in use, the valve is closed, which prevents blood from flowing back into the catheter. Therefore, this catheter does not require heparin as a flush solution or the use of a clamp when the cap or intravenous tubing is changed (Baranowski, 1993).

Long-Term Totally Implanted Devices

The second category of long-term venous catheters is totally implanted vascular devices (ports). These catheters are also surgically tunneled under the skin but possess a subcutaneous port, or reservoir, with a self-sealing septum that is implanted in the body. The septum is accessed by means of a noncoring, or Huber, needle through the skin (Fig. 4-2). The ports require less frequent maintenance, are much less noticeable, and facilitate optimal body image. Because the port is completely covered by the skin, the patient is able to more freely participate in activities, such as swimming and contact sports (Gullo, 1993).

Theoretically, patients with totally implanted vascular devices experience fewer infectious complications. However, variable infection rates have been reported when totally implanted catheters have been compared with partially implanted catheters. The results range from significantly lower infectious complications for totally implanted devices to comparable rates between the two catheter types (Groeger et al., 1993; LaQuaglia et al., 1992; Wiener et al., 1992). Table 4-1 provides a summary of the advantages and disadvantages of the long-term types of devices.

Short-Term Central Venous Nontunneled Catheters (Traditional, Peripherally Inserted Central Catheters [PICC], Midline Catheters)

Short-term central venous catheters provide central access, but they lack the features of a Dacron cuff and ex-

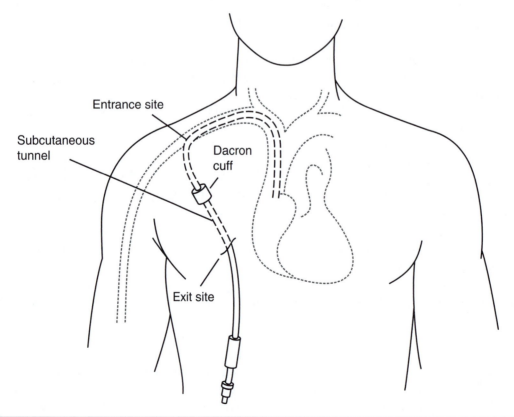

Figure 4-1 Pediatric Long-Term Central Venous Catheter Placement
Courtesy of Thomas Kenney.

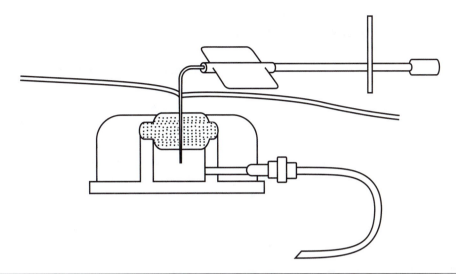

Figure 4-2 Totally Implanted Device (port)
Courtesy of Thomas Kenney.

tensive subcutaneous tunnel. The traditional short-term central venous catheters are those inserted directly into subclavian, jugular, or femoral veins and then sutured to the skin. These catheters are available with single- or multilumen capabilities.

A second type of short-term central venous catheter is the peripherally inserted central catheter (PICC). These catheters are placed in a variety of veins and are threaded to either a peripheral or a central tip location. Total parenteral nutrition can be administered only after the central tip location is verified by radiographic films. Peripheral parenteral nutrition is given through a line that does not have the tip centrally placed. Kearns, Coleman, and Wehner (1996) found that for PICCs placed in the upper extremity, advancing the catheter tip into a central vein reduced the occurrence of thrombosis. The PICCs do not require surgical insertion and have been placed in interventional radiology suites and by registered nurses in home, hospital, or clinic settings. PICCs are available in various lumen sizes ranging from 2F to 5F, with single-, double-, and triple-lumen styles. Knue, Doellman, Rabin, and Jacobs (2005) found that 3F catheters are suitable for administration or aspiration of blood samples. Bahruth (1996) was the first to report the vasoconstriction or vasospasm that resulted from the application of topical anesthetic cream before placement of a PICC.

Finally, midline catheters are inserted and cared for as PICCs. These catheters are shorter than PICCs and meet the access needs that arise for patients who need a catheter which will last longer than a peripheral line but do not need access to the central circulation (Anderson, 2004; Gorski & Czaplewski, 2004).

■ Care and Maintenance of Central Venous Catheters

Specific policies and procedures are required for the care and maintenance of vascular access devices. Controversy exists about the use of sterile technique versus clean procedures to change dressings and access totally implanted vascular devices. Discussion follows about the care and maintenance of central venous catheters.

Antiseptic Agents

The principles of the various antiseptic agents used for dressing change had traditionally been extrapolated from research that studied hand washing of hospital personnel using 70% alcohol and 10% povidone-iodine (Ayliffe, Babb, Davies, & Lilly, 1988; Rotter, Koller, & Wewalka, 1980). Other trials compared 2% chlorhexidine with these agents when used for catheter dressing changes (Larsen & Thurston, 1997; Maki, Ringer, & Alvarado, 1991). Kinirons et al. (2001) studied children who had epidural catheters and compared the use of chlorhexidine and povidone-iodine as skin preparation before epidural catheter insertion. This study documented that chlorhexidine reduced the risk of catheter colonization relative to the povidone-iodine group. The antiseptic agent should be applied using a circular motion, moving from the inside outward.

Topical Ointment

The use of topical antimicrobial ointment, such as 10% povidone-iodine or polyantibiotic ointment, is controversial. Some studies have reported that the ointment

Table 4-1	Comparisons of Long-Term Devices
Partially Implanted Devices	**Totally Implanted Devices**
Advantages	Advantages
No needle sticks	Few activity/clothing restrictions
Easy to initiate intravenous access	Less obvious to casual observer
Technically simple to place and remove	Improved body image
Device less expensive	Minimal care required
Can be removed at bedside/office setting with sedation	Fewer complications
Disadvantages	Disadvantages
Frequent flushing	Needle stick for each access
Dressing to maintain	Greater expense associated with placement
Cost and time required to care for line	Waiting time required when EMLA used
Catheter can be pulled on/broken	Requires a second operation for removal
Dressing change may be uncomfortable	Requires specific equipment (Huber needle) for access

decreases infection (Moran, Atwood, & Rowe, 1965; Norden, 1969), whereas other studies have not yielded these same conclusions (Maki & Band, 1981; Zinner et al., 1969). Polyantibiotic ointments that are not fungicidal have been shown to contribute to an increased risk of *Candida* colonization of central catheters (Maki & Band; Zinner et al.). Topical mupirocin (Bactroban) applied to the exit site is an effective antimicrobial against staphylococcal species. However, because it is not indicated for antimicrobial treatment against other organisms (*Physicians' Desk Reference*, 2006), the use of such ointments should be reserved for the treatment of organism-specific exit site infections.

Dressing Material

The use of transparent semipermeable dressings instead of the traditional dressing of gauze and tape is a growing trend. The transparent dressings (e.g., Tegaderm, OpSite, OpSite IV 3000) facilitate securing of the central venous catheter, which is a priority for pediatric patients. These dressings also allow for the visual observation of the exit site, less frequent dressing changes, and a greater ability for the patient to bathe or shower without saturating the exit site. The type of dressing material recommended has an impact on the desired frequency of dressing changes. The traditional dressing requires more frequent changes than the transparent dressing. Some researchers report that transparent dressings contribute to increased microbial colonization of the exit site and result in increased infection rates (Conly, Grieves, & Peters, 1989), whereas others have reported no difference in catheter coloniza-

tion and infection rates between the different dressing types used (Maki & Ringer, 1987). Two studies with pediatric subjects compared gauze dressings with transparent dressings and found no significant differences in the incidence of bacterial growth or positive skin cultures (Freiberger, Bryant, & Marino, 1992; Shivnan et al., 1991). The use of a highly permeable transparent dressing resulted in fewer catheter-related infections than the use of a traditional gauze and transparent dressing (Treston-Aurand, Olmsted, Allen-Bridson, & Craig, 1997). Taylor et al. (1996) found a significant increase in microbial growth for the transparent dressing group in their neonatal intensive care patients. However, because this microbial growth did not correlate with an increased sepsis rate, this study recommended the use of transparent dressings in children. Chambers et al. (2005) studied the use of a sustained-release chlorhexidine dressing in adult neutropenic patients with a central line. The incidence of exit-site infections, tunnel infections, and premature catheter removals was lower in the intervention group that used the sustained-release chlorhexidine dressings than in the group using a standard dressing protocol.

Flush Maintenance

The flush solution is yet another controversial issue for central catheter care. The recommended concentration, amount, and frequency of heparin used to maintain the patency of the central catheter and prevent thrombosis vary. Fry (1992) compiled a survey regarding flushing protocols for all intravenous catheters; the survey revealed a great variation in protocols ranging from a frequency of every 2 hours to every week, with the heparin concentration ranging from 10 to 1,000 units/mL. This survey provided minimal or no outcome evidence to support specific clinical practices. The use of the lowest possible concentration of heparin is recommended, and it is acceptable that the amount of flush should be double the volume needed to fill the catheter and add-on tubing (Intravenous Nursing Standards of Practice, 2000). Mechanical measures that use positive-pressure flushing techniques or closing the catheter clamp while maintaining pressure on the syringe plunger should be incorporated into the flushing maintenance regimen (Gorski & Czaplewski, 2004).

Heparin is not used with Groshong catheters because the pressure-sensitive valve eliminates the need for heparinization. Research has been conducted to suggest that 0.9% saline is as effective as heparin for peripheral catheters (Epperson, 1984; Goode et al., 1991). Rabe et al. (2002) conducted a study comparing flush solutions for central venous catheters in adult patients. The heparin-filled catheter group had fewer occluded catheters than the normal saline–filled group, demonstrating a prolonged patency in the heparin group. The practice of maintaining central venous catheters with saline has not been thoroughly tested in children. Future research will determine whether saline is an effective flush for central venous catheters, especially for catheters with small lumens.

Cleansing Catheter Junction/Cap

Sitges-Serra et al. (1984) documented that catheter sepsis originates from infected central venous catheter hubs, thus emphasizing the need for junctional care. The protocol for cleaning the catheter connection or infusion cap varies between the use of sterile versus aseptic procedures. Seventy percent alcohol and/or povidone-iodine may be used as antiseptic agents (Ruschman & Fulton, 1993). Mechanical barriers, such as sterile 2 × 2 gauze bandages may be used to decrease the potential for contamination when the catheter connection is opened. The Intravenous Nursing Standards of Practice (2000) report that the optimal time for changing the infusion cap is unknown. Their recommendation is to change the cap at least every 7 days and immediately if residual blood is observed in the cap or if the integrity of the cap may have been compromised.

In 1992, needleless systems were introduced to help make the environment safer for health care providers (Horner, 1998). Danzig et al. (1995) studied the occurrence of bloodstream infections of home intravenous infusion patients using one type of needleless system. The patients receiving parenteral nutrition had higher rates of infection than those receiving other therapies. The authors believed that the nutrient-rich parenteral nutrition solutions remained in the infusion cap and became contaminated with subsequent cap manipulations. Different product lines of needleless systems are available. The selection of a particular system should include consideration of the number of pieces required, which has a direct impact on the time and ease of assembly when using the system. Brown (2004) concluded that the best agents for hub care with needleless systems continue to be alcohol, povidone-iodine, and chlorhexidine.

Accessing an Implanted Port

The patient's skin over and surrounding the port must be prepared before the insertion of the noncoring, or Huber, needle. Insertion of the needle is referred to as "accessing" the implanted port. A Huber needle, which has a noncoring point, must be used because it slices the port septum, thus preserving its integrity. If a hypodermic needle is used, a cylindrical "core" is removed from the port septum with each use. An issue of controversy is whether sterile or clean gloves are necessary when a port is accessed. Long and Ovaska (1992) and Schulmeister (1987) found that no febrile episodes or septicemia occurred with either method.

After the needle placement is confirmed by blood aspiration and/or normal saline flush, the needle must be secured and stabilized to prevent needle dislodgment during use. Strips of tape may be used or a formal dressing applied (see "Dressing Material" discussion earlier). For continued intravenous access, the dressing and Huber needle must be changed, with a weekly change being the most commonly reported frequency. To maintain catheter patency, it is recommended that an implanted port be flushed with 5 mL of 100 units/mL of heparin after each use. The heparin flush can be effective for up to 1 month when the port is not accessed (Baranowski, 1993).

The psychological consequences and pain associated with the use of a needle to obtain vascular access is a definite disadvantage of the implanted port type of central venous catheter. The use of a topical anesthetic, such as eutectic mixture of local anesthetics (EMLA), helps minimize the pain and discomfort reported by patients. The EMLA cream should be applied and covered with a transparent dressing at least 1 hour before the port is accessed. McInally (2005) conducted an informal audit that discovered that the sensations of holding and pushing the port during accessing caused more discomfort for children than the needle going through the skin. Development and implementation of a preparation and distraction program with the child and family can help control anxieties and facilitate coping with the accessing procedure.

Potential Complications

Potential complications occurring with central catheters can be categorized into two groups: infectious and mechanical. Infections with central venous catheters occur as localized or systemic infections.

Infectious Complications

Localized Infections

Localized infections occur at the exit site of short- or long-term central venous catheters. The signs and symptoms include erythema, edema, drainage, and tenderness at the exit site or over the tunnel of the catheter; fever may be present. The most common organism involved is *Staphylococcus epidermidis*, but *Staphylococcus aureus*, *Pseudomonas* species, and *Mycobacterium* species may also be involved (Jones, 1998). Topical and/or systemic antibiotic therapy is needed in these cases. Clinicians may also determine that catheter removal or replacement is warranted for tunnel track infections or for exit site infections that recur when antibiotic therapy is concluded (Jones). If the exit site infection is caused by *Pseudomonas aeruginosa* or fungi, Shah, Smith, and Zaoutis (2005) recommended that the catheter be removed in adults and that removal be considered in children.

Systemic Infections

Historically, a positive blood culture meant immediate removal of the central venous catheter. More recently, depending on the type of organism isolated and the child's particular infectious history, systemic infections have been successfully treated with appropriate antibiotics through the catheter without requiring catheter removal. Many authors report the occurrences and circumstances regarding infectious complications in their patients. Wiener et al. (1992) analyzed the insertion and reason for removal of venous access devices for children with cancer. Infection was the most frequent complication-related reason for removal of a device. This study did not identify a difference between the number of partially implanted catheters and totally implanted devices removed because of infection. However, a large number of partially implanted catheters were inadvertently removed because of dislodgment and, therefore, could not acquire an infection. A weakness of this study was the inability to collect data on complications that occurred during the life of the catheter. The authors could not determine infection rates because they were only aware of the infections that were the reason for catheter removal. Jones, Konsler, Dunaway, Lacey, and Azizkhan (1993) also investigated pediatric

hematology-oncology patients with central venous catheters. They found a greater rate of catheter infection within the first 3 months after the device was placed and also noted that children younger than 2 years of age had an increased incidence of catheter infection. Kurkchubasche, Smith, and Rowe (1992) found that children with short bowel syndrome had a higher incidence of catheter sepsis (7.8/1,000 catheter days) than children without short bowel syndrome (1.3/1,000 catheter days). The children without short bowel syndrome had *Staphylococcus* species isolated from their blood cultures most of the time (88%). The short bowel syndrome group showed *Staphylococcus* in 38%, yeast in 23%, and gram-negative rods in 27% of cases. Buchman et al. (1994) reviewed the catheter-related infections of home parenteral nutrition adult and pediatric patients discharged from their institution. Their findings revealed that although the incidence of catheter infection was low for patients receiving home parenteral nutrition, there was a significantly greater occurrence of catheter sepsis and exit site infections in the children than in the adults.

Another consideration in the event of infection is the documented relationship between catheter-related sepsis and the presence of vascular thrombosis (Raad et al., 1994). Shah, Smith, and Zaoutis (2005) stated that when a thrombosis is present, the blood flow obstruction through a catheter promotes the colonization of microbes and evolution into an infection.

Mechanical Complications

Occlusion

Resistance to flow during flushing or attempts to administer intravenous fluid is characteristic of an occluded central venous catheter. It is imperative to determine the history and characteristics of this malfunction to decide whether the occlusion is caused by a clot or thrombus as opposed to being an intravenous medication or fluid precipitate. A perceived occlusion may be investigated radiographically. Stephens, Haire, and Kotulak (1995) radiographically examined 200 dysfunctional central venous catheters and found that 58% of the catheters were occluded as a result of a thrombus. Before any treatment, mechanical maneuvers should be tried, such as repositioning the patient and having the patient cough, deep breathe, and raise his or her arms above the head. The dressing should be removed to determine whether the catheter is kinked by the dressing or sutures, if present (Bagnall-Reeb, 1998).

A clotted catheter usually has a history of slight resistance over the previous few days, with flushing becoming increasingly difficult. The history may also reveal difficulty or inability to obtain blood samples from the catheter. Formerly, urokinase was the only approved thrombolytic agent that was effective in clearing catheters occluded by clot or thrombosis. However, since the US Food and Drug Administration removed urokinase from the market in 1999 (Hartnell & Gates, 2000), other thrombolytic agents have been used, including streptokinase and alteplase (tissue plasminogen activator or t-PA) (Hooke, 2000; McKnight, 2004).

Semba et al. (2002) reported on two phase III clinical trials using alteplase administered in up to two 2 mg/2 mL bolus doses. This study included 1,064 patients who were at least 2 years of age. Function was restored in the occluded catheters after one dose in 75% of the patients, and after two doses in 85% of the patients.

Low dose t-PA (1 mg/1 mL) was instilled in totally implanted devices (ports) to remove the catheter occlusion; a 92.9% success rate was achieved using an average t-PA dose of 2.29 mg. These patients all had documented fibrin sheaths present in their ports, causing their catheters to malfunction before the t-PA instillation (Whigham, Lindsey, Goodman, & Fisher 2002).

In contrast, in a catheter occluded with a precipitate, there is a sudden, complete inability to flush or infuse through the catheter. Drug or solution incompatibilities occur by inappropriate drug preparation or the mixing of incompatible medications or solutions. Evaluating the intermittent intravenous medications and the components of the intravenous solution should reveal the cause of the precipitate-occluded catheter. The clinician must know the chemicals involved in the precipitate when attempting to clear the catheter. Various precipitates and their treatments have been reported. Calcium phosphorus precipitates have been treated with 0.1 N hydrochloric acid (Hashimoto, Morgan, Kenney, Pringle, & Alcorn, 1986; Kupensky, 1995). Shulman, Barrish, and Hicks (1995) used a model to demonstrate that even a daily infusion of hydrochloric acid over an 8-week interval did not cause visible damage to central catheters. Pennington and Pithie (1987) reported experience using an ethanol solution to clear catheters occluded with lipid material associated with "three-in-one" (dextrose, amino acid, and lipid emulsion in same solution) parenteral nutrition. Werlin et al. (1995) also reported the efficacy of ethanol and hydrochloric acid to clear partially and totally implanted catheters.

Emergency Care of Broken/ Damaged Central Catheters

Should the central venous catheter become damaged or broken, the patient or caregiver must be prepared to clamp the catheter between the child and the damaged or broken area of the catheter. The patient or caregiver may be educated in performing a temporary repair by inserting the appropriate-sized blunt needle into the catheter lumen. A temporary repair kit can easily be assembled for the family/caregiver, which includes flushing supplies, sterile scissors, alcohol swabs, an appropriate-sized blunt needle, and a tongue depressor. The corresponding permanent repair kit is obtained from the manufacturer of the particular PICC. This permanent repair is performed by a member of the health care team.

Implanted Port-Specific Complications

Twiddler's Syndrome

Patients with the nervous habit of "twiddling" with their implanted ports may actually displace, curl, or kink the catheters. Twiddler's syndrome was originally associated with patients after pacemaker insertion, but it has also been reported in patients with implanted ports (Gebarski & Gebarski, 1984). Servetar (1992) first reported Twiddler's syndrome in a pediatric patient. The patient's port site was edematous and tender on one occasion but was resolving. Before a vesicant solution was administered, a chest radiograph film revealed the catheter had migrated out of the vein and the catheter had multiple revolutions in the subcutaneous tunnel. On questioning, the mother recalled noticing the patient playing with his port. This episode illustrates the need to observe for itching, scrubbing, or excess touching of the port and the need to obtain a history from the caregiver when the port area appears tender, to have changed location, or has signs of infection present.

Needle Dislodgment/Extravasation

The anatomic placement of the implanted port may be a factor in the phenomenon of needle dislodgment. A port placed in excessive adipose tissue, near breast tissue, and over the pectoral muscle near the axilla makes accessing the port more difficult. Movement of the arms and shoulders has the potential to cause accidental needle dislodgment when the port is placed in this position (Camp-Sorrell, 1998; Kurul, Saip, & Aydin, 2002). Another possible cause of catheter extravasation is migration of the catheter into a smaller vein (Ingle, 1995). Conditions that change intrathoracic pressure, such as coughing, sneezing, heavy lifting, and forceful flushing of the catheter, may result in catheter tip migration (Hadaway, 1998). The presence of a thrombus or fibrin sheath formation at the catheter tip is also associated with extravasation. The flow of infusate is obstructed at the catheter tip, which causes the infusate to flow back along the catheter into the subcutaneous tissue (Mayo & Pearson, 1995). The presence or absence of a blood return and patient discomfort should be assessed with each accessing. The port should flush easily without erythema or edema observed at the Huber needle site. If the device has a history of no blood return, a dye study should be obtained to evaluate the needle placement and catheter position before the port is used to infuse a vesicant (Chrystal, 1997). If it is uncertain whether needle dislodgment or extravasation has occurred, a physician should be consulted. Appropriate treatment of the suspected or known extravasation is determined by the type of infusate that was administered.

■ Conclusion

The use and maintenance of vascular access catheters constitute a rapidly growing and evolving area of health care. Many issues relevant to the care and maintenance of these catheters remain controversial. With continued research and outcome reporting, children requiring central venous access can safely receive a variety of medications and fluids through these devices.

■ Acknowledgment

The author wishes to thank Tom Kenney for his drawings and support during the preparation of this chapter.

■ Educational Materials

A Teaching Sheet for families of children with a central venous catheter is available (in English and Spanish) at www.apsna.org and www.jbpub.com. This teaching sheet may be downloaded free of charge and APSNA encourages its use with your patients and families.

References

Anderson, N. R. (2004). Midline catheters. *Journal of Infusion Nursing, 27*, 313–321.

Ayliffe, G. A., Babb, J. R., Davies, J. G., & Lilly, H. A. (1988). Hand disinfection: A comparison of various agents in laboratory and ward studies. *Journal of Hospital Infection, 11*, 226–243.

Bagnall-Reeb, H. (1998). Diagnosis of central venous access device occlusion: Implications for nursing practice. *Journal of Intravenous Nursing, 21*, S115–S121.

Bahruth, A. J. (1996). Peripherally inserted central catheter insertion problems associated with topical anesthesia. *Journal of Intravenous Nursing, 19*, 32–34.

Baranowski, L. (1993). Central venous access devices: Current technologies, use, and management strategies. *Journal of Intravenous Nursing, 16*, 167–194.

Brown, M. (2004). The impact of safety product use on catheter-related infections. *Journal of Infusion Nursing, 27*, 245–250.

Buchman, A. L., Moukarzel, A., Goodson, B., Herzog, F., Pollack, P., Reyen, L., et al. (1994). Catheter-related infection associated with home parenteral nutrition and predictive factors for the need for catheter removal in their treatment. *Journal of Parenteral and Enteral Nutrition, 18*, 297–302.

Camp-Sorrell, D. (1998). Developing extravasation protocols and monitoring outcomes. *Journal of Intravenous Nursing, 21*, 232–239.

Chambers, S. T., Sanders, J., Patton, W. N., Ganly, P., Birch, M., Crump, J. A., et al. (2005). Reduction of exit-site infections of tunneled intravascular catheters among neutropenic patients by sustained-released chlorhexidine dressings: Results from a prospective randomized controlled trial. *Journal of Hospital Infection, 61*, 53–61.

Chrystal, C. (1997). Administering continuous vesicant chemotherapy in the ambulatory setting. *Journal of Intravenous Nursing, 20*, 78–88.

Conly, J. M., Grieves, K., & Peters, B. (1989). A prospective, randomized study comparing transparent and dry gauze dressings for central venous catheters. *Journal of Infectious Diseases, 159*, 310–319.

Danzig, L. E., Short, L. J., Collins, K., Mahoney, M., Sepe, S., Bland, L., et al. (1995). Blood stream infections associated with a needleless intravenous infusion system in patients receiving home infusion therapy. *JAMA: Journal of the American Medical Association, 273*, 1862–1864.

Dudrick, S. J., Wilmore, D. W., Vars, H. M., & Rhoads, J. E. (1968). Long-term total parenteral nutrition with growth, development, and positive nitrogen balance. *Surgery, 64*, 134–142.

Epperson, E. L. (1984). Efficacy of 0.9% sodium chloride injection with and without heparin for maintaining indwelling intermittent injection sites. *Clinical Pharmacy, 3*, 626–629.

Freiberger, D., Bryant, J., & Marino, B. (1992). The effects of different central venous line dressing changes on bacterial growth in a pediatric oncology population. *Journal of Pediatric Oncology Nursing, 9*, 3–7.

Fry, B. (1992). Intermittent heparin flushing protocols: A standardization protocol. *Journal of Intravenous Nursing, 15*, 160–163.

Gabriel, J., Bravery, K., Dougherty, L., Kayley, J., Malster, M., & Scales, K. (2005). Vascular access: Indications and implications for patient care. *Nursing Standard, 19*(26), 45–52.

Gebarski, S. S., & Gebarski, K. S. (1984). Chemotherapy port "twiddler's syndrome": A need for preinjection radiography. *Cancer, 54*, 38–39.

Goode, C. J., Titler, M., Rakel, B., Ones, D. S., Kleiber, C., Small, S., et al. (1991). A meta-analysis of effects of heparin flush and saline flush: Quality and cost implications. *Nursing Research, 40*, 324–330.

Gorski, L., & Czaplewski, L. (2004). Peripherally inserted central catheters and midline catheters for the homecare nurse. *Journal of Infusion Nursing, 27*, 399–409.

Groeger, J. S., Lucas, A. B., Thaler, H. T., Friedlander-Klar, H., Brown, A. E., Kiehn, T. E., et al. (1993). Infectious morbidity associated with long-term use of venous access devices in patients with cancer. *Annals of Internal Medicine, 119*, 1168–1174.

Gullo, S. M. (1993). Implanted ports. Technologic advances and nursing care issues. *Nursing Clinics of North America, 28*, 859–871.

Hadaway, L. C. (1998). Major thrombotic and nonthrombotic complications: Loss of patency. *Journal of Intravenous Nursing, 21*, 143–160.

Hartnell, G. G., & Gates, J. (2000). The case of abbokinase and the FDA: The events leading to the suspension of abbokinase supplies in the United States. *Journal of Vascular and Interventional Radiology, 11*, 841–847.

Hashimoto, E., Morgan, D., Kenney, M., Pringle, K., & Alcorn, A. (1986). Blocked TPN catheters: Clots aren't the only culprit. *Journal of Parenteral and Enteral Nutrition, 10*, 17S.

Hooke, C. (2000). Recombinant tissue plasminogen activator for central venous access device occlusion. *Journal of Pediatric Oncology Nursing, 17*, 174–178.

Horner, K. A. (1998). Technology assessment of two needleless systems. *Journal of Intravenous Nursing, 21*, 203–208.

Ingle, R. J. (1995). Rare complications of vascular access devices. *Seminars in Oncology Nursing, 11*, 184–193.

Intravenous nursing standards of practice. (2000). *Journal of Intravenous Nursing, 21*, S1–S9.

Jones, G. R. (1998). A practical guide to evaluation and treatment of infections in patients with central venous catheters. *Journal of Intravenous Nursing, 21*, S134–S142.

Jones, G. R., Konsler, G. K., Dunaway, R. P., Lacey, S. R., & Azizkhan, R. G. (1993). Prospective analysis of urokinase in the treatment of catheter sepsis in pediatric hematology-oncology patients. *Journal of Pediatric Surgery, 28*, 350–357.

Kearns, P. J., Coleman, S., & Wehner, J. H. (1996). Complications of long arm catheters: A randomized trial of central vs. peripheral tip location. *Journal of Parenteral and Enteral Nutrition, 20*, 20–24.

Kinirons, B., Mimoz, O., Lafendi, L., Naas, T., Meunier, J., & Nordmann, P. (2001). Chlorhexidine versus povidone iodine in preventing colonization of continuous epidural catheters in children: A randomized, controlled study. *Anesthesiology, 94*, 239–244.

Knue, M., Doellman, D., Rabin, K., & Jacobs, B. R. (2005). The efficacy and safety of blood sampling through peripherally inserted central catheter devices in children. *Journal of Infusion Nursing, 28*, 30–35.

Kupensky, D. T. (1995). Use of hydrochloric acid to restore patency in an occluded implantable port. *Journal of Intravenous Nursing, 18*, 198–201.

Kurkchubasche, A. G., Smith, S. D., & Rowe, M. I. (1992). Catheter sepsis in short-bowel syndrome. *Archives of Surgery, 127*, 21–25.

Kurul, S., Saip, P., & Aydin, T. (2002). Totally implantable venous-access ports: Local problems and extravasation injury. *The Lancet Oncology, 3*, 684–692.

LaQuaglia, M. P., Lucas, A., Thaler, H. T., Friedlander-Klar, H., Exelby, P. R., & Groeger, J. S. (1992). A prospective analysis of vascular access device-related infections in children. *Journal of Pediatric Surgery, 27*, 840–842.

Larsen, L. L., & Thurston, N. E. (1997). Research utilization: Development of a central venous catheter procedure. *Applied Nursing Research, 10*, 44–51.

Long, M. C., & Ovaska, M. (1992). Comparative study of nursing protocols for venous access ports. *Cancer Nursing, 15*, 18–21.

Maki, D. G., & Band, J. D. (1981). A comparative study of polyantibiotic and iodophor ointments in prevention of vascular catheter-related infection. *American Journal of Medicine, 70*, 739–744.

Maki, D. G., Ringer, M., & Alvarado, C. J. (1991). Prospective randomized trial of povidone-iodine, alcohol, and chlorhexidine for prevention of infection associated with central venous and arterial catheters. *Lancet, 338*, 339–343.

Maki, D. G., & Ringer, M. (1987). Evaluation of dressing regimens for prevention of infection with peripheral intravenous catheters: Gauze, a transparent polyurethane dressing, and an iodophor-transparent dressing. *JAMA: Journal of the American Medical Association, 258*, 2396–2403.

Mayo, D. J., & Pearson, D. C. (1995). Chemotherapy extravasation: A consequence of fibrin sheath formation around venous access devices. *Oncology Nursing Forum, 22*, 675–680.

McInally, W. (2005). Whose line is it anyway? Management of central venous catheters in children. *Paediatric Nursing, 17*(5), 14–18.

McKnight, S. (2004). Nurse's guide to understanding and treating thrombotic occlusion of central venous access devices. *Medsurg Nursing, 13*, 377–382.

Moran, J. M., Atwood, R. P., & Rowe, M. I. (1965). A clinical and bacteriologic study of infections associated with venous cutdowns. *New England Journal of Medicine, 272*, 554–560.

Norden, C. W. (1969). Application of antibiotic ointment to the site of venous catheterization: A controlled trial. *Journal of Infectious Diseases, 120*, 611–615.

Pennington, C. R., & Pithie, A. D. (1987). Ethanol lock in the management of catheter occlusion. *Journal of Parenteral and Enteral Nutrition, 11*, 507–508.

Physicians' Desk Reference. (2006). Montvale, NJ: Thompson PDR.

Raad, I. I., Luna, M., Khalil, S. A., Costerton, J. W., Lam, C., & Bodey, G. P. (1994). The relationship between the thrombotic and infectious complications of central venous catheters. *JAMA: Journal of the American Medical Association, 271*, 1014–1016.

Rabe, C., Gramann, T., Sons, X., Berna, M., Gonzalez-Carmona, M. A., Klehr, H. U., et al. (2002). Keeping central venous lines open: A prospective comparison of heparin, vitamin C and sodium chloride sealing solutions in medical patients. *Intensive Care Medicine, 28*, 1172–1176.

Rotter, M., Koller, W., & Wewalka, G. (1980). Povidone-iodine and chlorhexidine gluconate containing detergents for disinfection of hands. *Journal of Hospital Infection, 1*, 149–158.

Ruschman, K. L., & Fulton, J. S. (1993). Effectiveness of disinfectant techniques on intravenous tubing latex injection ports. *Journal of Intravenous Nursing, 16*, 304–308.

Schulmeister, L. (1987). A comparison of skin preparation procedures for accessing implanted ports. *NITA: National Intravenous Therapy Association, 10*, 45–47.

Semba, C. P., Deitcher, S. R., Li, X., Resnansky, L., Tu, T., & McCluskey, E. R. (2002). Treatment of occluded central venous catheters with alteplase: Results in 1,064 patients. *Journal of Vascular Interventional Radiology, 13*, 1199–1205.

Servetar, E. M. (1992). A case of twiddler's syndrome in a pediatric patient. *Journal of Pediatric Oncology Nursing, 9*, 25–28.

Shah, S. S., Smith, M. J., & Zaoutis, T. E. (2005). Device-related infections in children. *Pediatric Clinics of North America, 52*, 1189–1208.

Shivnan, J. C., McGuire, D., Freedman, S., Sharkazy, E., Bosserman, G., Larson, E., et al. (1991). A comparison of transparent adherent and dry sterile gauze dressings for long-term central catheters in patients undergoing bone marrow transplant. *Oncology Nursing Forum, 18*, 1349–1356.

Shulman, R. J., Barrish, J. P., & Hicks, M. J. (1995). Does the use of hydrochloric acid damage silicone rubber central venous catheters? *Journal of Parenteral and Enteral Nutrition, 19*, 407–409.

Sitges-Serra, A., Puig, P., Linares, J., Perez, J. L., Farrero, N., Jaurrieta, E., et al. (1984). Hub colonization as the initial step in an outbreak of catheter-related sepsis due to coagulase negative Staphylococci during parenteral nutrition. *Journal of Parenteral and Enteral Nutrition, 8*, 668–672.

Stephens, L. C., Haire, W. D., & Kotulak, G. D. (1995). Are clinical signs accurate indicators of the cause of central venous catheter occlusion? *Journal of Parenteral and Enteral Nutrition, 19*, 75–79.

Taylor, D., Myers, S. T., Monarch, K., Leon, C., Hall, J., & Sibley, Y. (1996). Use of occlusive dressings on central venous catheter sites in hospitalized children. *Journal of Pediatric Nursing, 11*, 169–174.

Treston-Aurand, J., Olmsted, R. N., Allen-Bridson, K., & Craig, C. P. (1997). Impact of dressing materials on central venous catheter infection rates. *Journal of Intravenous Nursing, 20*, 201–206.

Werlin, S. L., Lausten, T., Jessen, S., Toy, L., Norton, A., Dallman, L., et al. (1995). Treatment of central venous catheter occlusions with ethanol and hydrochloric acid. *Journal of Parenteral and Enteral Nutrition, 19*, 416–418.

Whigham, C. J., Lindsey, J. I., Goodman, C. J., & Fisher, R. G. (2002). Venous port salvage utilizing low dose tPA. *Cardiovascular and Interventional Radiology, 25*, 513–516.

Wiener, E. S., McGuire, P., Stolar, C. J., Rich, R. H., Albo, V. C., Ablin, A. R., et al. (1992). The CCSG prospective study of venous access devices: An analysis of insertions and causes for removal. *Journal of Pediatric Surgery, 27*, 155–163.

Wilmore, D. W., & Dudrick, S. J. (1968). Growth and development of an infant receiving all nutrients exclusively by vein. *JAMA: Journal of the American Medical Association, 203*, 860–864.

Zinner, S. H., Denny-Brown, B. C., Braun, P., Burke, J. P., Toala, P., & Kass, E. H. (1969). Risk of infection with intravenous indwelling catheters: Effects of application of antibiotic ointment. *Journal of Infectious Diseases, 120*, 616–619.

Care of Children with Acute Pain: Operative, Procedural, and Traumatic

By Wendy Lord Mackey and Renee C.B. Manworren

■ Pain in Children: An Overview

Definition of Pain

The International Association for the Study of Pain Subcommittee on Taxonomy (1979) defines pain as "an unpleasant sensory and emotional experience associated with actual or potential tissue damage, or described in terms of such damage." According to McCaffery (1979), pain defies definition. However, she does offer a more liberal and operational definition by stating pain is "whatever the experiencing person says it is, existing whenever he says it does" (p. 11). Children are not small adults and may not demonstrate or even verbalize pain in the way adults do. This makes the job of assessing and controlling children's pain difficult.

Many factors may determine how a child responds to pain; these are developmental age, cognitive and developmental level, procedure or condition causing pain, coping style, advance preparation for the procedure or condition, gender, culture, temperament, past experiences with pain, expectations of pain, pain tolerance, parental response to pain, and type of pain (acute or chronic) (Burroughs, Maxey, Crawley, & Levy, 2002; Buskila et al., 2003; Cheng, Foster, & Hester, 2003; Finley

& Schechter, 2003; Kankkunen, Pietila, & Vehvilainen-Julkunen, 2004; Lea, 2005; McGrath & Hillier, 2003; Miaskowski, 1999, 2003; Neul et al., 2003; Rocha, Prkachin, Beaumont, Hardy, & Zumbo, 2003; Schechter, Berde, & Yaster, 2003; Unruh & Campbell, 1999; von Baeyer, Marche, Rocha, & Salmon, 2004). The experience of pain can be enhanced by fear, anxiety, depression, and many other factors. Therefore, it is imperative for the clinician to take into account what the procedure, treatment, or actual pain means to each child individually.

Pathophysiology of Pain

Pain is the result of stimulation of nociceptors from tissue damage. Nociceptors (or pain sensors) are free nerve endings located throughout the body in the skin, muscle, blood vessels, and organs. The transmission of the impulses occurs via two different types of afferent fibers, thereby creating two types of pain sensations. These fibers ascend to the dorsal horn of the spinal cord and are called A delta fibers and C fibers (Pasero, Paice, & McCaffery, 1999). A delta fibers are myelinated, thereby transmitting pain impulses very rapidly, resulting in sharp, localized sensations. The fibers are responsible for the withdrawal response from painful stimuli. C fibers are unmyelinated, smaller fibers. These fibers conduct impulses more slowly and are responsible for dull, diffuse, burning, aching pain. The afferent fibers transmit the nociceptive signals to the dorsal horn of the spinal cord. Cell bodies and dendrites from within the dorsal horn relay sensory messages to higher neuro centers, including the thalamus, cerebral cortex, limbic system, hypothalamus, areas of the frontal lobe, and cingulate gyrus (Fitzgerald & Howard, 2003). These higher centers warn the individual to recognize the pain experience and initiate an autonomic response, identify the location and quality of the pain experience, and initiate the emotional and behavioral responses to pain (Pasero, Paice, et al., 1999). The psychobiological aspect is an integral part of the pathophysiology of pain, with the affective and cognitive mechanisms of the experience often as important as the actual tissue damage.

■ Assessing Children's Acute Pain

Pain assessment requires obtaining a pain history, identifying potential sources of pain, assessing the patient's comfort and function with valid and reliable tools, evaluating pain relief interventions, and frequently reassessing the patient for pain. A pain history is an interview between a health care provider, the child, and the family to learn about the child's current and previous pain experiences. Ideally, the interview takes place before surgery or before an anticipated painful procedure. The interview provides an ideal opportunity to give the child and the family information regarding pain assessment and management strategies, as well as the general pain management plan. This is the time to answer any questions and correct misconceptions that the child and family may have about procedural or postoperative pain.

The initial pain assessment gathers information regarding the nature of the child's pain; the intensity, duration, quality, or description of the pain; and what alleviates or aggravates the pain (JCAHO, 2000). Assessment data is used to develop an individualized pain treatment plan. Continued reassessment is imperative to evaluate the efficacy of the pain management plan. Remind the child and family at regular intervals to report pain when it occurs so that the treatment plan may be further modified to provide optimal pain relief.

Cognitive development influences children's ability to report pain. Crying is widely accepted as a method of communicating pain. Cry patterns, facial expressions, and body movements are behavioral indicators of infant pain and, therefore, their pain language. Infants are behaviorally disorganized when agitated and distressed.

Cognitive development provides toddlers with greater communication skills and language to alert others to their pain. Toddlers may use unique words to denote pain, such as owie, boo-boo, and ache. Use terms specific to their language of pain when assessing toddlers. Children older than three years have the ability to distinguish and communicate pain intensity through the use of developmentally appropriate pain assessment tools (DiMaggio, 2002; Zempsky & Schechter, 2003). Reliable and valid pain assessment tools provide a method to standardize children's language of pain.

Adolescents have the ability to use abstract concepts and therefore easily quantify and qualify their pain experiences. However, some adolescents may have difficulty expressing their true feelings regarding pain and are developmentally egocentric in their thinking, and these developmental characteristics may hinder pain management. The adolescent may think that the clinician is aware of his or her pain and therefore may fail to report pain to the nurse. Consequently, it is equally important to assess for nonverbal indications of pain even when pain is denied.

The hierarchy of basic pain assessment techniques guides nurses in determining the presence and the intensity of children's pain (Manworren, Paulos, & Pop, 2004; Pasero, 2002). Self-report, presence of pathology or a condition associated with pain, behavior, proxy ratings, and, finally, physiological indicators of pain are ranked in descending order according to their importance and reliability for assessing pain. Factors that influence the pain experience, such as fear, must also be considered.

Self-Report

Self-report requires the child in pain to describe and score the intensity of pain experiences. Ask the child when the pain started, where it hurts, how much pain is being experienced, what does the pain feel like, a description of the quality (e.g., sharp, cramping, burning) of the pain, what relieves the pain, and what makes the pain worse. Self-report provides the most accurate estimate of an individual patient's pain location and severity.

By 2 years of age, most children can indicate the location of pain, although the description may be nonspecific because of vocabulary limitations. Ask patients to point to where it hurts with one finger to clarify the location of the pain. Children may have more than one site of pain, or the pain may radiate to other areas of the body, so question "do you hurt anywhere else?"

Children as young as 3 years of age are able to indicate the intensity of pain when provided with an appropriate tool (DiMaggio, 2002; Zempsky & Schechter, 2003). These tools allow children to discriminate the intensity of pain on a continuum from no pain to the most pain one could possibly experience. Self-report pain intensity rating tools are valid, reliable, easy to use, and therefore practical for clinical care. Pain intensity scales provide a standardized method of communicating pain intensity with the practitioner recognizing that children's pain ratings are personal and unique. The ratings are valid and meaningful when compared with the same child's pain rating at different times and occasions.

Pathology

The focus of this chapter on pain has been limited to the pain of surgery, procedures, and trauma. By definition, if a child has surgery, an invasive procedure, or trauma that causes or has the potential to cause tissue damage, the child experiences pain. Health care providers are obligated to assess, treat, and reassess this pain. In addition to, or in the absence of, self-report of pain, the nurse's pain assessment should consider whether the patient is experiencing a painful condition. Therefore, the nurse should be highly suspicious that postsurgical patients, patients having procedures that are painful, and children who are recovering from trauma are experiencing pain based on the pathology of the conditions.

Behavior

Children who are unable to provide a self-report of pain are also those patients who experience the greatest burden of pain. Preverbal, developmentally nonverbal, and unconscious or sedated children are more likely to experience pain from surgery, critical care procedures, and routine health maintenance requirements, such as physical therapy, immunizations, and blood tests, than healthy children.

Behaviors that are commonly used to identify presence of pain are facial expressions, vocalization, and posture/movement (Beacham, 2004; Gaffney, McGrath, & Dick, 2003; Johnston, Stevens, Boyer, & Porter, 2003). The inaccuracy and difficulty with behavioral observations are that they are not specific to pain; children may elicit similar behaviors for many other reasons. For example, a child who is crying may be in pain, may need to be changed, may be hungry, or may want to be held.

Objective pain scales rely on patients' behavioral and physiologic responses to alert clinicians to the potential for pain. Although observational pain assessment tools have been validated in some of these at-risk populations, the tools are not appropriate for all preverbal and nonverbal children or for all potential sources of pain. Behavioral and physiologic indicators of pain, including those quantified in observational pain scales, provide only an estimate of children's pain intensity. The gold standard for pain assessment, self-report, is just not possible with these high-risk patients. Objective pain assessment methods are indicated and appropriate only in the absence of self-report, for children who are unable to communicate or are preverbal, unconscious, or developmentally delayed.

Physiologic Changes

Pain can affect various physiologic indices, such as respiratory rate, heart rate, blood pressure, perspiration, and certain biological and hormonal measures. Once again, not one of these direct measures of the body's function is a specific indicator of pain. Using these responses as pain indicators is based on the principle that the perception of pain initiates a stress response. Furthermore, physiologic changes do not lend dependable and accurate information about the presence, intensity, or duration of pain, and there may be many reasons for variations in any of these parameters. A person experiencing acute pain may be tachycardic, tachypneic, and hypertensive, yet the absence of these physiologic changes cannot be interpreted as a lack of pain sensation. The body is often very quick to adapt to these physiologic changes and to establish a new equilibrium.

■ Pharmacologic Management of Pain

Pharmacologic interventions are the primary method of relieving and managing children's pain. The following is a summary of nonopioid analgesics, opioid analgesics, and coanalgesics, such as local anesthetics and sedatives.

Nonopioid Analgesia

This group of drugs includes acetaminophen, salicylates, and the nonsteroidal anti-inflammatory drugs (NSAIDs). All of these agents are thought to relieve pain by inhibiting prostaglandin synthesis. This phenomenon takes place in the central nervous system by acetaminophen and in the peripheral nervous system by NSAIDs (American Pain Society, 2003; Hutchison, 2004; Maunuksela & Olkkola, 2003). These drugs are the first-line analgesics for mild-to-moderate pain. The NSAIDS also provide an opioid-sparing effect when used in combination with opioids. Thus, NSAIDs limit the dose-related side effects and the risk of adverse opioid effects, like sedation and respiratory depression. Nonopioid analgesics all have an analgesic ceiling; that is, increasing the dose above the recommended therapeutic dosing range does not increase the analgesic effect.

Although unbridled use of acetaminophen results in liver toxicity, the incidence of side effects is low compared with that of NSAIDs. Side effects of NSAIDs include gastrointestinal irritation and ulceration, renal ischemia, electrolyte imbalances, and increased bleeding or potential for bleeding. Surgical patients must be well hydrated and hemodynamically stable before NSAIDs are introduced into the pain management plan.

Opioid Analgesia

Opioids are the mainstay for the treatment of acute moderate-to-severe pain, including postoperative pain, posttraumatic pain, sickle-cell pain, and cancer pain (American Pain Society, 1999, 2003, 2005). Opioid analgesics act centrally and peripherally as mu agonist opioids (Yaster, Kost-Byerly, & Maxwell, 2003). Opioids are further classified into three derivative classes on the basis of chemical structure: phenanthrenes (morphine, codeine, hydrocodone, oxycodone, and hydromorphone), benzomorphans (methadone), and phenylpiperidines (fentanyl and meperidine). Allergic reactions to opioids are rare, but if a patient exhibits an allergic reaction to one opioid, choose an opioid from another derivative class to limit the patient's risk of a subsequent allergic reaction. Opioid selection depends on the patient's condition, available routes, potential adverse effects, and environmental considerations, including the child's location and the expertise of the clinicians caring for the patient.

Right Route

Opioids are administered via the oral, buccal, sublingual, rectal, transdermal, subcutaneous, intramuscular, intravenous, and intraspinal routes. Dose is route dependent and all routes except oral avoid first-pass metabolism through the liver (Glen & St. Marie, 2002). Thus, in order for the same level of analgesia to be achieved, oral doses must be significantly higher than doses administered by other routes. Epidural and intrathecal administrations bypass systemic circulation, so these doses are significantly smaller than doses given by other routes. The goal is to administer safe and therapeutic doses to maintain a plasma level that is greater than the effective analgesic threshold and is less than the level of sedation and respiratory depression.

Opioids administered by the oral route are less expensive, have a longer duration of analgesia, and provide a more consistent blood level. The oral route is considered the preferred route for analgesic administration (APS, 2003). However, younger children may express difficulty swallowing pills, and the unavailability of palatable elixirs or chewable analgesics may prevent the use of this route for treating pain. Controlled-release oral opioids are not appropriate for the management of acute pain.

Patients that are unable to tolerate oral intake or swallow may benefit from buccal or sublingual administration of opioids. The rectal route is also an option, but drug absorption by this route is variable and unpredictable (DiMaggio, 2002). Most children older than 2 years resist this route of drug administration.

Transdermal administration of opioids is used to treat chronic pain, but this route is not appropriate for acute or procedural pain. Likewise, the subcutaneous route is often used for long-term opioid therapy at home for patients who lack intravenous access. Children recovering from surgery or being treated for the pain of a procedure require a functional intravenous line.

There is absolutely no physiologic reason to administer analgesics by injection (APS, 2003; DiMaggio, 2002). The intramuscular route provides unpredictable and erratic absorption. In addition, pain experienced by this route may dissuade the child from reporting pain. Therefore, it makes no sense whatsoever to treat pain by a painful route.

Intravenous administration of opioids provides prompt relief of severe pain and is the most reliable method of drug delivery (APS, 2003). Intermittent administration of intravenous opioids commonly produces fluctuating plasma drug levels, resulting in cycles of pain, comfort, and sedation. Continuous infusions are a practical and very therapeutic method of intravenous delivery; however, the American Pain Society warns that continuous infusions in opioid-naive individuals may result in an increased incidence of adverse effects without significant improvement in analgesia.

Intraspinal delivery of analgesia has become common practice in pediatric pain management (Desparmet, Hardart, & Yaster, 2003). This method entails delivery of a combination of preservative-free opioid and/or local anesthetic into the epidural or intrathecal space. Therapeutic success is dependent on the dermatomal level achieved and the cerebrospinal fluid concentration of the medications. A detailed discussion of epidural analgesia occurs later in the chapter.

Right Time

For most analgesics to be effective in controlling pain, steady-state blood levels must be maintained through around-the-clock administration. Yet, most analgesics are ordered on a PRN ("as needed") basis. Unfortunately, PRN is often interpreted to mean "as little as possible" as opposed to "as needed" to relieve and prevent pain. Analgesic administration should not be restricted to the child's report of pain or the parent's requests for analgesics; rather, doses should be provided in a timed manner to maintain comfort and prevent recurrent and severe pain (APS, 2003). If a child experiences pain before the next scheduled analgesic doses, the pain management plan must be revised.

Right Dose

Opioids do not have a ceiling effect; instead, analgesia increases with increased dosing, as do the risks of respiratory depression and other side effects. Doses of opioids are based on empiric evidence. Recommended initial pediatric doses are based on patient weight, but the doses must be adjusted for relief of pain and potential adverse events (APS, 2003; Schechter et al., 2003). Further modifications are required for children with disease processes that affect drug metabolism, and initial opioid doses in neonates and infants should be further reduced to 1/4 to 1/2 the recommended initial pediatric dose (APS; Goldman, Frager, & Pomietto, 2003; Launay-Vacher, Karie, Fau, Izzedine, & Deray, 2005; Schechter et al.; Stevens, 1999; Tobias, 2003; Yaster, Kost-Byerly, et al., 2003). Therefore, opioids must be titrated to provide optimal analgesic effect, yet minimize side effects. The use of patient-controlled analgesia (PCA), in which the child controls the amount and the timing of the drug administration, is based on this principal. A detailed discussion of PCA is presented later in the chapter.

Side Effects of Opioids

Opioid side effects are nausea/vomiting, pruritus, urinary retention, decreased gastrointestinal motility, including constipation or ileus, sedation, and respiratory depression (Ersek, Cherrier, Overman, & Irving, 2004; Plaisance & Ellis, 2002; Rothley & Therrien, 2002; Wheeler, Oderda, Ashburn, & Lipman, 2002; Yaster, Kost-Byerly, et al., 2003; Yaster, Tobin, & Kost-Byerly, 2003; Young-McCaughan & Miaskowski, 2001a & b). These side effects can often add to the patient's discomfort. Careful monitoring of the patient and anticipation of these effects avoid untoward complications. The side effects are primarily dose related and can be easily controlled with dose adjustments and various clinical antidotes.

Tolerance, dependence, and addiction are all phenomena associated with the use of opioids. Clearly defining these terms makes them easier to apply in clinical practice and to appreciate their true impact on patient care. According to the American Pain Society (1999), the following are recognized definitions:

Tolerance is a state of adaptation in which exposure to a drug induces changes that result in a diminution of one or more of the drug's effects over time.

Physical dependence is a state of adaptation that is manifested by a drug class-specific withdrawal syndrome that can be produced by abrupt cessation, rapid dose reduction, decreasing blood level of the drug, and/or administration of an antagonist.

Addiction is a primary, chronic, neurobiologic disease, with genetic, psychosocial, and environmental factors influencing its development and manifestations. It is characterized by behaviors that include one or more of the following: impaired control over drug use, compulsive use, continued use despite harm, and craving.

Coanalgesics

Local Anesthetics

Local anesthetics block the neural impulses along both central and peripheral nerve pathways (Glen & St. Marie, 2002; Yaster, Tobin, et al., 2003). To anesthetize an area, the anesthetic must be deposited directly into the area in which an effect is desired. In essence, the nerves bathe in the local solution and become "numb." Local anesthetics are extremely effective in obliterating pain sensation with minimal physiologic effect. They are primarily used to treat pain as part of a regional anesthetic technique, including topical application, local infiltration, peripheral nerve blocks, intravenous regional anesthesia (Bier blocks), and epidural or spinal anesthesia (APS, 2003, 2005; Pasero, 2003, 2004; Yaster, Tobin, et al.).

Injection and local infiltration of anesthetics are very uncomfortable for most people. Buffering the local anesthetic decreases the acidity of the solution and may decrease the burning sensation commonly described with its infiltration (Yaster, Tobin, et al., 2003). Buffering is simply performed by mixing one part (1 mL) bicarbonate with nine parts (9 mL) lidocaine. To decrease the discomfort from the needlestick, consider a topical anesthetic and use a small-gauge needle (30 gauge) when injecting the local anesthetic. Wound infiltration with local anesthetic before surgical wound closure effectively decreases postoperative pain and the amount of postoperative analgesics required to relieve pain. This technique should be considered for patients undergoing outpatient surgical procedures, such as hernia repairs. Epinephrine, a vasoconstrictor, is often added to local anesthetics. This agent decreases the vascular absorption of the local anesthetic, thereby increasing the duration of sensory block by almost 50% and decreasing peak plasma levels by 33% (Yaster, Tobin, et al.). Epinephrine is less effective when added to the other more lipophilic agents, like bupivacaine and ropivacaine. Solutions containing epinephrine should *never* be used in areas supplied by end arterials, such as the digits or the penis. Erroneous use of epinephrine may cause necrosis or ischemia to the injected area.

The most significant concern with the use of local anesthetics is the risk of toxicity. Local anesthetics can impact the function of any excitable membrane including the heart, brain, and the neuromuscular junction, when toxic levels are reached systemically (Yaster, Tobin, et al., 2003). Although routine clinical use of these agents at dosages below 0.4mg/kg prevents toxic systemic and tissue concentrations, the accidental intravascular or excessive extravascular administration can have catastrophic consequences on the cardiovascular and central nervous systems. Mild signs of central nervous system toxicity include tinnitus, light headedness, visual and auditory disturbances, restlessness, and muscular twitching. These symptoms may go undetected in infants and preverbal children and may not be spontaneously reported by other children. Severe side effects, such as seizures, arrhythmias, coma, cardiovascular collapse, and respiratory arrest, result as plasma levels rise. Fortunately, toxic reactions have rarely been reported in children.

Corticosteroids

Corticosteroids (most commonly prednisone and dexamethasone) do not have analgesic properties and are therefore considered coanalgesics. Corticosteroids are used to reduce swelling and thus the associated pain of rheumatologic disorders, nerve pressure pain, and pain from bone metastases and brain tumors (APS, 2005; Collins & Weisman, 2003). To reduce or relieve pain, corticosteroids must be used in combination with analgesics.

Anticonvulsants and Antidepressants

Acute, traumatic, and surgical pain are treated with conventional analgesics, like acetaminophen, NSAIDs, opioids, and anesthetics. Anticonvulsants and antidepressants, selective serotonin reuptake inhibitors, serotonin and norepinephrine reuptake inhibitors, and tricyclics have been successfully used to reduce chronic and neuropathic pain, which is beyond the scope of this chapter.

Sedatives

Anxiety and fear may exacerbate pain. Therefore, sedatives may be necessary to achieve optimal pain management. However, sedatives do not relieve pain, so they should be used in conjunction with analgesics, not in place of opioids when analgesia is needed. The goal of pain management is to relieve pain, not to render the child too sleepy to complain or resist.

Antiemetics and Antihistamines

Often used to treat postoperative and opioid-related nausea, vomiting, and pruritus, these medications may potentiate the sedative effects of opioids. However, they do not potentiate the analgesia. Carefully monitor sedation, respiration, and pain when patients are receiving opioids and these adjuvants.

■ Patient-Controlled Analgesia

Definition

Patient-controlled analgesia, or PCA, allows the patient to control analgesic administration. Because the only valid indicator of pain is the patient's subjective report, PCA provides a logical alternative to nurse-administered analgesics by eliminating the "middle man" (APS, 2003). PCA permits the patient to act on a pain experience and initiate analgesic treatment immediately upon sensation of pain.

The basic PCA system includes a programmable pump, a drug reservoir, and a handheld activation button. The patient is instructed to depress the button at the onset of pain to optimize pain relief. PCA delivers prescribed doses of medication intravenously or epidurally in response to the activation of the patient-controlled button. Each pump can be programmed with a lockout interval, a preset inactivation time interval, maximum dose per hour(s), and a dose limit. The pump is programmed as prescribed to prevent the administration of additional patient-activated doses until the patient can evaluate analgesic effectiveness, thus allowing for analgesic titration while preventing overdoses due to repetitive activation of the patient control device.

Delivery Methods

Most PCA devices have three ways to deliver analgesics: continuous infusion, interval dosing, or continuous basal infusion with interval dosing. The goal of the continuous infusion method is to maintain constant therapeutic analgesic levels. Interval dosing allows for small, prescribed amounts of analgesics to be given at frequent intervals. Requiring the patient to activate dosing limits the risks of sedation. The overall purpose of this method of pain control is to allow the patient a sense of control over his or her pain and to provide a more effective dosing method and pain control. Continuous basal infusion with intermittent dosing includes both of the aforementioned functions. The continuous basal infusion helps maintain a constant baseline level of comfort. When the patient feels pain or is preparing for a painful event (e.g., ambulation, dressing change), the basal infusion can be supplemented with periodic, patient-controlled, additional doses of analgesia. This method may be more effective in providing more consistent analgesic levels during sleep, but it may also increase the incidence of opioid-related side effects.

Patient Selection

PCA is only effective if used with the right patients. Researchers have explored the use of PCA with children as young as 3 years of age, but others question whether children this young are cognitively capable of appropriately using this technology (Berde & Solodiuk, 2003; Lehr & BeVier, 2003; Monitto et al., 2000). Rather than a strict age limit for PCA use, determine a patient's appropriateness for PCA using criteria that reflect the cognitive skills necessary to effectively activate this technology. The child should be able to physically activate the device and should be able to quantify pain in order to begin treatment in a timely manner and not allow pain to get out of control. He/she must be able to understand the relationship between pushing the button and medication delivery and be able to report unsatisfactory pain relief or adverse side effects. The patient should also understand the safety mechanism of the machine. Lastly, the child should be unable to tolerate oral medication, the preferred route for acute pain control because of the longer duration of pain relief with oral analgesics. To assess for appropriate and effective PCA use, the following questions should be asked: does the child push the button repeatedly to get one dose? Does the child reach the hourly lockout or consistently require several doses every hour to achieve pain relief? How hard is the child working to maintain or achieve comfort? Is the child able to rest and sleep? Does the child's self-report of pain, functional assessment, and PCA use indicate that pain is well controlled? This additional pain assessment data helps determine whether the child understands the machine and whether this technology is appropriately relieving the child's pain.

When a PCA pump is in a patient's room, anyone in the room can activate the PCA—even the little brother who is unable to understand that pushing the button administers an analgesic or the potential dangers of random or persistent PCA use. If someone other than the patient activates the PCA, this overrides the inherent safety of the device. An oversedated patient cannot self-administer PCA doses, but a well-meaning parent or visitor might. Thus, parent- or proxy-controlled analgesia remains an area of great controversy. The JCAHO (2004) recommends that family and visitors be taught to facilitate the patient's PCA use but not to push the button. Institutional guidelines for parent- or proxy-controlled analgesia must clearly delineate responsibilities and monitoring requirements (Lehr & BeVier, 2003).

■ Epidural Analgesia

Definition

Pain-relieving drugs, including opioids and local anesthetics, may be infused into the epidural, caudal, and intrathecal (spinal) spaces. The drugs are administered via a small-gauge flexible catheter for intermittent and/or continuous infusions, or via a small needle for a single-bolus administration. Epidural analgesia is the most commonly used regional technique for children's intra- and postoperative pain management after urologic, orthopedic, and general surgical procedures below the nipples (T-4 dermatomal level) (Desparmet et al., 2003).

Catheter Placement

Unlike adults, infants and children are usually sedated or anesthetized for epidural catheter placement (Desparmet et al., 2003). The ideal position for placement involves placing the patient in a lateral decubitus or sitting position with shoulders and hips squared, and hips and head flexed. In order to maintain an adequate airway in young infants, the position is modified by securing the chin upward, away from the chest. This position allows for the vertebral bodies to be well aligned and maximally separated. Catheter placement is confirmed by use of the loss-of-resistance technique, aspirating to assure lack of blood or CSF, test dosing with an epinephrine containing solution, and/or fluoroscopic confirmation. The desired location of the catheter tip is most frequently at the level of the surgical site or the dermatome level of the source of pain. Epidural catheters are covered with a sterile transparent occlusive dressing at the exit site. The site should remain visible through the dressing. The catheter is often taped up the patient's back to the shoulder or upper chest area for easy access and to avoid pressure areas at the hub site.

Contraindications to epidural catheter placement include: acquired or congenital bleeding disorders (risk of epidural hemorrhage), inability to place the catheter, infection at the catheter site, and hemodynamic instability (Desparmet et al., 2003). Postdural puncture headache, neurologic sequelae (caudal equina syndrome), pain at the catheter site and backache are potential complications of epidural catheter placement.

Anatomy and Physiology

All drugs administered into the epidural space must be preservative free because preservatives may cause neurotoxicity and severe spinal cord injury (Pasero, Portenoy, et al., 1999). Medications are administered into the epidural space as bolus doses (multiple or single shot), continuous infusions and by patient-controlled epidural analgesia (PCEA). Continuous infusions are the most popular delivery method. Also, local anesthetics, administered as a single shot caudal injection, are often performed prior to surgical incision and can provide prolonged postoperative analgesia for outpatient procedures.

Local anesthetics administered in the epidural space cut off pain signals in the dorsal root ganglion. The higher the concentration of local anesthetic administered, the greater the sensory block and potential for motor block. Careful attention must be given to assure that the overall dose of the local anesthetic administered is less than 0.4mg/kg/hr. The analgesic effects of local anesthetics and opioids are synergistic when administered epidurally and offer a higher therapeutic ratio when administered together versus independently.

Opioids administered into the epidural space, slowly diffuse into the cerebrospinal fluid, bind to the opioid receptors in the dorsal horn, thereby blocking substance P and transmission of the pain impulse (APS, 2003; Glen & St. Marie, 2002). Epidural opioid analgesic choice depends on the patient's age and history, the procedure, the location of the catheter tip, the dermatomal level or levels of the pain, and the preference of the physician and institution (Desparmet et al., 2003). Opioids that are more hydrophilic, such as morphine and hydromorphone, have an increased affinity to water and therefore a greater rostral spread (Pasero, Portenoy, et al., 1999). Rostral spread refers to the cephalic migration of a drug. The use of hydrophilic agents, such as morphine, are useful when the catheter tip lies well below the surgical site, or when the pain or surgical site involves many dermatomal levels. Thus, the risk of respiratory depression is greater when hydrophilic opioids are used, as opposed to lipophilic opioids. Lipophilic agents, such as fentanyl, are indicated when the catheter tip is at the dermatomal level of the pain and when patients are at high risk for respiratory depression.

Epidural analgesia provides profound pain relief, yet requires only a fraction of the opioid doses required with systemic administration. This decreases the incidence of opioid-related side effects. However, nurses must still monitor patients for unrelieved pain, epidural complications, level of consciousness, and other adverse effects. Although physiologic monitors can alert nurses to respiratory events, frequent, skilled, patient observations and assessments by nurses familiar and competent in the care of children receiving epidural analgesia are required (Berde & Solodiuk, 2003). Table 5-1 provides a summary of side effects of epidural analgesia with nursing considerations.

■ Biobehavioral Methods of Managing Acute Pain in Children

Biobehavioral or nonpharmacologic methods of pain control are an integral part of the care of children experiencing pain. Children require and desire coping mechanisms to guide them away from a frightening, unfamiliar, or painful situation. When used in conjunction with anesthetics and analgesics, these methods can reduce the distress of painful experiences. Biobehavioral techniques should be used with pharmacologic interventions, not instead of anesthetics and analgesics (APS, 2005). This section touches on a variety of behavioral methods, all of which contribute to the goal of comforting children.

Parental Presence

Separation from parents can be very stressful for the hospitalized patient and can contribute to the distress of pain (Broome & Huth, 2003; Finley & Schechter, 2003). Most hospitals have adopted very liberal policies concerning parental presence, including 24-hour rooming-in capabilities, and parental presence for procedures, anesthesia induction, and in the postanesthesia care unit (American Association of Critical Care Nurses, 2004; American Academy of Pediatrics & American Pain Society, 2001; American Heart Association, 2000; Emergency Nurses Association, 2001). The parents should be empowered to comfort and coach the child in coping strategies during such times (Broome , Rehwaldt, & Fogg, 1998; Kleiber & McCarthy, 1999; Melnyk, Small, & Carno, 2004).

Preparation

Control and predictability are vitally important to a child. The very nature of the hospital is one of little control. The child is submerged in an environment with different people, smells, noises, sounds, and activity. Creating an institutional philosophy incorporating the concepts and interventions identified in Table 5-2 help comfort the child and family and offer more predictability (Schechter, Blankson, Pachter, Sullivan, & Costa, 1997).

Table 5-1	Side Effects of Epidural Analgesia with Nursing Considerations	
Side Effect	**Cause and Effect**	**Care and Nursing Interventions**
Respiratory depression	• Too much opioid or local anesthetic (wrong dose, wrong concentration, or pump malfunction). • Accumulation of the opioid over a period of time. • Rostral spread of the opioid. Misplacement of the catheter in the intrathecal space or vasculature. • Concurrent administration of other opioids systemically. • There are two key times when the patient is at the greatest risk for this complication. The first is within the first hour of the injection or infusion caused by systemic absorption of the opioid. The second is 6 to 12 hours after initiation of the infusion secondary to cerebral migration of the drug.	• Hourly assessment of the patient's respiratory rate, rhythm, depth, and level of consciousness are indicated for the first 24 hrs. • Apnea monitors are the standard of care, especially in the younger age groups and high-risk patients. • Verify the drugs and doses and the infusion pump to identify any potential problems or issues. • If respiratory depression or distress occurs, it is essential to support respiration, notify the physician, and consider administering and titrating naloxone. • Ensure pain control. Management of the child's pain may continue with an epidural infusion once the respiratory crisis is resolved and the appropriate changes are made in the child's infusion or pump. • If respiratory depression is the result of a misplaced catheter, catheter removal by anesthesia is indicated.
Urinary retention	• May be caused by both local and opioid analgesia. • Patient may not feel the urge to void with bladder distention because of the sensory or motor block produced by the local anesthetic. • Opioids increase smooth muscle tone in the bladder and ureters and increase sphincter tone, causing bladder spasm, urgency, and difficult urination.	• Monitor the patient's intake and output. • Careful abdominal examinations assessing for bladder distention. • Urinary catheterization is indicated when the patient is unable to void.
Sensory and motor deficits	• Changes in sensation to the lower extremities, including motor weakness, motor blocks, tingling and numbness, may occur as a result of the effects of the local anesthetic.	• Safety is of vital importance to ensure that a child does not fall because of the alteration in sensation. • Careful explanations are essential to help children cope with this side effect and to help them understand that they will regain full feeling and movement of their extremities. • Concentration of the local anesthetic may be decreased or eliminated from the infusion to reverse this side effect.
Infection	Fortunately very rare.	• Meticulous aseptic technique is required during epidural placement and all subsequent care. • Nursing assessment should include a careful evaluation for infection (fever, drainage, redness, or tenderness at the exit site, nuchal rigidity) on a routine basis.

(continues)

Table 5-1 *(continued)*

Side Effect	Cause and Effect	Care and Nursing Interventions
		• The dressing should be occlusive but clear, allowing for frequent observation of the catheter exit site. • The frequency of dressing changes and tubing changes is controversial and depends on the institution's policy. However, all soiled or disrupted dressings should be changed. • When infection is suspected, the epidural catheter is pulled with the patient under anesthesia and is cultured. Antibiotics are prescribed as needed.
Spinal headache	• The result of dural penetration or leak. Cerebrospinal fluid leaks from the intrathecal space into the dura. • Symptoms include extreme headache, photophobia, tinnitus, diplopia, and increased discomfort in an upright position.	• Bedrest, hydration, and analgesia. • In some patients, an autologous blood patch is applied. Blood is injected through the catheter to seal the dural puncture and prevent further cerebrospinal fluid leak.
Pruritus and nausea or vomiting	• The opioid triggers a histamine release that causes the itchiness. • May be experienced anywhere on the body, most prevalently on the forehead and nasal region in children. • Stimulation of chemoreceptor trigger zone can result in nausea/vomiting.	• Often remedied by the administration of antipruritics or antiemetics. • Sometimes the infusion drugs or rate is changed to alleviate the problem. Continuous low-dose infusions of naloxone or intermittent doses of agonist/antagonists, like nalbuphine, may relieve opioid-related side effects of epidural opioid infusions.

Preparation enables a child to become acquainted with a situation or procedure before the event. Fear of the unknown is a very anxiety-provoking experience for a child. Any individual under stress has increased difficulty processing and coping with new experiences. Allowing children to visualize the environment or play with some of the equipment that will be used before the actual procedure increases their ability to cope (LaMontagne, Hepworth, Cohen, & Salisbury, 2003). Preparation also provides the child and family with time to develop and practice a coping plan in advance of the procedure (Gorski, Slifer, Kelly-Suttka, & Lowery, 2004).

Distraction Methods

Distraction methods are reality based, cognitive-behavioral techniques whereby the child focuses attention on an external object, separate from the pain, in order to maximize coping (APS, 1999; Piira, Hayes, & Goodenough, 2002; Hamrin, 2002). This method can implement one or a number of senses including visual, auditory, tactile, and taste, and may be used with any age group. Other techniques, such as breathing and relaxation, are often used in conjunction with distraction. Table 5-3 offers a variety of distraction tools with the corresponding age group for which they are most useful. The more unique and captivating the tool, the more distracting and effective the technique will be (Carlson, Broome, & Vessey, 2000; Hoffman, 2004; Piira et al.).

Breathing/Blowing Techniques

Controlled breathing and blowing techniques are powerful distraction tools with the added benefit of slowing down respirations and promoting relaxation. Implementation of this technique avoids the first response most children have to pain: breath holding. Deep breathing essentially consists of taking a long, deep breath in through the nose and then slowly blowing out through the mouth. Fantasy elements can be added to assist the child, such as blowing out pretend candles or the light of a flashlight, blowing up a pretend balloon, perhaps to help them float

Table 5-2	Increasing Control and Predictability in the Hospital Setting

Comfort Items: Allowing the child to have comfort items such as favorite toys or security items, pictures of family, friends or pets, musical tapes or videos; all may help make the environment more familiar and personal and less threatening. Allowing children to wear their own clothes and have their own bed linens may also help.

Comfort Measures: This includes providing a comfortable environment for the child. Ensuring the appropriate lighting, room temperature, and noise control. Making provisions for being held or rocked. Positioning is a very important aspect of comfort measures. A new theory is emerging called "positioning for comfort." This involves using various patient positions during procedures that promote the comfort of the child.

The Treatment Room: The treatment room is a place where any invasive procedure should take place. It provides the child with a sense of predictability. The child learns that when he or she enters that room, a procedure will take place. However, when the child leaves the room, he or she should feel safe again. The child's bed, on the other hand, should remain a safe place. Routine, noninvasive examinations, assessments, and vital sign checks will occur there, but nothing invasive or painful. Some children voice a preference to have certain things done in their bed, and these requests for the most part should be honored. For example, one child may prefer to have their central line dressing change performed in bed versus in the treatment room. The following passage basically sums it all up.

"There is a room where you have your IV done, the treatment room. Having your own room with friends, it's the thing in the hospital that's like your own home. It's a place for you to lie and stay and sleep. It can be nice and comfy. If you have an IV there, or even a finger stick, it doesn't feel like you're even at home! Only getting your IV out in your room is really okay." (Alex, age 7; personal interview).

Ensuring compliance with this concept and philosophy is very important. Although it does take a little more time to move the child from his or her room into the treatment room, in the end, it will benefit the child and health care team.

The Playroom: The playroom should be a child's safe haven. In our institution, the playroom belongs to the children. It is filled with fun things. Absolutely no procedures or examinations occur in the playroom. If it is necessary for a child to be examined or have vital signs while he or she is in the playroom, the child should leave and return once the intervention is completed. The only medical thing that occurs in the playroom is medical play and preparation. It is not uncommon to see children in the playroom giving a needle or intravenous to their doll, or playing with casting material or bandages.

away from the pain. Suggestive language such as, "blow away the owie," may also enhance the effectiveness of the technique. This technique can be used successfully even in the toddler years with the assistance of bubbles or other blow toys and activities. Creativity is the key.

Initially, most children do better if their coach breathes with them and encourages them. This offers a two-fold advantage to the coach (often the parent), whose tension and stress are controlled by the effects of the breathing as well as providing them with a tool effective in contributing to the management of the child's stress and pain (McDonnell & Bowden, 1989). When proficient, many children implement this technique independently. Breathing techniques assist in the management of pain and other discomforts, such as nausea. Using this technique in combination with other biobehavioral strategies such as imagery is encouraged.

Relaxation

Relaxation involves the voluntary relaxation of muscles in the body, thereby decreasing stress and anxiety and increasing coping abilities (Hamrin, 2002; McGrath, Dick, & Unruh, 2003). This technique strives to clear the mind and body of all internal and external influences. Numerous methods to induce relaxation include successive tension-relaxation methods, yoga-style breathing with suggestions for calmness, and guided release of tension from head to toe.

Guided Imagery

Imagery is a cognitive-behavioral technique that requires the child to create an image of something that is not actually present while in a relaxed state (Gerik, 2005). It draws on the child's active imagination, allowing the coach to guide the child through the painful, often frightening event, which leaves the child with feelings of security, control, and success (Huth, Broome, & Good, 2004). The child's attention is refocused away from the problem toward a new image. The image can be one that the child creates, an actual event (e.g., a birthday party or a baseball game), or a story portrayed and delivered by the coach. The incorporation of senses including sound, vision, taste, smell, movement, position, and touch brings the image to life. Some children want to

Table 5-3	Developmental Approaches with Distraction Resources					
Distraction Resource	**Newborn**	**Infant**	**Toddler**	**Preschool**	**School Age**	**Adolescent**
Music	X	X	X	X	X	X
Rattle, sound toys		X	X	X		
Bubbles		X	X	X	X	X
Magic wands			X	X	X	X
Videos		X	X	X	X	X
Party blowers			X	X	X	X
Stickers			X	X	X	X
I Spy books				X	X	X
Guided imagery				X	X	X
Travel games				X	X	X
Video games/computer						X
Massage	X	X	X	X	X	X
Magazine/book				X	X	X
Pinwheels			X	X	X	X
Musical/pop-up books			X	X	X	
View master			X	X	X	
Kaleidoscope			X	X		X
Virtual reality systems					X	X
Stress balls						X
Talking	X	X	X	X	X	X
Singing	X	X	X	X	X	X

vocally participate in the imagery, and others prefer to just listen. The child often needs support and coaching at least initially to participate in this method, especially when pain intensity increases. This method may be very effective for children who undergo repeated painful events.

Hypnosis

Hypnosis can be defined as the ability to focus attention and become absorbed in an altered state of consciousness whereby perceptions and sensations can be enhanced, modified, or changed (Butler, Symons, Henderson, Shortliffe, & Spiegel, 2005; Kuttner & Solomon, 2003). Hypnosis is an internal imaginative mind-body process. The goal of hypnosis in pain management is to empower the child to take control of the pain versus yielding to a passive role and state of helplessness. The key is to enable the child to focus attention on the task of undoing the pain, versus focusing on the pain itself. For example, empower the child to untie the pain knot or turn down the sensation of pain (Kuttner, 1997).

■ Sedation

Children may require sedation to help them hold still for a procedure, which may or may not be painful. Some procedures require a combination of analgesic or amnesic effects and sedation. In 1985, the American Academy of Pediatrics (AAP) developed guidelines for the use of depressant pharmacologic agents in children as a result of the increasing use of these agents in nontraditional clinical settings (American Academy of Pediatrics, 1985). The guidelines were revised in 1992, reaffirmed in 1995 and 1998, and had addendums added in 2001, to reflect an increased understanding of monitoring needs for children receiving sedation (American Academy of Pediatrics, 2002).

Definitions

Sedation is a physical state that is on a continuum that ranges from the awakened state to general anesthesia. One must be prepared to deal with situations when a child passes from one stage on the continuum into another. The American Academy of Pediatrics (2002) has defined the various states of sedation as follows. Mild sedation is the equivalent of anxiolysis. The term "conscious sedation" is confusing as originally used in the 1992 statement and has been replaced with the most current terminology of the American Society of Anesthesiologists, "moderate sedation" (American Society of Anesthesiology, 2004). Moderate sedation is a medically controlled, depressed level of consciousness that allows the patient to maintain protective reflexes and independently maintain a patent airway and the ability to respond to verbal or tactile stimuli. Deep sedation and general anesthesia refer to a medically controlled, depressed level of consciousness (or unconsciousness) from which the patient is not easily aroused (or unarousable). The patient may have partial or complete loss of protective reflexes, including airway maintenance, and is unable to respond purposefully to physical stimulation or verbal command. For purposes of monitoring, deep sedation and general anesthesia are virtually inseparable (AAP, 2002)

Equipment, Facilities, and Personnel

The practitioner and facility must be capable of safely treating any of the complications of conscious sedation, including vomiting, seizures, anaphylaxis, and cardiopulmonary arrest (American Academy of Pediatrics, 2001). An unfortunate number of deaths have occurred in the home or practitioner's office during sedation because rescue teams and proper equipment were not available. The AAP does not recommend sedation to be given in locations where the following minimal requirements are not readily available (AAP, 2002).

Minimal requirements include the availability of (1) monitoring equipment (pulse oximetry and blood pressure monitoring); (2) emergency equipment (emergency code cart including age-appropriate drugs and equipment to resuscitate an apneic patient, defibrillator, positive-pressure oxygen delivery system, suction equipment with appropriate catheters, supplies to initiate and maintain vascular access); (3) back-up emergency services with a protocol for implementation and use; and (4) qualified practitioners and personnel who are competent in providing pediatric life support and establishing intravenous access.

Patient Screening

Patients must have a responsible and competent person accompany them home after the procedure. (Often, two people are recommended, especially if one individual must drive or if the child is very young or developmentally delayed.) What is the child's medical condition? The American Society of Anesthesiologists physical status classification system (ASA classification) is used to identify appropriate candidates for sedation. Patients with a classification of I or II are often considered appropriate candidates (American Academy of Pediatrics, 1992). A health history and physical examination must be completed, including documentation of age and weight, allergies, drug use, relevant medical history and family history, review of systems, and vital signs. All pertinent laboratory results must be reviewed. An evaluation of the child's oral intake must be completed. It is also important to consider medications the child may be taking and to identify their potential impact on the procedure or drug interactions.

Perisedation Period

The practitioner(s) responsibilities include (1) the administration of the pharmacologic agents inducing sedation and (2) the treatment and monitoring of the patient undergoing the procedure. The practitioner must have a clear understanding of the pharmacokinetics of the drugs being administered, including onset time, duration, principal effect, side effects and their treatment, routes of administration, and dosing.

The support personnel responsibilities include (1) ongoing monitoring of appropriate physiologic parameters and (2) assisting in any supportive or resuscitative procedures required. The number of support personnel needed to be available depends on the procedure. It is always imperative to have the resources available to deal with an emergency situation. If the child should become deeply sedated, the level of vigilance must be increased to provide one-on-one observation, monitoring, and documentation of the patient's condition. Back-up personnel who are expert in airway management, emergency intubation, and advanced cardiopulmonary resuscitation must be available should complications arise (AAP, 2001). Personnel responsible for monitoring the child should not assist in the procedure (AAP, 2002).

■ The Prescription of Sedation

Whenever sedation is required for patient care, one must consider a number of factors pertaining to the patient and the procedure to choose an appropriate cocktail.

The Procedure

Where is the procedure being performed? What is the procedure being performed? Is it painful or nonpainful? This information is important to determine the need for analgesia. Does the procedure require the child to be motionless? The answer to this question is important in determining the level of sedation required and the appropriate drugs to use. How long will the procedure take? This information is helpful in determining the appropriate pharmacologic agent. If the anticipated procedure time is short, then short-acting agents, such as fentanyl and midazolam, may be used.

The Patient

What are the child's past experiences with sedation, and which agents were used? Data from patient screening (noted previously) should be taken into account, as well as the level of anxiety and agitation. This information helps determine whether an anxiolytic or amnesic agent is needed. One must consider the access routes that a patient has available for use. For example, if a child is NPO, oral administration may not be feasible. If a child has no vascular access, certain drugs are ruled out.

Postprocedure Care

Diligent monitoring of the patient's status after the procedure should continue until the child returns to a preprocedural level of functioning. Discrepancies between pre- and postlevel functioning must be carefully documented and justified at time of discharge. The child needs to be monitored in an environment where the appropriate medical personnel and equipment are readily available. Deep sedation may occur at any time after administration of sedatives in the child (AAP, 2002). Pulse oximetry monitoring until the child is fully awake is a sensitive and practical method of monitoring patients for adverse physiologic effects.

The American Academy of Pediatrics (1992) has outlined recommended discharge criteria, which are as follows: (1) the patient has satisfactory and stable cardiovascular function and airway patency, (2) the patient can be aroused easily and has intact protective reflexes, (3) the patient can talk if developmentally appropriate, (4) the patient can sit up unassisted if developmentally appropriate, (5) a child who is very young or developmentally compromised should return to his or her normal level of responsiveness, and (6) an adequate state of hydration exists.

Once the patient is considered medically safe for discharge, written instructions should be given to the accompanying adult. The instructions should outline information about who and when to call in an emergency, routine follow-up care, and diet. Ideally, two responsible adults should accompany the child on discharge.

■ Conclusion

Trauma, acute postoperative pain, and the pain of medical procedures hurt. Many scientific and technologic advances have significantly improved pain control for children. This chapter has provided an overview of pain assessment, management, and procedural sedation, with a focus on the pediatric surgical patient. Nurses caring for pediatric surgical patients use a variety of pain management strategies and techniques to achieve effective pain control and sedation.

■ Educational Materials

APSNA invites you to download the following diagnosis-related teaching tools (available in English and Spanish), for Chapter 5: Care of Children with Acute Pain: Operative, Procedural, and Traumatic at the APSNA Website (www.apsna.org) and the Jones and Bartlett Web site (www.jbpub.com): 1.) PCA 2.) Epidurals. These teaching materials are available free of charge and APSNA encourages their use for your patients and families.

References

American Academy of Pediatrics, Committee on Drugs. Section on Anesthesiology. (1985). Guidelines for the elective use of conscious sedation, deep sedation and general anesthesia in pediatric patients. *Pediatrics*, 76, 317–321.

American Academy of Pediatrics, Committee on Drugs. (1992). Guidelines for monitoring and management of pediatric patients during and after sedation for diagnostic and therapeutic procedures. *Pediatrics*, 89(6), 1110–1115.

American Academy of Pediatrics & American Pain Society. (2001). The assessment and management of acute pain in infants, children and adolescents. *Pediatrics*, 108(3), 793–797.

American Academy of Pediatrics, Committee on Drugs. (2002). Guidelines for monitoring and management of pediatric patients during and after sedation for diagnostic and therapeutic procedures: Addendum. *Pediatrics*, 110(4), 836–838.

American Association of Critical Care Nurses. (2004). Practice alert: Family presence during CPR and invasive procedures. *AACN News*, 21(11), 4 (www.aacn.org).

The American Heart Association. (2000). Guidelines 2000 for cardiopulmonary resuscitation and emergency care. *Circulation*, 102 (Suppl. 8), 158–165.

American Pain Society. (1999). *Guideline for the management of acute and chronic pain in sickle cell disease.* Glenview, IL: American Pain Society.

American Pain Society. (2003). *Principles of analgesic use in the treatment of acute pain and cancer pain* (5th ed.). Glenview, IL: American Pain Society.

American Pain Society. (2005). *Guideline for the management of cancer pain in adults and children.* Glenview, IL: American Pain Society.

American Society of Anesthesiology. (2004). *Continuum of depth of sedation: Definition of general anesthesia and levels of sedation/analgesia.* Published by ASA.

Beacham, P. S. (2004). Behavioral and physiological indicators of procedural and postoperative pain in high-risk infants. *Journal of Obstetric, Gynecologic, and Neonatal Nursing*, 33(2), 246–255.

Berde, C. B., & Solodiuk, J. (2003). Multidisciplinary programs for management of acute and chronic pain in children. In N. L. Schechter, C. B. Berde, & M. Yaster (Eds.), *Pain in infants, children and adolescents* (2nd ed.). Philadelphia: Lippincott Williams & Wilkins.

Broome, M. E., & Huth, M. M. (2003). Nursing management of the child in pain. In N. L. Schechter, C. B. Berde, & M. Yaster (Eds.), *Pain in infants, children and adolescents* (2nd ed., pp. 417–433). Philadelphia: Lippincott Williams & Wilkins.

Broome, M. E., Rehwaldt, M., & Fogg, L. (1998). Relationships between cognitive behavioral techniques, temperament, observed distress, and pain reports in children and adolescents during lumbar puncture. *Journal of Pediatric Nursing, 13*(1), 48–54.

Burroughs, V. J., Maxey, R. W., Crawley, L. M., & Levy, R. A. (2002). *Cultural and genetic diversity in America: The need for individualized pharmaceutical treatment.* National Pharmaceutical Council and National Medical Association. New York.

Buskila, D., Neumann, L., Zmora, E., Feldman, M., Bolotin, A., & Press, J. (2003). Pain sensitivity in prematurely born adolescents. *Archives of Pediatrics & Adolescent Medicine, 15*(7), 1079–1082.

Butler, L. S., Symons, B. K., Henderson, S. L., Shortliffe, L. D., & Spiegel, D. (2005). Hypnosis reduces distress and duration of an invasive medical procedure for children. *Pediatrics, 115*(1), 77–85.

Carlson, K. L., Broome, M., & Vessey, J. A. (2000). Using distraction to reduce reported pain, fear, and behavioral distress in children and adolescents: A multisite study. *Journal of the Society of Pediatric Nurses, 5*(2), 75–85.

Cheng, S. F., Foster, R. L., & Hester, N. O. (2003). A review of factors predicting children's pain experiences. *Issues in Comprehensive Pediatric Nursing, 26,* 203–216.

Collins, J. J., & Weisman, S. J. (2003). Management of pain in childhood cancer. In N. L. Schechter, C. B. Berde, & M. Yaster (Eds.), *Pain in infants, children and adolescents* (2nd ed., pp. 517–538). Philadelphia: Lippincott Williams & Wilkins.

Desparmet, J. F., Hardart, R. A., & Yaster, M. (2003). Central blocks in children and adolescents. In N. L. Schechter, C. B. Berde, & M. Yaster (Eds.), *Pain in infants, children and adolescents* (2nd ed., pp. 339–362). Philadelphia: Lippincott Williams & Wilkins.

DiMaggio, T. J. (2002). Pediatric pain management. In B. St. Marie (Ed.), *American society of pain management nurses: Core curriculum for pain management nursing* (pp. 367–411). Philadelphia: W.B. Saunders.

Emergency Nurses Association. (2001). *Presenting the option of family presence* (2nd ed., pp. 1–87). Des Plaines, IL: Emergency Nurses Association. (www.ena.org).

Ersek, M., Cherrier, M. M., Overman, S. S., & Irving, G. A. (2004). The cognitive effects of opioids. *Pain Management Nursing, 5*(2), 75–93.

Finley, G. A., & Schechter, N. L. (2003). Sedation. In N. L. Schechter, C. B. Berde, & M. Yaster (Eds.), *Pain in infants, children and adolescents* (2nd ed., pp. 563–577). Philadelphia: Lippincott Williams & Wilkins.

Fitzgerald, M., & Howard, R. F. (2003). The neurobiologic basis of pediatric pain. In N. L. Schechter, C. B. Berde, & M. Yaster (Eds.), *Pain in infants, children and adolescents* (2nd ed., pp. 19–42). Philadelphia: Lippincott Williams & Wilkins.

Gaffney, A., McGrath, P. J., & Dick, B. (2003). Measuring pain in children: Developmental and instrumental issues. In N. L. Schechter, C. B. Berde, & M. Yaster (Eds.), *Pain in infants, children and adolescents* (2nd ed., pp. 241–264). Philadelphia: Lippincott Williams & Wilkins.

Gerik, S. M. (2005). Pain management in children: Developmental considerations and mind-body therapies. *Southern Medical Journal, 98*(3), 295–302.

Glen, V. L., & St. Marie, B. (2002). Overview of pharmacology. In B. St. Marie (Ed.), *American society of pain management nurses: Core curriculum for pain management nursing* (pp.181–239). Philadelphia: W.B. Saunders.

Goldman, A., Frager, G., & Pomietto, M. (2003). Pain and palliative care. In N. L. Schechter, C. B. Berde, & M. Yaster (Eds.), *Pain in infants, children and adolescents* (2nd ed., pp. 539–562). Philadelphia: Lippincott Williams & Wilkins.

Gorski, J. A., Slifer, K. J., Kelly-Suttka, J., & Lowery, K. (2004). Behavioral interventions for pediatric patients' acute pain and anxiety: Improving health regimen compliance and outcomes. *Children's Health Care, 33*(1), 1–20.

Hamrin, V. (2002). Psychiatric assessment and treatment of pediatric pain. *Journal of Child and Adolescent Psychiatric Nursing, 15*(3), 106–117.

Hoffman, H. G. (2004). Virtual-reality therapy: Patients can get relief from pain or overcome their phobias by immersing themselves in computer-generated worlds. *Scientific American, 291*(2), 58–65.

Huth, M. M., Broome, M. E., & Good, M. (2004). Imagery reduces children's post-operative pain. *Pain, 110*(1-2), 430–448.

Hutchison, R. (2004). Cox-2-selective NSAIDs: A review and comparison with nonselective NSAIDs. *American Journal of Nursing, 104*(3), 52–55.

International Association for the Study of Pain, Subcommittee on Taxonomy. (1979). Pain terms: A list with definitions and notes on usage. *Pain, 6,* 249–252.

Johnston, C. C., Stevens, B. J., Boyer, K., & Porter, F. L. (2003). Development of psychologic responses to pain and assessment of pain in infants and toddlers. In N. L. Schechter, C. B. Berde, & M. Yaster (Eds.), *Pain in infants, children and adolescents* (2nd ed., pp. 105–127). Philadelphia: Lippincott Williams & Wilkins.

Joint Commission on Accreditation of Healthcare Organizations (JCAHO). (2000). *Pain assessment and management: An organizational approach.* Oakbrook Terrace, IL: The Commission 2 Volumes.

Joint Commission on Accreditation of Healthcare Organizations. (2004). *Sentinel event alert: Patient controlled analgesia by proxy.* Retrieved June 29, 2005, from http://www.jcaho.org/about+us/news+letters/sentinel+events+alert/sea_33.htm

Kankkunen, P., Pietila, A. M., & Vehvilainen-Julkunen, K. (2004). Families' and children's postoperative pain-literature review. *Journal of Pediatric Nursing, 19*(2), 133–139.

Kleiber, C., & McCarthy, A. M. (1999). Parent behavior and child distress during urethral catheterization. *Journal of the Society of Pediatric Nurses, 4*(3), 95–104.

Kuttner, L. (1997). Mind-body methods of pain management. *Child and Adolescent Psychiatric Clinics of North America, 6*(4), 783–784.

Kuttner, L., & Solomon, R. (2003). Hypnotherapy and imagery for managing children's pain. In N. L. Schechter, C. B. Berde, & M. Yaster (Eds.), *Pain in infants, children and adolescents* (2nd ed., pp. 317–328). Philadelphia: Lippincott Williams & Wilkins.

LaMontagne, L., Hepworth, J. T., Cohen, F., & Salisbury, M. (2003). Cognitive-behavioral intervention effects adolescents' anxiety and pain following spinal fusion surgery. *Nursing Research, 52*(3), 183–190.

Launay-Vacher, V., Karie, S., Fau, J. B., Izzedine, H., & Deray, G. (2005). Treatment of pain in patients with renal insufficiency: The world health organization three-step ladder adapted. *The Journal of Pain, 6*(3), 137–148.

Lea, D. H. (2005). Doing it better: Putting research into practice. Tailoring drug therapy with pharmacogenetics. *Nursing, 2005, 35*(4), 22–23.

Lehr, V. T., & BeVier, P. (2003). Patient-controlled analgesia for the pediatric patient. *Orthopaedic Nursing, 22*(4), 298–307.

Manworren, R. C. B., Paulos, C. L., & Pop, R. (2004). Treating children for acute agitation in the PACU: Differentiating pain and emergence delirium. *Journal of Perianesthesia Nursing, 19*(3), 183–193.

Maunuksela, E. L., & Olkkola, K. T. (2003). Nonsteroidal anti-inflammatory drugs in pediatric pain management. In N. L. Schechter, C. B. Berde, & M. Yaster (Eds.), *Pain in infants, children and adolescents* (2nd ed., pp. 171–180). Philadelphia: Lippincott Williams & Wilkins.

McCaffery, M. (1979). *Nursing management of the patient with pain* (2nd ed.). Philadelphia: J.B. Lippincott.

McDonnell, L., & Bowden, M. (1989). Breathing management: A simple stress and pain reduction strategy for use on a pediatric service. *Issues in Comprehensive Pediatric Nursing, 12*, 339–344.

McGrath, P. A., Dick, B., & Unruh, A. M. (2003). Psychologic and behavioral treatment of pain in children and adolescents. In N. L. Schechter, C. B. Berde, & M. Yaster (Eds.), *Pain in infants, children and adolescents* (2nd ed., pp. 303–316). Philadelphia: Lippincott Williams & Wilkins.

McGrath, P. A., & Hillier, L. M. (2003). Modifying the psychologic factors that intensify children's pain and prolong disability. In N. L. Schechter, C. B. Berde, & M. Yaster (Eds.), *Pain in infants, children and adolescents* (2nd ed., pp. 241–264). Philadelphia: Lippincott Williams & Wilkins.

Melnyk, B. M., Small, L., & Carno, M. (2004). The effectiveness of parent-focused interventions in improving coping/mental health outcomes of critically ill children and their parents: An evidence base to guide clinical practice. *Pediatric Nursing, 30*(2), 143–148.

Miaskowski, C. (1999). The role of sex and gender in pain perception and responses to treatment. In R. J. Gatchel & D. C. Turk (Eds.), *Psychosocial factors in pain* (pp. 401–411). New York: Guilford Press.

Miaskowski, C. (2003). Identifying issues in the management of pain in infants and children (Editorial). *Pain Management Nursing, 4*(1), 1–2.

Monitto, C. L., Greenberg, R. S., Kost-Byerly, S., Wetzel, R., Billett, C., Lebet, R. M., et al. (2000). The safety and efficacy of parent/nurse-controlled analgesia in patients less than six years of age. *Anesthesia and Analgesia, 91*, 573–579.

Neul, S. K. T., Elkin, T. D., Applegate, H., Griffin, K. J., Bockewitz, L., Iyer, R., et al. (2003). Developmental concepts of disease and pain in pediatric sickle cell patients. *Children's Health Care, 32*(2), 115–124.

Pasero, C. (2002). The challenge of pain assessment in the PACU. *Journal of Perianesthesia Nursing, 17*, 348–350.

Pasero, C. (2003). Lidocaine patch 5%: How to use a topical method of controlling localized pain. *American Journal of Nursing, 103*(9), 75, 77–78.

Pasero, C. (2004). Perineural local anesthetic infusion. *American Journal of Nursing, 104*(7), 89–93.

Pasero, C., Paice, J. A., & McCaffery, M. (1999). Basic mechanisms underlying the causes and effects of pain. In M. McCaffery & C. Pasero (Eds.), *Pain: Clinical manual* (2nd ed., pp.15–34). St. Louis, MO: Mosby.

Pasero, C., Portenoy, R. K., & McCaffery, M. (1999). Opioid analgesics. In M. McCaffery, & C. Pasero (Eds.), *Pain: Clinical manual* (2nd ed., pp.161–299). St. Louis, MO: Mosby.

Piira, T., Hayes, B., & Goodenough, B. (2002). Distraction methods in the management of children's pain: An approach based on evidence or intuition? *The Suffering Child 1*. Retrieved July 3, 2005, from www.thesufferingchild.net

Plaisance, L., & Ellis, J. A. (2002). Opioid-induced constipation: Management is necessary but prevention is better. American *Journal of Nursing, 102*(3), 72–73.

Rocha, E. M., Prkachin, K. M., Beaumont, S. L., Hardy, C. L., & Zumbo, B. D. (2003). Pain reactivity and somatization in kindergarten age children. *Journal of Pediatric Psychology, 28*(1), 47–57.

Rothley, B. B., & Therrien, S. R. (2002). Acute pain management. In B. St. Marie (Ed.), *American Society of Pain Management Nurses: Core Curriculum for Pain Management Nursing*. Philadelphia: WB Saunders.

Schechter, N. L., Berde, C. B., & Yaster, M. (2003). Pain in infants, children and adolescents: An overview. In N. L. Schechter, C. B. Berde, & M. Yaster (Eds.), *Pain in infants, children and adolescents* (2nd ed., pp. 3–18). Philadelphia: Lippincott Williams & Wilkins.

Schechter, N., Blankson, V., Pachter, L., Sullivan, C., & Costa, L. (1997). The ouchless place: No pain, children's gain. *Pediatrics, 99*(6), 890–893.

Stevens, B. (1999). Pain in infants. In M. McCaffery & C. Pasero (Eds.), *Pain: Clinical manual* (2nd ed., pp. 626–673). St. Louis, MO: Mosby.

Tobias, J. D. (2003). Pain management for the critically ill children in the pediatric intensive care unit. In N. L. Schechter, C. B. Berde, & M. Yaster (Eds.), *Pain in infants, children and adolescents* (2nd ed., pp. 807–840). Philadelphia: Lippincott Williams & Wilkins.

Unruh, A. M., & Campbell, M. A. (1999). Gender variation in children's pain experiences. In P. J. McGrath & G. A. Finley (Eds.), *Chronic and recurrent pain in children and adolescents* (pp. 199–241). *Progress in Pain Research and Management* (Vol. 13). Seattle, WA: IASP Press.

von Baeyer, C. L., Marche, T. A., Rocha, E. M., & Salmon, K. (2004). Children's memory for pain: Overview and implications for practice. *The Journal of Pain, 5*(5), 241–249.

Wheeler, M., Oderda, G. M., Ashburn, M. A., & Lipman, A. G. (2002). Adverse events associated with postoperative opioid analgesia: A systematic review. *The Journal of Pain, 3*(3), 159–180.

Yaster, M., Kost-Byerly, S., & Maxwell, L. G. (2003). Opioid agonists and antagonists. In N. L. Schechter, C. B. Berde, & M. Yaster (Eds.), *Pain in infants, children and adolescents* (2nd ed., pp. 181–224). Philadelphia: Lippincott Williams & Wilkins.

Yaster, M., Tobin, J., & Kost-Byerly, S. (2003). Local anesthetics. In N. L. Schechter, C. B. Berde, & M. Yaster (Eds.), *Pain in infants, children and adolescents* (2nd ed., pp. 241–264). Philadelphia: Lippincott Williams & Wilkins.

Young-McCaughan, S., & Miaskowski, C. (2001a). Definition of and mechanism for opioid-induced sedation. *Pain Management Nursing, 2*(3), 84–97.

Young-McCaughan, S., & Miaskowski, C. (2001b). Measurement of opioid-induced sedation. *Pain Management Nursing, 2*(4), 132–149.

Zempsky, W. T., & Schechter, N. L. (2003). What's new in the management of pain in children. *Pediatrics in Review, 24*(10), 337–348.

6

Caring for the Child with Technology Needs in the Home

By Kimberly Haus McIltrot

The discharge of children with complex health needs from the hospital to the home setting requires a collaborative relationship between the health care team, home care agencies, educational system, payers (insurance companies), and the family. A recent survey revealed that approximately 30% of children younger than 18 years of age have a chronic illness or disability, and many of these children require technologic support (Patterson & Blum, 1996). Apnea monitors, dialysis, infusion therapies, and ventilators are a few examples of technologic support being used in the home setting (Smith, 1995). The increased use of technology in the home requires an appropriate plan of care and knowledgeable caregivers. Experienced pediatric home care nurses are essential to provide education, assessment, and nursing care (Petit de Mange, 1998). Hospital costs are rising, health care benefits are changing, and home care is a viable alternative for families of children with complex needs (Schuman, 1997). This chapter discusses planning, funding, specific technologic services, educational issues, and family coping strategies related to providing care for the technology-dependent child in the home.

■ Developing a Plan of Care for Home

The goal of home care is to provide safe and effective medically necessary care in the home. This alternative to inpatient medical and nursing care includes nursing services, durable medical equipment (DME), rehabilitation services, social services, and educational support in the home. Discharge planning requires care coordination and anticipation of future needs. The health care team assists the family in accessing community supports and services needed to care for the child with technology needs at home (Goldberg, 1993). The role of the home care nurse is to educate and encourage independent caregiving by the parents and to provide a range of services, such as simple dressing changes, ostomy care, or infusion of intravenous antibiotics. The home care agency and nurse must partner with the parents and patients to improve compliance and therefore the outcome for the child (Jackson, 2005). Case managers are also responsible for ordering DME, such as wheelchairs and hospital beds, that facilitate the transition to the home.

Coordination of effective care for high-risk children involves case management and must use individualized care plans. Case managers assess progress toward stated goals, authorize and monitor referrals for related services, and provide family support and caregiver training. It is important to involve the family in the development of the plan of care to ensure its success. The family provides valuable feedback regarding the overall quality of the services and the effectiveness of the plan.

Not all situations are amenable to home care; guidance from health care professionals helps the family determine whether the technology regimens are realistic. The increase in the number of visiting doctors assessing the home environment may reduce hospitalizations and improve the plan of care (Jackson, 2005). Home care for young children has value because it allows the child to be in a "normal" environment. However, this can happen only if resources provided in the home lead to some semblance of normal life (Lindsay, 1999). Jennett's (1986) framework is a useful tool for determining whether technology in the home setting is appropriate. This tool evaluates the use of technology in the home by asking the questions: (1) Is it likely to be unsuccessful in achieving therapeutic purpose, given the child's condition? (2) Is it unnecessary? Could the therapeutic objective be met with simpler means? (3) Is it unsafe in that the complications of the technology outweigh the benefits? (4) Is it unkind in that the resulting quality of life for patient and family is poor? (5) Is it unwise? Does applying the technology deliver community resources that could better be used elsewhere?

After establishing that home care is a reasonable option for a child with complex health care needs, the health care team conducts a needs assessment and devises a discharge plan with the family. A complete needs assessment for children with complex health problems includes personal, physical, family, school, and community assessments (Guillett, 1998).

The discharge assessment should include the child's current level of function and a review of systems. The physical assessment should be focused on the systems affected by the illness, disability, or chronic condition (Guillett, 1998). Functional health patterns should be assessed, including cognitive-perceptual, activity-exercise, nutritional-metabolic, elimination, and sleep. Cognitive-perceptual patterns include language, visual acuity, hearing, fears and sensitivities, grade in school, and the parents' perception of the child's abilities. It is also important to note the therapies provided at school or in outpatient settings.

Home care providers assess the environment before discharging children with complex needs (Guillett, 1998). Evaluation of the environment includes consideration of the home, family, school, neighborhood, and community.

The home environment assessment includes safety, accessibility of the equipment, appropriate electrical hookups, and access to generators and telephone service. Structural changes, including larger doorways, ramps, and electrical rewiring, may be necessary to accommodate the needs of the child.

Assessment of the family as part of the home environment includes family members, folk health practices, values, knowledge level, health of the family members, coping skills, and support systems (Guillett, 1998). Nursing visits or shifts of nursing care may be needed to supplement the care family members provide. Social work consultations facilitate the family's coping with the stress of providing complex care in the home on a long-term basis.

Discharge information is often overwhelming for families. Before discharge, an educational and skills checklist should be completed. Table 6-1 illustrates necessary discharge information.

An educational or developmental assessment is essential in considering the whole child. Health care providers should encourage and facilitate regular school attendance to normalize the tasks of children; success in school is essential to the development of positive self-esteem. The health care provider needs to complete home tutoring forms for children who are absent for longer than 30 days or if a chronically ill child is expected to have intermittent absences related to hospitalization or medical

Table 6-1	Necessary Discharge Information

- Medical summary
- Medical discharge orders
- Nursing discharge orders
- Outline of child's typical day
- Medications, including action and use, dosage and frequency, route, side effects, and storage instructions
- Special treatment instructions
- Nutritional needs
- Instruction on use and maintenance of equipment
- When to call the doctor
- Phone numbers of physicians, utility companies (phone, gas, and electric), fire department, paramedics, nursing agencies, equipment companies, and pharmacy
- Home equipment and supply list
- Names and phone numbers of contact people at school
- Learning needs
- Rehabilitation needs (physical, occupational, and speech therapy)

visits. Referrals to local infant and toddler programs for chronically ill toddlers and preschoolers is essential to identifying delays in fine or gross motor skills, poor oral motor skills, or cognitive deficits.

Community resources vary greatly; therefore, an assessment of the availability of emergency services, transportation, neighborhood resources for respite care, support groups, and church supports is essential. Often, the services exist, but the health care providers and families must be creative in mobilizing the resources. For example, the fire department or first-responder teams may help transport or lift individuals in and out of apartments or housing.

Funding and Services

Reimbursement issues often affect decisions regarding home care. Insurance companies contract with specific home care agencies to provide DME and nursing services. Funding for portable equipment, formula, and enteral feeding supplies may be denied or severely limited. Specific equipment may be chosen because the insurance company will reimburse for it, but it may not be optimal; nursing services may be limited to visits only, not shifts of care (Zerwekh, 1995). Case managers identify resources available from the primary insurance company, and, if resources are limited, alternative payment mechanisms are pursued, such as blending state resources with commercial insurance or referrals to Medicaid waiver programs. All children are not covered by medical insurance, and, in fact, children are the largest group of uninsured or underinsured individuals in the United States (Mauldon, Leibowitz, Buchanan, Damberg, & McGuigan, 1994). These children rely on public support, but state laws governing social programs are not standardized between states. In addition, qualifications for federal programs are changing and becoming more restrictive, resulting in inconsistent funding of home care services. Case managers and social workers collaborate in discharge planning to identify financial resources that facilitate discharge to home and to assist with the complicated process of obtaining funding for services in the home setting. Table 6-2 reviews funding options for children without commercial insurance or as a supplement for an existing policy.

In the past, fee-for-service insurance programs allowed children with chronic or disabling conditions to receive care from tertiary care centers, specialty clinics, and specialists who were experienced in dealing with complex care issues. At present, commercial insurance plans, along with Medicaid, are shifting toward fully capitated arrangements with health maintenance organizations (HMOs). With capitation, each diagnosis is assigned

Table 6-2	Funding Options

1. Medicare: usually for the elderly but also includes children with renal failure
2. Medicaid: provides access to health care for families below the poverty level, which is determined by each state
3. Medicaid Waiver: established for children with many needs; does not consider family income
4. Supplemental Social Security: established by the states for children with long-term disabilities
5. Women, Infants, and Children (WIC): federal nutrition program that provides assistance with formula and food
6. Privately funded grants and special interest groups, e.g., the Lion's Club, Shriner's, Make a Wish Foundation
7. Nonprofit organizations, e.g., the American Heart Association, the American Cancer Society, the Muscular Dystrophy Association
8. Community funding, e.g., local churches and service organizations

a dollar amount for reimbursement, and the institution must then provide care within that assigned dollar amount unless there is an appeal for additional resources. Many children with chronic or disabling conditions are now receiving care in an HMO system designed to decrease the use of specialists (Mauldon et al., 1994).

The chronically ill child requires a health care network that includes primary care pediatricians, pediatric specialists, mental health care providers, hospitals, home agencies, and ancillary therapists. A mechanism to assess quality assurance or utilization review is an essential component of monitoring cost and quality outcomes for chronically ill children. To date, no outcome differences have been found between the HMO and fee-for-service groups in their efforts to reduce hospitalization rates and control hospital costs (Szilagyi, 1998). Refer to Table 6-3 for suggested questions for families to discuss with the plan provider about the network and care options when evaluating various plans.

Technology Services in the Home

Respiratory Support

Concomitant respiratory problems may be found in neonates or children with a surgical problem. Oxygen is provided in the home in liquid cylinders by way of nasal cannula, face mask, or ventilator. A portable oxygen tank is provided for clinic appointments or time away from

Table 6-3	Evaluating the Plan Provider

- What are the primary care provider's knowledge, expertise, and training to care for my child?
- What is the primary care provider's willingness to listen and learn from me the parent?
- What is my child's access to pediatric specialists? Is there an option for second opinions?
- What is the length of time that we have to wait for plan approval of a recommended service, and how long does it take to get appointments for the service?
- What level of communication can I expect between the health care providers and myself regarding my child's condition?
- Is adequate information about the coverage and grievance procedures available?

home. Periodic monitoring of oxygen saturations with a pulse oximeter may be required.

A respiratory therapist or nurse employed by the DME company instructs parents and caregivers on the correct operation of equipment and how to troubleshoot potential false-alarm situations and equipment malfunctions. Before discharge, families are instructed in basic cardiopulmonary resuscitation for infants and children, and the fire department is contacted to monitor the home for any gas leaks. Safety procedures, such as the safe storage of oxygen and no smoking, need to be observed in the home. The health care provider should ensure that DME companies and supply vendors provide 24-hour service to manage potential equipment failures. Discharge instructions include emergency phone numbers with providers familiar with the child and his or her specific needs.

Children with tracheostomies are another group of children requiring respiratory services at home. Stable ventilator-dependent children are also managed at home. Families and care providers undergo intensive training learning how to assemble ventilator circuits, operate controls, change settings, determine the correct source of alarms, clean and maintain equipment, set up and deliver breathing treatments, and perform emergency measures (Hilton & Gold, 1989). Home ventilator patients often have shift nursing care, and the family must adjust to the stress of having health care providers in their home environment for prolonged periods of time.

Nutritional Therapy

Children with congenital or acquired surgical problems, such as gastroschisis, necrotizing enterocolitis, or gas-

troesophageal reflux, may require supplemental nutritional therapy in the home. The child whose oral intake does not provide adequate calories for growth and development is an appropriate candidate for home parenteral or enteral nutrition therapy. The caregivers involved must learn to perform all the procedures for the administration of parenteral or enteral nutrition, in addition to the maintenance of a central venous catheter and gastrostomy, jejunostomy, or nasogastric tube.

Some children are unable to consume an adequate diet through the oral route because of problems with absorption or the inability to protect their airway. In this group of children, nutrition is provided by means of an enteral or parenteral route. The enteral route is preferred because it aids in adaptation of the gut to maximize absorption capability. Enteral feedings may be administered through nasogastric or gastrostomy tubes. Silicone elastomer (Silastic) and polyurethane nasogastric tubes are flexible and have a longer indwelling life than polyvinyl chloride tubes. The tubes need to be changed by a trained individual every 30 days (Young & White, 1992). Most parents prefer skin-level gastrostomy tubes that are more comfortable for the child and are difficult to dislodge. Skin level devices, known as buttons, interfere less than traditional gastrostomy tubes with the activities of daily living (Huth & O'Brien, 1987). Refer to Chapter 7 for further discussion of gastrostomy tubes.

Parenteral feeding is administered through a variety of devices that provide access to the central venous system. These devices require more meticulous care than enteral feeding tubes and can result in serious complications. Refer to Chapter 4 for further discussion of these devices and Chapter 3 for further information on parenteral and enteral feedings.

Several practical concerns should be considered regarding the physical environment of the home before discharge. A telephone is necessary so that the family has the ability to contact and follow the instructions of the health care providers if problems arise, especially during a nighttime infusion. A discussion of the layout of the home is required, in particular, the location of steps, the location of the bathroom in relation to the living and sleeping areas, and carpeting. Infants in an infant carrier can be placed in a small wagon with enteral pumps for easier movement throughout the home. Coat hangers can be used as portable infusion bag holders, which are convenient for cars and strollers. A baby monitor can be used to hear pump alarms when the child is sleeping and the parents are in another area of the home. A child receiving home total parenteral nutrition requires a separate refrigerator or space in the existing refrigerator for supplies, pumps with battery back-up for power outages, and a suitable area to store intravenous tubing. The family should notify the local electric company to put the household on a priority list for resumption of power in the event of an outage. Refer to Table 6-4 for home requirements for technology-assisted children.

The home equipment may differ from the hospital equipment, requiring more nursing support for the first few days of therapy. The home care nurse instructs and supervises the family in independent administration of infusions, such as intravenous antibiotics and fluid replacements. Infants require pumps that are not capable of free flow to prevent accidental overadministration. The connections should be taped along the enteral or parenteral line to prevent accidental dislodgment.

The time and attention required for complex medical therapies strain family relationships. The health care provider and the family need to encourage sibling involvement by asking for their help in bringing diapers or playing with the ill child. The family needs to make adjustments when one member has dietary restrictions. Compressing the infusion time of nutritional solutions, known as creating a window or cycling, helps normalize family activities. The window period, when infusions are off, allows the child to be free from equipment. The health care provider must assess the family schedule or routines to determine the optimal time for the window period. Many families prefer to infuse during the evening and night so that the window is during the daytime hours. Daytime windows facilitate the child's return to school or finding suitable child care providers for younger children (Loan, Kearney, Magnuson, & Williams, 1997).

Table 6-4	Home Requirements for Technology-Assisted Children

- Smoke detector
- Fire extinguisher
- Electrical service and outlets adequate to handle equipment
- Backup power source (generator or batteries)
- Telephone
- Heat
- Refrigeration for some medications and total parenteral nutrition
- Water
- Space for equipment and supplies
- Accessible entry and exit

Attending youth camps or family vacations can be less stressful if nutritional coordination is provided by regional and national vendors. Many families choose to travel with a 1-day supply of formula or total parenteral nutrition and rely on the delivery of additional equipment and solutions to the camp or vacation destination. This is convenient for the family, ensures safe storage of solutions, and enables the family to plan outings with ease.

■ Education

The technology-dependent child presents special challenges in educational planning and service provision in order to address his or her health care needs at school (Goldberg, 1993). The Individuals with Disabilities Education Act (IDEA) of 1990 mandates that state and local educational agencies serve all children with disabilities. Services included in these regulations are as follows: early identification and assessment of developmental delays, medical services, occupational therapy, parent counseling and training, physical therapy, school health services, and transportation (IDEA of 1990 Regulations 300.16). Congress also amended the IDEA to include assistive technology services and devices that are used to increase or improve the students' functional capabilities (IDEA of 1990 Regulations 300.5 and 300.6). The related services may be available only for students who have an individualized educational program (IEP) that documents the need for special services. However, technology-dependent children with special health care needs may not require specially designed instructions (Palfrey, Singer, Raphael, & Walder, 1990; Walker, 1987). These children can be protected under the Americans with Disabilities Act of 1990. This law prevents discrimination against an individual on the basis of their disability. The central component of this law requires that states provide education at the public expense. The education plan must meet the standards of the state educational agency, and related services must be provided in the least restrictive environment (Hamilton & Vessey, 1992). Often, the educational programs for students with complex health care needs are planned and implemented at the local level. Geiger and Schilit (1988) suggest that an individual be appointed to plan, administer, and coordinate integrated programming that increases communication and ensures the success of these programs.

Educators formally evaluate the abilities of the child with complex health care needs. Alternative response methods may be required in children with physical or cognitive deficits to obtain an accurate measure of their abilities. For example, a child with a tracheostomy or on a ventilator may have difficulty communicating verbally with the evaluator. The educational program developed should be accompanied by back-up strategies to deal with long absences from school caused by illness. The plan needs to be flexible and dynamic to encompass changes in the child's medical condition. Health care instructions with emergency plans are also developed individually for the child and the school. A successful program requires collaboration and communication between the family, medical personnel, and policy makers (Clatterbuck, Jones, Tumbull, & Moberly, 1998).

The role of the nurse or health care provider is one of educating families and school personnel about the child's condition and providing appropriate anticipatory guidance. Topics to address include clinical condition, medication and treatments, school readiness, lifestyle choices, promotion of self-esteem and coping strategies, and transition to adulthood (Vessey, 1997). The nurse can advocate for the family directly with the educational system or can recommend local or state advocacy groups for additional assistance.

■ Family Coping Strategies

Parents of children with complex health care needs require knowledge and skill in normal parenting issues and information specific to their situation. Parents must gain expertise in technologies while grieving for the "perfect" child of their dreams (Jenkins, 1996). The health care provider needs to support the parent through the grieving process. Moses (1993) described the five grieving stages as denial, anxiety, depression, anger, and guilt. Each of these stages has behaviors that can serve useful purposes for limited periods but are not helpful for extended periods. Denial of the child's handicap or illness can allow time for the parents to discover personal strengths that they can use to understand information and help offered by others. Anxiety can be used to mobilize and focus the parents' energies to cope with current demands. Depression is the most frequently identified behavior. It can provide a defining competence, values, capabilities, and potency. Anger can enable a parent to reassess and reconstruct beliefs concerning fairness and justice. Guilt may be the mechanism that enables the parents to reexamine and redefine their sense of meaning, importance, and responsibility within the context of the loss.

A supportive environment is necessary for parents to work through the grieving process. A nonjudgmental climate gives the parents permission to express emotions, to think, and to move through the stages of grief. The health care provider assists parents in using their existing support system and helps them inventory their resources so that they do not feel alone. The provider arranges follow-up communication and uses anticipatory guidance that builds on the parents' existing knowledge base, validates concerns, focuses on the future, and encourages developmental progress. The positive interactions between the child and parents should be reinforced, and the parents' ability to identify and respond to the child's special needs should be complimented (Jenkins, 1996). Parents who focus exclusively on the needs of the child with complex health care needs lose sight of their own needs or the needs of their other family members. Additional parental concerns include finances, altered career goals, and job sacrifices.

A source of support for families with medically complex children is the parents of other ill children. Networking often occurs informally during the child's hospitalization. Families exchange telephone numbers, addresses, or attend parent support groups. Diagnosis-related support groups are a valuable source of information and support for families with a child who has a newly diagnosed illness. Family Voices is a national grassroots clearinghouse for information and education regarding the health care needs of children with special needs. The purpose of this group is to give families a voice in the national health care reform debate. The group is also involved in managed care, Medicaid, access to specialty care, hospital policies, welfare reform, and corporate health policies at local, state, and federal levels (Arango, 1997). Many other information and support networks are available for families who have access to the Internet and electronic mail to obtain information about their child's diagnosis and treatment (Yerks, 1996). The Resource chapter in this textbook lists these family resources.

Caring for a technology-dependent child in the home stresses the parental relationship. Often, the parental relationship suffers because attention is focused on the technology-assisted child. Areas of difficulty include communication and information sharing, defining roles and responsibilities, and intimacy (Kahn, 1997). It is important for couples to communicate well, listen to each other, and learn to compromise. Home care may affect responsibilities if one spouse has to stop working. Frequently, one spouse has the primary responsibility of caring for the technology-assisted child. Both partners need to be valued for their roles. Companionship and sexuality are also important in the marital relationship, and time needs to be set aside to enjoy each other (Kahn).

Siblings act as support for each other in ordinary times and during crisis. Healthy siblings have both negative and positive perceptions of the impact of chronic illness on the family. They may feel loving, protective, jealous, angry, or a combination of feelings. Siblings need a safe environment to express these feelings. The parents need to reassure them that these feelings are normal and expected and that they are loved and are important members of the family (Kahn, 1997). Peer support groups can serve as a forum for discussion of many issues. Older siblings who have learned positive coping strategies serve as resources for children who have recently learned that their sibling has a chronic illness. Health professionals help siblings deal with misconceptions about the illness causes and consequences that may lead to a closer sibling relationship (Desiree & Jessee, 1996). Siblings need to be included in the family decision making when appropriate. Parents should schedule special events and outings for the siblings to spend special time together. In addition, support groups or camps for the siblings, such as Siblings of Cancer Patients, help them adjust to the situation.

Having health care professionals in the home can cause tension. The home is a private domain and is now open for public view. It is important for the health care provider and family to keep relationships on a professional basis. The health care provider should respect the family's cultural heritage, customs, religious beliefs, and health care practices (McNeal, 1998). Together, the health care provider and family should establish roles, rules, and responsibilities. Families must plan for the care of other children in the home because the health care provider is legally only responsible for the technology-dependent child. With good communication and planning, the family and health care provider can become a "team" and can provide optimal care (Kahn, 1997).

Respite care or child care that is provided by someone other than the parents may be difficult for the family to identify. Resources that some families have used as supports include schools, extended family members, community groups, such as church volunteers and hospice, and volunteer health care providers (Youngblood, 1994). Parents of technology-dependent children cope with the economic hardship of providing for their child's needs. Often, both parents must work outside of the home to meet their financial responsibilities. This necessitates pursuing day care services (Stutts, 1994). Finding acceptable day care services may be difficult when the child has special needs (Delaney & Zolondick, 1991). Medically fragile day care centers are few, and, if available, the services may not be covered by insurance. These day care centers

provide an alternative to home care or prolonged hospitalization. Parents who use these prescribed child care centers report fewer communicable diseases, lower monthly nursing costs, and improved coping levels (Stutts).

It is not always possible to care for the technology-dependent child in the home. Transfer to a long-term care facility, local hospital, or hospice program may be the best choice. It is important that the family does not feel like they have failed the child if an alternate site to the home is selected. The needs and well-being of the child and family unit are the first priority.

■ Conclusion

When the child with complex health care needs is able to be cared for at home, the child and family can concentrate on being a unit and integrating back into the community. Home health teams are an integral part of making home care of the technology-dependent child a safe and effective environment for meeting health care needs.

■ Acknowledgment

Thank you to Laura Phearman for her expertise in helping to write this chapter in the first edition of this textbook.

References

Arango, P. (1997). Family voices: Building voices for our children with special health care needs. *Pediatric Nursing, 23*(4), 400–402.

Burns, M., & Thornam, C. (1993). Broadening the scope of nursing practice: Federal programs for children. *Pediatric Nursing, 19*(6), 546–553.

Clatterbuck, C., Jones, D., Turnbull, H., & Moberly, R. (1998). Planning educational services for children who are ventilator assisted. *Children's Health Care, 27*(3), 185–204.

Delaney, N., & Zolondick, K. (1991). Day care for technology-dependent infants and children: A new alternative. *Journal of Perinatal and Neonatal Nursing, 5*, 80–85.

Desiree, D., & Jessee, P. (1996). Impact of a chronic illness in childhood: Siblings' preconceptions. *Issues in Comprehensive Pediatrics Nursing, 19*, 135–147.

Geiger, W., & Schilit, J. (1988). Providing appropriate education environments. In L. Sternberg (Ed.), *Educating students with severe or profound handicaps* (2nd ed., pp. 17–51). Rockville, MD: Aspen Publishers.

Goldberg, E. (1993). Getting off to a good start: Transition planning for children with chronic health conditions. *Network*, Summer, 9–10.

Guillett, S. (1998). Assessing the child with disabilities. *Home Healthcare Nurse, 16*(6), 403–407.

Hamilton, B., & Vessey, J. (1992). Pediatric discharge planning. *Pediatric Nursing, 18*(5), 475–478.

Hilton, T., & Gold, P. (1989). Hospital to home for the ventilator-assisted patient: The future is now! *Homecare Connection, 2*, 1–5.

Huth, M., & O'Brien, M. (1987). The gastrostomy feeding button. *Pediatric Nursing, 13*, 24, 1–245.

Jackson, S. (2005). HHAs must partner with patients to improve compliance, outcomes. *Sources in Homecare, 9*(4), 13–23.

Jackson, S. (2005). Polish up visiting MD relationships to boost referrals, reduce hospitalizations. *Sources in Homecare, 9*(5), 15–24.

Jenkins, R. L. (1996). Grieving the loss of the fantasy child. *Home Healthcare Nurse, 14*(9), 691–696.

Jennett, B. (1986). *Technology medicine: Benefits and burdens*. New York: Oxford University Press.

Kahn, P. (1997). *When your child is technology assisted: A home care guide for families*. Wolfeboro, NH: L & A Publishing/Training.

Lindsay, K. (1999). Challenges in pediatric home care. *Canadian Nurse, 95*(3), 61–62.

Loan, T., Keamey, P., Magnuson, B., & Williams, S. (1997). Enteral feeding in the home environment. *Home Healthcare Nurse, 15*(8), 531–536.

Mauldon, J., Leibowitz, A., Buchanan, J. L., Damberg, C., & McGuigan, K. A. (1994). Rationing or rationalizing children's medical care: Comparison of a Medicaid HMO with fee-for-service care. *American Journal of Public Health, 84*, 899–904.

McNeal, G. (1998). Diversity issues in the homecare setting. *Critical Care Nursing Clinics of North America, 10*(3), 357–368.

Moses, K. (1993). *Resource networks, crisis, trauma, and loss*. Evanston, IL: Consultation and Training Services.

Palfrey, J., Singer, J., Raphael, E., & Walder, D. (1990). Providing therapeutic services to children in special educational placements: An analysis of the related service provisions of public law 94-142 in five urban school districts. *Pediatrics, 85*(4), 518–524.

Patterson, J., & Blum, R. (1996). Risk and resilience among children and youth with disabilities. *Archives of Pediatric and Adolescent Medicine, 150*, 692–698.

Petit de Mange, E. (1998). Pediatric considerations in homecare. *Critical Care Nursing Clinics of North America, 10*(3), 339–346.

Schuman, A. (1997). Home sweet home: The best place for pediatric care. *Issues in Contemporary Pediatrics, 14*(3), 91–95.

Smith, C. E. (1995). Technology and home care. *Annual Review of Nursing Research, 13*, 137–167.

Stutts, A. (1994). Selected outcomes of technology dependent children receiving home care and prescribed child care services. *Pediatric Nursing, 20*(5), 501–507.

Szilagyi, P. (1998). Managed care for children: Effect on access to care and utilization of health services. *The Future of Children, 8*(2), 39–59.

Vessey, J. (1997). School services for children with chronic conditions. *Pediatric Nursing, 23*(5), 507–510.

Walker, D. (1987). Chronically ill children in schools: Programmatic and policy directions for the future. *Rheumatic Diseases of Childhood, 13*, 113–121.

Wells, N., & O'Neil, M. (1996). *Family perspective on managed care. Family voices pilot survey report*. Boston: Federation for Children with Special Needs.

Yerks, A. (1996). The internet and pediatric nursing: Guide to the information superhighway. *Pediatric Nursing, 22*, 11–14.

Young, C., & White, S. (1992). Tube feeding at home. *American Journal of Nursing, April*, 45–53.

Youngblood, A. (1994). Families with medically fragile children: An exploratory study. *Pediatric Nursing, 20*(5), 463–467.

Zerwekh J. (1995). High-tech home care for nurses. *Home Healthcare Nurse, 13*(1), 9–15.

Care and Management of Patients with Tubes and Drains

By Lynne D. Farber

The emphasis of this chapter is to provide general, practical information about common surgical tubes and drains. Clinicians caring for tubes and drains must learn how each device functions, the rationale for placement, and how to troubleshoot common problems.

Tubes and drains are used for many reasons: to remove fluids or gases from a cavity, to promote wound healing, to monitor leakage, or to facilitate access to an organ or cavity for irrigation or feedings (Ngo, Lam, & Deane, 2004). Understanding the rationale for tube or drain placement assists with the care of the device. In general, when a drain is no longer needed, the drain should be removed. Drains can be surgically placed to evacuate blood, pus, bile, urine, bowel contents, saliva, and lymph fluid.

■ Enteral Route of Nutrition

Nutritional support, by either the parenteral or the enteral route, is a crucial component of care for children with special health care needs. Overall, the enteral route is preferred, because it is associated with fewer infections and complications than the parenteral route. The enteral route preserves gastrointestinal mucosa and immunity, offers better metabolic control, is usually less expensive,

and has better long-term outcomes (ASPEN Board of Directors, 2002). Complications of gastric feeding include gastroesophageal reflux, aspiration, nasopharyngeal trauma, occlusion, dislodgement, metabolic complications, and nosocomial pneumonia.

■ Nasogastric and Orogastric Tubes

Nasogastric (NG) and orogastric (OG) tubes are bidirectional and can be used for drainage, enteral feeding, administering medications, aspiration for analysis, or to decrease bleeding (Noble, 2003; Yamaguchi, Mukai, Kinoshita, Ohtani, & Sawada, 2004). A NG tube is inserted through a nostril, down the nasopharynx and esophagus, and into the stomach. An OG tube is inserted into the mouth, down the esophagus, and into the stomach. Orogastric tubes are most often used in infants until the age of 4 to 6 months because they are obligate nasal breathers (Sasaki, Levine, Laitman, & Crelin, 1977).

Children with inadequate oral intake may need a temporary NG tube to instill feedings. NG/OG tubes can be helpful for children with adequate gastric function who require short-term feeding of four weeks or less. A small-bore NG feeding tube can be used for this purpose. If a child will need tube feeding for more than a few weeks, he or she will need a more permanent type of tube, placed surgically, endoscopically, or radiologically.

NG/OG Tube Size

Significant morbidity and even mortality can be associated with NG/OG tube placement (Ellett, Beckstrand, Flueckiger, Perkins, & Johnson, 2005). Proper tube selection (Table 7-1) is important. For example, it is crucial to place the appropriate-sized NG tube in a child who is predisposed to gastroesophageal reflux because a larger NG tube could interfere with the clearance of refluxed acid from the esophagus (Noviski, Yehuda, Serour, Gorenstein, & Mandelberg, 1999). A smaller-bored NG tube is usually tolerated better because there is less insertional trauma to the nasal mucosa and less damage while it is in place.

Complications

The main complications of NG tube insertion occur when placement is any place other than where the tube is intended (Ellett, Beckstrand, et al., 2005). It has been well documented that a misplaced feeding tube can cause esophageal perforation, or if it is placed in the airway: pneumothorax, hydrothorax, empyema, mediastinitis, and pneumonia (Kolbitsch, Pomaroli, Lorenz, Gassner, & Luger, 1997; Marderstein, Simmons, & Ochoa, 2004; McWey, Curry, Schabel, & Reines, 1988). When the NG or OG is inadvertently placed past the pylorus, malabsorption and weight loss may occur. The influx of a hyperosmolar formula, delivered directly into the jejunum, can present as abdominal cramping, hyperperistalsis, diarrhea, or other symptoms of dumping syndrome, because the jejunum usually relies on a continuous, controlled delivery of a relatively isotonic fluid.

Verification of NG Tube Placement

Safe and effective gastric feeding is contingent on optimal tube position upon insertion. Before tube feedings through any type of tube are begun, correct placement of the tube

must be verified. NG/OG tubes can be incorrectly placed or displaced over time. Studies in children have revealed that 21% to 43.5% of enteral tubes were incorrectly placed (Ellett, Croffie, Cohen, & Perkins, 2005; Ellett, Beckstrand, et al., 2005; Ellett & Beckstrand, 1999). To irrefutably confirm the position of any tube, injection under fluoroscopic visualization is required. Although an abdominal radiograph is the standard method used to confirm the position of nasogastric tubes (Ellett, 2004; Valk et al., 2001), it is not always deemed practical. The safety provided by multiple radiographs to determine gastric tube location must be balanced against the risk of accrued radiation exposure in addition to the accumulative medical cost.

Bedside NG/OG Confirmation

There are multiple bedside methods of confirming gastric tube placement: aspirating gastric tube contents and measuring the pH (Neumann, Meyer, Dutton, & Smith, 1995; Nyqvist, Sorell, & Ewald, 2005); testing bilirubin, pepsin, and trypsin levels; examining the visual characteristics of the aspirate (Metheny et al., 1994); placing the proximal end of the tube under water and observing for bubbles in synchrony with expirations; measuring the carbon dioxide level at the proximal end of the NG/OG tube (Burns, Carpenter, & Truwit, 2001; Howes, Shelley, & Pickett, 2005); auscultation for a gurgling sound over the epigastrium or left upper quadrant of the abdomen; measuring the landmarks from the Nose or mouth, to the Earlobe, to the Xiphoid process (NEX) (Ellett, 2004); and the graphic method utilizing a graph determining depth of gastric tube insertion based on patient height (Greenberg, Bejar, & Asser, 1993; Klasner, Luke, & Scalzo, 2002). Studies have cited that bedside sonography by clinicians is also a sensitive method to confirm weighted-tip NG tube placement (Vigneau, Baudel, Guidet, Offenstadt, & Maury, 2005). According to a nursing survey (Schiao & DiFiore, 1996), 98% of enteral tubes are placed using the NEX method to predict insertion distance.

Evaluation of Feeding Tube Aspirates

The appearance of aspirates (gastric, intestinal, tracheobronchial, and pleural fluids) differs, depending on tube. Gastric aspirates have different colors and vary from appearing cloudy and green, tan, off-white, bloody, brown, or clear, whereas small-bowel aspirates are primarily clear and yellow to bile colored (Ellett, 2004; Gharpure, Meert, Sarnaik, & Metheny, 2000). Thus, the ability to obtain gastric aspirates through a syringe is helpful but not a confirmation of correct tube placement. It may not be possible to obtain any aspirate, even when the tube is properly positioned in

Table 7-1	Approximation of NG tube size	
Age	**For Evacuation**	**For Feeding**
Newborn/Infant	8 French	5–6 French < 1500 gm
		8 French > 1500 gm
Toddler/ preschooler	10 French	8 French
School age	12 French	8–10 French
Adolescent	14–16 French	10–12 French

the GI tract if one or more of the tube orifices are not in a pool of fluid. Also, the lack of aspirate may be a mechanical problem, since the flexible small-bore tubes may collapse when negative pressure is applied with a syringe.

The Auscultatory Method

If no aspirates are obtained, the auscultatory method is a commonly employed bedside method to confirm intragastric placement. Air is insufflated through the gastric tube, generating an audible whooshing sound that can be heard during auscultation through a stethoscope placed over the upper middle part of the abdomen, or epigastrium. Unfortunately, studies in adult patients have demonstrated that the sound of injected air can be heard over the epigastric area, regardless of tube location: in the stomach, esophagus, duodenum, proximal jejunum, respiratory tract, or lung (Metheny, Dettenmeier, Hampton, Wiersema, & Williams, 1990).

Current literature cites that incorrect feeding tube placement leads to significant morbidity and mortality as well as incorrect decisions about advancement of enteral feeding. Radiography provides the only reliable and valid evidence of correct placement. Visual inspection between gastric aspirates and other types of aspirated fluids is subjective, and the auscultation method is not considered safe practice for detecting tube misplacement. pH testing is not considered reliable, because gastric fluid may not be capable of being aspirated. Fluids with pH greater than 6 may not be conclusive for gastric placement (because both intestinal and pulmonary placements can have pH values above 6.0). Use of a CO_2 monitor shows potential for detecting respiratory placements; however, this requires further research in children (Ellett, 2004). In addition, this method cannot differentiate between esophageal, gastric, and intestinal tube placement, thereby limiting its clinical value.

NG Tube Placement

Before placement of a nasogastric tube, educate and prepare the family member by discussing the process and expected outcomes (Sacchetti, Lichenstein, Carraccio, & Harris, 1996). If able, allow the family member to play a supportive role. The actual placement of the tube can induce gagging or vomiting; therefore, suction should always be available.

Before nasogastric intubation, position infants and unresponsive children supine, with their head turned toward the side. Always ensure nasal patency before insertion of the tube.

For intubations of older children who will cooperate, the child sits upright or lies in the left lateral decu-

bitus position (left side down). Measure the NG tube by placing the distal end of the tube at the tip of the nose and extending it to the earlobe and down to the area between the xiphoid process and the umbilicus. Mark the estimated needed length of the NG tube by wrapping a piece of tape around the tube. With the child's neck partially flexed, the lubricated tube is inserted through a nostril, aimed straight back, and then guided gently down to the nasopharynx. As the tip reaches the posterior pharyngeal wall, the patient should sip water through a straw, when able. If the patient begins to cough or have respiratory difficulty, the tube may errantly lie in the trachea and should be withdrawn immediately. Do not force the tube if an obstruction is encountered. If the procedure is felt to be successful, confirm placement of tube and secure with tape.

Before placing an OG or NG tube in an infant, it is beneficial to use a pacifier with sucrose for comfort. Other comforting measures include swaddling, containment, or facilitated tucking. As with all procedures, expertise evolves with time and experience. It is appropriate to use water-soluble lubricant before insertion. In pediatric patients, care should be used to tape the tube away from the alae or nares to avoid alar necrosis (Fig. 7-1). Children have experienced irreversible disfiguring consequences related to improperly secured tubes (Fig. 7-2). The NG tube is for short-term use of not more than 2 weeks because it could cause necrosis of the nasal septum. Many nasogastric tubes can be replaced at home after the caregivers have been properly trained. Radiologic verification should be obtained whenever there is concern about feeding tube position.

Removal of NG/OG Tube

Clean technique is used for NG tube removal. If applicable, the clinician should turn off suction and remove tape from the nose or face. If the child is able to sit, place him or her in semi-Fowler's position or higher to decrease the risk of aspiration. Have suction available at the bedside. Recommend that the child close his or her eyes to minimize irritational tearing. If the child will cooperate, ask the child to hold his or her breath and proceed to pull the tube out in a gentle, steady motion.

■ Nasoduodenal and Nasojejunal Tubes

Although most patients tolerate gastric feedings, patients with histories of gastroparesis, recurrent aspiration of gastric contents, severe gastroesophageal reflux disease,

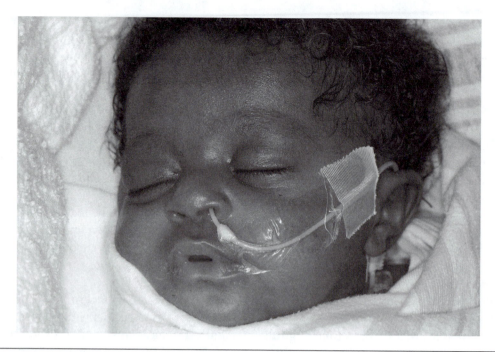

FIGURE 7-1 Proper nasogastric tube placement.

esophageal dysmotility with vomiting, and delayed gastric emptying often benefit from postpyloric feeding (Fortunato, Darbari, Mitchell, Thompson, & Cuffari, 2005). Nasoduodenal and nasojejunal tubes allow indirect access to the duodenum or jejunum, respectively, to provide enteral feedings. A nasoduodenal tube is inserted through the nose into the duodenum. It is used for administering formula or medication. Nasoduodenal and nasojejunal placements require a finer-bore tube and are prone to accidental removal or occlusion. This situation

is generally related to the administration of a viscous formula, medication, or the lack of adequate tube flushing (Reising & Neal, 2005). In critically ill children, small-bowel feedings have been shown to allow a greater amount of nutrition when compared to gastric feedings (Meert, Daphtary, & Metheny, 2004).

Postpyloric Feeding Tube Placement

Current techniques for the placement of postpyloric feeding tubes are complex and time consuming. Many tech-

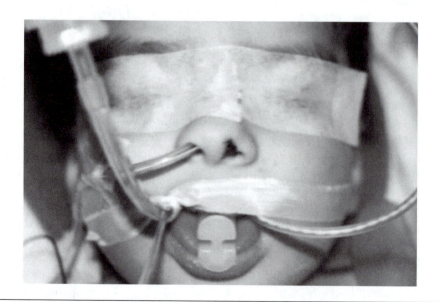

FIGURE 7-2 Alar necrosis.

niques have been described in the literature, including the use of stylets, weighted tube tips, magnets, mechanical manipulations of the tube during placement, as well as prokinetic drugs and abdominal radiography. The most common conventional method of placement involves turning the patient onto his or her right side in addition to the use of prokinetic drugs (metoclopramide or erythromycin) to promote transpyloric passage (Joffe, Grant, Wong, & Gresiuk, 2000). These tubes often require fluoroscopic or radiographic assistance for passage through the pylorus. Endoscopic placement of a jejunal feeding tube is common because it allows placement under direct vision.

A gold color of feeding tube aspirate has a strong predictive value for small bowel placement (Metheny, Eikov, Rountree, & Lengettie, 1999). Gharpure et al. (2000) cited that a pepsin concentration of ≤ 20 mcg/mL and a trypsin concentration ≥ 50 mcg/mL was a good predictor of intestinal placement in neonates. Because there are no currently available routine bedside tests for measuring pepsin and trypsin, clinical application is limited. It is also more difficult to aspirate liquid from postpyloric tubes.

Complications of Postpyloric Tube Placement

Risks of nasoduodenal placement include gastroesophageal reflux with aspiration because the tubes often recoil into the stomach. Duodenal placement is difficult to maintain and is prone to duodenogastric reflux of feed. Research focusing on small-bowel feeds cite that they do not prevent aspiration of gastric contents. Ideal positioning for postpyloric feedings is into the distal duodenum or jejunum. Tubes placed with stylets may have higher rates of complications, specifically enterocutaneous fistulae, perforation of the gastrointestinal tract requiring surgical repair, and inadvertent positioning in the respiratory system.

Dumping Syndrome

Jejunal feedings are best tolerated as low-volume, continuous infusions. Too rapid infusion of formula into the jejunum may result in a complication called "dumping syndrome" (Peters, Simpson, & Tolia, 1997). Symptoms may include postprandial nausea, vomiting, diarrhea, cramps, diaphoresis, palpitations, and flushing. The dumping syndrome is a physiologic response to an altered movement of large amounts of hyperosmotic partially digested food into the proximal small bowel. Circulating blood volume may be reduced by this rapid fluid shift. Early dumping occurs when symptoms start 10 to 30 minutes after eating, whereas late dumping appears 60 or 90 minutes after eating. Treatment may involve decreasing the rate of enteral infusion or changing the formula.

■ Nasogastric Tubes for Decompression

Nasogastric decompression after abdominal surgery can be traced to 1921, when Dr. Levin introduced the nasogastric tube. A Levin tube or a Salem sump tube is used to decompress the stomach in the treatment of gastric atony, ileus, or obstruction; to remove ingested toxins; and to obtain a sample of gastric contents for analysis (volume, acid content, blood). The intended use of these devices is to hasten the return of bowel function, prevent pulmonary complications, diminish the risk of anastomotic leakage, increase patient comfort, and shorten length of hospital stay. Recent studies suggest that the placement of these tubes should be selective rather than routine (Dinsmore et al., 1997; Nelson, Tse, & Edwards, 2005).

The Levin tube and Salem sumps (Fig. 7-3) are commonly inserted for gastric decompression or drainage. The Salem sump tube is a radiopaque tube that is used to remove gastric contents. The Salem sump has two lumens: one for drainage and one for venting or sumping. The drainage tube should be connected to low continuous suction. The air vent should be left open, *never* clamped or covered. By sumping air into the gastric lumen, this air vent prevents damage to the gastric mucosa and ensures effective gastric drainage. To prevent clogging of the air vent, inject air as needed to clean the vent of secretions. Common errors are to tie the vent in a knot to prevent backflow of gastric contents or to insert the opening of the vent into a collection container to prevent soiling of linen. Blocking the vent by plugging or covering it negates the function of the tube and may precipitate complications, such as reflux.

Management of the Salem sump tube requires flushing the vent and main lumen with 5 to 15 mL of air (less with a neonate, more with a larger child) every 2 to 4 hours and as necessary to ensure patency. It is necessary to clamp the vent closed when the main channel is being flushed. The "whistler," or vent, is patent when it whistles continuously while it is connected to continuous suction.

The single-lumen Levin tube is connected to low intermittent suction, *not continuous suction*, because this tube does not have a vent lumen, and intermittent suction allows the stomach wall to fall away from the tube periodically. Children with Levin and Salem sump tubes need frequent mouth care for comfort.

■ Surgical Gastrostomy

A gastrostomy involves the creation of a new opening into the stomach. A small incision is made in the skin and

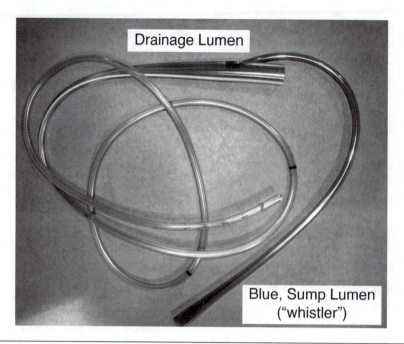

FIGURE 7-3 Salem sump tube.

stomach wall, and a feeding tube is inserted into the stomach. Gastrostomy feeding is well tolerated if the stomach is structurally and functionally able to act as a reservoir as well as a propulsive and digestive organ. The lower esophageal sphincter should have adequate tone and function to allow food to flow into the stomach and prevent reflux back into the esophagus. Good gastric function necessitates coordinated contraction, normal antroduodenal progression, and adequate emptying of liquids. The method of insertion and the choice of tube are often dependent on the indication for the gastrostomy as well as the preference of the surgeon.

Indications

Gastrostomy tubes (G-tubes) are inserted for temporary or permanent reasons. They may be placed in children with birth defects of the mouth, esophagus, or stomach; swallowing dysfunction; malnutrition; need for medication administration; or aspiration of feedings while eating. The patient's underlying disease and available medical expertise must be considered in the decision of type of placement (operative, percutaneous endoscopic, or radiographically guided gastrostomy).

The surgical gastrostomy was conceived in 1837 by the Norwegian surgeon Egeberg and was later implemented in 1876 by Verneuil in Paris (Walker, 1984). For most of the 20th century, an open Stamm gastrostomy placement has been the method of choice. Laparoscopic, endoscopic, and radiologic placements have also been developed.

Stamm Gastrostomy

A Stamm gastrostomy can be performed either by the open or the laparoscopic method. The open Stamm gastrostomy is typically performed under general anesthesia. A short, midline incision is made above the umbilicus, or, alternatively, a left upper-quadrant transverse incision is made. The stomach is decompressed with a NG tube if the esophagus is patent. One to three concentric purse string sutures are placed on the midbody of the stomach, typically on its front surface. A gastrostomy tube (de Pezzer, Malecot, MIC® tube [Kimberly-Clark Health Care, Neenah, WI]), Foley catheter, or primary low-profile balloon device is passed through this incision and into the stomach through the center of the purse strings. The first purse-string suture is tied and the tube is infolded into the second purse string as that suture is tied to create a serosa-lined tract. The stomach is usually sewn to the anterior abdominal wall. The G-tube may be secured to the skin with nonabsorbable temporary sutures. Surgeons should avoid placing the tube too close to the costal margin because this may cause significant discomfort and/or chondritis.

The gastrostomy is usually kept to gravity drainage until gastrointestinal function resumes (24 to 48 hours), and then oral and/or tube feedings can be started. After 3 to 6 weeks (surgeon dependent), the tract is considered healed and mature enough for a tube change (Fig. 7-4). If the primary tube was a de Pezzer or Malecot tube, the

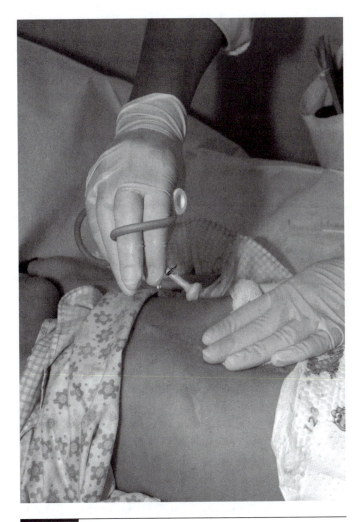

FIGURE 7-4 Removing the de Pezzer catheter.

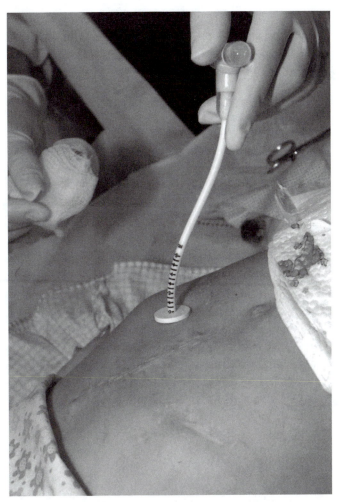

FIGURE 7-5 Use of gastrostomy measuring device.

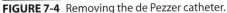

child will need to be correctly sized for a skin level device (Fig. 7-5).

If the tube is inadvertently pulled out before the tract is believed to be mature, a smaller tube (Foley catheter, 1 French size smaller) should be immediately placed into the stoma, and the caregiver should immediately contact their pediatric surgeon or nurse clinician/practitioner. The patient should not be fed or given fluids or formula until the physician has verified the position of the tube.

Laparoscopic G-Tube Placement

Laparoscopic gastrostomy tube placement typically uses a laparoscope to view the operative site. The scope is connected to a video camera and surgically introduced through the patient's umbilicus with images digitally projected onto a video monitor in the operating suite. A surgeon may make additional small incisions to introduce additional instruments. The operation involves the insertion of a port (typically called a trocar), so that carbon dioxide can be introduced into the abdomen for creation of pneumoperitoneum. Diagnostic laparoscopy is then performed to expose the anterior wall of stomach and the site of tube insertion.

The site of insertion should be at least 2 cm away from the costal margin, if possible. A low-profile balloon gastrostomy tube of appropriate French size and stem length may be placed directly into the stomach through a gastrotomy incision. Some surgeons also place purse-string and/or anchoring fascial sutures to secure the anterior gastric wall to the abdominal wall. The surgical field is then inspected for any inadvertent bowel injury or excessive bleeding. The instruments are removed, and wounds are closed with absorbable sutures.

Laparoscopy allows a quick and relatively simple technique of gastrostomy placement under direct vision in even small newborns. Several authors have suggested that the laparoscopic placement of a low-profile G-tube is associated with less morbidity, permits earlier enteral nutrition, and has a cosmetic advantage over the traditional "open" approach (Tomicic, Luks, Shalon, & Tracy, 2002;

Wadie & Lobe, 2002). The laparoscopic placement of a low-profile device also eliminates the need for a second procedural anesthetic and has become the new gold standard for gastrostomy tube placement.

Postoperative Care Interventions

Surgically placed tubes require good pain control, similar to any other procedure that creates an incision. Postoperative care also involves monitoring vital signs, assessing the incision site or sites for signs of infection, and stabilizing the gastrostomy tube.

If possible, convert all enteral drugs to the intravenous route until the postoperative ileus has resolved. Many surgeons permit immediate tube use for small-volume medication administration and clamp the tube for 1 hour. Nonessential enteral medications may be held until enteral feedings are restarted.

Children receiving enteral feedings often experience transient nausea and/or delayed gastric emptying after surgery. If the child's stomach does not empty, feedings are retained and eventually regurgitated, and the child becomes at risk for aspiration. Passing flatus is a cue that the postoperative ileus has resolved, and feedings may be initiated. Metoclopramide (starting dose 0.1mg/kg) either intravenously or via feeding tube is often helpful for increasing gastric motility. Erythromycin may also be administered via the feeding tube for improved gastric motility.

Enteral feedings can usually be initiated once the postoperative adynamic ileus has resolved. Typically, the tube is placed to gravity drainage for 24 hours, and then Pedialyte or a similar clear electrolyte solution is started as a continuous infusion via pump. Enteral feeding rates should be advanced gradually because rapid rate increases can cause abdominal discomfort, diarrhea, or intolerance. After several hours of clear electrolyte solution is infused, the feedings can usually be changed either to half-strength or directly to full-strength formula. If the child is also receiving intravenous fluids, increases in the rate of tube feeding should correspond to a decrease in the parenteral fluids. It is important to flush the enteral tube with water before and after each feeding, as well as before and after each medication administration to avoid clogging the device.

Children with postoperative retching can be initially managed by continuous feedings via pump infusion as well as frequent or continuous venting of the stomach. Children with neurodevelopmental disorders, such as cerebral palsy, are more prone to retching and gagging. If the retching persists, consider a foregut motility disorder and consult a pediatric gastroenterologist.

If the child has received laxatives for bowel management before surgery, it is important to restart this management as soon as feedings are initiated. Constipation is a preventable common side effect of opioids.

Site Care

The exit site should be assessed daily, and any redness, drainage, or skin breakdown should be noted. The stoma site may be cleansed with half-strength hydrogen peroxide, saline, or water for 1 to 2 weeks to remove crusts and exudates. In premature infants or neonates, saline or water is usually sufficient to clean the stoma site. After the first 2 weeks, soap and water are adequate for ongoing site care. It is important to thoroughly dry the skin after the soap is rinsed off with warm water. If the stoma site is clean and dry, it usually does not require a dressing. For low-profile balloon devices, rotate the tube 90 to 180 degrees once a day to prevent the balloon from adhering to the gastric wall.

Low-Profile or Skin Level Gastrostomy Tubes

The components of a low-profile gastrostomy tube include the internal portion within the stomach, the external button that lays on the skin, and the extension sets. There are two basic types of low-profile gastrostomy tubes: a balloon device or a device with a soft silicone dome (mushroom style). Both devices (Fig. 7-6) have one-way valves to prevent formula from leaking from within the tube shaft, and a plug to seal the tube between feedings. Extension tubing is attached to the device to administer enteral feedings or medication. It is important to remove the extension set from the device when a feeding is not in progress. This is a good time to clean the extension sets. A good cleanser can be made with half-strength white vinegar and water, rinsing each extension set afterwards with warm water.

There are two important measurements of a child's low-profile device; the French size and the stem length. The French-size measurement relates to the diameter of the gastrostomy device, whereas the stem length is usually measured in centimeters. As the child gains weight, the length of the tube should be increased to prevent pressure necrosis on the surrounding skin.

Balloon Devices

Although many companies make a variety of sizes, they generally range from 12 to 24 Fr and 0.8 to 4.5 cm in stem length. A few examples of brands of low-profile balloon devices are: MIC-KEY G® low-profile (Kimberly-Clark Health Care, Neenah, WI), the AMT Mini® (Applied Medical Technology, Inc. Cleveland, OH), and the NutriPort® (Kendall-Tyco Healthcare Group, Mansfield, MA). Important features of improved gastrostomy devices

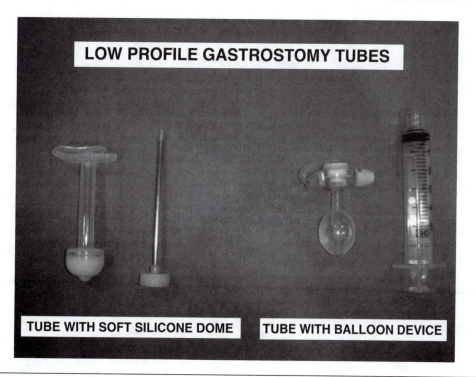

LOW PROFILE GASTROSTOMY TUBES

TUBE WITH SOFT SILICONE DOME   TUBE WITH BALLOON DEVICE

FIGURE 7-6 Two types of low-profile gastrostomy devices.

include a recessed distal tip, tapered distal tip for ease of insertion, clearly marked feeding and balloon ports, and a well-designed button that allows air to circulate around the stoma.

The gastrostomy tube is placed in the stoma, and then the balloon is inflated with water (Figs. 7-7 and 7-8). The amount of water is typically determined by the size of the child's stomach. For example, a premature infant may need only 1 to 2 mL of water in the balloon, whereas an older child usually has 5 mL. The tube should rotate easily, with 1/8th of an inch or approximately 3 to 4 mm between the abdomen and the device.

After the initial postoperative period, placements of subsequent gastrostomy tubes are usually not painful. It is helpful to teach a parent to place his or her tongue against the inside of his or her cheek and equate that feeling to what the stoma feels like to their child. This often helps decrease the overall anxiety associated with learning tube replacement.

A 5-cc syringe is necessary to exchange a balloon skin level device. Apply a small amount of water-soluble lubricant (K-Y® jelly or Sugilube®) to the stem of the tube before insertion. Balloon device replacement can be easily taught to caregivers with the use of a doll with a similar balloon device before the patient is discharged from the hospital. The balloon device usually lasts 4 to 6 months or can be exchanged when it is broken or outgrown

(Michaud et al., 2004). In this author's facility, approximately 85% of children use a balloon skin-level device.

Tubes with Soft Silicone Domes

The gastrostomy tube with a soft silicone dome is an option for children who frequently pull out their tubes, caregivers who are unable to exchange the devices at home, or adolescents that prefer the aesthetics of a device with a flat or less obvious appearance. The Bard Button® (Bard Access Systems, Salt Lake City, UT) is flatter because the one-way valve is within the stomach. The softer, flatter silicone tube is an advantage for children with chest/abdominal brace or casts, because the tube does not tend to rub or get caught as frequently as the balloon device. The disadvantages of this tube include the following: it is more difficult and painful to replace, it has limited size availability, the extension tubing does not lock in place, and it requires a separate decompression extension set to vent the stomach or bypass the one-way valve. A study comparing the balloon device (MIC-KEY®) with the Bard Button® stated that valve incompetence and flap damage were the most common cause of removal of the Bard Button® (38%), whereas balloon rupture was the major cause of removal of MIC-KEY® device (44%).

A pediatric surgery physician or nurse practitioner places the soft silicone dome device using an obturator.

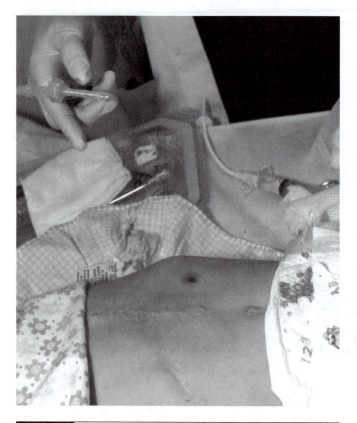

FIGURE 7-7 Placing skin-level device.

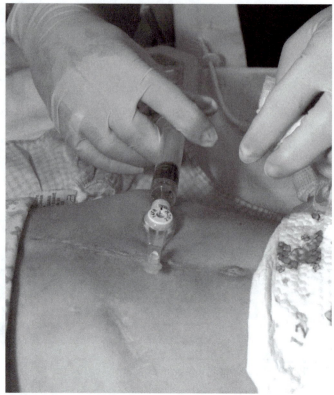

FIGURE 7-8 Adding water to balloon.

This procedure can be performed in the clinic with or without conscious sedation, but it is important that adequate local anesthetic is applied before removal or replacement. The average exchange time is 1 year unless the device malfunctions or there is a significant increase or decrease in weight.

The Bard Button® (Bard Access Systems, Salt Lake City, UT), Ross Stomate® (Abbott Laboratories, Abbott Park, IL), and the Entristar® (Tyco Healthcare, Mansfield, MA) are examples of devices with soft silicone domes. Our institutional experience has been that the Bard Button® has proved to be less easily dislodged by patients and is less prone to complications.

Troubleshooting Complications

Short-term problems, such as local inflammation, granulation tissue, leakage, and mechanical problems are not uncommon and typically respond to local measures. Caregivers should be reassured that most complications are low-acuity, "nuisance" problems that can be managed safely at home. Preventive education, which involves keeping tension off the stoma site by securing the tubes as well as keeping the site clean and dry, is essential. Our institution has found that comprehensive preoperative teaching, which includes a 30-minute video, significantly enhanced caregiver competence while decreasing the reliance on clinicians for low-acuity problem solving.

Leaking

If the gastrostomy tube is leaking, it is important to apply a barrier cream (e.g., zinc oxide) to the surrounding skin until the cause of the leak is determined and corrected. If gauze is needed for leakage, it is important to apply one pad and change it frequently to keep the site dry. If the tube has a gastric balloon, check the amount of water in the balloon because it might be underinflated or broken.

If the drainage is excessive in the early postoperative period, a tube study should be performed to rule out migration of the tube from the stomach back into the tract. If the de Pezzer or Malecot tube has pulled back into the subcutaneous tissue, a Foley catheter, Corpak Gastrostomy Tube® (Viasys Healthcare, Conshohocken, PA), or MIC® (Kimberly-Clark/Ballard Medical Products, Draper, UT) gastrostomy tube (long tube with balloon) should be gently inserted into the tract after the initial tube is removed. If nothing is placed in the tract, it will close over and reoperation will be required. If the initial gastrostomy surgery was performed less than 3 to 4 weeks earlier, a tube study is necessary before feeding the child to ensure that the tube is in the stomach.

Children with profuse leaking may require a temporary transpyloric tube to allow the gastrostomy site to heal. Continuous leaking causes increased erythema, excoriation, and breakdown to the stoma. If a child develops abdominal distention and discomfort after surgery, suspect a postoperative ileus and obtain an abdominal x-ray study.

If the one-way valve on the tube is not functioning on a tube that has been in place more than 3 to 4 weeks, the tube should be exchanged. If the gastrostomy stoma tract has enlarged, it is often helpful to reduce or downsize the track by replacing the balloon device with a smaller-sized Foley catheter (two French sizes smaller) for 24 to 48 hours. Encouraging the patient to sleep on his or her right side after tube feedings may also reduce the probability of leakage.

Appropriate Fit
Children receiving enteral feeding often gain weight quickly, necessitating a longer-length device. A sizing or measuring device (see Fig. 7-5) is helpful to determine the appropriate length or size in centimeters. In order to determine the correct fit of the tube, it is necessary to measure the child lying down as well as sitting upright, if possible. The child's caregivers may require a new prescription for the new gastrostomy tube size each time a new tube is placed.

Erosion
Gastrostomy erosion is a breakdown of the epidermis or outer layer of the skin, usually caused by physical abrasion or inflammatory processes. This situation can be prevented simply by avoiding tension on the gastrostomy site. Unsecured extension sets are often the primary preventable cause for gastrostomy leakage. The tube should not be taped tautly to the side but should come straight up out of the stoma. Gauze and tape can be used to prevent tension on the healing site. This author often secures the tubes with tape over the rib area, so that in the case of an accidental tug, the stoma is not traumatized. There are also drain tube attachment devices that secure the tube, such as the Hollister® tube attachment device. This may be changed every 4 to 5 days or as necessary.

Hypergranulation Tissue
Granulation tissue is beefy red, friable, inflamed epithelial tissue surrounding the gastrostomy tube. When this tissue progresses beyond the level of the wound bed, it is called hypergranulation tissue. This abnormal tissue formation is one of the most common complications (67%) of patients with gastrostomy tubes. Hypergranulation (also known as "proud flesh") often occurs in wounds that are healing by secondary intention, or from the bottom up. In this situation, there is an overgrowth of fibroblasts and endothelial cells preventing wound healing, often with associated weeping and bleeding. The appearance of granulation tissue is often noted in the initial postoperative period.

Treatment consists of destruction of the hypergranulation tissue by chemical cautery with silver nitrate sticks, sharp debridement, or 0.1% triamcinolone cream. Silver nitrate application is a skill that can be taught to competent caregivers. Before silver nitrate is applied to the granulation tissue, lidocaine (Xylocaine) 2% jelly may be applied as a topical anesthetic. This author also applies Calmoseptine ointment to the area surrounding the granulation tissue for skin protection, primarily to avoid the silver component of the treatment from staining or tattooing the normal skin surrounding the granulation tissue. Treatments with silver nitrate sticks are usually administered once per day until the site is healed. The treated area should be covered with one layer of gauze and changed when wet. Alternatively, triamcinolone cream 0.1% can be applied three times a day to the affected tissue or until the granulation tissue is healed. Trials of triamcinolone cream 0.5% cream have also been successful for the short-term treatment of granulation tissue. Both techniques are usually effective and well tolerated in children. Hypergranulation tissue is often a clue that the simple rules of "clean and dry" and "no tension to the site" need to be reinforced. Potential causes of granulation tissue are tension or friction at the gastrostomy site (Nelson, 1999) or an incorrectly fitted gastrostomy device. The origin of the granulation tissue must be corrected or the granulation tissue may recur.

■ Endoscopic Feeding Tubes

Current available endoscopic techniques include percutaneous endoscopic gastrostomy (PEG), jejunostomy, and gastrojejunostomy (PEG-J). Careful selection of patients is important to minimize the complications and morbidity of each intervention. Tubes that are placed in the stomach are easier to replace and allow continuous-pump or bolus feedings. Tubes that are sited in the small intestine are prone to dislodgement and are difficult to replace. Small-bowel feedings need to be administered as a continuous infusion via pump.

Percutaneous Endoscopic Gastrostomy (PEG)
The PEG is a minimally invasive technique, initially developed for children with an inability to swallow. It was

first introduced at the American Pediatric Surgical Association meeting in Florida in 1980. PEG insertion is performed by any of the following three techniques: the Ponsky-Gauderer (pull) technique (on string), the Sacks-Vine (push) technique (over wire), and the Russell (introducer) technique. The most commonly performed are the pull and push techniques.

The basic elements common to all techniques are gastric insufflation to approximate the stomach to the abdominal wall, percutaneous placement of a tapered flexible tube into the stomach, and passage of a guidewire or suture into the stomach (Seldinger technique), placement of the gastrostomy tube, and confirmation of proper position. Mushroom or bumper catheters are usually placed with these methods (Fig. 7-9).

Postoperative Care

Use clean technique or good hand washing before handling a PEG tube. The site should be cleansed daily or as needed with half-strength hydrogen peroxide, saline, or water for 1 week and patted dry. After the first week, site care consists of soap and water, with the site gently patted dry after cleansing. Site care can usually be performed in the shower 48 hours after initial placement, or in a bathtub or submerged after 1 week. If there is stoma drainage, a clean dressing, 2 × 2 or a similar size, should be applied to the site and changed when wet or soiled. The site should be checked daily for redness or leaking at the insertion site. Proper tube securement prevents tugging or tension at the stoma. Keeping the site clean and dry and avoiding tension at the stoma site prevent most site complications.

PEG tubes usually have an external bolster or disk that sits on the skin, which prevents the tubing from migrating back into the stomach or intestine. Rotate this bolster daily to prevent skin breakdown. This bolster should lay 1/8th of an inch (approximately 3 to 4 mm) above the skin, preventing undue tension against the abdomen. One should be able to place a US dime under the bolster. The tube should be flushed with water before and after every feeding and medication. PEG tubes may be exchanged every 18 to 24 months or as needed for malfunction.

Initiating Enteral Feedings

A team approach is essential to ensure appropriate nutrition, development of potential oromotor skills, and oral intake of nutrition whenever possible. Appropriate consultations would include a registered dietician to establish nutritional goals and a speech therapist for feeding/swallowing evaluation. Social workers or Discharge Care Coordinators should be consulted early to help coordinate home health supplies, equipment, and nursing assistance. Unfortunately, some health care insurers may not pay for important medical supplies, such as nutritional supplements, unless they are the only source of patient nutrition. Other supplies are usually paid for, as long as there are ongoing nurse visits to the home. It is important to help families compare costs because there are lifetime caps with many health care insurance policies.

Enteral feedings can be initiated once the postoperative adynamic ileus has resolved. Enteral feeding rates should be advanced gradually because rapid increases can cause abdominal discomfort, diarrhea, or intolerance. After several hours of Pedialyte or a similar clear electrolyte solution, the feeding can be changed either to half-strength or directly to full-strength formula. If the child is also receiving intravenous fluids, an increase in the rate of tube feeding should correspond to a decrease in the rate of parenteral fluids. Many children can be discharged 1 to 2 days after surgery.

Complications

PEG complications may be more significant than other gastrostomy tube placements and include cellulitis, peristomal leakage, bleeding, skin or gastric ulceration, gastrocolic fistula, pneumoperitoneum, ileus, dislodgement of tube, peritonitis, tube occlusion, and early tube extrusion, or "buried bumper" (Chang, Ni, & Chang, 2003; Crosby & Duerksen, 2005; Segal et al., 2001; Zamakhshary

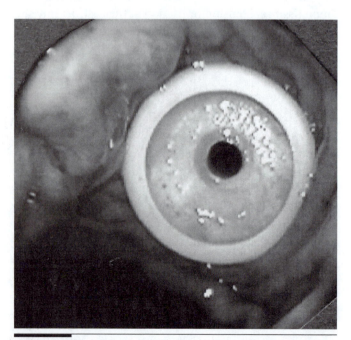

FIGURE 7-9 Percutaneous endoscopic gastrostomy positioned in stomach.

et al., 2005). If the tube is accidentally dislodged during the first 2 weeks, it typically requires replacement. It is important to educate the patient and family that a slight in-and-out movement of the tube is normal and helps prevent complications resulting from an overly tight abdominal bolster.

With a PEG tube, the stomach is not surgically sutured to the abdominal wall. However, adhesions usually develop over time, securing the stomach to the abdominal wall. There are currently no published studies that indicate a safe waiting period after PEG placement for tube replacement. If the PEG is dislodged within 3 months of its insertion, place a Foley catheter or low-profile balloon device in the track to prevent closure. After such a replacement, a tube study should be performed before feeding the patient to ensure that the stomach has not separated from the abdominal wall.

Troubleshooting

Lack of adequate water flushes before *and* after medications and feedings, coagulation of formula, pill fragments, kinked tubing, and precipitation of incompatible medications cause feeding tube obstructions. When attempting to remove the obstruction, it is helpful to withdraw any enteral solution remaining in the tube with a 60-mL syringe. Irrigating the tube with 5 to 15 mL of warm water using a 60-mL syringe and alternating gentle pressure followed by suction often relieves the obstruction. If unsuccessful, carbonated water can also be instilled into the tube and clamped for 30 to 60 minutes. After the dwell time is completed, the tube can be unclamped and gently flushed. If the tube is unclogged, flush with water until clear.

If the occlusion is caused by formula, several institutions advocate using Clog Zapper® enzyme solution. This product contains papain, amylase, and cellulase that can unclog protein and starch obstructions. After mixing the enzyme solution with water in a 10-mL syringe, 2 to 5 mL is gently instilled in the obstructed tube and clamped for 30 to 60 minutes. After the dwell, the tube is unclamped and gently flushed. Once the enteral tube is unobstructed, it should be flushed with water until clear. Because Clog Zapper® has not been evaluated for drug-related occlusions, alkalinized enzyme solutions should be used for precipitates from medications (Beckwith, Feddema, Barton, & Graves, 2004).

For medication-related occlusions, a pancreatic enzyme (Viokase) can be mixed with both sodium bicarbonate tablet (crushed) and sterile water and instilled in the tube as directed by the institution. The sodium bicarbonate powder/Viokase solution is inserted into the clogged feeding tube lumen until resistance is met and then is allowed to dwell approximately 20 minutes. After the dwell time is completed, it is helpful to agitate the obstruction by gently pushing and withdrawing the plunger in a back-and-forth motion. If the tube becomes unclogged, flush with water until clear. A 30-cc or larger syringe is advised to avoid excess pressure and possible rupture of the feeding tube.

Before administering any medication via the enteral tube, the clinician should evaluate the tube type, tube location in the gastrointestinal tract, site of drug action and absorption, and effects of food on drug absorption. Bioavailability may increase with intrajejunal administration of drugs that have extensive first-pass metabolism, such as opioids, tricyclics, beta blockers, and nitrates. Medications intended for buccal and sublingual dosage forms may be ineffective when given enterally. Many drugs should be administered on an empty stomach. For these medications, it is important to discontinue the enteral feeding 30 minutes before and after the medication administration if the medication is administered via a gastrostomy tube (Beckwith et al., 2004).

Liquid medications should always be used, when possible. Sustained-release, enteric-coated, or microencapsulated products should *not* be crushed or administered through the feeding tube (Beckwith et al., 2004). Crushing negates the sustained-release properties, resulting in erratic blood levels. Enteric coatings do not crush well, often clogging the tube with small bits of medications.

If the PEG is obstructed and unable to rotate freely, suspect a buried bumper, which occurs when there is complete growth of gastric mucosa over the internal bolster, flange, or bumper. This complication necessitates a medical evaluation and possibly endoscopy to relieve the obstruction.

Partial dislodgment of a gastrostomy tube may cause infusion of enteral feedings into the peritoneum and cause peritonitis and sepsis. If the tube is accidentally dislodged, teach caregivers to insert a replacement tube (Foley or gastrostomy tube with a balloon) into the stoma to prevent closure. Again, feeding is never initiated in a newly placed gastrostomy until the gastric placement of the tube is confirmed.

Discharge Instructions

Discharge instructions should include a list of common problems that might need the attention of the patient's physician, nurse, or nurse practitioner. Possible problems are postoperative fever; redness, edema, leakage, bleeding, or pus around the tube; change in tube length of more than two numbers (if the tube has markings); clogged tube that cannot be cleared; or dislodged tube. The patient's caregiver should be given telephone numbers for urgent contact with the pediatric surgery team after discharge from the hospital.

Percutaneous Endoscopic Gastrojejunostomy

A variation of the PEG is the PEG-J (Fig. 7-10). The PEG-J feeding tube is usually a safe and useful method to provide postpyloric feeds for children intolerant to gastrostomy tube feeds. PEG-J feedings are indicated for children with pulmonary aspiration, severe gastroesophageal reflux, inability to access upper gastrointestinal tract, gastric dysfunction, neurogenic dysphagia, and failure of antireflux surgery (Godbole et al., 2002). An advantage of the dual-lumen PEG-J tube is simultaneous gastric decompression during small intestinal feedings.

Careful selection of patients is important to minimize the complications and morbidity of this intervention. Although children may gain adequate weight, the inabil-

ity to bolus formula necessitates continuous pump feeding for at least 12 to 14 hours per day and water flushes every 4 to 6 hours.

PEG-J Procedure

A pediatric surgeon, endoscopist, or interventional radiologist using conscious sedation or general anesthesia may perform PEG-J insertions. This procedure involves placing a portion of the PEG tube in the gastric position and passing a thinner jejunostomy tube portion through the pylorus. Intubating the jejunum is often difficult because of the angulation of the gastrostomy track. The jejunostomy tube passes through the pylorus and extends past the ligament of Treitz.

Postoperative Care

Postoperative care plans are surgeon and facility dependent. The goals should be adequate caregiver educa-

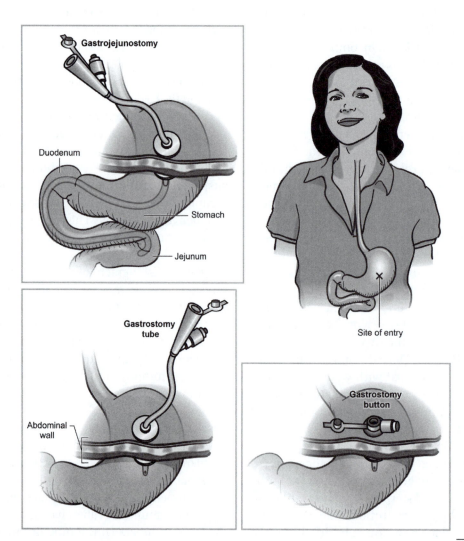

FIGURE 7-10 Types of gastrostomy tubes.

tion and preparation for discharge, toleration of feedings, and adequate pain control. PEG-J tubes are usually placed to gravity drainage on postoperative day zero for 24 hours. On postoperative day 1, Pedialyte or a similar clear electrolyte solution is started at a slow, continuous infusion rate via pump and advanced every 4 hours until a goal rate is reached. Once formula is initiated, the child should be monitored for abdominal distention and discomfort because the jejunum is not a reservoir and may respond poorly to distention. If intolerance develops, the infusion rate may be reduced to the previously tolerated rate, or the formula may be diluted to half strength until the desired rate is achieved. When the desired rate is tolerated, the formula may be advanced to full strength. The tube must be flushed with 10 to 20 mL of water every 4 to 6 hours to avoid clogging. It is necessary to flush with water before and after each feeding or medication administration. Whenever possible, administer medications in a syrup or suspension form. It is not necessary to check small-bowel residuals because they are inaccurate and are of no clinical value. If there is suspicion that the feeding tube is malpositioned, discontinue the feeding immediately and obtain a radiographic tube study.

Complications

Complications of PEG-J are essentially the same as those of the PEG. Although PEG-J is intended to reduce gastroesophageal reflux and pulmonary aspiration, several studies have found that PEG-Js are associated with higher rate (50%–85%) of tube dysfunction (Simon & Fink, 2000) and do not completely eliminate the risk of pulmonary aspiration (Kadakia, Sullivan, & Starnes, 1992). PEG-J tubes have a higher incidence of obstruction, migration, dislodgment, leakage, and intussusception than gastrostomy tubes (Friedman, Ahmed, Connolly, Chait, & Mahant, 2004). Because of the frequent need for tube maintenance and replacement of PEG-J feeding tubes, this tube may not be the most feasible clinical option in providing long-term (> 1 month) enteral access. Future studies are needed to develop innovative percutaneous jejunostomy tube placement techniques that facilitate long-term enteral access.

■ Surgical Jejunostomy Tubes

Surmay performed the first surgical jejunostomy in 1878. Placement of a jejunostomy tube may be indicated for children who have failed or are not candidates for antireflux procedures or have gastric dysmotility or gastroparesis (Neuman & Phillips, 2005). This surgical option allows direct access to the jejunum for enteral feedings. There are many techniques used to place jejunostomy tubes: Witzel, Stamm, Marwedel, needle catheter technique, and laparoscopy. The Witzel procedure, which creates a serosal tunnel on the antimesenteric border, may be associated with complications of tube dislodgment and obstruction due to narrowing of the intestinal lumen (Neuman & Phillips) and the oblique trajectory of the tube into the bowel.

Several recent reports have described the creation of Roux-en-Y feeding jejunostomies, via either minilaparotomy or laparoscopic techniques, and have advocated these procedures for use in patients with severe foregut dysfunction (Gilchrist, Luks, DeLuca, & Wesselhoeft, Jr., 1997; Godbole et al., 2002; Neuman & Phillips, 2005; Yoshida, Webber, Gillis, & Giacomantonio, 1996). They appear to be gaining popularity, particularly in the management of neurologically impaired children who have one or more failed Nissen fundoplications.

Roux-en-Y Procedure

The proximal jejunum is transected and then approximated in an end-to-side fashion to jejunum roughly 5 to 6 cm distal to the transection site. The Roux limb (blind-ending "stump" of jejunum) is then brought up to the anterior abdominal wall and secured to the undersurface of the abdominal wall with sutures. A MIC-KEY gastrostomy button (or similar enteral feeding tube) is placed within the lumen of the Roux limb of the jejunum. This procedure allows easy exchange of the low-profile device without radiologic assistance. It also eliminates the potential for obstruction of the functional bowel lumen.

Initiation of Enteral Feeds

When a jejunostomy is established for feeding purposes, many physicians await resolution of postoperative adynamic ileus as a sign of anastomotic healing before initiating enteral feedings. In the past, jejunal feeds have been predominantly elemental, hydrolyzed, and less viscous because of the narrow lumen of tubes needed to pass the pylorus. Most children can and do tolerate a standard isotonic polymeric formula via a pump-controlled infusion (Ford, Hull, Jennings, & Andrassy, 1992).

Complications

Jejunostomy complications include obstruction, wound infection, peritoneal leakage, accidental dislodgment, diarrhea, intussusception, and volvulus (Braghetto et al., 2005; Gilchrist et al., 1997; Linke, Eble, & Berger, 1998; Neuman & Phillips, 2005; Yoshida et al., 1996). The most common reported postoperative complications were clogging and dislodgment of the jejunostomy tube.

A careful surgical history is necessary before replacement of a gastrostomy or jejunostomy tube. Jejunostomy tube balloons should have only 2 to 3 cc of water in the balloon because they lie within the jejunum. It is not always visually apparent to a clinician whether the tube lies in the stomach or the jejunum (Fig. 7-11). Accidental overfilling of the balloon could cause bowel-wall pressure necrosis, intestinal perforation, and peritoneal leakage. The surgeon should determine how much water would be placed in the balloon inside the Roux limb, and all caregivers should strictly adhere to this amount.

■ Surgical Drain Overview

Various devices are used to drain purulent materials, blood, or serum from body cavities. Basic surgical drain care begins by understanding the rationale for the drain,

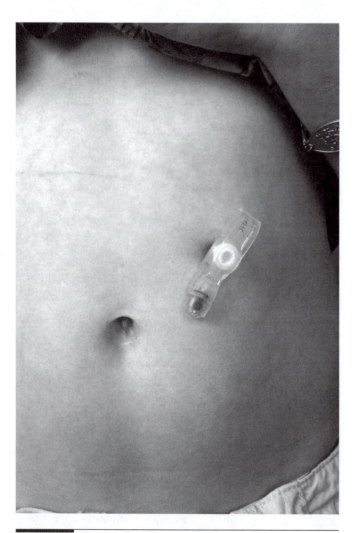

FIGURE 7-11 G-tube or J-tube?

and how it should function. Generally, drains can be classified as open or closed, and active or passive. Drain complications can include infection, hemorrhage, kinking, and hernia.

Open drains, such as the Penrose drain or the corrugated drain, lie within a cavity or space, creating a tract to allow fluids to drain by gravity around the drain onto the skin or dressing. A disadvantage of an open drain is the potential for bacterial contamination of the tubing (Noble, 2003). Drains should be considered two-way streets because bacteria can travel back into the surgical area. This is the primary reason to remove drains as soon as possible. Whenever possible, drains should be placed through a small incision separate from the primary incisions.

Closed drains allow airtight drainage of a cavity, usually by a soft, pliable drain that is connected to negative-pressure suction with reservoirs to collect drainage. Closed drains have advantages over open drains because they are associated with lower infection rates, and they allow accurate measurement of drainage output. A closed system also protects the surrounding skin from irritating effluent. Examples of closed drains are Hemovac® and Jackson-Pratt® drains.

Any tubes that drain by gravity are considered passive drains, whereas those that use suction are considered active drains. Examples of passive-gravity drains include the Penrose drain and the Foley and Malecot catheters.

Active drainage surgical tubes have an expandable chamber to create low-pressure suction. Examples of active drainage systems are the Jackson-Pratt® drain and the spring-activated Hemovac® device. The tubing in each of the aforementioned devices has drain holes through which the drainage is extracted into the tube. The act of compressing and sealing the device creates a vacuum or suction. Care involves monitoring the amount of drainage and emptying the reservoir before it is more than 50% filled. The amount and color of the drainage should be recorded and the device recompressed to continue the evacuation of wound drainage. Disadvantages of active surgical or suction drains are that they can cause tissue collapse around the drain, can cause tissue erosion if suction is high, and may promote anastomotic leaks and/or retard healing of an existing fistula (Ngo et al., 2004). If there is a sudden increase in the drain output, this may signify a complication such as an anastomotic leak or erosion into adjacent organs, and a physician should be notified.

Proper function of any drain depends on the appropriate size and length placed by the surgeon or radiologist. The physiology of drain function is often related to Poiseuille's law, in which drainage flow is directly proportional to the suction pressure applied to the drain and to the fourth power of the drain radius. Flow is inversely proportional to the viscosity and length of the drain; consequently, decreasing the length of the drain by 50% should double the flow (Ngo et al., 2004).

Fluid may stop flowing through the drain for several reasons: fluid production ceases; cavity being drained has been evacuated; drain holes are clogged with tissue or clots; drain lumen is cracked, blocked or kinked; or suction pressure source has been inactivated or disconnected (Ngo et al., 2004). It is important to troubleshoot possible blockages or identify drain malfunction before removing the drain. Most importantly, drains must be firmly secured at the exit site to prevent accidental dislodgment.

Penrose Drain

The Penrose drain, named for the American gynecologist Charles Bingham Penrose (1862–1925), is a passive, flat, single-lumen drain (Fig. 7-12). This gravity drainage device may be made of either latex or silicone. The tubing is available in different widths (1/4 inch, 1/2 inch, 3/4 inch, 1 inch). The softness of this device minimizes wound irritation. It is radiopaque to facilitate placement verification. The Penrose drain functions as a track for drainage when there is a pressure gradient between the cavity being drained and the outside.

Gauze dressing usually covers a Penrose drain. This dressing should be changed as necessary to keep the skin dry and maintain skin integrity. If the output is high, the drainage on the dressing may need to be calculated to reflect accurate total body fluid monitoring. The drain is removed when the output has markedly decreased or ceased. Some surgeons "crack" the drain and remove it incrementally to allow the tract to close by secondary in-

tention (deeper to more superficial). It is helpful to place topical lidocaine cream for 30 minutes to 1 hour as a topical anesthetic before drain removal (Fig. 7-13), especially if sutures need to be removed. Gauze dressing may also be necessary after drain removal until the wound heals by secondary intention.

A Penrose drain is an option for fragile neonates with necrotizing enterocolitis. The drain decompresses the peritoneal cavity of gas, necrotic debris, and stool and can often be placed at the bedside with the use of local anesthesia and sedation. The incision is made in the right lower quadrant, and the Penrose drain is placed into the peritoneal cavity. The peritoneal cavity is irrigated with normal saline to remove any further contaminating material. The infant is sustained with total parenteral nutrition and treated with antibiotics. The drain is then left in place for 1 to 2 weeks and removed when the bowel has recovered (Wu et al., 2002). The indications, use, and care of such drains vary among individual surgeons.

Jackson-Pratt® Drain

Jackson-Pratt drains are closed systems that are rectangular in cross-section. Many Jackson-Pratt drains are placed interoperatively or by an interventional radiologist. The Jackson-Pratt is also known as a bulb drain because it has a soft, squeeze bulb or "grenade" at the end of the plastic tubing (Fig. 7-14). The squeeze bulb on the end of the tube creates suction when it is compressed and sealed. Care involves daily dressing changes and evaluation of effluent. Should the drain become clogged, the fluid in the tubing can be squeezed between your thumb and index finger while moving your finger along the tubing towards the suction bottle. This is called "milking" the tubing, which helps dislodge debris from the tubing. These drains

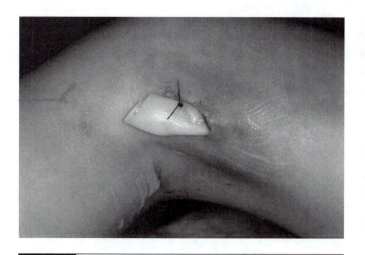

FIGURE 7-12 Penrose drain after the removal of a foreign body in leg.

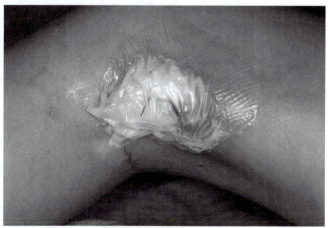

FIGURE 7-13 Topical 4% lidocaine cream administered before drain removal.

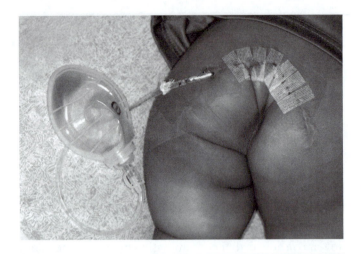

FIGURE 7-14 Insertion of a Jackson-Pratt drain after removal of sacrococcygeal teratoma.

are often managed in an outpatient setting. When the drain is ready to be removed, sutures need to be cut (Fig. 7-15) and the suction bulb decompressed or opened. The tube should be removed with gentle, steady traction, with gauze being held over the exit site (Fig. 7-16).

Urinary Drainage Tubes

Urinary drainage tubes are soft tubes, composed of either silicone or latex. These drainage tubes may have one, two, or three lumens. Single lumen tubes are used to access the bladder for the collection of a sterile urine sample, or bladder decompression. Clean intermittent catheterization (CIC) is commonly used for patients who are unable to void, such as the population of children with neurospinal dysraphism, and neurogenic bladders. The Foley catheter, a double lumen, straight-tip catheter, is a commonly used device, as it allows drainage of urine through one lumen while the second lumen leads to a balloon that is filled with water. This balloon secures the tube in the bladder. Triple lumen catheters allow both irrigation and drainage of the bladder. Contraindications to urinary catheter tube insertion include pelvic fracture, urethral injuries, perineal ecchymoses, and blood at the urinary meatus.

Complications of Urinary Drainage Tubes

Catheter-associated urinary tract infection is the most common nosocomial infection, especially with long-term indwelling catheters. The incidence of genitourinary complications associated with the long-term use of CIC in children is low. The use of prophylactic antibiotics for children who intermittently catheterize is not necessary and may be detrimental due to the increased rate of infection associated with resistant organisms. Other common complications of urinary drainage tubes are mis-

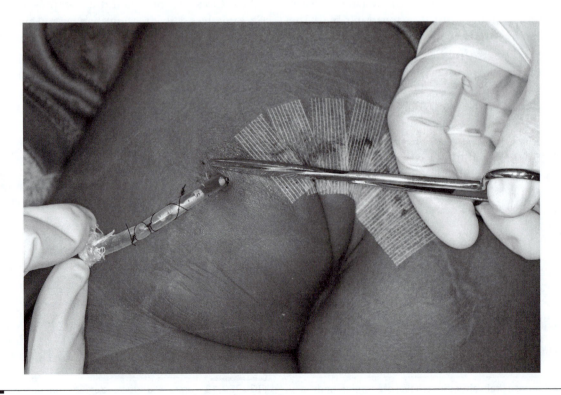

FIGURE 7-15 Suture removal before Jackson-Pratt drain removal.

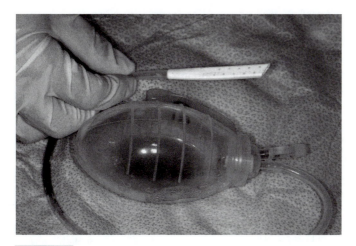

FIGURE 7-16 Jackson-Pratt drain.

placement, bladder or urethral trauma, catheter encrustation, catheter blockage, bladder spasms, balloon rupture, leakage, and retained catheter.

Rectal Tubes

Tubes placed transanally for the purpose of repeated enemas or irrigations may be used for the management of constipation or colitis. The tubes vary in diameter, stiffness, and number of side holes. The placement should be performed with a gentle steady pressure in order to negotiate the rectal "valves" as well as the tortuosity of the colon. A child with severe colitis, coagulopathy, or immunosuppression may have higher risks of complications, such as perforation, bleeding, and infection.

Reports of routine postoperative rectal irrigations have significantly decreased the incidence and severity of enterocolitis in children after surgical correction of Hirschsprung's disease (Marty et al., 1995). Rectal irrigations are typically administered as 10-cc/kg warm saline infusions over 1 to 2 minutes, followed by gentle aspiration. (See Chapter 20, Table 20-2 for detailed protocol for rectal irrigations.) Leaving a rectal tube in place for extended periods (> 24 hours) may increase the risk for pressure necrosis and bowel perforation.

■ Conclusion

The insertion and care of many pediatric surgical tubes and drains are procedures that are commonly managed by nurses; however, there are wide variations in practice. Nursing procedures should evolve from scientific data, yet many practices are based on hospital tradition. With the development of evidence-based medicine, current practices and biases should be challenged and new approaches evaluated. Progress in this routine aspect of surgical care is promising and should help minimize avoidable morbidity.

■ Educational Materials

APSNA invites you to download the diagnosis-related teaching tool "Gastrostomy" for Chapter 7, Care and Management of Patients with Tubes and Drains, at the APSNA Web site (www.apsna.org) and the Jones and Bartlett Web site (www.jbpub.com). All teaching materials are available in English and Spanish and are free of charge. APSNA encourages their use for your patients and families.

References

ASPEN Board of Directors. (2002). Guidelines for the use of parenteral and enteral nutrition in adult and pediatric patients. *Journal of Parenteral and Enteral Nutrition, 26*(1 Suppl.), 1SA–138SA.

Beckwith, C. M., Feddema, S. S., Barton, R. G., & Graves, C. (2004). A guide to drug therapy in patients with enteral feeding tubes: Dosage form selection and administration methods. *Hospital Pharmacy, 39*(3), 225–237.

Braghetto, I., Papapietro, K., Csendes, A., Gutierrez, J., Fagalde, P., Diaz, E., et al. (2005). Nonesophageal side-effects after antireflux surgery plus acid-suppression duodenal diversion surgery in patients with long-segment Barrett's esophagus. *Diseases of the Esophagus, 18*(3), 140–145.

Burns, S. M., Carpenter, R., & Truwit, J. D. (2001). Report on the development of a procedure to prevent placement of feeding tubes into the lungs using end-tidal CO_2 measurements. *Critical Care Medicine, 29*(5), 936–939.

Chang, P. F., Ni, Y. H., & Chang, M. H. (2003). Percutaneous endoscopic gastrostomy to set up a long-term enteral feeding route in children: An encouraging result. *Pediatric Surgery International, 19*(4), 283–285.

Crosby, J., & Duerksen, D. (2005). A retrospective survey of tube-related complications in patients receiving long-term home enteral nutrition. *Digestive Diseases and Sciences, 50*(9), 1712–1717.

Dinsmore, J. E., Maxson, R. T., Johnson, D. D., Jackson, R. J., Wagner, C. W., & Smith, S. D. (1997). Is nasogastric tube decompression necessary after major abdominal surgery in children? *Journal of Pediatric Surgery, 32*(7), 982–984; discussion 984–985.

Ellett, M. L. (2004). What is known about methods of correctly placing gastric tubes in adults and children? *Gastroenterology Nursing, 27*(6), 253–259; quiz 260–251.

Ellett, M. L., & Beckstrand, J. (1999). Examination of gavage tube placement in children. *Journal of the Society of Pediatric Nurses, 4*, 51–60.

Ellett, M. L., Beckstrand, J., Flueckiger, J., Perkins, S. M., & Johnson, C. S. (2005). Predicting the insertion distance for placing gastric tubes. *Clinical Nursing Research, 14*(1), 11–27; discussion 28–31.

Ellett, M. L., Croffie, J. M., Cohen, M. D., & Perkins, S. M. (2005). Gastric tube placement in young children. *Clinical Nursing Research, 14*(3), 238–252.

Ford, E. G., Hull, S. F., Jennings, L. M., & Andrassy, R. J. (1992). Clinical comparison of tolerance to elemental or polymeric enteral feedings in the postoperative patient. *Journal of the American College of Nutrition, 11*(1), 11–16.

Fortunato, J. E., Darbari, A., Mitchell, S. E., Thompson, R. E., & Cuffari, C. (2005). The limitations of gastro-jejunal (G-J) feeding tubes in children: A 9-year pediatric hospital database analysis. *American Journal of Gastroenterology, 100*(1), 186–189.

Friedman, J. N., Ahmed, S., Connolly, B., Chait, P., & Mahant, S. (2004). Complications associated with image-guided gastrostomy and gastrojejunostomy tubes in children. *Pediatrics, 114*(2), 458–461.

Gharpure, V., Meert, K. L., Sarnaik, A. P., & Metheny, N. A. (2000). Indicators of postpyloric feeding tube placement in children. *Critical Care Medicine, 28*(8), 2962–2966.

Gilchrist, B. F., Luks, F. I., DeLuca, F. G., & Wesselhoeft, C. W., Jr. (1997). A modified feeding Roux-en-Y jejunostomy in the neurologically damaged child. *Journal of Pediatric Surgery, 32*(4), 588–589.

Godbole, P., Margabanthu, G., Crabbe, D. C., Thomas, A., Puntis, J. W., Abel, G., et al. (2002). Limitations and uses of gastrojejunal feeding tubes. *Archives of Disease in Childhood, 86*(2), 134–137.

Greenberg, M., Bejar, R., & Asser, S. (1993). Confirmation of transpyloric feeding tube placement by ultrasonography. *Journal of Pediatrics, 122*(3), 413–415.

Howes, D. W., Shelley, E. S., & Pickett, W. (2005). Colorimetric carbon dioxide detector to determine accidental tracheal feeding tube placement. *Canadian Journal of Anaesthesia, 52*(4), 428–432.

Joffe, A. R., Grant, M., Wong, B., & Gresiuk, C. (2000). Validation of a blind transpyloric feeding tube placement technique in pediatric intensive care: Rapid, simple, and highly successful. *Pediatric Critical Care Medicine, 1*(2), 151–155.

Kadakia, S. C., Sullivan, H. O., & Starnes, E. (1992). Percutaneous endoscopic gastrostomy or jejunostomy and the incidence of aspiration in 79 patients. *American Journal of Surgery, 164*(2), 114–118.

Klasner, A. E., Luke, D. A., & Scalzo, A. J. (2002). Pediatric orogastric and nasogastric tubes: A new formula evaluated. *Annals of Emergency Medicine, 39*(3), 268–272.

Kolbitsch, C., Pomaroli, A., Lorenz, I., Gassner, M., & Luger, T. J. (1997). Pneumothorax following nasogastric feeding tube insertion in a tracheostomized patient after bilateral lung transplantation. *Intensive Care Medicine, 23*(4), 440–442.

Linke, F., Eble, F., & Berger, S. (1998). Postoperative intussusception in childhood. *Pediatric Surgery International, 14*(3), 175–177.

Marderstein, E. L., Simmons, R. L., & Ochoa, J. B. (2004). Patient safety: Effect of institutional protocols on adverse events related to feeding tube placement in the critically ill. *Journal of the American College of Surgery, 199*(1), 39–47; discussion 47–50.

Marty, T. L., Seo, T., Sullivan, J. J., Matlak, M. E., Black, R. E., & Johnson, D. G. (1995). Rectal irrigations for the prevention of postoperative enterocolitis in Hirschsprung's disease. *Journal of Pediatric Surgery, 30*(5), 652–654.

McWey, R. E., Curry, N. S., Schabel, S. I., & Reines, H. D. (1988). Complications of nasoenteric feeding tubes. *American Journal of Surgery, 155*(2), 253–257.

Meert, K. L., Daphtary, K. M., & Metheny, N. A. (2004). Gastric vs. small-bowel feeding in critically ill children receiving mechanical ventilation: A randomized controlled trial. *Chest, 126*(3), 872–878.

Metheny, N., Dettenmeier, P., Hampton, K., Wiersema, L., & Williams, P. (1990). Detection of inadvertent respiratory placement of small-bore feeding tubes: A report of 10 cases. *Heart and Lung, 19*(6), 631–638.

Metheny, N. A., Clouse, R. E., Clark, J. M., Reed, L., Wehrle, M. A., & Wiersema, L. (1994). pH testing of feeding-tube aspirates to determine placement. *Nutrition in Clinical Practice, 9*(5), 185–190.

Metheny, N. A., Eikov, R., Rountree, V., & Lengettie, E. (1999). Indicators of feeding tube placement in neonates. *Nutrition in Clinical Practice, 14*, 307–314.

Michaud, L., Guimber, D., Blain-Stregloff, A. S., Ganga-Zandzou, S., Gottrand, F., & Turck, D. (2004). Longevity of balloon-stabilized skin-level gastrostomy device. *Journal of Pediatric Gastroenterology and Nutrition, 38*(4), 426–429.

Nelson, L. (1999). Wound care. Points of friction. *Nursing Times, 95*(34), 72, 75.

Nelson, R., Tse, B., & Edwards, S. (2005). Systematic review of prophylactic nasogastric decompression after abdominal operations. *British Journal of Surgery, 92*(6), 673–680.

Neuman, H. B., & Phillips, J. D. (2005). Laparoscopic Roux-en-Y feeding jejunostomy: A new minimally invasive surgical procedure for permanent feeding access in children with gastric dysfunction. *Journal of Laparoendoscopic & Advanced Surgical Techniques. Part A. 15*(1), 71–74.

Neumann, M. J., Meyer, C. T., Dutton, J. L., & Smith, R. (1995). Hold that x-ray: Aspirate pH and auscultation prove enteral tube placement. *Journal of Clinical Gastroenterology, 20*(4), 293–295.

Ngo, Q. D., Lam, V. W., & Deane, S. A. (2004). *Drowning in drainage. The Liverpool Hospital survival guide to drains and tubes.* Sydney: Liverpool Hospital.

Noble, K. A. (2003). Name that tube. *Nursing, 33*(3), 56–62; quiz NO63.

Noviski, N., Yehuda, Y. B., Serour, F., Gorenstein, A., & Mandelberg, A. (1999). Does the size of nasogastric tubes affect gastroesophageal reflux in children? *Journal of Pediatric Gastroenterology and Nutrition, 29*(4), 448–451.

Nyqvist, K. H., Sorell, A., & Ewald, U. (2005). Litmus tests for verification of feeding tube location in infants: Evaluation of their clinical use. *Journal of Clinical Nursing, 14*(4), 486–495.

Peters, J. M., Simpson, P., & Tolia, V. (1997). Experience with gastrojejunal feeding tubes in children. *The American Journal of Gastroenterology, 92*(3), 476–480.

Reising, D. L., & Neal, R. S. (2005). Enteral tube flushing. *American Journal of Nursing, 105*(3), 58–63; quiz 63–54.

Sacchetti, A., Lichenstein, R., Carraccio, C. A., & Harris, R. H. (1996). Family member presence during pediatric emergency department procedures. *Pediatric Emergency Care, 12*(4), 268–271.

Sasaki, C. T., Levine, P. A., Laitman, J. T., & Crelin, E. S., Jr. (1977). Postnatal descent of the epiglottis in man. A preliminary report. *Archives of Otolaryngology, 103*(3), 169–171.

Schiao, S. Y., & DiFiore, T. E. (1996). A survey of gastric tube practices in level II and level III nurseries. *Issues Comprehensive Pediatric Nursing, 19*(3), 209–220.

Segal, D., Michaud, L., Guimber, D., Ganga-Zandzou, P. S., Turck, D., & Gottrand, F. (2001). Late-onset complications of percutaneous endoscopic gastrostomy in children. *Journal of Pediatric Gastroenterology and Nutrition, 33*(4), 495–500.

Simon, T., & Fink, A. S. (2000). Recent experience with percutaneous endoscopic gastrostomy/jejunostomy (Peg/J) for enteral nutrition. *Surgical Endoscopy, 14*(5), 436–438.

Tomicic, J. T., Luks, F. I., Shalon, L., & Tracy, T. F. (2002). Laparoscopic gastrostomy in infants and children. *European Journal of Pediatric Surgery, 12*(2), 107–110.

Valk, J. W., Plotz, F. B., Schuerman, F. A., van Vught, H., Kramer, P. P., & Beek, E. J. (2001). The value of routine chest radiographs in a paediatric intensive care unit: A prospective study. *Pediatric Radiology, 31*(5), 343–347.

Vigneau, C., Baudel, J. L., Guidet, B., Offenstadt, G., & Maury, E. (2005). Sonography as an alternative to radiography for nasogastric feeding tube location. *Intensive Care Medicine, 31*(11), 1570–1572.

Wadie, G. M., & Lobe, T. E. (2002). Gastroesophageal reflux disease in neurologically impaired children: The role of the gastrostomy tube. *Seminars in Laparoscopic Surgery, 9*(3), 180–189.

Walker, L. G., Jr. (1984). L. L. Staton, M.D., and the first successful gastrostomy in America. *Surgery, Gynecology & Obstetrics, 158*(4), 387–388.

Wu, C. H., Tsao, P. N., Chou, H. C., Tang, J. R., Chan, W. K., & Tsou, K. I. (2002). Necrotizing enterocolitis complicated with perforation in extremely low birth-weight premature infants. *Acta Paediatrica Taiwan, 43*(3), 127–132.

Yamaguchi, T., Mukai, S., Kinoshita, E., Ohtani, H., & Sawada, Y. (2004). Treatment of gastric hemorrhage by pulverized omeprazole and antacid: Concomitant administration via a nasogastric tube. *International Journal of Clinical Pharmacology and Therapeutics, 42*(11), 594–596.

Yoshida, N. R., Webber, E. M., Gillis, D. A., & Giacomantonio, J. M. (1996). Roux-en-Y jejunostomy in the pediatric population. *Journal of Pediatric Surgery, 31*(6), 791–793.

Zamakhshary, M., Jamal, M., Blair, G. K., Murphy, J. J., Webber, E. M., & Skarsgard, E. D. (2005). Laparoscopic vs. percutaneous endoscopic gastrostomy tube insertion: A new pediatric gold standard? *Journal of Pediatric Surgery, 40*(5), 859–862.

8

Care of the Child with an Ostomy

By Valerie E. Rogers

It is increasingly common for nurses to care for children with ostomies. Many children with gastrointestinal (GI) disorders, and some children with urinary tract disorders, return from surgery with a stoma to divert the stream of feces or urine. Living with an ostomy is a life-altering experience. Nurses can make an incredible difference in the adjustment of a child and his or her family to living with a stoma through their positive attitude, their skillful care of the child, and their knowledgeable guidance of the family toward independence in care. This chapter reviews ostomies and their management to help nurses provide care and teaching to pediatric surgical patients with a stoma and their families.

■ What Is a Stoma?

Fecal diversions, commonly called stomas or ostomies, are employed as a surgical technique with increasing frequency. A fecal stoma is a diversion of the GI tract fashioned by bringing part of the bowel up through an incision in the abdominal wall. An incision is made into the bowel and it is then turned inside out (everted), in a process called "maturing" the stoma. The bowel is then sutured to the skin of the abdomen. The function of a fecal stoma

is to divert stool from entering the distal bowel. Diversion may be required to protect a surgical anastomosis or suture line from exposure to feces, to relieve a distal bowel obstruction, or to allow bowel rest and decompression. One of the primary goals in creating a stoma is to preserve all possible bowel length and to minimize the risk of short-bowel syndrome. Although a stoma can be created at any point in the GI tract, this chapter limits discussion of fecal stomas to those of the small and large intestine.

Urinary diversions, or urostomies, are also called *ostomies*. A urostomy is a surgically created opening into the urinary tract—specifically into the bladder, ureter, or kidney. Urostomy stomas are similar in appearance to fecal stomas. The primary goals of a urostomy are decompression of the urinary tract and preservation of renal function. Unlike fecal stomas, urostomies are becoming uncommon in children. Several recent advances account for this trend. Improvements in surgical technique now allow primary repair of many congenital urinary tract anomalies that formerly required diversion. Temporizing measures, such as the insertion of drainage catheters, are being increasingly used to relieve urinary tract obstruction in lieu of surgery. Clean intermittent self-catheterization has demonstrated its effectiveness in managing neurogenic bladder in place of urostomy. Finally, surgical techniques that more closely mimic normal urinary elimination, such as bladder augmentation, have become more acceptable to patients (Hendren, 1998).

Although stomas may be present for weeks or months, most ostomies in children are temporary. Once the disease process necessitating a stoma is stable or surgical correction of an anomaly has been performed and growth is acceptable, the ostomy is "taken down" or closed. Table 8-1 lists the common reasons for children to have an ostomy and the age at which ostomy surgery is commonly performed. As can be seen by this list, most stomas are created during the newborn period as a result of congenital anomalies. However, there are almost as many indications for a stoma as there are children with an ostomy. Many of the conditions leading to ostomy surgery are discussed in detail in other chapters of this text.

■ Preoperative Considerations

The Importance of Preoperative Teaching

Most stomas in children are created during emergency surgery. Unfortunately, opportunities for preoperative preparation of a family in this situation are limited, and teaching and support measures must be initiated after surgery. However, patients experience less stress and better adjustment to a stoma when preoperative teaching can be instituted. When the possibility of surgery that might result in a stoma arises, preoperative preparation of the patient and family should begin.

Preoperative teaching can begin with a simple explanation of the GI or genitourinary system and of the child's disease process. Nurses can clarify explanations given by the surgeon and answer the family's questions about surgery. The possibility of the child coming back from surgery with a stoma can be gently introduced. Many people are unfamiliar with stomas, so pictures and printed materials given to the family are helpful. Ostomy equipment manufacturers have a wide variety of educational materials in the form of pamphlets, videos, and coloring books that they provide as a courtesy for patients. Several of these educational materials are geared to children.

If a wound, ostomy, and continence (WOC) nurse or enterostomal therapy nurse is available, it is valuable to have them meet with the family before surgery. Besides answering questions regarding the function and care of a stoma, they can bring samples of pouches and other ostomy equipment to show the family. The WOC nurse can also mark a stoma site on the patient's abdomen, a task that must be performed while a patient is awake. Stoma

Table 8-1	Indications for Ostomies by Age Group[a]	
	Fecal Stoma	**Urinary Stoma**
Newborn/Infant	Anorectal malformations (imperforate anus, cloaca)	Bladder exstrophy
	Cloacal exstrophy	Epispadias
	Hirschsprung's disease	Cloacal exstrophy
	Intestinal atresias (duodenal, jejunal)	Deteriorating renal function
	Intestinal pseudo-obstruction (congenital)	Hydronephrosis
	Intussusception	Myelomeningocele
	Malrotation with midgut volvulus	Posterior urethral valves
	Meconium ileus (complicated)	Prune belly syndrome
	Necrotizing enterocolitis	
Toddler/Preschool	Hirschsprung's disease (late diagnosis)	Myelomeningocele
School Age/Adolescent	Crohn's disease	Myelomeningocele
	Familial adenomatous polyposis	
	Intestinal transplant	
	Ulcerative colitis	
All Age Groups	Appendicitis (perforated with peritonitis)	Trauma
	Chronic intestinal pseudo-obstruction, acquired	Tumor
	Trauma	
	Tumor	

[a]Diagnoses are listed under the most common age groups but may be seen in other age groups.

placement is important in determining a patient's quality of life after stoma surgery, and preoperative stoma marking by a WOC nurse has been shown to decrease ostomy-related complications (Bass et al., 1997).

Choosing a Site for the Stoma

Preoperative stoma site marking is one of the best measures to minimize stoma complications after surgery. A stoma that is located in a crease or other hard-to-pouch site on the abdomen is poorly positioned and can shorten the length of time a pouch can be worn (Barr, 2004)—the "wear time" of the pouch. A child must be awake during the process of marking the stoma site so that the rectus muscle and the normal bulges and creases of the abdomen can be identified.

Several considerations are important in choosing a stoma site. Stomas should be placed through the rectus muscle to minimize the likelihood of prolapse. The outlines of the rectus muscle can be identified when a child is supine and flexes his or her head toward the chest or coughs. Stomas should be sited away from abdominal landmarks, such as the costal margins, the anterior iliac crests, and the umbilicus. This ensures an adequate area for pouch adhesion. The stoma site should, when possible, be placed away from scars and other irregularities that provide an uneven pouching surface. Although infants sometimes have stomas above the umbilicus, beyond infancy, stomas are placed below the waistline so that clothing can easily hide the pouch. When a stoma is marked on an obese child, the site needs to be visible to the child over any large abdominal bulges, so that he or she can see and care for the stoma as independently as his or her age allows.

After a tentative stoma site is marked with the child in the supine position, the site should be observed while the child sits, stands, and bends to be sure that the stoma will not be positioned in a skin crease. A pouch can be placed over the proposed site to ensure adequate pouching surface and placement below the waistline and to ensure that the pouch is not too near bony prominences or the groin. Patients should be allowed input about their stoma placement if their age allows, because they will be living with and caring for their ostomy.

■ Postoperative Considerations

The type of stoma and anatomic location (e.g., the part of the bowel in which the stoma is located) are important elements of information in the initial postoperative assessment of a child returning from surgery. This infor-mation gives clues to the expected appearance, size, and shape of the stoma as well as to the volume, color, consistency, and erosive potential of the stool or urine coming from the stoma (the effluent). This information can be found in the operative note or in the progress notes on the patient record.

Anatomic Location of the Stoma

Stomas are named for their anatomic location in the GI or genitourinary tract. Fecal stomas placed in the colon are called *colostomies*. A colostomy can either be in the ascending, transverse, descending, or sigmoid colon and is named accordingly. A stoma in the small intestine is called an *ileostomy* if placed in the ileum, a *jejunostomy* if placed in the jejunum, or a *duodenostomy* if placed in the duodenum. Urinary stomas are called *vesicostomies* if they are placed in the urinary bladder (sometimes called the vesical), *ureterostomies* if they are created from one or both ureters, or *pyelostomies* if they open into the renal pelvis. A nephrostomy, which provides short-term drainage through a tube placed into the kidney, is not a stoma and is not discussed in this chapter.

Occasionally, children have a urinary diversion known as an *ileal conduit*, which is a type of permanent diversion of the upper urinary tract. It is fashioned by dissecting a short segment of the ileum from the small bowel while maintaining its connection to the mesentery. One end of the ileal segment is brought through the abdominal wall as a stoma, and the other end is sutured closed. The ureters are dissected from the bladder and anastomosed to the displaced segment of ileum, which then acts as a conduit to drain urine from the kidneys and out the stoma. Although this technique of urinary diversion is still commonly used in adults, its use in children has largely been replaced by surgical techniques such as bladder augmentation.

A fecal stoma is generally bright, beefy red similar to the inside of the cheek. A ureterostomy is pale pink. In the immediate postoperative period, a stoma may be tense and edematous and may appear slightly dusky due to venous stasis (Weber, 2003). Stoma color rapidly improves with circulatory support, oxygenation, and a decrease in postoperative edema. A dark or black stoma indicates ischemia or necrosis of the stoma, and the surgeon must be notified. Stomas can change color with crying, appearing either more pale or darker than usual. This is a normal occurrence, and color returns once the child stops crying. Postoperative swelling of the stoma resolves over 6 to 8 weeks, and the stoma gradually decreases in size.

Stoma size is dictated by the size of the organ from which it is made. A colostomy is the largest stoma. An ileostomy is smaller than a colostomy, because the lumen of the small bowel is smaller than the lumen of the colon. A ureterostomy is smaller than a fecal stoma because of the narrow lumen of the ureter. Any disease process that changes the size of the organ from which a stoma is created also affects the stoma size. A child with a greatly distended colon, for example, a toddler with delayed diagnosis of Hirschsprung's disease, can have a surprisingly large stoma initially.

Output from a new stoma must be measured and assessed for color and consistency. A urinary stoma should produce urine immediately. Lack of urine output through the stoma is an emergency, and the surgeon must be notified. The urine may be slightly blood-tinged during the first 24 to 36 hours following surgery. If the urostomy is an ileal conduit, the urine also contains mucus from the bowel employed in the anastomosis. Fecal stomas, in contrast, may not produce gas or stool for 24 to 72 hours after surgery until the bowel resumes function. A fecal stoma may produce small amounts of serous fluid or stool in the immediate postoperative period, but it is the passage of gas that indicates that the GI tract is patent from the mouth to the stoma. Initially, a patient may produce large amounts of gas from the stoma. This can be distressing to patients, and they should be assured that the gas problems resolve once the bowel resumes its normal functioning.

Once the bowel resumes function, effluent from a fecal stoma is likely to be high output and liquid until inflammation from the surgery subsides and the child begins to eat solid foods. The more proximal (closer to the stomach) the stoma is located, the higher volume and more liquid the effluent will be, because a greater volume of the bowel's absorptive surface area has been bypassed. Output from the small bowel is bilious (green) initially. Jejunostomy output remains liquid and green.

Volume of output can be quite variable, depending on the disease process, the amount of bypassed bowel, the age of the child, the child's formula tolerance, and other factors. Estimates of normal ileostomy output vary between authors. Minkes and Langer (2000) propose 10 to 15 mL/kg/day as an average ileostomy output. Doubling of the expected stoma output, or effluent in excess of 20 to 30 mL/kg/day, is considered to be abnormal, and fluid replacement is recommended. Harrison and Boarini (2004) suggest a formula of 1 mL/kg/hour as an acceptable ileostomy output and consider 30 mL/kg/day as the upper acceptable limit of output for advancing feedings. In the surgical neonate, Quigley, Hansen, and Puder (2003) consider output equal to or greater than 2 mL/kg/hr as abnormal and necessitates volume replacement. Ultimately, the child's surgeon must make the decision as to what is acceptable stoma output for a patient. If questions regarding output arise, the surgeon or pediatric surgery nurse practitioner should be consulted.

Over time, stool from an ileostomy or colostomy thickens. A distal colostomy eventually produces stool that is similar in consistency to the child's stool before surgery. An ileostomy, which bypasses the colon where water is absorbed from the stool, produces less formed stool than that produced by the child before surgery. Over a period of months, however, the distal ileum assumes some absorptive function, and stool adopts the consistency of oatmeal or toothpaste.

Stoma Construction

Stomas are constructed as either end or loop stomas. An end stoma is created by completely dividing the involved organ, such as the bowel or ureter. The proximal end of the organ is brought out through the abdominal wall and matured to create a stoma. An end stoma is constructed when total diversion of stool or urine from the distal portion of the organ is required. When a fecal stoma is created, the distal end of the bowel can also be brought out through the abdominal wall to create a second stoma, called a *mucous fistula*, which is created when the distal bowel requires decompression. It is essentially a nonfunctioning stoma because it is disconnected from enteral intake. However, the mucous fistula intermittently discharges mucus that continues to be produced by the bowel mucosa.

If the proximal and distal ends of a divided bowel are brought up to the abdominal wall through the same opening in the fascia so that they are positioned in close proximity to one another, they are called a *double-barrel stoma*. If the two stomas are brought up to the abdominal wall through separate incisions and are separated on the abdomen, they are called a *proximal stoma* with mucous fistula (Fig. 8-1). In common usage, however, a proximal stoma and mucous fistula are often referred to as a *double-barrel stoma*. If decompression of the distal bowel is not required, the distal end of the bowel can be sutured closed and left in the abdomen. The distal bowel is then called a Hartmann's pouch. The only opening of a Hartmann's pouch is through the anus. As with the mucous fistula, the mucosa of the Hartmann's pouch continues to produce mucus, and patients intermittently expel dark mucus resembling stool from the rectum.

A loop stoma is created by bringing a continuous loop of bowel or ureter out through an opening on the abdominal wall. A support bridge, such as a plastic retention rod or a ring constructed from a red rubber catheter, is placed beneath or around the loop to support it above skin level. A transverse incision is made partially through

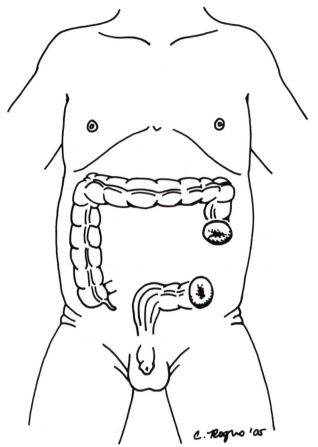

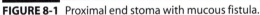

FIGURE 8-1 Proximal end stoma with mucous fistula.

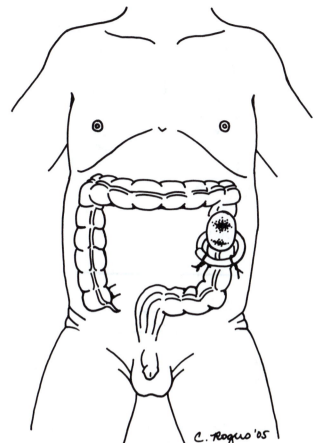

FIGURE 8-2 Loop stoma with retention ring.

the organ, and it is matured to form a stoma with two openings or lumens—the proximal or functioning lumen and the distal lumen or mucous fistula (Fig. 8-2). This is in contrast to the end stoma, in which the bowel or ureter is completely divided. As a consequence of bringing both ends of the organ up to the abdomen, the loop stoma is oval. A loop stoma is not considered totally diverting of the fecal or urinary stream, but it is easier to take down, so it is often used when a stoma is temporary. The support bridge is left in place for 7 to 14 days, at the discretion of the surgeon, until the stoma is healed and is unlikely to slip down below skin level.

Ostomy Equipment

A wide variety of pouches (sometimes called appliances) and ostomy supplies are available for children with ostomies. The pouch and all products used to maintain an ostomy are called a *pouching system*. These products are intended to protect the stoma and the peristomal skin from damage, to promote patient comfort, to be easy to use, and to provide a secure fit with predictable wear time.

Pouches

Pouches come in a large assortment of sizes, shapes, and styles to fit the smallest infant to the largest adult as well as to fit any size, shape, or type of stoma. They are constructed of two parts: the pouch or container that catches the effluent or output from the stoma, and the skin barrier or wafer that holds the pouch securely to the skin. When these two parts are permanently attached, the pouch is called a *one-piece pouch*. Figure 8-3 identifies the components of a one-piece ostomy appliance. An appliance having a pouch that is constructed as a separate component from the skin barrier is called a *two-piece pouch*. The two pieces are joined either by plastic rings that snap together, called flanges, or by rings of flexible adhesive called "adhesive coupling." Pressure is required to join the flanges of a two-piece appliance, and consequently, this style of pouch is usually avoided on postoperative patients.

Urinary pouches are different from fecal pouches in several ways. They have a tap through which urine is emptied from the pouch rather than having a tail with pouch closure, as do fecal pouches. The tap is a small, round

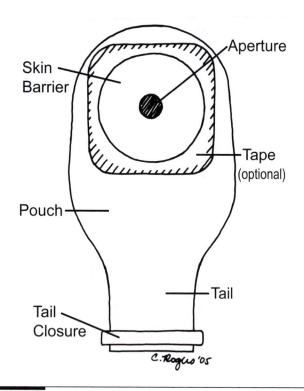

Skin Barrier

Aperture

Tape (optional)

Pouch

Tail

Tail Closure

C. Rogers '05

FIGURE 8-3 Anatomy of a pouch.

opening similar to a spigot. The tap can be connected to a nighttime drainage system, such as a urinary collection bag, so children do not have to empty their pouches during the night. A urinary pouch has an antireflux valve within the pouch just below the aperture; this valve allows urine to pass into the distal pouch and inhibits it from flowing back toward the stoma.

The skin barrier of a pouch is composed of adhesives, softeners, and hydrocolloid (similar to hydrocolloid wound dressings). Adhesives aid the skin barrier in adhering to the skin. Softeners are oils that soften the skin barrier and allow it to mold or "flow" into the normal irregularities of the abdominal surface. Hydrocolloids absorb moisture released from the skin and the stoma while continuing to adhere to the peristomal skin. As the hydrocolloid absorbs moisture, it swells and eventually breaks apart, signaling the need to change the pouch. Skin barriers vary in their moisture-absorbing capacity, depending on whether they are regular-wear or extended-wear skin barriers. Compared with regular-wear skin barriers, extended-wear skin barriers absorb moisture more slowly and provide greater adhesion. Application of the two types of skin barriers differs. Regular-wear skin barriers should be warmed with the hand and pressed onto the skin after application, whereas extended-wear skin barriers only require pressure to enhance the skin barrier seal (Colwell, 2004).

Skin barriers come in either a flat or a convex shape. Flat skin barriers have a level skin contact area and are used with a peristomal plane (area around the stoma) that is flat, and with a stoma that protrudes beyond the skin surface. A flat skin barrier is the shape that suits most children because children have few skin folds and firm abdomens. Convex skin barriers provide an outward curve along the skin contact area. When used with a flush or retracted stoma, convex skin barriers push against the peristomal skin and help the stoma project into the pouch. Several levels of convexity are available, depending on the amount of pressure needed to push the stoma out into the pouch. They include shallow, having less than 1/16-inch depth to the curve of the skin barrier; moderate, having greater than 1/16 inch but less than 1/4 inch of depth; and deep, with a curve greater than 1/4 inch deep (Rolstad & Boarini, 1996). Convexity should never be used on a stoma before the mucocutaneous suture line is healed, or before at least 7 days have passed (Rolstad & Boarini). Premature pressure exerted by a convex skin barrier can cause separation of the suture line.

Skin barriers are available with apertures, or openings, that are either cut to fit or precut by the manufacturer. The decision about which to use is based on whether the stoma is expected to change in size. Cut-to-fit skin barriers are always used after surgery because normal postoperative swelling of the stoma subsides over 6 to 8 weeks, and the stoma gradually shrinks in size. They are also used for infants, whose stomas grow as they grow. Precut apertures are useful for older children whose stomas are stable in size. See Table 8-2 for further discussion of options in pouches, as well as their advantages and disadvantages and tips for their use.

Pouching Accessories

Numerous accessory products are available to support children in caring for their ostomies. Although some children can apply a pouch and never have another thing to do until their weekly pouch change, many children need more than just the pouch to maintain an acceptable wear time. Table 8-3 describes various products that are useful for improving pouch wear time and gives the advantages and disadvantages, as well as some examples of each type of product. Space does not allow consideration of each of these products, but several are discussed in the section on ostomy challenges and complications.

Despite the wide variety and availability of ostomy accessory products, nurses caring for children with stomas must carefully consider the necessity of every product that is used on a child. This is an especially important consideration in caring for neonates and premature in-

Table 8-2 Options in Stoma Appliances: Advantages, Disadvantages, and Usage Tips

Pouch Option	Advantages	Disadvantages	Tips
Fecal pouch	Large tail opening for emptying thick stool Some styles have built-in gas filters, different lengths for different outputs, regular or extended-wear skin barrier Choice of one- and two-piece pouches	Liquid stool prematurely erodes most barriers Limited sizes for preschool and school ages	Preschool and school-aged children may need small or "mini" adult pouch
Urinary pouch	Tap-style pouch closure; antireflux valve minimizes urine backflow Can be attached to nighttime urine collector or leg bag Choice of one- and two-piece pouches	Liquid stool with solid components may not pass through antireflux valve or tap-style pouch closure	Useful with high-output liquid stool Disable antireflux valve if stool cannot pass through Thread nighttime drainage tube through pajamas to minimize kinking
One-piece	Flexible Low profile Minimum application steps	Entire pouch/skin barrier must be removed to change Difficult to center opaque pouch over stoma (can't see)	Use on postoperative patients with tender incisions Easy for younger child to use No pouch detachment from skin barrier for athletes or active children
Two-piece	Can change pouch without changing skin barrier Different size pouches can be used on the same skin barrier Easy to center skin barrier over stoma without pouch	Higher profile than one-piece pouches Plastic flanges on skin barrier and pouch require pressure to snap together Risk of leakage or pouch detachment if flanges are not secure Plastic flange may lacerate prolapsed stoma	Limited use on postoperative patients Change pouch size depending on activity With active infant or toddler, can change pouch instead of emptying it Flexible adhesive coupling replaces flange on some styles Can be used postoperatively
Flat skin barrier	Flexible Low profile	Effluent from flush or retracted stoma may undermine barrier	Use with a level peristomal plane, protruding stoma
Convex skin barrier	Helps push a flush or retracted stoma into the pouch Helps project stool from skin level (off-centered) stoma lumen into the pouch Helps flatten loose or uneven peristomal skin (flabby, obese, skin folds)	Cannot be used postoperatively after stoma surgery Long-term use can cause pressure ulcers	Shallow, moderate, and deep convexity available Use of ostomy support belt improves adherence

(continues)

Table 8-2 *(continued)*

Pouch Option	Advantages	Disadvantages	Tips
Drainable	Empty as needed Output can be measured	Wearer must manipulate stool out the tail to empty	Integrated Velcro©-like pouch closure eliminates plastic closure Insurance generally covers cost of 20 pouches/month
Nondrainable (closed-end)	No need to empty pouch Less aggressive skin barrier avoids skin irritation with frequent pouch changes	Must change entire pouch when full Not practical for hospital use Best with limited number of daily bowel movements Frequent pouch changes = greater expense	Some children prefer for school use Insurance generally covers cost of 60 pouches/month
Regular-wear skin barrier	Easier to remove Less expensive	Erodes with liquid effluent or high skin moisture	Warmth and pressure after application improves adhesion
Extended-wear skin barrier	Longer wearing Higher level adhesion	More expensive Adhesion may be too aggressive for fragile skin	Apply pressure after application to improve adhesion Not suitable when frequent skin barrier removal is required
Cut-to-fit aperture	Use when stoma size is changing (postoperatively, growing infant) Can custom cut aperture for irregularly shaped stoma	Requires extra step of cutting aperture when changing pouch	Fit should be at mucocutaneous junction to avoid skin exposure to effluent
Precut aperture	Saves step of cutting aperture	Stoma must be round Stoma must fit precut measurements Stoma size must be stable	Use measuring device in stoma box to determine aperture size before ordering Order sample pouch from manufacturer to test aperture size
Gas filter	Allows slow escape of air from pouch with flatulence Charcoal filter deodorizes escaping gas Built into some pouches, or can be added on to pouch without built-in filter	Loses deodorizing effectiveness when wet Ineffective filter may necessitate premature pouch change	Use manufacturer-supplied filter cover (sticker) when bathing Loose stool can wet filter Add-on (stick-on) filter must be pierced with pin to vent May require daily repiercing

Table 8-3   Accessories for Stoma Care

Accessories/Examples[a]	Description	Advantages/Tips for Use	Disadvantages
Absorption Crystals			
Ile-Sorb Absorbent Gel Packets, Cymed Ostomy Co., Berkeley, CA NuSorb Absorption Granules, NuHope Laboratories, Inc., Pacoima, CA	Crystals or granules added to pouch to absorb liquid Absorbs excess liquid from stool to minimize skin barrier erosion	Improves pouch wear time with liquid stool Decreases sloshing of liquid effluent	Changes output measurement
Adhesive Agents			
Medical Adhesive Spray, Hollister Inc., Libertyville, IL Skin Tac :H" (latex-free), Torbot Group, Inc., Cranston, RI	Bonding agent that increases adhesion of skin barrier	Can improve pouch wear time Come as wipes, spray After application, allow to dry before pouching	Some contain latex Creates an aggressive bond that can cause epidermal stripping with removal
Adhesive Removers			
Detachol, Ferndale Laboratories, Ferndale, MI AllKare Adhesive Remover Wipe, ConvaTec, Princeton, NJ	Dissolves adhesives to ease removal	Decreases pain and trauma of adhesive/ skin barrier removal Must remove from skin with soap and water after use Limit use in preterm infants	Most contain alcohol and petroleum distillates; skin absorption can cause toxicity; toxic epidermal necrolysis can occur in all age groups after use[b]
Belt			
(Manufacturer of belt should match manufacturer of ostomy pouch)	Elastic strip, attaches to belt loops on 2-piece pouch Supports pouch at 3- and 9-o'clock positions Wider hernia support belts (custom sized) available to stabilize the entire peristomal plane	Supports pouch to improve wear time (active child, obesity, soft abdomen); some manufacturers have infant/child sizes; helps maintain contact of convex pouch to skin; hernia support belt useful to provide pouch support on active child who fails other options, or with peristomal hernia	One-piece pouches do not have belt loop attachments; migrates up to waistline when stoma is low on abdomen—may dislodge pouch; wider hernia support belt not for use on infants (may restrict abdominal excursion, respirations)
Ostomy Paste			
	Soft skin barrier in a tube Fills peristomal irregularities to level pouching surface	Use smallest volume required to achieve pouch adhesion Use paste-filled syringe to apply small amounts on infants To promote alcohol evaporation before application, apply to pouch and air dry 1 to 2 minutes	Do not apply to entire skin barrier (not an adhesive) Contains alcohol (absorbed through skin); burning sensation when applied to irritated skin; wear time > 24 hours to decrease trauma with removal; caution with use in infants due to alcohol, aggressive adhesion; does not withstand urine

(continues)

Table 8-3 *(continued)*

Examples[a]	Description	Use/Application	Considerations
Ostomy Powder			
Stomahesive Powder, ConvaTec; Premium Powder, Hollister, Inc.	Skin barrier in powder form; Absorbs fluid beneath pouch to minimize pouch disruption by moisture	Lightly dust denuded skin with 1 or more layers to contain drainage; lightly pat powder with alcohol-free skin sealant to improve pouch adhesion; apply minimum required for moisture absorption	Should not be inhaled by infants (do not remove excess by blowing); Excess application may loosen pouch
Pouch Deodorant			
m9 and Adapt Lubricating Deodorant, Hollister, Inc.	Substance placed within pouch to neutralize odor of stool, urine	Safe for contact with stoma; Add to pouch after each pouch change or emptying	Increases cost of stoma care; Caution with use in infants
Skin Barrier Supplements			
Eakin Cohesive Seals, ConvaTec; Strip Paste, Coloplast Corp., Marietta, GA; Adapt Barrier Rings and Strips, Hollister, Inc.	Skin barrier similar to that on pouches; may improve pouch wear time; can create shallow convexity on flat skin barrier	Come as flat washers (rings) and strips, triangular washers and strips (for convexity); apply to pouch skin barrier to slow erosion from effluent; place pieces in abdominal irregularities to level peristomal plane	Expensive; Adds extra steps in pouching routine
Skin Sealants			
Cavilon No-Sting Skin Barrier Film (alcohol-free), 3M Healthcare, St. Paul, MN; No-Sting Skin Prep (alcohol-free) Wipes and Skin Prep Skin Barrier Wipes, Smith & Nephew, Inc., Largo, FL	Also called skin barrier wipes; Provides protective film on skin	Decrease skin damage with frequent adhesive removal; air dry before covering, to allow chemicals to evaporate; with excess perspiration, oily skin, & humidity may improve pouch wear time; on preterm infants, use with caution and only use alcohol-free brand	Many brands contain alcohol; usually reduces skin barrier (pouch) adhesion by preventing contact between skin and skin barrier; can cause chemical dermatitis; Cavilon = water insoluble; No-Sting Skin Prep = water soluble
Waterproof Tape			
HyTape the Original Pink Tape (latex-free), HyTape International, Patterson, NY; Pink Tape, NuHope Laboratories, Inc.	Zinc-based, waterproof tape; Gentle adhesive	Adheres to slightly moist skin; Use to waterproof skin barrier in areas exposed to moisture, urine; Skin barrier can be "picture-framed" with tape during swimming, bathing	Use of tape on infant skin, particularly premature infants, should be minimized due to the risk of epidermal stripping

From "Pediatric Ostomy Care, Best Practice Document," by the Wound, Ostomy and Continence Nurses Society (in review). Copyright 2005 by the WOCN Society. Adapted with permission.
[a]Examples are not inclusive of all products in the category.
[b]From Ittmann & Bozynski (1993).

fants. The immature epidermis, underdeveloped dermal and subcutaneous layers, and large body surface area to weight ratio of premature infants, in particular, result in absorption of products through the skin (Nachman & Esterly, 1971; Lund, 1999). Transcutaneously absorbed chemicals that are insignificant to an older child can be toxic to a preterm infant. Products that contain alcohol, such as ostomy paste and skin sealants, or those that contain petroleum distillates, such as adhesive remover, have the potential to cause systemic toxicity (Darmstadt & Dinulos, 2000; Harpin & Rutter, 1982; Ittmann & Bozynski, 1993; Mydler, Wasserman, Watson, & Knapp, 1993; Schick & Milstein, 1981), allergic reactions, or skin irritation. Products with aggressive adhesion such as ostomy paste, bonding agents (adhesive agents), and tape can strip the epidermis with removal (Irving, 2001; Lund et al., 1997). These products should be used sparingly (Association of Women's Health, Obstetric and Neonatal Nurses & National Association of Neonatal Nurses, 2001) and only when pouching without their use has failed. Sometimes, shorter pouch wear time is preferable to unnecessary exposure to chemicals, irritants, and adhesives if the skin remains intact (Rogers, 2003). Pouching should be initiated with minimal use of accessory ostomy products, and products can be added or changed until wear time is acceptable, peristomal skin is protected, and the child and family feel confident reentering their life outside the hospital.

Care of an Ostomy

Nurses should be comfortable with basic stoma care skills so that they can teach children and their families how to care for an ostomy. Basic skills include emptying and removing a pouch, care of the stoma and peristomal skin, application of a new pouch and care of a mucous fistula. These "survival skills" of ostomy care (Erwin-Toth & Doughty, 1992) are reviewed, as well as differences between caring for a fecal and a urinary stoma.

Emptying a Pouch

Emptying the ostomy appliance is the first skill acquired by a child and his or her family. It is the skill that is performed most frequently and soonest after surgery. Emptying a pouch is easy to do and allows the family to begin hands-on care rapidly during the postoperative period. After surgery, of course, output is measured and recorded.

The pouch should be emptied when it becomes one-third to one-half full. Measurement of the fullness of a pouch includes gas. A pouch that is full of air pulls the skin barrier away from the skin and causes the pouch to leak. Excessive weight of its contents can also pull off the

pouch. If the child is old enough to evacuate on the toilet, he or she can empty the pouch while sitting on the toilet. The child can sit a little farther to the back of the toilet seat than normal and empty the pouch between his or her legs. The pouch can be worn at an angle toward the crotch to make it easier to empty into the toilet. Tip the pouch tail upward before opening the pouch closure, so that the contents do not spill out. Open and remove the pouch closure and drain the pouch contents into the toilet or measuring container. To prevent backsplash of toilet contents, strips of toilet paper can be laid onto the surface of the toilet water and the pouch contents emptied onto the toilet paper. When the pouch is empty, lift up the tail and wipe the outside of the pouch with toilet paper. Wipe inside the tail, at least up to the level of the pouch closure, to prevent a detectable odor and leakage onto clothes, and refasten the pouch closure. An infant's pouch can be emptied into his or her diaper during diaper changes. The pouch can be angled laterally during its application to make it easier to empty into the diaper. Very small infants sometimes wear a pouch with a tap-style tail. A syringe can be fitted onto the tap and the contents pulled into the syringe for measurement.

Excessive output may require intravenous fluid replacement. Families should be warned not to empty the contents of the pouch into the toilet before measurement. Standard precautions require health care personnel to wear gloves when caring for a stoma. At home, however, gloves are not needed by the child or family for stoma care any more than gloves are needed for changing a diaper or toileting in the normal way.

Deciding When to Change a Pouch

Wear times for every child and every stoma are different. Among premature infants and infants who have undergone recent stoma surgery, initially wear time may only be a few hours. Factors such as fragile or gelatinous skin, a flush or retracted stoma, multiple stomas, presence of an umbilical cord, and a small abdomen with limited pouching surface often lead to multiple daily pouch changes. An appropriate goal for these infants may be a 12- to a 24-hour wear time. Normal wear time for infants with established stomas is 2 to 3 days. Older children can generally go 3 to 5 days between pouch changes. Activity level, amount of perspiration, abdominal contours, anatomic location of the stoma, and volume and consistency of effluent all influence wear time. Some children, particularly adolescents, do all they can to prolong the life of their pouch because of a strong dislike of changing their appliance. Provided there is not a leak, and the stoma and surrounding skin remain in good condition, they can safely extend the interval between pouch changes. However, they should be encouraged to change their appliance at least every 7 days in order to inspect the stoma and the peristomal skin.

Personal preference often causes children to change their pouches before they show signs of deterioration. Although intact pouches contain effluent completely and are odor proof when they are closed, some people feel cleaner if their pouch is changed every 2 to 3 days. Anticipatory changing can also be useful. For example, if a child's pouch tends to leak on the fourth day, it can routinely be changed every third day to avoid accidents at inconvenient times. Finally, planned times for pouch changes can make the routine more convenient. The best time for a family to spend time on a pouch change may be after the evening bath, when the pressing responsibilities of a busy schedule are winding down. Alternately, it may be easier to change the pouch when stoma output is minimal, such as in the morning after awakening and before eating, or 2 to 3 hours after a meal.

Regardless of anticipated wear time, pouches should be changed immediately if they leak. Never patch a leaking appliance because stool can quickly damage the peristomal skin. Signs of leakage include odor from a closed pouch, visible erosion of the skin barrier around the stoma, or effluent on clothing or bedding with a pouch that is still closed.

Removing a Pouch

Before removing the pouch on a new stoma, be aware of the presence of any devices in or around the stoma. Patients sometimes return from surgery with a temporary device in their stoma, such as a retention ring or rod to support a loop ostomy, or a stent to support a ureteral anastomosis. These devices are removed when the incisions have healed. Pouching techniques require modification to incorporate these devices into the pouch.

Pouches should never be pulled off, because aggressive removal can traumatize peristomal skin. Before removing, empty the pouch to prevent spilling the effluent. Use a damp cloth or paper towel to help separate an edge of the skin barrier from the skin, or rub a finger inward over the edge to curl up an edge. Gently lift the skin barrier with one hand while pushing the skin down and away from the skin barrier with a finger or a damp cloth held in the other hand. Work your way around the entire skin barrier, loosening it to the stoma. If the pouch has a tape border, the tape can be lifted in the same manner. This method of pouch removal is time consuming, but preserving skin integrity beneath the pouch is critical for proper adhesion of the next pouch.

If the skin barrier adheres aggressively to the skin or if there is hair on the skin, adhesive remover may be required. Once the pouch has been removed, wash the peristomal skin and stoma with warm water and a soft cloth or soft paper towels. The use of soap is not generally necessary. If adhesive remover was used, however, the residue should be removed with soap and water because adhesive remover is not water soluble. Adhesive remover should be used with caution on small infants because of the risk of percutaneous absorption. Although every remnant of skin barrier does *not* need to be scrubbed from the skin before application of the next pouch, all effluent should be removed so that it does not harm the skin. If soap is used, it should not contain moisturizers, and the skin should be rinsed thoroughly with water before the pouch is reapplied. Moisturizers in commercial infant wipes may impede pouch adhesion.

Stomas do not contain pain fibers, so cleaning around the stoma should not hurt once the incision is healed. The stoma is very vascular, and it is normal for it to bleed slightly with manipulation. Only continuous bleeding from the stoma, from the stoma lumen, or from the incision needs to be reported to the surgeon. When the stoma is active—in other words, produces effluent during pouch changing—soft paper towels, gauze, or a small cloth can be wrapped around the stoma to prevent effluent from getting on cleaned skin. Dry the skin well before applying the new pouch. Although hair dryers have sometimes been recommended for this purpose, they can burn the skin and should be used with caution (Deans, Slater, & Goldfarb, 1990), and then only on the "cool" setting.

Pouch changing time is a good time to assess the stoma. Important observations to be made during the stomal assessment are included in Table 8-4. These observations should be documented on the patient record while the patient is in the hospital. The family should continue assessing the stoma after discharge, although they do not need to record this information.

Preparing a New Pouch

In the case of a child having more than one stoma, the stomas can generally be pouched within the same appliance. For example, a mucous fistula positioned close to a proximal stoma is easily pouched together with the proximal stoma. However, there are notable times when stomas must be pouched separately. Fecal and urinary stomas are always pouched using separate appliances, except at the discretion of the surgeon. A proximal stoma may require a separate pouch from the mucous fistula if crossover of stool from the proximal to the distal bowel must be avoided, such as after repair of a high anorectal malfor-

Table 8-4	Assessing the Stoma

Observations of stomal integrity and function should include

1. What color is the stoma?
2. Does the stoma protrude or retract? How far? Is this a change?
3. Is there a stomal laceration (white line near base of the stoma)?
4. Is there excessive bleeding? If so, where and how much?
5. Is the mucocutaneous junction intact? If not, where is the separation, how long, and how deep?
6. What is the condition of the peristomal skin?
7. What are the volume, color, and consistency of the effluent?

mation. If questions arise when multiple stomas are pouched, the surgeon should be consulted.

Because most children use cut-to-fit pouches, the first step in applying a new pouch is cutting the aperture to fit the stoma. The skin barrier should fit up to the mucocutaneous junction in order to avoid exposing skin to damaging effluent. The skin barrier is soft when warmed and does not harm the stoma if it is fitted properly. The aperture should not be smaller than the skin-level diameter of the stoma, or part of the stoma will be trapped under the skin barrier, resulting in a poor fit and potentially lacerating the stoma.

Using the measuring guide that comes with every box of ostomy pouches, measure the stoma diameter at the mucocutaneous junction. Trace the pattern onto the paper backing of the skin barrier, and cut the aperture with blunt-tipped scissors to avoid puncturing the front of the pouch. Before removing the paper backing, place the skin barrier over the stoma to test the size, and trim to fit. Irregular or oval stomas require custom fitting. The paper backing can be saved as a template for the next pouch change, but keep in mind that stomas decrease in size over the weeks following surgery and grow as children grow. A template needs to be compared regularly to the stoma(s) and modified accordingly before cutting the pouch.

An appliance may better fit a child's abdomen if the aperture is not cut directly in the center of the skin barrier. To shift the pouch away from a crease in the groin or the iliac crest, for example, the aperture needs to be cut either below the center of the skin barrier (to raise the pouch above a crease) or to the right or left of the skin barrier center (to shift the pouch away from a bony prominence). When the placement of the aperture is modified away from center, the aperture must include the starter hole or the starter hole must be covered with a piece of skin barrier so that effluent does not come in contact with the skin in that area.

Preparing the Pouching Surface

A pouch adheres more securely to the abdomen if the area around the stoma is level. Ostomy products can be used to level the irregularities of the peristomal plane. Pieces of skin barrier supplement washers, or strips can be used to fill creases in the skin or can be positioned circumferentially around a stoma to level the peristomal plane and to protect from undermining (leakage) of effluent under the skin barrier.

Ostomy paste, a softened skin barrier that comes in a tube, can also be used to level the peristomal plane. Because of the strong adhesiveness and alcohol content of ostomy paste, its use is generally reserved for older children. Ostomy paste is not meant to be used as an adhesive and should *never* be spread over the entire skin barrier to improve adhesion. Similar to skin barrier supplement washers and strips (see Table 8-3), ostomy paste should be used to fill irregularities in the pouching surface. When the paste is applied circumferentially around the aperture, the mouth of the tube of paste can be held close to and perpendicular to the skin barrier as the paste is squeezed out. This creates a flat strip of paste and minimizes the amount of paste coming out of the tube. Because ostomy paste dissolves in the presence of urine, it is not recommended in areas that may come in contact with urine.

Occasionally, ostomy paste may be more effective than skin barrier supplements on infants. Although it should not be used as a first-line product, use of ostomy paste may be preferable to sustaining skin damage from undermining of effluent. When ostomy paste is used on infants, application can be minimized by squeezing paste into a syringe and applying the paste in a thin line directly from the syringe. To do this, remove the plunger from a small, needleless syringe. Squeeze paste into the barrel of the syringe and replace the plunger. Ostomy paste should be used only when wear time is expected to be at least 24 to 48 hours. Oils and moisture from the skin begin to loosen the adhesion of the ostomy paste and help make pouch removal less traumatic.

Applying the Pouch

The skin barrier of a pouch molds to the skin more easily if it is warmed before application. It can be warmed between the hands or against the skin for a minute or two before it is placed on the child. Alternately, if an infant is being pouched, the new pouch can be placed beneath the infant, allowing the skin barrier to be warmed by body heat while the old pouch is removed and the peristomal surface is prepared. Warming under a radiant warmer poses a risk of overheating the skin barrier and burning the skin on application.

When a new pouch is applied, the peristomal skin should be completely dry. Before making contact with the skin, angle the pouch so the tail points in the desired direction. Check the stoma to be sure that no part of it is trapped under the skin barrier. Press the skin barrier onto the skin, starting from the stoma and moving outward, smoothing out wrinkles and securing good contact with the skin. Warm the skin barrier for a minute or two by placing one or both hands over the pouch, and press the skin barrier firmly onto the skin. This is a good activity for the children themselves to perform. Warmth and pressure ensure good contact between the skin barrier and the skin and can make a significant difference in wear time. If pouch adhesion is a problem, children may need to avoid strenuous activities for 15 to 30 minutes after applying the pouch. This quiet time allows the skin barrier to warm and enhance its adhesion to the skin. See Table 8-5 for a brief review of the procedure for changing a child's appliance.

Managing a Stoma without a Pouch

Fecal Stoma

Fecal ostomies are sometimes cared for without a pouch. Parents may choose to maintain their infant's stoma by di-apering because they do not want to bother with a pouch. Small infants may not maintain a pouch seal because of immature skin, or because of denuded and weepy peristomal skin. Measures can be instituted to protect and heal the skin until pouching is once more an option. Generally, it is safer to use a nonpouching method with colostomies than with small-bowel stomas. Stool from the small bowel contains proteolytic enzymes that are damaging to the skin.

There are several options for protecting intact skin from effluent when a nonpouching approach is used for stoma care. One option is to apply an alcohol-free skin sealant to the peristomal skin once a day. Another option is to maintain a layer of petrolatum-, dimethicone-, or zinc-oxide–based barrier (diaper rash) ointment on the skin around the stoma. A combination of the two options, with the skin sealant first being covered over with barrier ointment, can be used if skin irritation develops. If the stoma is positioned low on the abdomen, an oversized diaper usually can contain the effluent. On a small, hospitalized infant on bed rest, fluffed gauze can be placed around the stoma to collect effluent. The gauze can be weighed for an approximate idea of output.

Most over-the-counter barrier ointments do not adhere to skin that has become denuded and weepy. Ostomy powder, a powdered form of the ingredient in skin barriers, can be dusted over denuded areas and barrier ointment applied over the powder. Ostomy powder absorbs moisture from denuded skin and improves adherence of the ointment. Several commercially manufactured barrier ointments are formulated to adhere to damaged or denuded skin and are listed in Table 8-6. Many of these commercial products contain ingredients similar to those in ostomy powder and can be used in place of petrolatum- or zinc oxide–based ointments.

Barrier ointments do not need to be removed and replaced at each diaper change, or even daily. Barrier

Table 8-5	Steps for Changing an Ostomy Pouch
1.	Empty pouch.
2.	Remove pouch: lift skin barrier while pushing skin down and away from barrier.
3.	Clean skin with soft cloth and warm water. Dry well.
4.	Assess stoma and skin.
5.	Measure stoma and cut aperture to size.
6.	Level irregular pouching surface with skin barrier strips, washers, paste.
7.	Remove paper backing from skin barrier and apply pouch over stoma.
8.	Firmly press skin barrier into place from inner to outer edge.
9.	Close pouch tail with pouch closure.
10.	Apply warmth and pressure to skin barrier for 1 to 2 minutes.

Table 8-6	Barrier Products for Severely Irritated Skin	
Manufacturer	**Product[a]**	**Caution**
Boudreaux, Dr. George L., P.D.	Boudreaux's Butt Paste	Contains boric acid Not for use on small infants
Calmoseptine, Inc.	Calmoseptine Ointment	
Coloplast Corporation	Critic-Aid Anorectal Skin Paste	
ConvaTec	Sensi-Care Protective; Barrier Skin; Protectant	
Healthpoint, Ltd.	Xenaderm	Prescription; contains balsam of Peru (capillary stimulant) and trypsin (mild débrider); anecdotal experience in children only
Johnson & Johnson	Previcare Extra Protective Ointment	
3M Health Care	Cavilon Durable Barrier Cream	Do not use with denuded skin Pouch and tape adhere better when cream applied sparingly to underlying skin
Medcon Bio Lab Technologies, Inc.	Ilex Skin Protectant Paste	Petrolatum layer over top decreases sticking to diaper
Smith & Nephew	Secura Extra Protective Cream (EPC)	Contains karaya

[a]Remove adhesive ointments with mineral oil to avoid causing skin damage.

ointment does not damage skin and in fact, protects the skin from damaging contact with stool and urine. When changing the diaper, wipe stool from the surface of the barrier ointment gently and reapply barrier ointment where needed. Scrubbing to remove the barrier ointment may damage the skin. If barrier ointment must be removed, a cotton ball soaked in mineral oil or baby oil dissolves the barrier ointment. Commercial barrier ointments can stick to diapers aggressively, requiring reapplication of the barrier ointment with every diaper change. A light dusting of ostomy powder or a coating of petrolatum on top of the barrier ointment minimizes its tack.

Urinary Stoma

Urinary diversions on infants are frequently maintained without a pouch. Ureterostomies are flush with the skin, and vesicostomies are low on the abdomen. Both types of stomas are difficult to pouch, so effluent is usually contained in a child's diaper. Basic skin care during diaper changes and a barrier ointment are usually adequate to manage a nonpouched urostomy. Skin around the stoma can be protected with petrolatum. To contain urine and to protect the child's clothing, the diaper may need to be larger than the size the child would normally wear. Urinary stomas above the diaper line, such as pyelostomies, may require a urinary pouch. If acceptable to the surgeon, the pouch can be left open at the bottom and allowed to drain continuously into the diaper.

Mucous Fistula

A mucous fistula that is positioned close to the functional stoma can be pouched within the same appliance as the proximal stoma. Mucous fistulas that are not conveniently near the proximal stoma do not generally need to be pouched. However, they must be protected from drying and trauma. An infant under a radiant warmer, for example, should have the mucous fistula covered with a nonadherent dressing. Water-soluble lubricant can be applied, if needed, to keep the gauze from adhering to the stoma. Petrolatum-impregnated gauze may loosen adhesion of the pouch and is generally not used once pouching is instituted. The mucous fistula on an infant can often be left uncovered inside a diaper. If it becomes irritated or becomes a play object of the infant, the mucous fistula may need to be covered with a small dressing or adhesive bandage.

Beyond Basic Ostomy Care: Managing Complications

Sometimes, caring for an ostomy requires skills beyond the basic ostomy care skills discussed in the previous paragraphs. Complications following ostomy surgery are surprisingly common, often exceeding 50% (Chandramouli, Srinivasan, Jagdish, & Ananthakrishnan, 2004; Gauderer, 1998; Patwardhan, Kiely, Drake, Spitz, & Pierro, 2001). Consequently, nurses caring for children with ostomies should be prepared to identify and manage some of the common complications. These include laceration of the stoma, mucocutaneous separation, stomal necrosis, obstruction, peristomal hernia, peristomal skin breakdown and infection, and prolapse and retraction of the stoma. Suggestions for nursing management of common ostomy challenges are included in this section.

Stomal Complications

Laceration

Lacerations can occur when a stoma is traumatized. A laceration appears as a white or yellow line in the stomal mucosa, usually at the base of the stoma. Bleeding is unusual but, if present, can usually be managed by applying pressure until hemostasis is achieved. Pain is not usually a clue to the presence of a laceration because the stoma does not contain pain fibers. Most often, lacerations are shallow, and identifying and correcting the cause allow it to heal without treatment.

Impact to the stoma during sports, although rare, can lacerate the stoma. However, sports participation is strongly encouraged among children with ostomies. During activities in which high-impact contact with the stoma is a possibility, protective padding should be placed over the stoma. Occasionally, adolescents with heavy body hair can achieve good contact between the skin and skin barrier only by shaving of the peristomal hair. Clipping excess hair with scissors or removing hair with an electric razor is preferable to using a straight-edge razor, but any hair removal should be performed with caution near the stoma.

Pouching equipment is by far the most common cause of stomal laceration. An aperture that is smaller than the diameter of the stoma can trap part of the stoma under the skin barrier during pouch application or can cut into the stoma at its point of contact with the stoma. This is a mistake most commonly made in caring for infants, for whom caregivers continue to use the same aperture pattern they were given in the hospital, despite growth of the stoma as the infant has grown. Weekly measurement of the stoma in growing children allows correction to be made in the size of the aperture as the stoma grows. When a two-piece pouch is used, an elongated or prolapsed stoma can be pinched within the plastic flange when the two pieces of the pouch are connected, causing a laceration. Alternately, a prolapsed stoma can hang over the plastic flange of a two-piece pouch and sustain a laceration if the stoma is pinched between the clothing and the flange. Change to a one-piece pouch may be required.

Mucocutaneous Separation

During surgical creation of a stoma, the bowel is brought through an incision in the abdominal wall, everted to form a matured stoma, and sutured to the skin. This suture line, called the *mucocutaneous junction*, heals in a week or two. Excessive tension on the suture line before healing can cause dehiscence of the suture line known as *mucocutaneous separation*. Conditions favoring the development of mucocutaneous separation include obesity and those resulting in poor wound healing, such as corticosteroid therapy, malnutrition, and diabetes. Separation can occur over a small area of the mucocutaneous junction or involve the entire circumference of the stoma.

Treatment of a mucocutaneous separation is comparable to the treatment of any wound. The wound or defect in the suture line should be kept clean, moist, and protected from effluent. During pouch changes, the defect should be irrigated thoroughly with normal saline to remove stool and debris. The wound can then be filled with an absorptive substance, such as ostomy powder, or a soft, absorptive wound dressing, to absorb drainage from the wound and to level the pouching surface. If the defect is large, a piece of solid skin barrier or a hydrocolloid dressing can be cut to fit closely around the stoma and placed over the filled defect to cover it. Before applying the pouch, a "bead" or strip of ostomy paste can be applied around the stoma to prevent effluent from tunneling under the dressing and into the wound. The stoma can then be pouched. The aperture of the pouch should not be enlarged to incorporate the mucocutaneous separation within the aperture. The mucocutaneous separation gradually fills with granulation tissue and becomes skin covered.

Necrosis

Stoma necrosis results from ischemia of the stoma. It is most often noticed within the first 24 hours following surgery, although it may occur as many as 3 to 5 days after surgery. The color of an ischemic stoma varies from dark red to purple to black, and the stoma feels flaccid. Necrosis can involve the entire stoma or just a small area. Ischemia leading to necrosis of the stoma can result from surgical technique, tension on the mesentery, or trauma to the stoma during surgery (Barr, 2004; Colwell, 2004). Necrosis of the stoma occurs more frequently in obese patients and in those who are acutely ill. Because of this, neonates with a diseased bowel are often left unpouched for the first 24 to 48 hours after surgery so the stoma can be observed (Quigley et al., 2003). Surgical consultation is required if stomal necrosis occurs, and reoperation may be necessary. If necrosis does not extend to the fascia, however, surgical intervention is not indicated, and close observation and gentle handling of the stoma may be all that is required. Necrotic stomal mucosa eventually sloughs. Stenosis or retraction of the stoma is common after healing of a stoma with extensive necrosis.

Obstruction

Mechanical obstruction of the bowel proximal to the stoma with fibrous food is a problem specific to ileostomies. Bulky, nondigestible residue from high-fiber foods can become lodged in the lumen of the small intestine at the point at which the ileostomy angles upward toward the stoma. Inadequate chewing of food, inadequate fluid intake while eating, and eating large volumes of high-fiber food all contribute to obstruction. Symptoms are acute and include abdominal pain and cramping, abdominal distention, nausea, and vomiting. High-pitched bowel sounds occur early in the obstruction as the bowel attempts to push its contents past the obstruction, but become hypoactive as the bowel becomes distended and atonic. Stool and gas output from the stoma are minimal or absent. The stoma may swell.

If a patient shows signs of an obstruction while still in the hospital, he or she should be given nothing by mouth (NPO), and the surgeon should be notified immediately. At home, caretakers can institute the following measures to relieve the obstruction for a short time if the child is otherwise stable before calling the surgeon or going to the emergency room. Intake of all solid food should be discontinued. If the child is not vomiting, having him or her drink warm, clear liquids sometimes help the obstruction to pass. The child can be placed into a warm bath in a knee-chest position. The abdomen can be gently massaged. The pouch should be removed if the stoma becomes edematous. If the pouch is replaced, the aperture should be enlarged to accommodate the enlarged stoma. Notify the surgeon within an hour if the blockage does not pass or immediately, if symptoms progress, or if the child is in severe pain or is vomiting.

The problem of food obstruction is best managed preemptively, with education before hospital discharge. Teach children to eat slowly and to chew their food thoroughly. Drinking adequate fluids during meals helps flush food through the bowel. Postoperatively, high-fiber foods should be introduced into the diet one at a time and in small amounts to test the patient's tolerance of each food item. Surgeons may have specific foods that they recommend patients avoid for the duration of their ileostomy, such as popcorn and nuts. However, most foods are well tolerated if precautions are followed.

Bowel obstruction following stoma surgery can be caused by etiologies other than food blockage. Adhesions from previous abdominal surgeries are a common cause of small-bowel obstruction. Bowel strictures resulting from Crohn's disease, necrotizing enterocolitis, and other bowel diseases can result in complete or near-complete bowel obstruction. Adynamic obstruction, or ileus, results from loss of peristalsis rather than blockage and can occur with illness, infection, following narcotic administration or abdominal surgery, or with severe electrolyte imbalance (Turnbull, 2003). Bowel obstruction is an emergency, and patients must call the surgeon and seek medical care quickly. Untreated obstruction can result in significant fluid and electrolyte shifts and bowel perforation.

Prolapse

Prolapse of a stoma occurs when the bowel telescopes out through the lumen. Prolapse can be continuous or it can be intermittent, retracting when a child is quiet. It can occur with any fecal stoma, but it happens more frequently from the nonfunctioning lumen of a loop ostomy (Barr, 2004; Minkes & Langer, 2000; Weber, 2003). One of the suspected etiologies of stomal prolapse is the presence of a large defect in the fascia. This occurs when the bowel decreases in size after surgery. Poor support of the fascia is another cause of prolapse and occurs when a stoma placed outside the rectus muscle or through weak abdominal muscles, such as with premature infants. Increased intra-abdominal pressure from forceful coughing, crying, or pregnancy is also thought to contribute to prolapse.

If the prolapse does not progress and the bowel remains well perfused with good output, neither reduction nor surgical correction of the prolapse is attempted. Given the temporary nature of stomas in children, additional surgeries are avoided if possible, and closure of the stoma corrects the problem. Until stoma takedown, however, the prolapsed bowel is at risk of ischemia, obstruction, bleeding, and trauma, and the stoma must be monitored closely.

Measures must be instituted to protect a prolapsed stoma. A pouch can damage a prolapsed stoma, so the pouching system should be reevaluated. A larger and longer pouch may be required to accommodate the length of the stoma. Use of two-piece pouches with plastic flanges should be discontinued. There is a risk of strangulation of the stoma inside the plastic flanges, as well as laceration of the stoma if it becomes trapped between the two flanges or between the flange and clothing.

The stoma diameter may also be wider than it was before the prolapse, and a larger skin barrier may be needed to accommodate the wider stoma. The aperture, when cut to fit over the widest part of the stoma, may not cover all peristomal skin. This leaves skin exposed to effluent. An aperture sized to fit the skin-level diameter of the stoma can be cut in the center of a sheet of hydrocolloid (skin barrier) dressing. A slit cut from the aperture to the outer edge of the hydrocolloid dressing allows the dressing to be placed around the stoma to cover exposed skin. The pouch is then applied over the top. A skin barrier supplement can also be used to cover exposed skin. Alternately, the aperture can be cut to fit the circumference of the stoma at skin level, and radial slits can be made around the circumference of the aperture (Fig. 8-4). Radial slits in the skin barrier allow the aperture to expand as it is placed over the stoma and to fit up to the mucocutaneous junction when flush with the skin. The skin beneath the radial slits must be protected from effluent leaking beneath the slits by placing either a skin barrier supplement or a thin layer of ostomy paste on the skin beneath the radial slits.

Retraction

Retraction of a stoma occurs when the stoma is pulled back below skin level. Complete retraction occurs when the stoma descends below the level of the fascia and is a surgical emergency. If retraction is incomplete, and the stoma continues to function, however, no surgical intervention is required. Retraction can occur with excessive tension on the mesentery and occurs commonly in obese children who have a thick abdominal wall. It can also occur with premature removal of the retention ring in a loop stoma or after healing of a large mucocutaneous separation. Stoma necrosis can result in retraction if a large area of the stoma is involved.

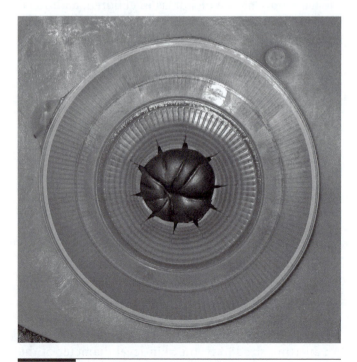

FIGURE 8-4 Radial slits around aperture of a skin barrier.

Patients with retracted stomas have problems with persistent leakage under the skin barrier, shortened pouch wear time, and peristomal skin breakdown (Barr, 2004). These problems occur because the stoma does not protrude beyond the skin and is therefore unable to project effluent into the pouch. To maintain a secure pouch seal, pouching techniques require modification. A convex skin barrier can help push the stoma out beyond the skin and project effluent forward into the pouch, especially on an obese patient. An ostomy belt can be added to a convex pouch to exert pressure on the pouch and improve contact between the skin barrier and the skin. A bead of ostomy paste applied around the aperture or an adhesive agent applied to the skin barrier may be required to improve pouch adherence. A skin sealant, applied to the skin before pouch application, may be needed to protect peristomal skin from effluent. Absorption crystals or cotton balls may need to be added to the pouch to thicken the stool and decrease the chance of leakage.

Small infants present a difficult problem in maintaining pouch seal with a retracted stoma. A piece of skin barrier supplement rolled into a rope and placed around the aperture of a pouch can provide a small amount of convexity. Leveling the pouching surface to ensure good pouch adherence is imperative. This is one of the situations in infants in which ostomy paste may be needed to prevent tunneling of effluent beneath the pouch. Frequent pouch changes may also be needed to observe peristomal skin, and if skin breakdown occurs, a nonpouching option can be used.

Peristomal Complications

Hernia

A peristomal hernia, also called a *parastomal hernia*, occurs when the defect in the fascia is larger than the bowel. The excess space between the fascial ring and the bowel allows another loop of bowel to herniate through the fascia and enter the subcutaneous layer of skin. This creates a bulge in the skin adjacent to the stoma. When the child lies down, the bulge often disappears, as the bowel reduces into the abdomen.

One of the common causes of peristomal hernias in children is a decrease in the size of the bowel after ostomy surgery. This situation can occur in delayed diagnosis of Hirschsprung's disease, for example, when the proximal bowel has become grossly distended due to inadequate passage of stool beyond the aganglionic or diseased segment of bowel. Once the bowel obstruction is relieved, the bowel decompresses and returns to its normal size, leaving behind a large defect in the fascia.

Placement of a stoma outside the rectus muscle and immaturity of abdominal muscles also contribute to the development of peristomal hernias. This is common in premature infants who undergo emergency surgery for necrotizing enterocolitis. The fragile viability of the diseased bowel limits the surgeon's choice of stoma location. Less-than-optimal stoma location, combined with weak abdominal muscles and increased abdominal pressure from crying, feeding, and bowel distention, predispose preterm infants to development of peristomal hernias. Other factors contributing to peristomal hernia formation include infection of the mucocutaneous junction, significant weight gain or loss, and suboptimal surgical technique (Gray, Colwell, & Goldberg, 2005).

The bulge created by a peristomal hernia causes problems in applying and maintaining the seal of an ostomy appliance. Furthermore, the herniated bowel is at risk of becoming incarcerated in the hernia sac. However, because stomas in children are generally temporary, peristomal hernias are not repaired surgically unless the bowel becomes incarcerated. Instead, they are managed clinically until the stoma can be closed.

Nursing management of peristomal hernias includes adaptation of the pouching system and education of the family regarding complications. A flexible pouch should be used to pouch a stoma with a peristomal hernia. Flexibility allows the skin barrier to mold to the contours of the bulge created by the hernia. A one-piece pouch is generally used in this situation. If the stoma is observed to enlarge when the hernia sac is enlarged, radial slits can be made in the skin barrier to allow expansion of the aperture and prevent constriction of the stoma. The skin beneath the radial slits must be protected from effluent by application of a skin barrier supplement or a thin layer of ostomy passed directly beneath the radial slits. Convexity is not used to manage a peristomal hernia. The addition of an ostomy belt, or alternately a hernia belt on a child beyond infancy, may help stabilize the pouch on the uneven surface created by the hernia.

Skin Breakdown

Skin beneath a pouch can sustain damage in several ways, including mechanical trauma, exposure to chemicals or irritants, allergy to ostomy products, and skin infection. In order to treat the problem, the cause of the skin breakdown must be identified. Mechanical trauma of peristomal skin is usually caused by improper removal of the pouch. Proper technique for pouch removal must be followed with every pouch change. Adhesive agents, such as ostomy paste, can result in damage to the epidermis during removal of the appliance, particularly on a child with fragile skin or one requiring frequent pouch changes. Once skin is denuded, pouch adhesion is difficult to achieve, predisposing to undermining and compounding skin breakdown. Adhesive agents should be reserved for those instances in which pouch wear time for a child is unacceptably short with the use of basic pouching techniques. On premature infants, the decision to use ostomy paste should be made on an individual basis, but in any case, it should be used with extreme caution because of the risk of epidermal stripping and percutaneous absorption of ingredients.

Chemical or irritant dermatitis results from exposure of the skin either to chemicals or to effluent. Ostomy products containing chemicals include adhesive remover, skin sealant, ostomy paste, and soap. These products should be used on an "as needed" basis. Products used for dissolving adhesives or cleaning the skin should be thoroughly removed from the skin before pouching. Products that are designed to remain on the skin beneath the pouch, such as skin sealant, should be allowed to dry completely before reapplication of the pouch.

Undermining of effluent beneath a skin barrier exposes skin to damaging fecal enzymes and can occur for many reasons. An aperture can be cut too small for a stoma, redirecting effluent beneath the skin barrier. It can also be cut too large for the stoma, leaving skin exposed. The skin barrier can dissolve with exposure to effluent, particularly liquid effluent, leaving the peristomal skin exposed. Improper placement of either the pouch (too close to the bend of the leg or waistline) or the stoma (too close to anatomic landmarks) can result in difficulty with pouch adhesion. An irregular pouching surface that has not been leveled properly will not hold a pouch well. Excessive perspiration or oil on the skin can loosen the skin barrier. Finally, a very active child, or one who plays with the pouch, may pose challenges to pouch adhesion.

If dermatitis is discovered beneath the skin barrier, check to be sure that the aperture is sized correctly. The location of the aperture may need to be changed to shift the pouch away from bendable areas of the body. Examination of the skin barrier, when removed, may reveal areas where leakage is occurring. Watch the child while the pouch is off, in a lying, sitting, and standing position, to determine whether the peristomal skin surface changes with movement and needs to be leveled differently. Sometimes, skin folds or creases can be seen during these maneuvers that may not be noted in the supine position. Bending the legs of an infant up toward the abdomen can help define abdominal creases.

The skin barrier can be changed to an extended-wear skin barrier or can be reinforced with the addition of a skin barrier supplement around the aperture. The pouch can be changed to a more flexible one-piece style, or alternately to a less flexible two-piece appliance. Absorption crystals or cotton balls may need to be added to the pouch to sequester liquid in the stool and decrease the chance of leakage. Excessive perspiration or oil can be absorbed with a light dusting of ostomy powder. Patting skin sealant over the powder helps seal in the powder and improves pouch adhesion. The pouch of an active child can be supported with the addition of an ostomy belt. Some children tuck their appliances into stretchy, biker-style shorts to support the pouch during sports to help prevent disruption of the pouch seal.

Allergy to the skin barrier or other ostomy products is easily identified because the shape of the skin reaction matches the shape of the skin barrier. Not all skin barriers are alike, and generally, switching to a different brand of product resolves the allergy. As always, limit use of products under the skin barrier to the absolute essentials for maintaining adequate pouch adhesion.

Skin infection is usually caused by yeast. *Candida* commonly colonizes the skin and can proliferate on moist skin beneath a pouch. Cutaneous candidiasis can be identified by the presence of a bright red papular or pustular rash with satellite lesions, accompanied by itching. Often, the skin is denuded and weepy, creating difficulty maintaining a pouch seal. Treatment requires application of a topical antifungal powder. Antifungal creams are avoided because they can impair adhesion of the pouch. Antifungal powder is sprinkled lightly onto the rash and spread evenly with a gloved finger. If the skin is moist, ostomy powder can be sprinkled over the antifungal powder. For the first day or two after treatment, antifungal powder should be applied once a day, or with each pouch change if more frequent than daily. As the rash improves, the frequency of pouch removal with application of antifungal powder can be decreased to every other day. Occasionally, a fungal infection is serious enough for oral antifungal agents to be considered.

Complication of Stoma Closure: Perianal Dermatitis

Takedown or closure of a stoma does not necessarily signal an end to complications but often brings about its own complication of severe perianal dermatitis. This complication is particularly reported in children with Hirschsprung's disease (Cano, Briones, Jové, & Rodellas, 1994; Rodriguez-Poblador, González-Castro, Herranz-Martínez, & Luelmo-Aguilar, 1998; Tamaki & Yokomori, 1987). Although this condition is not fully understood, there are several factors that may contribute to perianal dermatitis after stoma closure. Perianal skin is poorly prepared for its initial exposure to stool. Before stoma takedown, a child may never have passed stool through the anus, or months may have passed since the child's last stool contacted perianal skin. Skin that has not been exposed to stool is thought to be more sensitive to its damaging effect than is skin that has been repeatedly exposed. Decreased stool transit time from postoperative bowel edema and inflammation, as well as loss of bowel during surgery, can result in malabsorption and stool that contains more bile salts, fecal enzymes, and a higher pH than normal stool (Lund, 1999).

After a child's stoma is taken down and before his or her first stool is passed, measures should be instituted to protect perianal skin from exposure to stool. A continuous barrier of petrolatum-, dimethicone-, or zinc oxide–based barrier ointment should be maintained around the anus. If perianal skin breakdown occurs, ostomy powder can be sprinkled over excoriated areas and a barrier ointment applied over the top. Alternately, a commercial barrier ointment can be applied to denuded skin (Table 8-6). These products do not require routine removal from the skin but can be left in place and reapplied as needed. To prevent commercial barrier ointments from sticking to the diaper, they can be covered with a layer of petrolatum or sprinkled with ostomy powder. If removal of the barrier ointment is desired to assess skin integrity or to air dry the perineum, a cotton ball soaked with mineral oil or baby oil can be used to dissolve the ointment.

Children who are not toilet trained should have their diapers changed promptly to limit exposure to urine or stool. Perianal cleansing should be performed gently, with patting rather than rubbing of the skin and avoidance of harsh soaps. If perianal skin is already painfully excoriated, a squeeze or spray bottle filled with warm water can be used to rinse away stool and urine. A mineral oil–soaked cotton ball can be used to remove dried stool. Compresses of Burow's solution can be applied to soothe inflamed skin and to help dry exudate. Burow's solution contains aluminum salts and has a mild astringent effect (Sussman & Bates-Jensen, 2001). Irritated skin is at risk for developing secondary infection, particularly with *Candida albicans*. Any rash that develops on the perianal skin should be assessed and topical antifungal therapy instituted, if appropriate.

Teaching and Discharge Planning

Teaching Points

In order to continue care after discharge, children and their families need information and teaching related to the stoma and all of the aspects of life that will be touched by the presence of the child's ostomy. Frequently asked questions relate to bathing, appropriate clothing, dietary changes, medications, participation in sports and other activities, and managing the school attendance of a child who has an ostomy. Although space does not permit discussion of developmental considerations, ostomy care and teaching should always be appropriate to the developmental level of the child.

Bathing

Children who have a fecal ostomy can bathe or shower either with the pouch on or off. Bath water does not harm the stoma, nor is it harmful for water to enter the stoma. Many parents choose to give their child a bath while the pouch is off during a pouch change. During a shower, children can turn the showerhead so that the full force of the water is not aimed directly at the stoma. Soap should not contain moisturizers, because moisturizers prevent good adhesion of the skin barrier. The skin should be completely dry when the pouch is replaced. The skin barrier generally withstands soaking in the tub for short periods, if the child bathes with the pouch in place, but it can be bordered with waterproof tape before bathing if the edges tend to lift during the bath. The pouch should be dried thoroughly after bathing to avoid maceration of the skin beneath the pouch. Hair driers on the "cool" setting can be used cautiously to dry the cloth backing that is present on some pouches, but they should be aimed away from the skin. The use of hair driers is not recommended with infants because of the risk of burning the skin (Deans et al., 1990). Bathing may be allowed with a urinary stoma if the water level is maintained below the level of the stoma. However, infants with a urostomy should receive the approval of the surgeon before being placed in a tub of water without wearing their pouch.

Clothing

Little modification is required to clothe a child with a stoma. The exception to this is in the postoperative period, when children with tender abdominal incisions are likely to be more comfortable wearing loose clothing. Infants and small children who play with or remove their pouches can be placed in one-piece snap-in-the-crotch shirts or overalls to keep their hands away from the pouch. Otherwise, any normal infant wear is acceptable. The pouch can be placed either inside or outside of an infant's diaper. However, urine in the diaper may erode the skin barrier, especially in the case of boys whose urine stream points up toward the pouch. The edge of the skin barrier inside the diaper can be reinforced with either waterproof

tape or transparent film dressing. Belts can be worn either above or beneath the stoma but should not be worn directly over the stoma. Many adolescent girls successfully continue to wear fitted clothing after ostomy surgery without causing problems to their stomas. A pouch that is inconspicuous under tailored clothing, such as a low-profile, one-piece pouch, can be worn discretely, and frequent pouch emptying prevents a tell-tale bulge.

Children with a urinary stoma who wear a pouch connect their pouch to a nighttime drainage system during sleep. Often, young children are restless sleepers and become entangled in the drainage tubing or kink the tubing so that it does not drain. The nighttime drainage tubing can be threaded through a leg of a child's pajama bottoms to prevent entanglement, and the drainage container can be positioned at the foot of the bed. A second option to stabilize the drainage tubing makes use of a pair of girl's tights or panty hose. Cut a leg off the tights at the level of the panty and remove the toe to create a long, stretchy tube. Pull the tube onto the child's leg, and thread the drainage tubing inside and up the length of the tube before connecting the drainage tubing to the pouch.

Dietary Considerations

Children with ostomies can usually resume their normal diets after ostomy surgery, with few exceptions. A child with an ileostomy is at risk for developing a food obstruction. Eating slowly, chewing food thoroughly, drinking adequate fluids with meals, and avoiding a large amount of high-fiber food at one sitting generally prevent this problem. Foods can affect stool consistency and gas production. Table 8-7 lists some common offending foods (Bryant & Fleischer, 2003; Erwin-Toth & Doughty, 1992; Floruta, 2001; Floruta, 2004).

The colon absorbs nine-tenths of the effluent that passes the ileocecal valve (Erwin-Toth & Doughty, 1992). Because a stoma causes stool to bypass part of this absorptive surface, fluid is lost in the effluent that would otherwise be reabsorbed. Furthermore, loss of the colon, as with an ileostomy, results in fluid and sodium losses two to three times that of normal (Minkes & Langer, 2000). Therefore, dehydration is a particular risk in a child with an ileostomy. Children must be taught to drink larger-than-normal volumes of fluids throughout the day, especially during hot weather or during illness. They are encouraged to keep a bottle of water or a sport drink with them during activities and school, so that they can continually replenish their fluids. Families must be taught the signs of dehydration, including increased thirst, dry mouth, concentrated or dark urine, decreased urine output, loss of appetite, lethargy or faint feeling, sunken eyes,

Table 8-7	Food Effects on Ostomy Output		
Gas and Odor	**Food Obstruction**	**Loosens Stool**	**Thickens Stool**
Asparagus	Apple skins	Apple or prune juice	Applesauce, unsweetened
Beans (dried, string)	Celery	Beans (dried, string)	Bananas
Broccoli	Chinese vegetables	Caffeine	Cheese (if no lactose
Cabbage	Citrus fruits	Chocolate	intolerance)
Carbonated drinks	Coconut	Citrus	Cooked carrots
Cauliflower	Corn	Milk (lactose intolerant)	Marshmallows
Cucumber	Dried fruits (raisins, dates)	Nuts	Oatmeal
Dairy products	Grapes	Popcorn	Pasta
Dried fruits	Meat casings (bologna, hot	Raw fruits and vegetables	Peanut butter
Eggs	dogs)	Refined sugar	Potatoes without the skin
Fish	Mushrooms	Spicy or greasy foods	Pretzels
Garlic	Nuts, peanuts	Sugar-free products containing	Rice
Onions	Pineapple	sorbitol and mannitol	Tapioca
Spicy foods	Popcorn		White bread
	Seeds from fruits and		Yogurt
	vegetables		

abdominal cramps, muscle cramps, and confusion as dehydration progresses. If children with a stoma, particularly an ileostomy, become ill and cannot drink adequately, the physician must be notified. Intravenous fluid replacement may be required.

Children with urostomies, like those with ileostomies, need to drink extra fluid throughout the day. Keeping the urine dilute helps maintain an acid pH of the urine to prevent bacterial growth, and it also flushes bacteria from the urinary tract. Families should be familiar with the symptoms of a urinary tract infection, including fever, strong-smelling urine, blood in the urine, cloudy urine, back pain, nausea or vomiting, confusion, and fatigue.

Medications

Administration of oral medications is an area of concern in children with an ileostomy. Because a large part of the bowel is bypassed, extended-release or enteric-coated medications may not be absorbed. The prescribing doctor and the pharmacist need to be alert to the fact that the child does not have a colon, and prompt-acting formulations, such as solutions, suspensions, gelatin capsules, and uncoated tablets should be prescribed (Turnbull, 2005). Never crush medications to speed absorption unless instructed to do so by a pharmacist.

Activities and School Attendance

After the convalescent period, stomas generally do not prevent children from doing the things they did before

surgery. Children with fecal ostomies can swim in a pool or lake with their pouches on. Those with a urinary stoma need to discuss swimming with their surgeon, and if this activity is approved, they are restricted to swimming in a chlorinated pool. Swimmers may prefer to wear a two-piece appliance. During swimming, a small, discrete, nondrainable pouch can be worn. After swimming, the pouch can be replaced with a larger, drainable model. Covering the edge of the skin barrier with waterproof tape or transparent film dressing before swimming helps extend the life of the skin barrier and helps prevent accidental dislodgment. When participating in contact sports, if the surgeon allows these activities, the stoma should be protected with padding. Rapid movements and perspiration during sporting activities can create challenges in maintaining a pouch seal. An ostomy belt or a hernia belt can be worn to stabilize the pouch during these activities. Biker-style shorts can also be worn to stabilize the pouch. Children can keep a change of clothing and pouching equipment on hand in case of a leak. The coach should be made aware of the child's ostomy, as with any medical condition.

Once children have recovered from their surgery and are at least competent in emptying their pouch, they can return to school. A change of clothing and pouching equipment should be kept in a backpack in the child's locker or in the school office. Teachers and the school nurse should be aware of a child's stoma, and the nurse or another adult at the school should receive instructions on caring for the ostomy should the child require assistance during school hours. However, planned pouch changes before anticipated times of leakage can help prevent the need for pouch changes at school. A private bathroom, such as the teacher's bathroom, should be designated as a place a child can go to attend to his or her ostomy privately. Room deodorizer and pouch deodorant (a deodorant placed into a pouch to decrease effluent odor) can be tucked into a child's backpack and used when emptying the pouch to minimize embarrassing odor. Some children prefer to use a nondrainable pouch at school. When the pouch requires emptying, the old pouch can be snapped off and a new pouch applied. The old pouch can be sealed in a plastic bag and disposed of. A pouch with a gas filter may be useful at school to allow the slow and inconspicuous release of gas from the pouch and to increase the time between emptying the pouch.

Planning for Discharge

Before the child goes home from the hospital, caregivers should be provided the opportunity to perform all aspects of caring for their child's ostomy. Older children should also be provided the opportunity to care for their stoma. Besides the survival skills discussed previously, important teaching points to be covered with the family before discharge include

- Reason for the surgery and the ostomy
- Usual pattern and consistency of stoma output
- Potential problems that may develop with the stoma
- Symptoms of dehydration and obstruction
- Guidelines for seeking medical care, including names and phone numbers of the surgeon and WOC nurse
- Guidelines for diet and medications
- Supplies needed in caring for the stoma, including where and how to obtain supplies
- Discussion on ways in which the stoma will affect family life and how they can be managed, including bathing, clothing, activity, school or day care arrangements, travel, sibling preparation, emotional adjustment, and any topic about which the family has questions

A discharge teaching sheet can be kept on the patient's chart as a guide to ensure that all necessary teaching is completed before discharge (see Appendix A).

Families can be given the opportunity to view videos of stoma care in the hospital and should receive a variety of educational materials to read before leaving the hospital. These materials go home with the family and can be referred to when questions arise and there are no health care professionals around to provide answers. A prescription for all ostomy supplies, with the diagnosis written on the script, should be provided to the family to ensure coverage by third party payers (Gill & Giordano, 2003). Home ostomy supplies should be arranged before discharge so that families do not have to wait to have their supplies delivered after discharge. Nevertheless, because delays can occur with insurance coverage or delivery of supplies, patients should be discharged with enough supplies for three pouch changes or at least 1 week, if their frequency of pouch changes in the hospital has been more often than every other day.

Short hospital stays result in little time for the family or child to become competent or comfortable with ostomy care skills. Home nursing visits can be helpful during the first week or two after discharge to reinforce ostomy care skills and to allow the family time to become comfortable with stoma care under the watchful eyes of an experienced nurse. Home visits should be arranged before the child is discharged.

■ Conclusion

Children generally adapt well to having a stoma. Families need to feel confident that they have learned the survival skills of caring for a stoma, that they will be able to obtain needed supplies, and that they will have resources at their disposal to seek help when they have questions or problems after discharge. Support and teaching by nurses can have a huge impact on the child's and the family's adaptation to the stoma, and to the unrestricted return to their life.

■ Acknowledgments

I would like to thank my daughter, Carolyn R. Rogers, who is a student at the University of Pittsburgh School of Medicine, for her persistence and hard work in creating the drawings in this chapter, all of which are her own original artwork.

I would also like to acknowledge Gail Garvin, for her many contributions toward advancing the care of children with ostomies and wounds, including authorship of the chapter Caring for Children with Ostomies and Wounds in the first edition of this textbook.

■ Educational Materials

APSNA invites you to download the diagnosis-related teaching tool "Ostomy" (available in English and Spanish) for Chapter 8 "Care of the Child with an Ostomy" at the APSNA Web site (www.apsna.org) and the Jones and Bartlett Web site (www.jbpub.com). All teaching materials are available free of charge and APSNA encourages their use for your patients and families.

References

Association of Women's Health, Obstetric and Neonatal Nurses, & National Association of Neonatal Nurses. (2001). *Evidence-based clinical practice guideline: Neonatal skin care*. Washington, DC: AWHONN.

Barr, J. E. (2004). Assessment and management of stomal complications: A framework for clinical decision making. *Ostomy Wound Management, 50*(9), 50–67.

Bass, E. M., Del Pino, A., Tan, A., Pearl, R. K., Orsay, C. P., & Abcarian, H. (1997). Does preoperative stoma marking and education by the enterostomal therapist affect outcome? *Diseases of Colon and Rectum, 40*(4), 440–442.

Bryant, D. E., & Fleischer, I. R. (2003). Routine management of the patient with an ostomy. In C. T. Milne, L. Q. Corbett, & D. L. Dubuc (Eds.), *Wound, ostomy, and continence nursing secrets* (pp. 308–318). Philadelphia: Hanley & Belfus.

Cano, L. R., Briones, V. G. P., Jové, R. P., & Rodellas, A. C. (1994). Perianal pseudoverrucous papules and nodules after surgery for Hirschsprung's disease. *The Journal of Pediatrics, 125*(6), 914–916.

Chandramouli, B., Srinivasan, K., Jagdish, S., & Ananthakrishnan, N. (2004). Morbidity and mortality of colostomy and its closure in children. *Journal of Pediatric Surgery, 39*(4), 596–599.

Colwell, J. C. (2004). Stomal and peristomal complications. In J. C. Colwell, M. T. Goldberg, & J. E. Carmel (Eds.), *Fecal & urinary diversions: Management principles* (pp. 308–325). St. Louis, MO: Mosby.

Darmstadt, G. L., & Dinulos, J. G. (2000). Neonatal skin care. *Pediatric Clinics of North America, 47*(4), 757–782.

Deans, L., Slater, H., & Goldfarb, I. W. (1990). Bad advice, bad burn: A new problem in burn prevention. *Journal of Burn Care Rehabilitation, 11*(6), 563–564.

Erwin-Toth, P., & Doughty, D. B. (1992). Principles and procedures of stomal management. In B. G. Hampton & R. A. Bryant (Eds.), *Ostomies and continent diversions: Nursing management* (pp. 29–104). St. Louis, MO: Mosby.

Floruta, C. V. (2001). Dietary choices of people with ostomies. *Journal of Wound, Ostomy, and Continence Nursing, 28*(1), 28–31.

Floruta, C. V. (2004). Nutritional resources. In J. C. Colwell, M. T. Goldberg, & J. E. Carmel (Eds.), *Fecal & urinary diversions: Management principles* (pp. 476–477). St. Louis, MO: Mosby.

Gauderer, M. W. L. (1998). Stomas of the small and large intestine. In J. A. O'Neill, M. I. Rowe, J. L. Grosfeld, E. W. Fonkalsrud, & A. G. Coran (Eds.), *Pediatric surgery* (5th ed., pp. 1349–1359). St. Louis, MO: Mosby.

Gill, F. T., & Giordano, K. H. (2003). Preparing children with special needs for discharge: Gastrointestinal tubes and stomas. In P. Mattei (Ed.), *Surgical directives: Pediatric surgery* (pp. 19–24). Philadelphia: Lippincott Williams & Wilkins.

Gray, M., Colwell, J. C., & Goldberg, M. T. (2005). What treatments are effective for the management of peristomal hernia? *Journal of Wound, Ostomy, and Continence Nursing, 32*(2), 87–92.

Harpin, V., & Rutter, N. (1982). Percutaneous alcohol absorption and skin necrosis in a preterm infant. *Archives of Disease in Childhood, 57*(6), 477–479.

Harrison, B., & Boarini, J. (2004). Pediatric ostomies: Pathophysiology and management. In J. C. Colwell, M. T. Goldberg, & J. E. Carmel (Eds.), *Fecal & urinary diversions: Management principles* (pp. 207–239). St. Louis, MO: Mosby.

Hendren, W. H. (1998). Diversion and undiversion. In J. A. O'Neill, M. I. Rowe, J. L. Grosfeld, E. W. Fonkalsrud, & A. G. Coran (Eds.), *Pediatric surgery* (5th ed., pp. 1653–1670). St. Louis, MO: Mosby.

Irving, V. (2001). Reducing the risk of epidermal stripping in the neonatal population: An evaluation of an alcohol-free barrier film. *Journal of Neonatal Nursing, 7*(1), 5–8.

Ittmann, P. I., & Bozynski, M. E. (1993). Toxic epidermal necrolysis in a newborn infant after exposure to adhesive remover. *Journal of Perinatology, 13*(6), 476–477.

Lund, C. (1999). Prevention and management of infant skin breakdown. *Nursing Clinics of North America, 34*(4), 907–920.

Lund, C. H., Nonato, L. B., Kuller, J. M., Franck, L. S., Cullander, C., & Durand, D. J. (1997). Disruption of barrier function in neonatal skin associated with adhesive removal. *The Journal of Pediatrics, 131*(3), 367–372.

Minkes, R. K., & Langer, J. C. (2000). The pediatric ostomy. In W. A. Walker, P. R. Durie, J. R. Hamilton, J. A. Walker-Smith, & J. B. Watkins (Eds.), *Pediatric gastrointestinal disease: Pathophysiology, diagnosis, management* (3rd ed., pp. 1877–1884). Hamilton, Ontario, Canada: BC Decker.

Mydler, T. T., Wasserman, G. S., Watson, W. A., & Knapp, J. F. (1993). Two-week-old infant with isopropanol intoxication. *Pediatric Emergency Care, 9*(3), 146–148.

Nachman, R. L., & Esterly, N. B. (1971). Increased skin permeability in preterm infants. *The Journal of Pediatrics, 79*(4), 628–632.

Patwardhan, N., Kiely, E. M., Drake, D. P., Spitz, L., & Pierro, A. (2001). Colostomy for anorectal anomalies: High incidence of complications. *Journal of Pediatric Surgery, 36*(5), 795–798.

Quigley, S., Hansen, A. R., & Puder, M. (2003). Ostomy diversions and management. In A. R. Hansen & M. Puder (Eds.), *Manual of neonatal surgical intensive care* (pp. 260–277). Hamilton, Ontario, Canada: BC Decker.

Rodriguez-Poblador, J., González-Castro, U., Herranz-Martínez, S., & Luelmo-Aguilar, J. (1998). Jacquet erosive diaper dermatitis after surgery for Hirschsprung's disease. *Pediatric Dermatology, 15*(1), 46–47.

Rolstad, B. S., & Boarini, J. (1996). Principles and techniques in the use of convexity. *Ostomy Wound Management, 42*(1), 24–32.

Rogers, V. E. (2003). Managing preemie stomas: More than just the pouch. *Journal of Wound, Ostomy, and Continence Nursing, 30*(2), 100–110.

Schick, J. B., & Milstein, J. M. (1981). Burn hazard of isopropyl alcohol in the neonate. *Pediatrics, 68*(4), 587–588.

Sussman, C., & Bates-Jensen, B. M. (2001). Index to topical antiseptics. In C. Sussman & M. B. Bates-Jensen (Eds.), *Wound care: A collaborative practice manual for physical therapists and nurses* (2nd ed., pp. 662–665). Gaithersburg, MD: Aspen.

Tamaki, K., & Yokomori, K. (1987). Diaper dermatitis with granuloma following surgery for Hirschsprung's disease. *Journal of Dermatology, 14*(3), 262–265.

Turnbull, G. B. (2003). Patient teaching: Intestinal obstruction. *Ostomy Wound Management, 49*(9), 20–21.

Turnbull, G. B. (2005). The issue of oral medications and a fecal ostomy. *Ostomy Wound Management, 51*(3), 14–16.

Weber, T. R. (2003). Intestinal stomas. In M. M. Ziegler, R. G. Azizkhan, & T. R. Weber (Eds.), *Operative pediatric surgery* (pp. 657–660). New York: McGraw-Hill Professional.

Appendix 8A	Parent Teaching Record for Ostomy Care				

Return Demonstration	Person Taught	Date/Initials	Person Taught	Date/Initials
Empties pouch				
Prepares new pouch				
Removed old pouch				
Cleanses peristomal skin				
Assesses stoma and peristomal skin				
Applies new pouch				
Connects urinary pouch to nighttime drainage system				

Verbal Expression of:	Person Taught	Date/Initials	Person Taught	Date/Initials
When to empty pouch				
When to change pouch				
Normal appearance of stoma and peristomal skin				
Diet and fluid modifications				
Reason for stoma and anatomic location (e.g., colon, bladder)				
When to contact health care provider for problems				
Where/how to obtain ostomy supplies				

Given Copy of:	Receiving Person	Date/Initials
Educational materials		
Surgeon name/telephone number, time frame for follow-up		
Home nursing company name/telephone number		
Manufacturer and order number of ostomy pouch and supplies		
Name/telephone number of ostomy supplier		
WOC nurse name/telephone number		

Document the name of the person *receiving* instructions. The person *providing* instruction should sign at the bottom of the page and date/initial each teaching point.

Provider signatures:

_____

From Wise, B.V., McKenna, C., Garvin, G., & Harmon, B.J. (2000). *Nursing Care of the General Pediatric Surgical Patient* (p. 277). Gaithersburg, MD: Aspen Publishers, Inc. Copyright 2000 by the American Pediatric Surgical Nurses Association. Adapted with permission.

Bowel Management

By Frances T. Gill and Linda J. Haga

Bowel management is a program designed collaboratively by the pediatric surgical nurse, the pediatric surgeon, and the family to allow the child to evacuate the bowel regularly and effectively, or to prevent complications of Hirschsprung's disease. The surgical patient with constipation or fecal soiling poses multiple challenges for the team entrusted with his or her care. Bowel management encompasses rectal irrigations for children who have had surgical repair for Hirschsprung's disease and disordered evacuation in children with anorectal malformations. Patients who have spina bifida, sacral agenesis, behavioral disorders, or varied issues with constipation may also benefit from a structured plan. These may be children who have been lost to follow-up for prolonged periods of time, often resurfacing for care at times of toilet training or entry into school. At presentation, a constellation of symptoms may be described. Although their stories are varied, the messages are similar. These are children at risk for social isolation, decreased self-esteem, and impaired school performance.

The hallmark of a good bowel management program is daily consistency, family diligence, and a supportive care provider who makes careful assessments, provides timely clinical changes, and gives generous praise for small successes. This chapter gives the clinician a guide to coordinate an effective plan using varied techniques to support optimal outcomes for each child and family.

■ Presentation

Achieving a normal bowel movement requires three interrelated functions: normal colonic motility to transport fecal contents into the rectum, intermittent evacuation of stool, and retention of stool between evacuations (Weinberg & Boley, 2005). Children born with anorectal malformations or Hirschsprung's disease lack some or all of these functions. This lack manifests as an absence of social continence or the ability to control when and where bowel emptying occurs. A bowel management plan, using a combination of diet, medications, and/or enemas, is often necessary to help the child achieve social continence.

When the child first presents for evaluation, a detailed history and physical examination are obtained. Before the evaluation, parents should be encouraged to acquire all operative records, radiology reports, and discharge summaries for their child. Encouraging parents to coordinate these reports in a binder or computer program creates an organized method for documenting their child's history and progress.

During the initial meeting, an objective checklist may assist the practitioner in identifying pertinent data in the clinical interview process (Table 9-1). The family is also asked to fill out a questionnaire about their child's bowel habits. After the interview and questionnaire are completed, it is imperative to discuss the level of commitment that will be needed from all participants in the bowel management program, including the care team, the parents, and the child. Because bowel management is a lifelong reality for these children, an honest discussion of the program allows the family to decide whether they are willing to embark on a journey that will potentially change some basic activities of their family life. Because improvement is the norm, realistic hope is provided to the family in order to ensure agreement from all. The fact that this program will not provide a rapid answer must be stressed.

The physical examination should include an overall assessment with focus on the abdomen. A rectal examination should be performed to evaluate the caliber of the rectum while revealing the tone of the vault, retention of stool, or palpation of an anal stricture. Anal strictures can be from previous surgeries or may be congenital. If a stricture is present, anal dilatations need to be started and gradually increased to the caliber of normal stool. After the initial rectal examination, it is possible to gauge the size of the dilator that is needed by comparing the care provider's finger size to the size of the dilator. Because graduated sizes are available (3/4 to 15/16 and above), the initial size can be chosen. The parents need to be taught the proper method of anal dilatation. This is often a source of great anxiety and fear for them. Clearly demonstrating the technique and requiring return demonstration is important, reinforcing that adequate lubrication and gentle pressure are needed. Guiding the parent's hand during their first dilatation attempt can be beneficial and can significantly decrease his or her anxiety. Determining that the dilator is passing through the area of structure is key. Many parents start dilatations timidly and fail to pass through this area, thus leading to further stricture formation. Noting that the parents are helping their child and preventing further complications are important points to stress.

Table 9-1	Bowel Management Interview		
Name:	Date:		
Date of birth:			
Birth weight:	Current weight:		
Diagnosis:			
Associated past medical history:			
Surgical procedure/s:			
Past stooling history:			
Current stooling history:			
Characteristics of stools:	Frequency of stools:		
Straining:	Smearing:		Accidents:
Appetite:			
Diet history (typical 24-hour food/fluid intake):			
Medications:			
Allergies:			
Past therapies attempted:			
Successes/failures:			
Social concerns:			
What is your goal today?			
What are your fears?			
What is your expectation of the bowel management program?			
Comments?			

■ Beginning the Bowel Management Plan

After determining that the patient has significant issues with constipation and/or fecal soiling that have failed previous treatments, the program can be developed. The goal will be for the child to empty the colon daily; one to two stools per day are optimal. Multiple small stools and smears denote an ineffectual evacuation pattern and are not acceptable. A radiograph of the abdomen is obtained before treatment begins to give the care provider a baseline picture of the amount of retained stool in the colon. This also allows the family to visualize the problem. From the outset, families should be partners in the care of the child. Viewing the x-ray study and receiving education on the structure and function of the normal gastrointestinal tract can improve their understanding and compliance with the frequent follow-up examinations that are necessary and expected. Regular abdominal films provide objective data on the progress of the bowel program that guide changes in therapy and allow early troubleshooting of problems. Parents are encouraged to call the care provider frequently, especially for decreased bowel movements, abdominal distention, alterations in appetite, vomiting, straining, or smearing. A structured method of collecting this clinical information in an ongoing manner assists the care provider in evaluating patient progress (Table 9-2). It is important to ensure easy access to these data, either online or in a binder that can provide the basis for phone consultations or on-the-spot treatment changes.

Diet

Analyzing the family diet history is a key element in the construction of a plan for the patient with constipation. In today's culture, children's diets are often filled with high-fat, low-fiber convenience foods. Fruits and vegetables are often lacking. Sugary fruit juices and sodas lead the list of patient favorites. Fiber, a key element in the healthy diet, is usually far below the recommended daily requirement (10–30 g, depending on age). Restructuring the eating habits of the patient must include the entire family. An insightful way to understand family nutritional patterns is to have them document a 1-week account of all meals, snacks, and fluid intake. This provides an effective educational starting point for the nurse and clinical dietician attempting to restructure learned dietary habits.

In infancy, the addition of pureed pure prunes or diluted prune juice (1:1) provides a laxative effect without the institution of medication. The Nutra/Balance® products provide 10 g of fiber per 8-ounce juice box. Two-ounce cookies provide 3 g of fiber each. Both come in a variety of flavors (see Product Information). Changing from white bread to wheat bread and from white rice to brown are small changes that will begin the process (Table 9-3).

Table 9-2	**Bowel Management Follow-Up Visit**
Name:	
Date:	
Contact number:	
Age:	
Recent issue:	
Current diet:	
Current fluid intake:	
Current medications:	
Current enema schedule:	
Current results:	
Clinical goal:	
Changes:	
Pharmacy number:	
Recheck plan:	
Comments:	

Table 9-3	Dietary Tips	
Foods to Include		**Foods to Avoid**
Beans		Apples
Blackberries		Banana
Boysenberries		Carbonated beverages
Bran cereal		Crackers
Brown rice		Excessive cheese
Fruits with skin		Excessive milk
Multigrain cereals		Peanut butter
Nuts (age permitting)		Pretzels
Oatmeal		Sugary fruit juices
Pears		Tea
Popcorn (age permitting)		White bread
Potato with skin		White rice
Prunes		White pasta
Raspberries		
Water		
Whole grain flour (baking)		
Whole wheat bread		
Whole wheat pasta		

Sufficient water intake is important at all times, especially during times of high heat and humidity or increased physical activity. Families should know that the first place the body takes fluid during early dehydration is the bowel. If this occurs, even well-tuned bowel management can fail. Training the child to bring water along on outings helps prevent these problems. Purchasing a special cup may entice the child to want to drink. Often, school officials must be notified to allow the child to drink water during the day or to go to the restroom when needed. A note from the care provider is often required.

When diet alterations alone do not produce daily bowel movements, medications are added to the regimen. Results of an abdominal x-ray study are used to guide drug choices. If the x-ray study demonstrates a significant collection of stool in the rectosigmoid segment of the colon, an enema helps prevent abdominal cramping before the institution of stimulant laxatives. Based on the degree of fecal retention, one phosphate enema (Fleet) daily for 3 days facilitates evacuation. Parents must be cautioned to only use one enema per day to avoid dehydration and electrolyte imbalance (Fledderman, 2001). For severe fecal retention throughout the colon, the osmotic effect of polyethylene glycol (Miralax [GlycoLax]) facilitates evacuation. Senna preparations (Senokot, Little Tummies) act as a stimulant to enhance the propulsion of the bowel, thus increasing stool passage. Based on the pharmacologic action and patient tolerance, a combination of medications may be needed to obtain an adequate effect (Table 9-4).

After diet and laxative doses have been optimized, a follow-up x-ray study demonstrates the level of success of the bowel management plan. In some children, these changes do not provide optimal fecal cleanliness (Fig. 9-1). This is the time to discuss patient and family compliance. An enema program may need to be instituted for selected patients. Before beginning, a water-soluble contrast enema serves a twofold purpose: demonstrating the caliber of the colon and assisting with therapeutic evacuation of stool.

Enemas

Children with anorectal malformations who have failed management with optimized medications often need to receive daily enemas to have social continence (see Anorectal Malformations in Children, Chapter 21). Some centers require a successful enema regime before evaluation for an antegrade continence enema procedure (ACE).

Antegrade Continence Enema Procedure

Malone, Ransley, and Kiely (1990) first described the ACE procedure, which uses the appendix to create a conduit

Table 9-4 Medication and Enema Template

Drug	Dosage	Mechanism	Side Effects	Drug Interaction	Contraindication	Considerations
Milk of Magnesia	Oral <2 yrs: 0.5 mL/kg/dose 2–5 yrs: 5–15 mL/day 6–12 yrs: 15–30 mL/day >12 yrs: 30–60 mL/day	Osmotic effect on colon promoting evacuation	Nausea, vomiting, cramping, diarrhea, hypermagnesemia, hyperphosphatemia	Decreased effect of tetracyclines, digoxin, indomethacin, iron salts	Intestinal obstruction, fecal impaction, renal failure, R/O appendicitis	May be given in divided doses. Give with fluid. Good for short-term use for constipation.
Miralax	Oral: 0.8 g/day	Osmotic effect on colon promoting evacuation	Perineal rash, nausea, vomiting, diarrhea	None	Intestinal obstruction, fecal impaction, colitis, R/O appendicitis	Give with 4–8 ounces of water or juice.
Senokot	Oral: 1 mo–1 yr: 1.25–2.5 mL; max. 5 mL/day 1–5 yrs: 2.5–5 mL; max. 20 mL/d 5–15 yrs: 5–10 mL; max. 20 mL/day	Stimulates peristalsis	Rash, nausea, vomiting, diarrhea, abdominal cramps	None	R/O appendicitis, intestinal obstruction, fecal impaction	Encourage increased fluid intake.
Glycerin	Rectal: <6 yrs: infant suppository or Babylax bid >6 years: 1 adult suppository	Fluid drawn to colon; lubricates rectum, stool easier to pass	Local irritation	None	None	Good to use in treating infants with constipation.
Fleet enema®	Rectal: 2–8 years: 1 pediatric enema daily >8 yrs: 1 adult enema	Osmotic effect on colon promoting evacuation	Local irritation; prolonged use may cause hyperphosphatemia, hypernatremia, hypocalcemia	None	R/O appendicitis or intestinal perforation	Never administer >1 per day; avoid prolonged use.
Normal saline enema	Rectal: 10–20 mL/kg all ages, at room temperature	Osmotic effect on colon promoting evacuation	Local irritation	None	R/O appendicitis or intestinal perforation	May use Foley catheter to help child retain enema fluid.
Lomotil	Oral solution: 2–12 years: 0.3–0.4 mg/kg/day in 4 divided doses Tablets: 13–16 years: 2 tablets tid	Slows or inhibits peristalsis	Dizziness, drowsiness, euphoria, sedation, nausea, vomiting, cramps, dry mouth	Ambenonium, arbutamine, digoxin	Contraindicated: <2 yrs of age, hypersensitivity to atropine, diarrhea caused by enterotoxin-producing bacteria	Adjust dose according to number of stools; monitor liver function if used for prolonged periods. *(continues)*

Table 9-4 *(continued)*

Drug	Dosage	Mechanism	Side Effects	Drug Interaction	Contraindication	Considerations
Imodium	Oral: 2–6 yrs: 1 mg tid 6–8 yrs: 2 mg bid 8–12 yrs: 2 mg tid > 12 years: up to 16 mg per day	Inhibits peristalsis of intestine	Sedation, rash dizziness, nausea, vomiting, cramps, constipation, dry mouth	Increased toxicity: CNS depressants, phenothiazines, TCAs	Diarrhea resulting from enterotoxin-producing bacteria	Adjust dose according to number of stools.
Fiber supplements —Metamucil —Benefiber	Oral: 3–11 yrs: ½–2 tsps/4 oz fluid 1–2 times daily > 12 years: 1–2 tsps/4 oz juice/fluid 2–4 times daily	Pulls water into the intestine: promotes peristalsis	Diarrhea	Affects: Coumadin, potassium-sparing diuretics, salicylates, tetracyclines, nitrofurantoin	Fluid intake should be increased while on fiber supplements.	Metamucil tends to be thick and grainy.

CNS, central nervous system; R/O, rule out; TCA, tricyclic antidepressant.

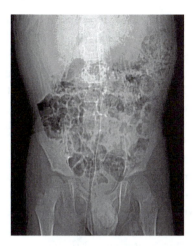

FIGURE 9-1 Flat plate of the abdomen: retained stool.

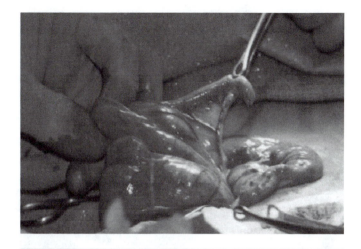

FIGURE 9-2 Identifying the appendix.

from the skin to the large bowel for the administration of enema solution. This process involves the creation of a stoma, which provides access to colon cleansing through the ascending segment, thus optimizing evacuation through the anus while the child is seated on the toilet. Antegrade enemas flush a longer segment of colon than is possible with conventional retrograde enemas.

Initially, this procedure is performed by resecting the appendix on its vascular pedicle with a generous cuff of cecum left at the base. The cecal defect is closed and the distal end of the appendix amputated. The appendix is then inverted and the distal end anastomosed to a mucosal opening in the cecum. The submucosal tunnel and the seromuscular layers of the cecum are closed over it, thus creating a nonrefluxing channel (Malone, Ransely, & Kiely, 1990). An indwelling catheter (i.e., 10-French Mentor® Self-Cath coudé catheter olive tip with guide stripe) is left in place for 2 to 4 weeks to allow the tract to mature and the mucosal skin junction to heal. It is advisable to discharge the child with a catheter one size smaller, in case of local edema or stricture formation. Figures 9-2 to 9-4 demonstrate the intraoperative identification of the appendix, the intubation of the appendix, and the use of the catheter to check the patency of the ACE through the completed stoma.

Over the years, many revisions have been made to this initial technique. Levitt, Soffer, and Peña (1997) described a method that plicated the cecum around the appendix, thus creating a one-way valve mechanism while leaving the appendix in its native position. The cecum is mobilized and the appendix is externalized at the umbilicus, creating an inconspicuous stoma. Children without an appendix have a neoappendix fashioned from a 2.5-cm segment of ileum. The indwelling catheter should be left in place at least 4 weeks after the creation of the

neoappendix. Most recently, this procedure has been performed using a laparoscopic approach with great success.

Candidates for the ACE procedure must be chosen carefully; the ACE is not a panacea or a cure for the problems related to constipation or fecal soiling. Rather, it is an alternative for delivering enemas and encouraging self-care and increased independence. The positive psychological effects of the ACE procedure are well documented. Increased psychological function, improved self-esteem, self-reliance, control, independence, and security, as well as decreased practical and emotional strain, have been demonstrated (Aksnes et al., 2002).

Before surgery, children require a standard bowel preparation. After surgery, a prescribed schedule is followed to allow titration of the ACE irrigant to the desired effect. The first irrigation of 50 to 100 cc of normal saline solution can be performed on either the first or the second

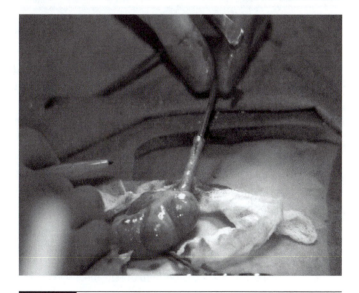

FIGURE 9-3 Intubating the appendix.

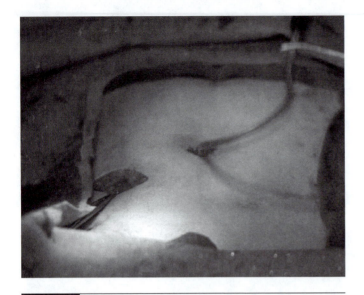

FIGURE 9-4 Checking the patency of the antegrade continence enema procedure.

postoperative day. Rectal enemas can continue to maintain cleanliness. The schedule is adjusted daily to provide increasing volumes through the ACE while decreasing the rectal irrigant. Daily increases of 100 cc are usually well tolerated. Most children receive a maximum volume of between 500 and 1000 cc per day.

A hypertonic saline solution can be used at home to increase the irritant content of the irrigant and thus the effectiveness of the enema. The saline solution is concentrated by mixing three level teaspoons of noniodized salt in 1000 cc of warm water. Emphasis on proper mix-

ing must be stressed. Use of a graduated medicine cup provides safety with the salt measurement. To prevent devastating complications, only adults who have been instructed in the preparation of the saline solution should mix the solution. After parent teaching, a return demonstration is performed. A written guideline is given to the family, a signed copy of which should be added to the patient's medical record (Table 9-5).

If the child continues to have fecal soiling, adding an additional irritant product (e.g., glycerin, castile soap, phosphate enema) to the saline irrigant may increase the effectiveness of the enema. Polyethylene glycol (Miralax) can also be used through the ACE if fecal leakage persists (Kokoska, Keller, & Weber, 2001). Glycerin can be used in small volumes and mixed one part to one part saline (Fledderman, 2001).

Enemas are usually performed on a daily basis because skipping days may predispose the child to stool retention with subsequent soiling. Consistent timing of enemas each day also increases the effectiveness of the program. Having the child start the enema after dinner uses the normal physiologic function of the gastrocolic reflex, which is present after ingesting a meal. Enemas given near bedtime also prevents fecal soiling at night (Kokoska et al., 2001).

If children experience cramping, nausea, headache, or sweating during the enema, treatment with 4 to 8 ounces of an electrolyte drink (e.g., Gatorade) before and after the procedure can replace potential electrolyte losses and increase patient tolerance. If symptoms persist, the par-

Table 9-5	**Instructions for Administration of Antegrade Enemas**

1. **Gather supplies:** Lubricant, catheter size # _____, gravity bag, noniodized table salt, medication measuring cup, 4 cups of warm tap water, diversional activities (television, video games, books, schoolwork)

2. **Mix the solution:** Measure the salt VERY carefully using the medicine cup to the #15. This is the same as 3 teaspoonfuls. If using a spoon, ALWAYS use a baking teaspoon *only*. Close the clamp on the enema bag. Add 4 cups (1000 cc) of warm tap water to the bag and mix in the salt.
   Mix gently. NOTE: At times, you may be advised to add other products to the saline solution. Do not add anything without the direction of your health care provider.

3. **Give the enema by ACE or Chait cecostomy tube:** Connect the gravity bag to the catheter, flush out the air, and close the clamp. With your child seated on the toilet or potty chair (make sure his/her feet touch the ground!), lubricate the catheter. Insert the catheter *gently*. Have the child sit on the toilet or potty chair for 30 to 45 minutes.

4. **Troubleshooting:** If you have trouble with the catheter, STOP! Remove the catheter, re-lubricate the tip, and try again. If you still have trouble *do not continue*.
   Call the office at:_____ or "On Call Physician" at _____.
   If your child has headache, cramps, or vomiting, give 4 to 8 ounces of Gatorade before and after the enema. If the problem continues, call the office. Flashback of stool from the site means you may need to increase the solution or add another ingredient. Call the office for more information.

ents should call the surgical office for advice. In some cases, a serum electrolyte panel may be necessary. Questioning the family about preparation of the irrigant should be completed and the proper method reinforced.

Providing the child a comfortable space to evacuate the enema increases effectiveness and compliance. Setting up games, television, or computers on a low table over the toilet or commode chair helps the child accept the time required for evacuation more easily. Figure 9-5 shows a child holding the tube in the ACE stoma.

Complications

The most common postoperative complication is stricture formation within the ACE tract. The patient experiences an inability to easily pass the catheter through the stoma. Attempts to pass a smaller caliber catheter should be attempted, and if unsuccessful, evaluation by the surgery team is warranted. If the stoma is tightly closed, passing a small feeding tube (5 Fr) may be possible and sufficient to allow access for progressive dilatation by the health care team. Slowly increasing the size to an 8- or 10-Fr catheter is optimal.

In some cases, stool may leak from the stoma. In this case, increasing the volume of irrigant may be necessary to facilitate a more complete colonic cleansing. Protecting the peristomal skin with a petroleum- or zinc-based cream is important. An abdominal x-ray study may help gauge the degree of bowel cleansing and compliance. The formation of granulation tissue around the stoma is also common and can be treated with triamcinolone (Kenalog) cream 0.5% three times a day. Rare complications of the ACE procedure can include volvulus, perforation of the conduit, and wound dehiscence.

Studies have documented the positive effects of the ACE procedure. Levitt, Soffer, and Peña (1997) reported

that 19 of 20 patients in their series were completely clean after surgery. Aksnes et al. (2002) reported significant improvement in self-esteem and psychosocial function within 6 months of surgery. Numerous anecdotal stories describe positive lifestyle changes by children and families (Crawley-Coha, 2004; Gill, 2003).

■ Cecostomy/Chait Button

An alternative to the ACE procedure is the percutaneous cecostomy. Chait, Shlomovitz, and Connolly (2003) described accessing the cecum with the assistance of fluoroscopic guidance. Selected patients require a bowel preparation before the procedure and are instructed to follow a prescribed preoperative fasting regimen. Prophylactic intravenous antibiotics are given and a topical anesthetic applied to the right lower quadrant of the abdomen approximately 1 hour before the procedure. Local anesthesia, along with intravenous sedation, may also be given, although general anesthesia may be warranted in some cases.

Many centers perform cecostomies laparoscopically. The cecostomy procedure fashions a tract between the skin and the bowel that accommodates a cecal tube. A temporary cecostomy tube (C tube) is then inserted into the cecum at the right lower quadrant of the abdomen, thus providing easy access for enema self-administration. Immediately after placement, the tube should be flushed with 10 cc of warm tap water twice daily. Enemas are begun within a few days, using a gravity-type feeding bag with a roll clamp. Tube adapters may be needed to provide an adequate fit for the bag and tube connection (Fig. 9-6).

Six weeks after the procedure, the more permanent Chait Trapdoor™ Cecostomy tube (Cook®) is inserted under fluoroscopy. This is a nonlatex tube that utilizes a small, flat-lying access site that is nearly undetectable under clothing (Fig. 9-7). The Chait Trapdoor™ Cecostomy (Cook®) tube comes in two sizes: pediatric and adult. After the first change, the tubes are usually replaced annually on an elective basis.

The most common complications of the cecostomy procedure include granulation tissue at the insertion site, infection, discomfort, and dislodgment or blockage of the tube. Difficulty opening or closing the device has also been reported.

Parents should be instructed to wash the area with warm soap and water. Antibiotic ointments can be used for the first week after insertion. Granulation tissue can be treated topically with triamcinolone (Kenalog 0.5%)

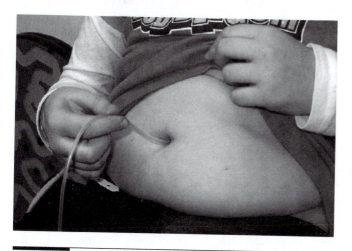

FIGURE 9-5 The antegrade continence enema procedure.

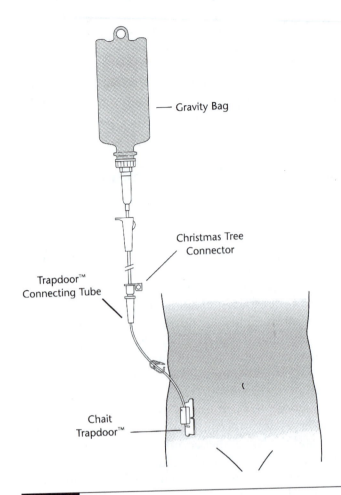

FIGURE 9-6 Cecostomy enema administration.

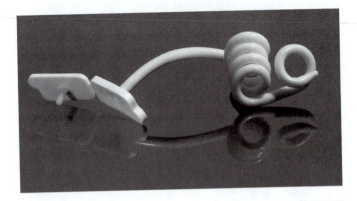

FIGURE 9-7 Chait trapdoor cecostomy tube (Cook Critical Care, Bloomington, IL).

cream. Warm water flushes may relieve blockage of the tube, but if dislodgment is suspected, the patient should be evaluated by the surgical team as soon as possible.

■ Prevention

The most effective way to treat constipation in children is through prevention strategies. At the time of diagnosis, parents should be told clearly that bowel management will be a long-term process. Having a surgical procedure does not eradicate the need for strict attention to the child's bowel function and diet. The health care team stresses that the vision for the child is to grow, thrive, and live a full, happy life, although special needs will exist. Early attention to diet, exercise, and stooling patterns prevents escalated problems in the future. If these patterns are less than optimal, bowel dilatation can occur, leading to an overstretched and underfunctioning colon. The overall goal of the bowel management program is social continence and the prevention of retained stool. Close, ongoing follow-up by the family with the bowel management team maximizes the opportunity to achieve this goal.

Rectal Irrigations

Children with Hirschsprung's disease frequently require specialized bowel care to prevent the devastating complication of enterocolitis (see Chapter 20). These children require rectal irrigations to flush the bowel. Parents need to understand that bowel irrigations are performed differently than enemas. The child should be positioned either over the parent's lap or on his or her left side. A second person may be helpful to support the child through the procedure while providing diversional activities and comfort. A 14- to 24-Fr nonlatex catheter attached to a 60-cc catheter tip syringe should be lubricated with water-soluble lubricant and inserted into the rectum, approximately 3 to 5 inches, or until stool or flatus is expelled. Warmed saline solution (2 level teaspoons of noniodized salt in 1000 cc of warm water) should be gently instilled into the rectum and then slowly pulled back into the syringe. This process should be performed until a volume of 10 cc per kilogram of weight has been instilled. If it is difficult to pull back the liquid, the catheter should be repositioned because adherence to the bowel wall is possible. If clogging of the catheter tip with stool is problematic, it may need to be removed and flushed before continuing the irrigation. During this procedure, the child should be assessed frequently for nausea, vomiting, or abdominal distention.

In some cases, children who have undergone endorectal pull-through surgery for Hirschsprung's disease are started on prophylactic saline irrigations to prevent enterocolitis. Irrigations are performed twice a day for 3 months and once daily for 3 months. Studies have shown a significant reduction in enterocolitis in this population if this regimen is followed (Marty, Seo, Sullivan, Matlak, Black, & Johnson, 1995).

Conclusion

Tackling a bowel management plan for children is a challenging issue for all involved. Identifying a dedicated care provider with a special interest in this patient population is a key aspect to the success of any program. Although this position can be time consuming and demanding, the personal and professional rewards are immeasurable. Children's lives will be greatly improved through these efforts. Woven into each child's story is hope, hope that he or she will be able to live a "normal" life, go to sleepover parties, swim, play sports, date, and go on to college. The possibilities are endless. Being an integral part of this process combines the art and the science of nursing at its best.

Acknowledgments

This chapter is dedicated to the children and families who demonstrate the courage to enter into a bowel management plan and the surgical nurses who care for them and give them hope.

Educational Materials

APSNA invites you to download the diagnosis-related teaching tool "Bowel Management" (available in English and Spanish), for Chapter 9 "Bowel Management" at the APSNA Web site (www.apsna.org) and the Jones and Bartlett Web site (www.jbpub.com). All teaching materials are available free of charge and APSNA encourages their use for your patients and families.

References

Aksnes, G., Diseth, T. H., Helseth, A., Edwin, B., Stange, M., Asfos, G., et al. (2002). Appendicostomy for antegrade enema: Effects on somatic and psychological functioning in children with myelomeningocele. *Pediatrics, 109*(3), 484–489.

Chait, P., Shlomovitz, E., & Connolly, B. (2003). Percutaneous cecostomy: Updates in technique and patient care. *Radiology, 227,* 246–250.

Crawley-Coha, T. (2004). Cecostomy for antegrade continence enemas in children. *Journal of Wound Ostomy Care Nursing, 31*(1), 23–29.

Fledderman, M. (2001). Pediatric enema solutions. *Pull-thru Network News, 10*(2), 1–3.

Gill, F. T. (2003). Antegrade continent enema (ACE) procedure. *American Pediatric Surgical Nurses Association Sutureline Independent Study, 11*(3), 1–3.

Kokoska, E. R., Keller, M. S., & Weber, T. R. (2001). Outcome of the antegrade colonic enema procedure in children with chronic constipation. *The American Journal of Surgery, 182,* 625–629.

Levitt, M. A., Soffer, S. Z., & Peña, A. (1997). Continent appendicostomy in the bowel management of fecally incontinent children. *Journal of Pediatric Surgery, 32*(11), 1630–1633.

Malone, P. S., Ransley, P. G., & Kiely, E. M. (1990). Preliminary report: The antegrade continence enema. *Lancet, 336,* 1217–1218.

Marty, T. L., Seo, T., Sullivan, J. J., Matlak, M. E., Black, R. E., & Johnson, D. G. (1995). Rectal irrigations for the prevention of postoperative enterocolitis in Hirschsprung's disease. *Journal of Pediatric Surgery, 30*(5), 652–654.

Weinberg, G., & Boley, S. (2005). Anorectal continence and management of constipation. In K. Ashcraft, G. Holcomb, & J. Murphy (Eds.), *Pediatric surgery* (4th ed., pp. 518–526). Philadelphia: Elsevier Saunders.

Common Outpatient Pediatric Surgical Procedures: Inguinal and Umbilical Hernias, Hydroceles, Undescended Testes, and Circumcision

By Mary Ellen Connolly and Carmel A. McComiskey

Pediatric surgical procedures are performed in a variety of settings: tertiary teaching facilities, children's hospitals, community hospitals, and free-standing surgicenters. Regardless of the site, all children and their families should be offered the same standard of care that is developmentally sensitive and family focused, ensures appropriate pediatric pain management strategies, and causes minimal inconvenience and/or morbidity.

Although most outpatient surgery is considered straightforward and relatively minor by care providers of all levels, parents do not consider any procedure performed on their child to be minor. For that reason, all children and their families deserve preoperative preparation and education. This results in decreased patient and caregiver anxiety, improved compliance, decreased readmissions, and few postoperative telephone calls. In addition, because the opportunity to provide teaching is limited, both perioperative instructions and postoperative educational material should be provided at the initial encounter. This chapter reviews the surgical management and nursing care of children undergoing repair of a hernia, hydrocele, undescended testicle, and circumcision.

Preoperative testing is generally not necessary in the pediatric age group, although a recent anesthesia practice survey (Patel, DeWitt, & Hannallah, 1997) reported that hemoglobin testing is still performed by 27% to 48% of the respondents, indicating that policies are slow to change. Many centers do not routinely perform laboratory investigations and have liberalized feeding regimens for both children and adults. Clear liquid diet up to 2 hours before anesthesia induction is common practice. A liberal preoperative clear liquid diet allows for a more comfortable preoperative experience without an increased risk of aspiration or regurgitation (Brady, Kinn, O'Rourke, Randhawa, & Stuart, 2005).

Minimal physical preparation is necessary beyond these usual anesthetic recommendations. Premedication should be offered to children older than 6 months of age to decrease separation anxiety. Parent-accompanied anesthetic induction is also offered in some centers where anesthesiologists are comfortable with parental presence and the physical design of the operative area is suitable for visitors.

Inguinal Hernias in Children

Description/Pathophysiology of the Hernias

A hernia is the protrusion of tissue through an abnormal opening. An indirect inguinal hernia (congenital) exists when the peritoneal contents enter the processus vaginalis through the internal ring and follow the spermatic cord in boys or the round ligament in girls (Fig. 10-1). The contents are usually bowel but may include ovary or fallopian tube in girls (Borkowski, 1994; Hutson, Beasley, & Woodward, 1992). The contents emerge at the external ring and extend into the scrotum or the labia. Nearly all inguinal hernias in children are indirect (Hutson et al., 1992). These hernias arise lateral to the inferior epigastric vessels in contrast to a direct hernia, which is medial to these vessels and bulges through a weakened posterior wall of the inguinal canal.

Direct inguinal hernias are rarely seen in children. The incidence is 1% of all pediatric hernias. They occur occasionally in infants with bronchopulmonary dysplasia and in children with cystic fibrosis as a result of prolonged ventilation (O'Neill, Grosfeld, Fonkalsrud, Coran, & Caldamone, 2003).

Incidence

Although few population-based studies have been performed, the incidence of inguinal hernias in children is estimated to be between 10 and 20 per 1000 live births.

The ratio of males to females is 4:1. Approximately 55% to 70% of inguinal hernias are diagnosed on the right side, 30% on the left, and 10% bilaterally (Skinner & Grosfeld, 1993). The higher incidence of right-sided hernias is thought to be related to the later descent of the right testis and delayed closure of the processus vaginalis on the right side. The incidence of inguinal hernia is greater in premature infants. The incidence of hernia in premature infants weighing less than 1500 gm is reported to be as high as 30% (Gill, 1998; Skinner & Grosfeld). Other conditions that influence the incidence include a positive family history, an undescended testis, hypospadias, ascites, the presence of a ventriculoperitoneal shunt, and ventilatory support increasing intraabdominal pressure. Hernias are also more common in children with connective tissue disorders because of the fragility of the peritoneal tissues (O'Neill et al., 2003).

Clinical Presentation of Hernias in Children

Generally, the infant or child has a history of an obvious bulge at the internal or external ring or within the scrotum. The differential diagnosis in males includes hydrocele, retractile testis, undescended testis, varicocele, and testicular tumor. Often, the hernia bulge is not present when the child visits the primary care provider and is often difficult to produce, even when the child is crying or straining. Many practitioners attempt to palpate the hernia sac over the cord structures in the inguinal region. The sliding sensation of the sac and cord structures over the pubic bone is known as a positive "silk glove sign." This is a suggestive, but not a diagnostic, finding. Occasionally, if the hernia cannot be demonstrated at the surgical office visit, an operation is still planned if the primary

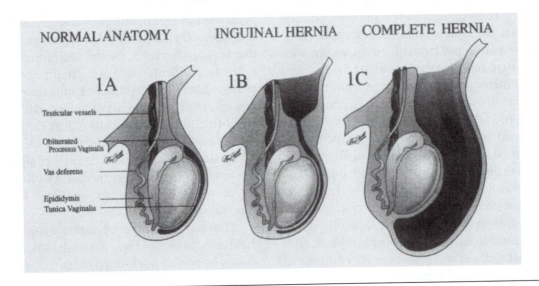

FIGURE 10-1 Inguinal hernia.

care physician has demonstrated the hernia and is a known, reliable observer (O'Neill et al., 2003).

Surgical Management

Elective surgical repair is recommended for all hernias, with surgery planned as soon as possible (Hutson et al., 1992). Repair of the inguinal hernia is necessary because of the danger of bowel strangulation and ischemic injury to the gonad. Incarceration and potential strangulation can occur when a piece of the bowel extrudes through the ring and cannot be reduced. The term "incarceration" refers to the condition when the bowel is stuck through the ring and cannot be reduced. Strangulation of the bowel occurs when the blood supply is compromised. When the hernia contents are not reducible, surgical intervention is emergent. Strangulation occurs most frequently in the first 6 months of life (Hutson et al.). The incidence of strangulation is reported between 9% and 20%. Children with a strangulated hernia have a firm, hard, and tender mass in the inguinal region. The mass can be erythematous or blue. The children are fussy, are often inconsolable, and can have vomiting and abdominal distention.

An incarcerated hernia requires reduction. Parents can be instructed to reduce the hernia at home with gentle pressure on the contents, gradually emptying the sac. This procedure is most successful when families administer acetaminophen, elevate the swollen groin, and calm the child. If the hernia sac remains tense, the child should be taken to the emergency department. Often, the hernia spontaneously reduces during the ride to the hospital. Sedation can be used to reduce hernias that are still incarcerated on arrival at the hospital. When this is successful, repair is performed within 24 to 48 hours. Emergency surgery is planned once an irreducible hernia is identified because of the risk of strangulation (O'Neill et al., 2003).

Various rationales influence contralateral exploration. To decrease the risks of anesthesia and incarceration, contralateral groin exploration is sometimes recommended. Traditionally, routine contralateral exploration was not performed because of the risks of extended anesthesia time and the potential for injury to the testes and vas deferens. Laparoscopy has become an increasingly popular tool for exploratory surgery. Laparoscopic exploration adds minutes to the surgery procedure without the addition of a second incision. There is minimal risk of injury to the testes or vas deferens. Exploration is frequently recommended for girls and for children under 2 years of age who are considered at high risk for a contralateral hernia (Geisler et al., 2001).

The procedure to repair a hernia is an inguinal herniorrhaphy. The goal of the operation is a high ligation of the patent processus vaginalis (Borkowski, 1994). Herniorrhaphy performed by open technique is the standard in most pediatric surgery practices. However, laparoscopic repair and laparoscopic exploration of the contralateral side are also performed. Spurbeck, Prasad, and Lobe (2005) reported that minimally invasive herniorrhaphy in children is a safe alternative to traditional hernia repair surgery. The laparoscopic approach results in a superior cosmetic outcome, with no increased risk of hernia recurrence when compared with the traditional open approach.

Complications

The hernia repair itself is an uncomplicated operation, with minimal blood loss. Complications include wound infection (1%–2%), hernia recurrence (< 1%), and injury to the vas deferens or ilioinguinal nerves (< 1%) (Skinner & Grosfeld, 1993).

Nursing Interventions and Expected Outcomes

Postoperative Care

Postoperative pain is managed by the use of ilioinguinal nerve blocks or by single-dose caudal or epidural anesthetic, administered during the procedure. Local anesthetic administered as a single dose is reported to manage postoperative pain for at least 6 and as long as 24 hours after surgery (Fisher et al., 1993). Discomfort at home is managed with the addition of acetaminophen or ibuprofen. Opioids are usually not necessary for postoperative pain control.

Patient education is an important nursing responsibility and has been shown to prevent or at least reduce negative responses to surgery, improve pain management, and achieve an optimum experience for the child and family. Children and parents who are properly educated have decreased anxiety and feel an improved sense of control over the situation (Bar-Mor, 1997; Brewer & Lampert, 1997). Other postoperative concerns are urinary retention and constipation (Linden & Engberg, 1994). Urinary retention is a temporary postoperative concern and does not usually require intervention; it is a side effect of the caudal anesthetic and resolves spontaneously within 6 to 8 hours. Constipation is easily managed with increased clear liquids by mouth and stool softeners or suppository, if necessary.

Infants usually return to normal feeding and sleep habits within 24 to 48 hours. Recommendations regarding activity vary by practice. Although school-aged children may return to normal routines after 2 to 3 days, contact sports should be restricted for at least 2 weeks.

Yaster, Sola, Pegoli, and Paidas (1994) recommended a full 2-week recovery before toddlers ride tricycles and a full 4- to 6-week recovery period for contact sports.

Umbilical Hernias in Children

Description of the Hernia

Umbilical hernias occur when the fascial ring, which surrounds the umbilical cord and vessels, fails to close after birth. The skin and the peritoneum are intact. A hernia occurs when a loop of bowel protrudes through the ring (Fig. 10-2) (Gill, 1998; Rowe, O'Neill, Grosfeld, Fonkalsrud, & Coran, 1995).

Umbilical hernias are present in approximately 20% of all newborns. Most umbilical hernias close spontaneously by 3 years of age. In the United States, an increased incidence of umbilical hernias occurs in African-American infants compared with Caucasian infants. The incidence is equal among boys and girls. It is considered an isolated problem in otherwise healthy children, but the incidence is higher in children with Down syndrome, hypothyroidism, and Beckwith-Weidemann syndrome (Gill, 1998; Rowe et al., 1995).

Incarceration occurs when a piece of bowel gets stuck through the opening. This can cause compromise to the blood supply. Incarceration is rare but is reported (Keshtgar & Griffiths, 2003). Vransky and Bourdelat (1997) reported four cases of incarcerated umbilical hernia over a 5-year period.

Clinical Presentation of Hernias in Children

Umbilical hernias present as a bulging at the umbilicus. The skin becomes stretched. The bulge is more prominent when the infant cries and usually reduces spontaneously when the infant relaxes, leaving the redundant skin.

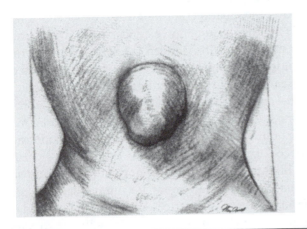

FIGURE 10-2 Umbilical hernia.

On physical examination, one can detect the size of the defect by placing a finger into the umbilicus and palpating the fascial ring. The diameter of the hole varies from 1 mm to 3 cm. Because most of these hernias close spontaneously, no treatment is indicated in the first 2 to 3 years of life.

Surgical Management

Surgical repair is performed for the following reasons: incarceration, persistence of a hernia beyond the age of 3 years, and large defects. The incision is made within an infraumbilical skin crease and is extended down to the rectus fascia and linea alba. The neck of the sac is dissected, and then the sac is freed from the overlying skin. The redundant sac is excised, and then the defect in the linea alba is closed transversely, usually in two layers. The umbilical skin is then tacked down to the fascia, and the wound is closed. A pressure dressing is placed over the wound (Rowe et al., 1995).

Nursing Interventions and Expected Outcomes

Preoperative Care

Preoperative nursing care emphasizes parental teaching and reassurance that most umbilical hernias spontaneously resolve. Families should be informed that the bulge often becomes larger before the defect closes. In addition, parents may be worried that the skin may rupture. Finally, families should be discouraged from taping coins over the bulge to facilitate early closure because this does not speed closure or prevent incarceration and may cause ulceration and infection to the skin (Rowe et al., 1995).

Postoperative Care

A large sponge dressing is applied with pressure in the operating room to minimize hematoma; the dressing remains intact for at least 48 hours. Children are ready for discharge from the outpatient setting when they are hemodynamically stable, breathing normally, and tolerating clear liquids. Pain at home is managed with acetaminophen or ibuprofen. Children can resume normal activity and return to day care within 2 to 3 days. Unsupervised play and contact sports should be delayed for 2 weeks.

Hydroceles

Description of the Hydrocele

A hydrocele (Fig. 10-3) is a painless cyst formed by the tunica vaginalis that contains fluid. Hydroceles occur when fluid accumulates in or above the scrotum via a patent processus vaginalis connected to the peritoneal cavity. The

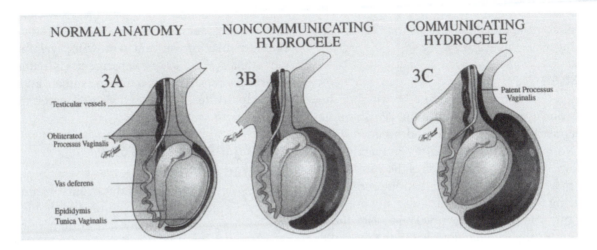

NORMAL ANATOMY   NONCOMMUNICATING HYDROCELE   COMMUNICATING HYDROCELE

3A — Testicular vessels, Obliterated Processus Vaginalis, Vas deferens, Epididymis, Tunica Vaginalis

3B

3C — Patent Processus Vaginalis

FIGURE 10-3 Hydrocele.

hydrocele is usually located in front of the testis. The testis can usually be palpated without difficulty. When the hydrocele is large or tense, the scrotum can be transilluminated (Hutson et al., 1992). Transillumination (shining a small light source through it) differentiates the hydrocele from tumor, varicocele, and blood.

Clinical Presentation of Hydroceles

In male infants, both unilateral and bilateral hydroceles are common in the first few months of life. They are painless, often large, and usually resolve spontaneously by 1 year of age. If the hydrocele persists, there is usually a narrow communication with the peritoneal cavity (communicating hydrocele). The fluid is reabsorbed while the child is lying down and reaccumulates in the scrotum by gravity after ambulation and upright activity during the course of the day. Therefore, caregivers report a change in size, smaller in the morning and after naptime. This type of hydrocele rarely disappears spontaneously and may continue to increase in size. Therefore, surgery is recommended (Hutson et al., 1992). The differential diagnosis includes inguinal hernia, tumor, testicular torsion, and varicocele.

Surgical Management

If the hydrocele is still present at 1 year of age, it is repaired electively. The repair is similar to a hernia repair. In addition to high ligation, a portion of the excess sac down to and around the testis is removed. The fluid may persist for several weeks or months.

Nursing Interventions and Expected Outcomes

Postoperative Care

Postoperative care is the same as discussed previously for an inguinal hernia.

■ Undescended Testis

Pathophysiology

Cryptorchidism is the failure of the testis to descend into the scrotum during gestation. The mechanism of the descent is not fully understood, although it is generally regarded to be hormonally directed, and the level of descent is believed to be related to the long-term quality of the testis (the lower the testis, the more normal the histologic findings) (O'Neill et al., 2003). The diagnosis is made on the basis of the physical examination when there is an inability to palpate the testes or to bring them into a normal scrotal position.

Failure of testicular descent by 6 months to 1 year of age requires surgical correction (Hutson, 1998). The testis requires the cooler environment of the scrotum (96° F) to develop and function correctly (produce male hormones and sperm). An increased risk of infertility and cancer is found later in life if the testis is exposed to the warmer environment of the body. It is unclear why males with cryptorchidism are at greater risk for testicular tumors later in life. However, placing the testis in the scrotum and performing regular self-examination results in early detection of cancer. If the testis is abnormal at the time of surgery, it is removed (Hutson).

Incidence

Cryptorchidism occurs more commonly in premature males (33%) than in term males (3%). Maternal exposure to estrogens during the first trimester and ordinal rank (first child) are additional risk factors. Descent continues during the first year of life. The postnatal peak in androgen production during the first 6 months of life mediates continued descent of the testis. By age 1, the incidence of cryptorchidism decreases to 0.7% to 0.8% (Kelalis, King, & Belman, 1992).

Classification

Undescended testes are classified first by whether they are palpable during physical examination. Palpable testes are either retractile, ectopic, or truly undescended within the canal. Nonpalpable testes are either intraabdominal or absent (Fig. 10-4). The examination of the testes should take place in a warm, relaxed examination room. Begin by first placing the thumb and index finger of one hand on the scrotum and palpating gently. Then, place the index finger of the opposite hand medial to the iliac spine and move the finger gently over toward the pubis.

Retractile testes are most commonly palpated in the canal or scrotal infundibulum. They are not undescended but rather withdraw secondary to an active cremasteric reflex. Surgical intervention is not indicated unless the testes do not remain in the scrotum (O'Neill et al., 2003). Ectopic testes descend outside the external ring and then are misdirected to the abdominal wall, medial thigh, or perineum. This occurs as a result of a mechanical obstruction of the path of descent (Hutson et al., 1992). Undescended testes may be intraabdominal, intracanalicular, or emergent (just outside the ring). Both the length and the fixation of the spermatic vessels cause arrest of the descent. The testes may move and intermittently become palpable. The higher the testis, the more severe the degree of maldevelopment (Kelalis et al., 1992). Absent testes are uncommon.

Surgical Management

The treatment of an undescended testis is to surgically fix the testis in the scrotum. This is called an *orchidopexy* or *orchiopexy*. The optimal time of surgical intervention is at 6 months of age (Hutson & Hasthorpe, 2005). The goal of the procedure is to improve fertility, to reduce the

risk of malignancy, to correct associated hernias, to prevent testicular torsion, and to provide psychological support (Kelalis et al., 1992). Laparoscopy is frequently used in primary repair and as a tool to evaluate and explore a nonpalpable testis (Schleef, von Bismarck, Burmucic, Gutmann, & Mayr, 2002).

Nursing Interventions and Expected Outcomes

The long-term follow-up of this group of patients is important. Careful testicular examination should be part of the yearly primary care physical examination. All adolescent males should be taught to perform testicular self-examination.

Postoperative Care

Postoperative care is the same as discussed previously for an inguinal hernia.

■ Circumcision

The decision about whether to circumcise the newborn boy is greatly debated among family members. It is usually a decision made on the basis of either religious or cultural preferences. Many parents make the decision without seeking a medical opinion. When parents' opinions differ, they seek information from other sources. Proper information regarding the foreskin is necessary when advice is given.

In its summary, the American Academy of Pediatrics (1999) offers the following advice: "Existing scientific evidence demonstrates potential medical benefits of newborn circumcision; however, these data are not sufficient to recommend routine neonatal circumcision." All studies that have examined the relationship between urinary tract infection (UTI) and circumcision have shown an increased incidence of urinary tract infection in uncircumcised males. However, the risk is low. In addition, the American Academy of Pediatrics (AAP) reviewed the existing literature regarding the incidence of penile cancer and circumcision and found a threefold greater incidence among uncircumcised men related to the development of phimosis in uncircumcised men. However, the studies did not examine whether or not effective hygiene would prevent phimosis. Finally, the relationship between sexually transmitted diseases, including human immunodeficiency virus, and circumcision were reviewed. Although there is an increased incidence of sexually transmitted diseases in males who are not circumcised, behavioral risk factors were found to be more important.

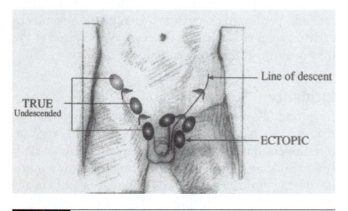

FIGURE 10-4 Undescended testes.

The American Academy of Pediatrics recommends that providers give unbiased information regarding the risks and benefits of the procedure and suggests that the decision about whether to circumcise the normal newborn boy rests with the parents. Ethnic, religious, and cultural traditions are valid factors in the decision making. When circumcision is elected in the newborn period, it should be performed with local analgesia.

The foreskin (prepuce) is the skin that covers the glans. It is lightly adherent to the glans at birth and remains so throughout infancy. Spontaneous separation of the foreskin from the glans occurs with the shedding of normal skin cells (smegma) by the foreskin during infancy. This continues throughout childhood.

The normal foreskin needs no special care other than normal bathing. As the foreskin normally separates from the glans, perform gentle retraction during bathing. This is not recommended before 1 to 2 years of age.

There are three medical indications for circumcision: phimosis, paraphimosis, and balanitis (Hutson et al., 1992). Phimosis is stenosis of the opening of the foreskin. This occurs as a result of forceful attempts at retraction of the foreskin. Paraphimosis occurs in older boys when the foreskin gets pulled behind the glans and cannot be brought back. This causes constriction and swelling of the glans, and it is very painful. Local anesthesia and often general anesthesia are necessary before manual reduction of the foreskin can be performed. A circumcision is then performed to prevent recurrence. Balanitis is an infection of the foreskin. Usually resulting from phimosis, balanitis can also occur when the foreskin is not retracted and contamination occurs. Topical antibiotic ointment or systemic antibiotics are used to reduce inflammation (Hutson et al.). Elective circumcision is planned when the infection and inflammation have resolved.

Surgical Intervention

Circumcision is most commonly performed with local anesthesia in the newborn period. After the dorsal penile nerve block is placed, the circumcision can be performed with the use of a clamp, such as a Gomco clamp which is left on for several minutes. The foreskin is then excised and the clamp is removed. When the Plastibell® device is used, a suture is used to tie off the foreskin, and the disposable ring is left on until it falls off. This takes approximately 9 days and occurs when the skin necroses (Cuckow, 1998). The wound is wrapped with petroleum gauze, and antibiotic ointment may be applied for several diaper changes to protect the wound and prevent sticking to the diaper.

Circumcision is considered a more significant surgical procedure in the older boy for a variety of reasons: the need for general anesthesia, increased incidence of postoperative bleeding, and finally, developmental sensitivity to prepare the boy for surgery on his penis. The surgery is usually performed in a freehand manner. Hemostasis is achieved with cautery, and the wound is secured with absorbable sutures.

Complications

Complications are rare; however, the most common is bleeding. Others include meatal ulceration, stenosis, urinary retention, and postcircumcision phimosis.

Postoperative Care

Postoperative care includes the use of petroleum gauze or a transparent dressing on the wound to prevent sticking to the diaper or the underwear. Careful cleansing and antibiotic ointment application to the wound are important to provide comfort and to prevent infection. Pain control is achieved with oxycodone, ibuprofen, or acetaminophen. Parents are often concerned about the degree of erythema and swelling and should be reassured that this will resolve after 5 to 7 days.

■ Conclusion

When outpatient surgery is efficiently planned and children and families are both physically and developmentally prepared, short stay surgery is safe, recovery is fast, and children return to normal living within days.

■ Educational Materials

APSNA invites you to download the diagnosis-related teaching tools "Hydrocelectomy," "Inguinal Hernias," "Orchidopexy," and "Umbilical Hernia" for Chapter 10, Common Outpatient Pediatric Surgical Procedures, at the APSNA Web site (www.apsna.org) and the Jones and Bartlett Web site (www.jbpub.com). All teaching materials are available in English and Spanish and are free of charge. APSNA encourages their use for your patients and families.

References

American Academy of Pediatrics. (1999). Circumcision policy statement. American academy of pediatrics. *Pediatrics, 103*(3), 686–693.

Bar-Mor, G. (1997). Preparation of children for surgery and invasive procedures: Milestones on the way to success. *Journal of Pediatric Nursing, 12*(4), 257–259.

Borkowski, S. (1994). Common pediatric surgical problems. *Nursing Clinics of North America, 29*, 551–562.

Brady, M., Kinn, S., O'Rourke, K., Randhawa, N., & Stuart, P. (2005). Preoperative fasting for preventing perioperative complications in children. The Cochrane Database of Systematic Reviews, Issue 2. Art. No.: CD005285. DOI: 10.1002/14651858.CD005285.

Brewer, S. L., & Lambert, C. S. (1997). Preparing children for same-day surgery: Innovative approaches. *Journal of Pediatric Nursing, 12*(4), 252–255.

Cuckow, P. M. (1998). Circumcision. In M. D. Stringer, P. D. E. Mouriquand, K. T. Oldham, & E. R. Howard (Eds.), *Pediatric surgery and urology: Long term outcomes* (pp. 616–623). Philadelphia: WB Saunders.

Fisher, Q. A., McComiskey, C. M., Hill, J. L., Spurrier, E. A., Voigt, R. W., Savarese, A. M., et al. (1993). Postoperative voiding interval and duration of analgesia following peripheral or caudal nerve blocks in children. *Anesthesia and Analgesia, 76,* 173–177.

Geisler, D. P., Jegathesan, S., Parmley, M. C., McGee, J. M., Nolen, M. G., & Broughan, T. A. (2001). Laparoscopic exploration for the clinically undetected hernia in infancy and childhood. *American Journal of Surgery, 182*(6), 693–696.

Gill, F. T. (1998). Umbilical hernia, inguinal hernias, and hydroceles in children: Diagnostic clues for optimal patient management. *Journal of Pediatric Health Care, 12*(5), 231–235.

Hutson, J., & Hasthorpe, S. (2005). Testicular descent and cryptorchidism: The state of the art in 2004. *Journal of Pediatric Surgery, 40,* 297–302.

Hutson, J. M. (1998). Undescended testes. In M. D. Stringer, P. D. E. Mouriquand, K. T. Oldham, & E. R. Howard (Eds.), *Pediatric surgery and urology: Long term outcomes* (pp. 603–615). Philadelphia: WB Saunders.

Hutson, J. M., Beasley, S. W., & Woodward, A. A. (1992). *Jones' clinical paediatric surgery.* Oxford, England: Blackwell Scientific Publications.

Kelalis, P. P., King, L. R., & Belman, A. B. (1992). *Clinical pediatric urology.* Philadelphia: WB Saunders.

Keshtgar, A. S., & Griffiths, M. (2003). Incarceration of umbilical hernia in children: Is the trend increasing? *European Journal of Pediatric Surgery, 12*(1), 40–43.

Linden, J., & Engberg, J. B. (1994). Nursing discharge assessment of the patient postinguinal herniorrhaphy in the ambulatory surgery setting. *Journal of Post Anesthesia Nursing, 9,* 14–19.

O'Neill, J., Grosfeld, J., Fonkalsrud, E., Coran, A., & Caldamone, A. (2003). *Principles of pediatric surgery.* Philadelphia: Mosby.

Patel, R. I., DeWitt, L., & Hannallah, R. S. (1997). Preoperative laboratory testing in children undergoing elective surgery: Analysis of current practice. *Journal of Clinical Anesthesia, 9*(7), 569–575.

Rowe, M. I., O'Neill, J. A., Grosfeld, J. L., Fonkalsrud, E. W., & Coran, A. G. (1995). *Essentials of pediatric surgery.* St. Louis, MO: Mosby.

Schleef, J., von Bismarck, S., Burmucic, K., Gutmann, A., & Mayr, J. (2002). Groin exploration for nonpalpable testes: Laparoscopic approach. *Journal of Pediatric Surgery, 37*(11), 1552–1555.

Skinner, M. A., & Grosfeld, J. L. (1993). Inguinal and umbilical repair in infants and children. *Surgical Clinics of North America, 73,* 439–448.

Spurbeck, W. W., Prasad, R., & Lobe, T. E. (2005). Two year experience with minimally invasive herniorrhaphy in children. *Surgical Endoscopy, 19,* 551–553.

Vransky, P., & Bourdelat, D. (1997). Incarcerated umbilical hernia in children. *Pediatric Surgery International, 12*(1), 61–62.

Yaster, M., Sola, J. E., Pegoli, W., & Paidas, C. N. (1994). The night after surgery. Postoperative management of the pediatric outpatient—Surgical and anesthetic aspects. *Pediatric Clinics of North America, 41*(1), 199–218.

Special Considerations in the Care of the Neonate

II

Fetal Surgery

*By Lori J. Howell, Susan R. Miesnik,
Kelli B. Young*

The focus of this chapter is to describe those fetal diagnoses that may be considered for prenatal surgery. In most cases, detection of a fetal anomaly leads to a change in the timing, mode, or location of delivery to improve the maternal-infant outcome. For a few severely affected fetuses, fetal surgery may be the best option. Each of these anatomic malformations presents with a spectrum of severity, and only those fetuses with life-threatening or severely debilitating anomalies are considered candidates for fetal surgery (Table 11-1).

The incidence, embryology, prenatal diagnosis, and in utero repair of anatomic malformations are described. In addition, the role of the surgical nurse providing preoperative, intraoperative, and postoperative nursing care is presented, as is the role of a center for fetal diagnosis and treatment. Maternal teaching sheets for open fetal surgical procedures and shunting procedures are also presented. Postnatal repair is detailed elsewhere in the appropriate chapters in this text.

◼ Fetal Congenital Diaphragmatic Hernia

Congenital diaphragmatic hernia (CDH) occurs in about 1 in 2,400 live births, with left-sided hernias occurring about seven times more frequently than right-sided hernias. CDH occurs when the pleuroperitoneal canal fails to close and the abdominal viscera migrate into the thoracic cavity, compressing the existing fetal lung and preventing normal pulmonary development (Fig. 11-1). Advances have been made in the care of these challenging infants, including extracorporeal membrane oxygenation (Bartlett et al., 1986; Stolar, Dillon, & Reyes, 1988), high-frequency oscillatory ventilation (Tamura et al., 1988), nitric oxide, and liquid ventilation. In one prospective study, despite optimal postnatal care, fetuses with isolated CDH diagnosed before 25 weeks' gestation had a mortality rate of 58% (Harrison, Adzick, Estes, & Howell, 1994).

Prenatal Diagnosis and Indication for Fetal Surgery

Because the prognosis of CDH is not universally fatal, selecting the most severely affected fetuses with CDH is critical. It now appears that liver herniation into the chest is a predictor of poor outcome in fetal CDH (Albanese et al., 1998). Liver herniation is detected by following the umbilical vein and ductus venosus above the level of the diaphragm with color-flow Doppler ultrasonography.

Table 11-1 **Conditions Amenable to Fetal Surgery**

Congenital Anomaly	Prenatal Effects	Postnatal Outcome	Fetal Surgical Procedure	Postnatal Surgical Procedure
Congenital diaphragmatic hernia	Lung hypoplasia	Pulmonary failure	Tracheal occlusion	CDH repair
Congenital cystic adenomatoid malformation	Lung hypoplasia Hydrops, death	Pulmonary failure Death	Open fetal lobectomy Shunt placement	Lobectomy
Sacrococcygeal teratoma	Hydrops, death Maternal mirror syndrome		EXIT procedure Tumor debulking	Complete resection
Urinary tract obstruction	Hydronephrosis Oligohydramnios	Renal & pulmonary failure	Vesicoamniotic shunt Fetoscopic laser	± Urethral valve ablation
Neck masses	Pulmonary hypoplasia Airway obstruction Polyhydramnios	Asphyxia Prematurity	EXIT procedure	± Tumor resection
Myelomeningocele*	Hydrocephalus; lower extremity involvement		Open fetal repair	

Abbreviations: CDH, congenital diaphragmatic hernia; EXIT, ex utero intra partum treatment.
*Currently performed in an NIH prospective randomized trial U10 HD41666.

Ultrafast fetal magnetic resonance imaging is an even better technique to detect liver position and does not require maternal sedation or fetal paralysis to prevent motion artifact (Hubbard, Adzick, Crombleholme, & Haselgrove, 1997). The use of sonographic determination of the lung/head ratio (LHR) is also used as a predictor of survival in fetal CDH (Metkus, Filly, Stringer, Harrison, & Adzick, 1996). The LHR is a measurement of the right lung at the level of the atria expressed as a ratio to the head circumference, where an LHR less than 1 is associated with 90% mortality. Careful sonographic evaluation is also important to rule out such syndromes as Fryns' syndrome. This is an autosomal recessive condition with multiple defects, including CDH, and is associated with mental retardation in those who survive but is generally lethal because of the severe pulmonary hypoplasia associated with CDH (McPherson, Ketterer, & Salsburey, 1993). A chromosome analysis is completed by amniocentesis, chorionic villus sampling, or percutaneous umbilical blood sampling to rule out abnormalities such as trisomy 13, trisomy 18, and mosaic tetrasomy 12-p (Bergoffen, Prunett, & Campbell, 1993). Fetal surgery is not offered when a chromosomal abnormality is detected. A fetal echocardiogram is performed to rule out structural heart disease. Thus, a mother is considered a candidate for fetal surgery for CDH when her fetus has an isolated CDH with liver herniation into the chest, has an LHR less than 1, and is less than 26 weeks gestation. In addition, the fetus must have a structurally normal heart by fetal echocardiogram and no chromosomal abnormality. Only the most severely affected fetuses are considered candidates for prenatal surgery because of additional risk to the mother as an innocent bystander trying to help her fetus.

Initially, the standard postnatal CDH repair was offered prenatally. The results observed in the surviving infants prompted a National Institutes of Health (NIH)-sponsored trial of complete repair in utero (Harrison et al., 1997). Data from this trial indicated that fetal surgery was successful in fetuses without liver herniation, but no better than standard postnatal care (Harrison et al.). For those with liver herniation, complete repair was not feasible because the umbilical vein became kinked and resulted in fetal death. Subsequently, a new strategy of tracheal occlusion to accelerate lung growth was applied to fetal sheep and later clinically (Hedrick, Estes, Sullivan, Adzick, & Harrison, 1994; Wilson, DiFiore, & Peters, 1993). A comparison of postnatal CDH with fetoscopically occluded tracheas indicated a benefit to performing the procedure fetoscopically and described 75% survival in this latter group with an LHR from 0.7 to 1.4 (Harrison et al.). These preliminary data demonstrated the fetoscopic tracheal occlusion technique to have great promise and formed the basis for a 1999 NIH-sponsored clinical trial comparing fetoscopic tracheal occlusion with standard postnatal care for fetuses with an LHR < 1.4. Results from this trial in-

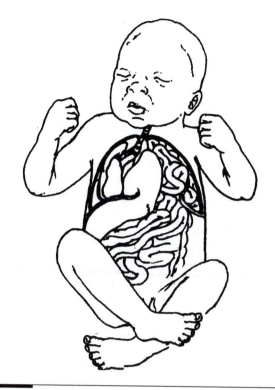

Figure 11-1 Fetus with severe left-sided congenital diaphragmatic hernia.
Source: Center for Fetal Diagnosis and Treatment, Children's Hospital of Philadelphia.

dicated that mortality was equivocal for fetal and postnatal repair. However, the issue of morbidity is under evaluation. The group at The Children's Hospital of Philadelphia reported a 33% survival in 15 fetuses who underwent open tracheal occlusion in fetuses with a predicted mortality in excess of 90% (based on LHR < 1.0) when fetal tracheal clip application was performed at 26 weeks' gestation (Flake, 1996). However, the authors noted that survival remains compromised by pulmonary function and prematurity. The outcome of severely affected CDH fetuses appears to be somewhat improved by tracheal occlusion, but more work is needed to achieve consistent lung growth and decrease the effects of prematurity.

Fetal Surgery Technique for CDH

The goal of fetal surgery in the fetus with a severe CDH is to improve pulmonary hypoplasia. The therapeutic strategy for fetal CDH is to promote lung growth by impeding the normal egress of lung fluid by tracheal occlusion. The lungs enlarge and push the viscera back into the abdomen (Hedrick, Estes, et al., 1994; Wilson et al., 1993). The use of fetoscopic balloon placement into the trachea and decompression of the balloon before delivery make a vaginal delivery possible. At delivery, bronchoscopy of the neonate's airway is performed, exogenous

surfactant is instilled if the fetus is premature, and the airway is intubated. Umbilical lines are placed, the cord is clamped and cut, and the neonate is taken to the adjacent operating room for the remainder of the resuscitation. Once the neonate's condition is stabilized, a standard repair of the CDH is performed usually several weeks later, often with a synthetic patch because these diaphragmatic defects are typically quite large. At present, this technique is applied clinically in Europe (Deprest et al., 2006). Ongoing laboratory work into the fetal biology of lung growth is being actively pursued.

Fetal Lung Lesions

There are two types of thoracic masses, congenital cystic adenomatoid malformation of the lung (CCAM) and bronchopulmonary sequestration (BPS), that are sometimes amenable to prenatal resection. CCAM is a benign pulmonary lung mass characterized by an overgrowth of the terminal bronchioles that form various-sized cysts (Adzick, Harrison, Crombleholme, Flake, & Howell, 1998). CCAMs develop during the first 6 weeks of gestation and generally arise from one lobe. CCAMs are classified into two types on the basis of the size and distribution of the cysts. Macrocystic lesions contain a single or multiple cysts that are greater than 5 mm on ultrasound. Microcystic masses appear on ultrasound as solid masses (Adzick, 2003; Adzick & Kitano, 2003). BPS is a mass of abnormal lung tissue that receives an anomalous blood supply from a feeding vessel off the aorta and does not communicate with the tracheobronchial tree by normally related bronchi. BPSs may be intralobar (90%) or extralobar (10%) (Bianchi, Crombleholme, & D'Alton, 2000). A recent report describes a "hybrid" mass that has histologic findings similar to that of a CCAM, with an anomalous blood supply (Cass et al., 1997). Both types of masses may compromise lung growth and thus lead to lung hypoplasia.

Prenatal Diagnosis of a Thoracic Mass and Indication for Fetal Surgery

The diagnosis of a fetal thoracic mass is made by ultrasonography. The differential diagnoses include CDH, bronchogenic/neuroenteric cysts, bronchial atresia, pleural effusions (usually an infectious origin), and congenital high airway obstruction (CHAOS) (Hedrick, Ferro, et al., 1994). Prenatally detected CCAM and BPS have a much higher mortality than those diagnosed after birth. The mortality underestimation occurs because some fetuses die in utero, whereas others with large masses resulting in pulmonary hypoplasia require urgent removal in the delivery room and do not survive resuscitation and transfer to a tertiary center. Those fetuses with fetal hydrops caused by large mass compression have a dismal prognosis without prenatal intervention (Adzick et al., 1998).

Once a diagnosis of a fetal CCAM is made, ultrasonographic surveillance to detect tumor growth leading to hydrops is critical. The sonographic determination of the CCAM volume ratio (CVR) is useful as an indicator of fetuses at risk for developing hydrops (Crombleholme et al., 2002). The CCAM volume ratio is calculated using the formula for a prolate ellipse (height times length and width × 0.52). To account for gestational age, this result is divided by the head circumference to determine the CVR. A CVR greater than 1.6 at initial presentation accurately predicts an increased risk of the fetus for developing hydrops.

The ability to provide this prognostic information to families is very reassuring and enables identification of those patients who require close observation and possible fetal intervention. Serial sonography is often performed several times per week for large masses. If the mass appears to regress in size or to stabilize, the frequency of the ultrasonography is decreased. However, for masses that increase in size, the heart may become displaced, impede venous return, and result in fetal hydrops. Fetal hydrops is a precursor of fetal death and is the only indication for fetal surgery (Adzick et al., 1998). Typically, fetal hydrops is demonstrated by the following progression of findings: fetal ascites, placentomegaly, and skin and scalp edema.

Chromosome analysis is not necessary to proceed with fetal surgery because there appears to be no abnormal chromosomal association with CCAM. A large CCAM also can have maternal health implications, known as the "maternal mirror syndrome." This pre-eclamptic state can be life threatening to the mother as she mirrors the condition of the sick fetus. Fetal surgery does not cure this maternal hyperdynamic state, and if the mother chooses to continue the pregnancy without fetal surgery in the face of a hydropic fetus, she must be closely monitored for hypertension, proteinuria, and edema (Adzick et al., 1993).

Fetal Surgery Technique for CCAM

For the hydropic fetus less than 32 weeks' gestation that presents with a large macrocystic CCAM, decompression of the mass through long-term fluid drainage may be achieved with thoracoamniotic shunt placement (Wilson et al., 2004). Six to 10% of fetuses with BPS experience pleural effusions (Johnson & Hubbard, 2004). This population may also require the insertion of a thoracoamniotic

shunt for long-term drainage of the effusion. Shunt placement is best accomplished as an outpatient procedure using maternal sedation with morphine sulfate and diazepam (Fig. 11-2). Careful ultrasound evaluation before shunt placement is essential in identifying fetal and placental position. Once the approach is decided upon, the mother's skin is anesthetized using a local anesthetic agent, and a stab wound is made in the maternal abdomen. Under continuous ultrasound guidance, the shunt trocar is advanced through the mother's abdomen, uterine wall, and fetal chest wall and into the cystic component of the CCAM. The shunt is then advanced through the trocar until the proximal end is placed in the cysts. The trocar is then removed from the fetal chest, and the distal end of the shunt is deployed in the amniotic fluid (Keswani, Wilson, & Johnson, in press). The mother is monitored for uterine activity and recovered from sedation for a few hours before being discharged. Uterine contractions are aggressively treated with tocolytic medications and intravenous fluids.

For the hydropic fetus with a CCAM diagnosed before 32 weeks' gestation, fetal surgery may be considered (Fig. 11-3). Fetal surgery involves maternal-fetal general anesthesia, laparotomy, hysterotomy, and fetal exposure of the presenting side of the CCAM. A fetal thoracotomy and lobectomy are then performed. Operative time is usually quite short, and blood loss is typically minimal. The fetus is then returned to the womb to await delivery.

Unlike fetal surgery for CDH, cesarean delivery is performed by an obstetrician with neonatal resuscitation immediately available. Prenatal surgery has dramatically improved the outcome for fetuses with hydrops associated with CCAM. In one reported series, 13 hydropic

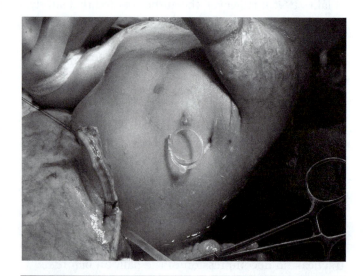

Figure 11-2 Thoracoamniotic shunt in place at delivery.
Source: Center for Fetal Diagnosis and Treatment, Children's Hospital of Philadelphia.

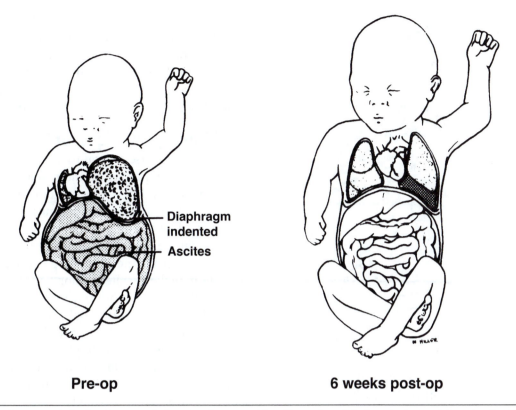

Pre-op

6 weeks post-op

Figure 11-3 Fetal anatomy in hydropic congenital cystic adenomatoid malformation of the lung before and 6 weeks after fetal surgery.
Source: Center for Fetal Diagnosis and Treatment, Children's Hospital of Philadelphia.

CCAM fetuses underwent fetal surgery, and eight survived with an excellent quality of life (Adzick et al., 1998; Flake & Howell, 1998).

The fetus with a large CCAM may experience severe pulmonary compromise at the time of delivery. To minimize the risk of inadequate ventilation caused by the mass effect, delivery can occur using an ex utero intra partum treatment (EXIT)-to-CCAM resection approach. The EXIT procedure is performed using maternal general anesthesia to provide for optimal uterine relaxation. A maternal laparotomy and hysterotomy are performed. The fetal head, shoulders, thorax, and one arm are delivered through the hysterotomy. To reduce the risk of premature placental separation, uterine volume is maintained by the trunk and lower extremities of the fetus remaining in the uterus. Continuous amnioinfusion with warmed saline or lactated Ringer's solution also contributes to maintenance of uterine volume. An infant airway is established and secured, peripheral intravenous access is obtained, and oxygen saturation monitoring is begun. A thoracotomy is performed, the CCAM is resected, and ventilation of the infant is initiated. Throughout the procedure, continuous fetal echocardiography is monitored, and additional intravenous fluids, blood products, and/or medications are administered to the infant

as indicated. After the resection the infant is delivered, the umbilical cord clamped, and the baby is taken to the neonatal intensive care unit. In one small series of five patients, an 80% overall survival rate was reported (Hedrick, 2003).

■ Fetal Sacrococcygeal Teratoma

Sacrococcygeal teratoma (SCT) is the most common tumor found in the newborn, with a reported incidence of 1 in 35,000 to 40,000 live births (Pantoja, Llobet, & Gonzalez-Flores, 1976). Fetal SCT is a tumor arising from the presacral space that may grow to massive proportions. Teratomas are embryonal neoplasms derived from totipotential cells that contain tissue from two or three germ cell layers (ectoderm, endoderm, and mesoderm) (Flake, 1993). SCTs arise from the coccyx bone. The American Academy of Pediatrics Surgical Section suggests four classifications according to location (Altman, Randolph, & Lilly, 1974). Type I tumors are external with little presacral component (Fig. 11-4). Type II tumors have more external than intrapelvic components, whereas type III tumors, although obvious externally, have more internal components. A type IV tumor is located entirely within

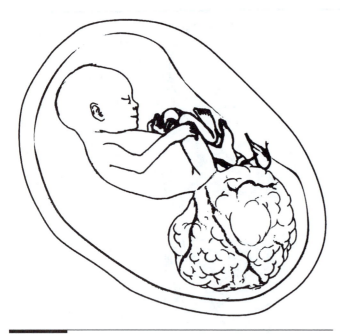

Figure 11-4 Fetus with huge type 1 sacrococcygeal teratoma.
Source: Center for Fetal Diagnosis and Treatment, Children's Hospital of Philadelphia.

the pelvis and may go unrecognized until symptomatic. These tumors are also classified according to histologic findings. Type I histologic findings are mature and well differentiated and may contain endodermal, mesodermal, or ectodermal tissue. These tumors are usually benign. Type II histologic findings are immature and contain embryonal elements and may become malignant. Type III histologic findings are malignant and contain elements of the yolk sac (Altman et al.).

Prenatal Diagnosis of SCT and Indication for Fetal Surgery

Fetal SCT is diagnosed by prenatal ultrasonography. As with other fetal diagnoses, most fetal SCTs can be managed with routine prenatal care. For fetuses with large SCTs who show no signs of hydrops, a cesarean section is recommended to prevent dystocia, tumor rupture, and exsanguination (Flake, 1993). Preterm delivery caused by polyhydramnios may affect morbidity and mortality. The mechanism of polyhydramnios in SCT is not completely understood, but the condition seems to accompany the development of placentomegaly and may be the first sign that the tumor is affecting the fetus (Holzgreve, Flake, & Langer, 1990). Fetal SCTs are followed with serial ultrasonographic studies using color and power Doppler ultrasonography to identify fetuses with large, vascular lesions who are at risk for fetal death due to high-output cardiac failure. Ultrasonography is useful to determine fetal hemodynamics, such as inferior vena caval dilation and increased cardiac output as well as placen-

tal thickness, as a predictor for fetal hydrops. As with other fetal conditions that result in poor placental perfusion and endothelial cell injury, maternal mirror syndrome may be seen (Flake). The indication for fetal SCT resection is a type I SCT with hydrops, evidenced by placentomegaly and increased combined ventricular output.

Fetal Surgery Technique for SCT

The presumed cause of fetal hydrops is a vascular steal by the teratoma, placing an increased workload on the fetal heart (Flake, 1993). Emergency debulking of the tumor is performed as a palliative measure to reduce the cardiac workload. The mother and fetus receive a deep inhalational anesthetic. A maternal laparotomy and hysterotomy are performed, allowing exposure of the fetal buttocks with the attached tumor. Because the tumor can be larger than the fetus, uterine relaxation is critical. The anus is identified, and the fetal skin is incised posterior to the anorectal sphincter to avoid injury to the continence mechanism. A tourniquet is then applied to the base of the tumor and cinched down gradually to the vascular pedicle. Tumor debulking is then performed with a stapler. Care is taken to avoid tumor rupture. The entire fetal procedure typically is performed in less than 15 minutes with minimal blood loss (Flake). Delivery is performed by obstetricians, with neonatal resuscitation immediately available. Once the neonate is stabilized, a complete resection of the mass, including the coccyx, is performed. Of the four fetal SCT resections performed at the Children's Hospital of Philadelphia, three have survived (Adzick, Crombleholme, Morgan, & Quinn, 1997; Hedrick, 2003).

■ Obstructive Uropathy

Obstructive uropathy refers to multiple conditions that may cause an obstruction in the urinary system, such as ureteropelvic junction obstruction, posterior urethral valves, ureterocele, megaureter, multicystic kidney, duplex collecting system, and prune belly syndrome (Fig. 11-5). Most of these anomalies require surgery after birth. Most fetuses with obstructive uropathy are male, but obstructions in females do occur and tend to be associated with complex cloacal abnormalities (Tsao & Albanese, 2003). The most common cause of obstruction in the male is posterior urethral valves, with a reported incidence of 1 in 5,000 to 8,000 (Casale, 1990). Obstruction of the fetal urinary tract may result in renal damage that ranges from hydronephrosis to renal dysplasia (Lebowitz & Griscom, 1997). The obstruction leads to a decrease

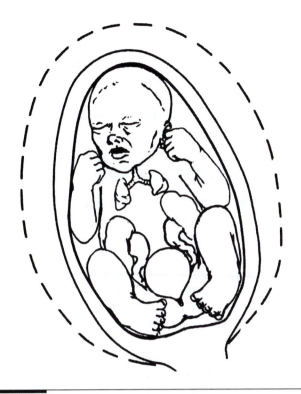

Figure 11-5 Fetus with obstructive uropathy.
Source: Center for Fetal Diagnosis and Treatment, Children's Hospital of Philadelphia.

or absence of amniotic fluid, resulting in fatal pulmonary hypoplasia, Potter's facies, and contractures (Harrison, Ross, Noall, & de Lorimier, 1983).

Prenatal Diagnosis of Obstruction Uropathy and Indication for Fetal Surgery

Ultrasonographic evaluation and urine sampling of fetuses with obstructive uropathy have helped explain the natural history of this process and formulate selection criteria for intervention. Ultrasonographic examination indicating poor renal function is evidenced by the development of cortical cysts and renal echogenicity indicating renal dysplasia. Poor renal function is likely to be present when elevated fetal urinary electrolytes (sodium and chloride) and $beta_2$-microglobulin are noted (Freedman et al., 1997). Fetal urine sampling techniques involve three percutaneous aspirations of the fetal bladder, usually 48 to 72 hours apart. The first and second urine samples can be stale and the results unreliable. The third aspiration provides the most reliable indicator of kidney function and damage (Johnson & Freedman, 1999). The indications for fetal intervention include bilateral obstructive uropathy, known onset of oligohydramnios, normal male chromosomes, favorable urine electrolytes and $beta_2$-microglobulins, and the absence of renal echogenicity and cortical cysts.

Fetal Surgery Technique for Obstructive Uropathy

At present, the most widely accepted method for decompressing the fetal urinary tract is the use of a double pig-tailed catheter placed percutaneously with sonographic guidance. However, the catheter lumen can become occluded, migrate, or injure the fetus during placement. Most recently, fetoscopy has been performed to ablate the valves using a yttrium-aluminum-garnet laser through an antegrade approach (Quintero, Morales, Allen, Bornick, & Johnson, 2000). Despite the treatment techniques developed for obstructive uropathy, reliable ways of predicting long-term renal function are still needed.

■ Giant Neck Masses

Giant fetal neck masses, such as cervical teratomas, hygromas, and hemangiomas, as well as anomalies such as congenital high airway obstruction (CHAOS), can case airway obstruction at delivery. CHAOS is characterized by a blockage at the laryngeal level or laryngeal atresia. Fetal neck mass disorders can result in profound hypoxia and even death due to the inability to obtain an airway after birth. Although fetuses with these conditions do not undergo fetal surgery in the classic sense (i.e., the fetus is not returned to the womb after the operation), they can undergo multiple procedures for up to an hour while they are still attached to the placental circulation (Howell, Burns, Lenghetti, Kerr, & Harkins, 2002).

Prenatal Diagnosis of Giant Neck Masses and Indications for Fetal Surgery

Accurate diagnosis of these anomalies with prenatal ultrasonography and ultrafast fetal magnetic resonance imaging (Fig. 11-6) ensures appropriate preparation for a planned delivery to rule out anomalies, establish fetal growth, and detail characteristics of the fetal airway anatomy (Hubbard, Crombleholme, & Adzick, 1998). A complete obstetric history and physical and genetic evaluation are also performed. For example, polyhydramnios caused by esophageal compression of the neck mass causes distention of the uterus and may lead to preterm labor. Genetic abnormalities, such as 69XXX, or syndromes, such as Fraser's syndrome, may be associated with CHAOS (Hedrick, Ferro, et al., 1994). A triploidy chromosomal abnormality, 69XXX, is characterized by marked lateral physical asymmetry and syndactyly and is often associated with a myelomeningocele. Fraser's syndrome is an autosomal recessive disorder in which laryngeal atresia and renal agenesis are common findings. These conditions

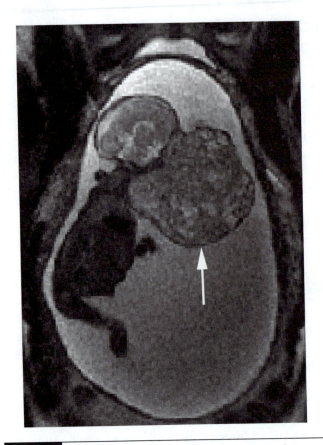

Figure 11-6 Ultrafast fetal magnetic resonance imaging of giant cervical teratoma.
Source: Center for Fetal Diagnosis and Treatment, Children's Hospital of Philadelphia.

are usually fatal in pregnancies that reach full term. A fetal echocardiogram is performed to rule out structural abnormalities and to identify impending hydrops.

Fetal Surgery Technique for Giant Neck Mass

The EXIT procedure is a technique first described for the delivery of a fetus in which tracheal occlusion had been performed in cases of severe CDH (Bealer et al., 1995; Skarsgard et al., 1996). This technique is now used successfully to secure a fetal airway in near-term infants with giant neck masses (Bouchard et al., 2002). Maternal-fetal anesthesia is provided to enhance uterine relaxation, a crucial point to preserve utero-placental circulation. A maternal laparotomy and an amniotic fluid reduction are performed through a uterine trocar for patients with severe polyhydramnios. When possible, a lower-uterine-segment hysterotomy is performed to expose the fetal head, neck, and thorax. A classical caesarean delivery is necessary when extension of the head and neck cannot be obtained because of tumor size. The head, neck, thorax, and one arm are then delivered. Fetal pulse oximetry continuously monitors the fetal heart rate and

hemoglobin saturation. Multiple procedures can be performed for up to an hour before the cord is clamped and subsequent delivery is achieved. These procedures may include laryngoscopy, bronchoscopy, intubation, exogenous surfactant instillation, placement of umbilical lines, and, in rare instances, tumor resection (Fig. 11-7).

■ Patient Selection Process

When a fetal abnormality amenable to fetal intervention is diagnosed, the prospective parents have three choices. If the gestation is before 24 weeks, termination of the pregnancy may be an option. After 24 weeks, continuation of the pregnancy and providing for the best postnatal care may be the parents' decision. For some, intervening before birth may be the option selected. Parents need to be supported regardless of their decision to minimize feelings of guilt later.

An evaluation for fetal surgery consists of outpatient diagnostic tests and a review of results by a multidisciplinary team (Fig. 11-8). A detailed sonographic survey is performed to confirm the diagnosis, detect any additional fetal abnormalities, and assess the presence and severity of hydrops. A fetal echocardiogram is performed to assess any structural abnormalities of the heart and in certain diagnoses, such as SCT, to assess subtle hemodynamic changes. Ultrafast fetal magnetic resonance imaging is a newer modality that provides striking anatomic detail and is particularly useful for diagnostic dilemmas and confirmation of liver position in CDH fetuses. If genetic karyotyping is not performed at the referring institution, an amniocentesis, chorionic villus sampling, or percutaneous blood sampling is obtained to rule out chromosomal abnormalities associated with certain fetal diseases. Rapid karyotyping can be performed for emergency problems by fluorescence in situ hybridization. This diagnostic procedure provides information about chromosomes 13, 18, and 21, as well as gender.

Finally, an informed consent conference is held with the family, fetal/pediatric surgeon, obstetric specialists, fetal and obstetric anesthesiologists, social worker, and nurse coordinator to review the test results and explain the available options for the pregnancy. All of these services should be coordinated so that the family can learn of their fetus' anomaly and options in an unhurried, comprehensive manner. The informed consent conference provides an in-depth description of the fetal surgery procedure, results from the procedure, maternal risks, potential benefits, and alternatives. If the family opts for a planned delivery and postnatal surgery, the

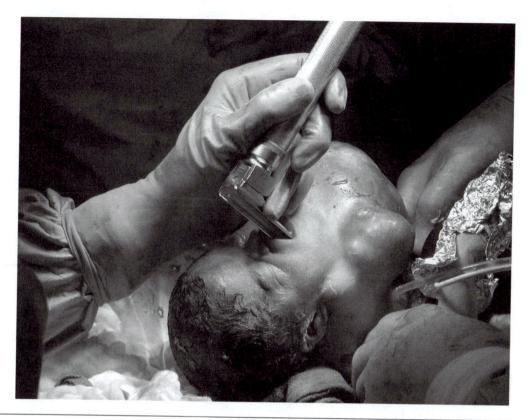

Figure 11-7 Intubation during ex utero intra partum treatment procedure for a neonate with giant cervical teratomas.
Source: Center for Fetal Diagnosis and Treatment, Children's Hospital of Philadelphia.

surgeon counsels the parents regarding the anomaly, the surgical repair, and the anticipated neonatal course. Arrangements are then made for maternal transport and planned delivery at the tertiary center. If the fetus has a fatal defect that is not amenable to fetal or postnatal surgery or if the parents opt to terminate the pregnancy, the parents receive counseling from the reproductive geneticist. Follow-up telephone and written consultation is provided immediately to the referring physician.

■ Maternal-Fetal Management

Preoperative

Once the complete evaluation indicates that the mother and fetus are candidates for fetal intervention and the parents choose to proceed, the preoperative process is arranged. The mother undergoes an electrocardiogram, chest x-ray, and laboratory studies, including a complete blood count with differential, a metabolic profile, and a type and cross-match for two units of packed red blood cells. An order is placed for 50 mL of O-negative packed red blood cells to be available intraoperatively for the fetus. An advance practice nurse completes the preoperative history and physi-

cal and anesthesia evaluation. Preoperative instruction is provided, including fasting for 8 hours before surgery, use of an antibacterial soap for a preoperative shower, and administration of indomethacin, 50 mg by mouth 2 hours before surgery to promote uterine relaxation. Additional preparation includes a tour of the obstetric and neonatal units, the scheduled time of surgery, and the expected preoperative arrival time. Additional questions and concerns that the family may have are answered.

Perioperative

When the mother arrives the morning of the surgery, vital signs, fetal well-being, and uterine activity are assessed. Support stockings are placed to prevent an embolic event. The patient is brought to the operating room for the planned procedure. The specific intervention determines the anesthetic to be used. Fetoscopic procedures are performed under regional anesthesia with maternal sedation. Open fetal surgical procedures, including EXIT procedures, are performed with the mother under general anesthesia, and epidural analgesia is used for postoperative pain management.

Upon the mother's arrival in the operating room, an epidural catheter is placed. If the mother is to receive a general anesthetic, the anesthetic induction and intuba-

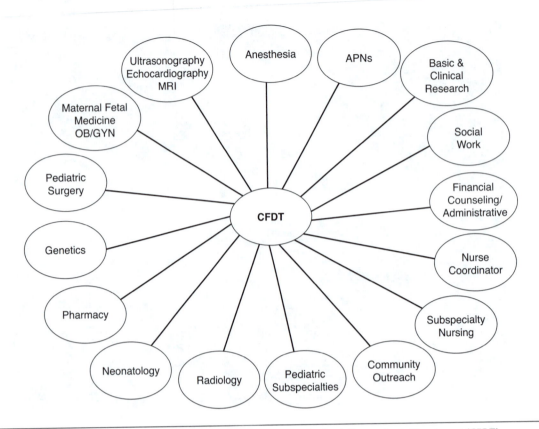

Figure 11-8 The expertise of many different specialists is required by a center for fetal diagnosis and treatment (CFDT).
Source: Center for Fetal Diagnosis and Treatment, Children's Hospital of Philadelphia.

tion are then initiated. Once the mother is anesthetized, a Foley catheter is inserted into the bladder, and the sequential compression device to prevent embolic events is activated. For open fetal cases, an arterial line, additional peripheral intravenous lines, and a nasogastric tube are also placed. The mother is prepped and draped for the fetal surgery. Ultrasound assessment is then made to confirm that there has been no change from the preoperative evaluation and to mark the placental edges.

If fetoscopic surgery is to be performed, the procedure is undertaken as previously described. If open fetal surgery is to be performed, a low transverse maternal laparotomy is then made. If the placenta is anterior, the uterus must be lifted up so that the hysterotomy can be made on the posterior aspect of the uterus. If the placenta is posterior, the hysterotomy is made on the anterior side of the uterus. The hysterotomy is performed using a specially devised stapler, with care being taken to avoid the placenta (Harrison & Adzick, 1993).

The arm of the fetus is brought out, and a miniaturized fetal pulse oximeter is applied and secured with a transparent dressing and foil. The affected portion of the fetus is then exteriorized, and the fetal surgery, as described in the preceding sections, is performed. The pulse oximetry is removed, and the hysterotomy is closed with reinfusion of warmed normal saline with an antibiotic substituted for the previously removed amniotic fluid. The maternal abdomen is then closed, and a transparent dressing is applied to allow for the postoperative sonographic evaluations.

Postoperative

The mother is awakened, and the nasogastric and endotracheal tubes are removed in the operating room. She is then transported to the Labor and Delivery unit, where intensive maternal and fetal monitoring are provided for 48 to 72 hours. Magnesium sulfate is administered as a bolus of 6 g over 20 minutes before the mother leaves the operating room, and a basal infusion rate of 2 to 4 g/hour is then initiated. Indomethacin is administered every 6 hours for the first 48 hours after surgery as an additional tocolytic. Intravenous antibiotic therapy is administered for 24 hours after surgery. Careful fluid management is critical to avoid hypovolemia, which leads to poor uterine perfusion, or hypervolemia, which can induce pulmonary edema when magnesium sulfate is used for tocolysis. Patient-controlled epidural analgesia is used for pain management.

Daily ultrasonographic surveillance is performed for fetal well-being and amniotic fluid volumes. A daily echocardiogram is also performed while the mother is taking indomethacin to assess ductal constriction and tricuspid regurgitation of the fetal heart. Once uterine activity is controlled, usually on postoperative day 1, the monitoring lines are removed, and the tocolysis is weaned to oral nifedipine. The epidural and Foley catheters are usually removed on postoperative day 2, and the mother is transferred to the antepartum unit. Pain management is accomplished using oral narcotics and acetaminophen. By this time, the mother is able to be out of bed to go to the bathroom, and if she is able to tolerate fluids, her diet may be advanced.

The mother typically remains in the hospital for 4 to 5 days. Plans are made for discharge to the nearby Ronald McDonald House by the social worker or the advanced practice nurse. Modified bed rest is recommended for the first 2 to 3 weeks after surgery, after which progression to a moderate activity level can be recommended if the mother's condition permits. Oral tocolysis is maintained for the duration of the pregnancy. In most surgery cases, the mother and her support person remain near the hospital for weekly sonographic evaluations and obstetrical care visits for the remainder of her pregnancy.

■ The Fetal Diagnosis and Treatment Center

A center for fetal diagnosis and treatment provides a coordinated approach to the care for the mother and fetus with an anomaly, using the many necessary specialists and state-of-the-art facilities required (Howell & Adzick, 2003). Because the center focuses on maternal-fetal problems, this model offers a systematic approach for diagnosing and providing treatment options; thus, expert, coordinated, efficient, and compassionate care is offered to parents facing a decision about their unborn child.

The institutional setting for the center must be able to provide a combination of clinical and basic science research with complex antepartum, intrapartum, and postpartum clinical care for the maternal-fetal patient. An active maternal transport system and high-risk obstetrical and neonatal units are essential. A neonatal resuscitation room adjacent to the operating suite must be available to provide immediate neonatal resuscitation and surgical intervention to critically ill newborns as necessary. In addition to the setting, numerous items have required adaptation, including special surgical instruments, specially devised staplers, atraumatic retractors, the level I intrauterine

warming device, fetal medications, and fetal intravenous access equipment (Harrison & Adzick, 1993).

In addition to the necessary medical specialists, nurses trained in the management of high-risk obstetric patients are crucial, and education about fetal surgery should be provided on an ongoing basis. A center should provide community education regarding the most current information related to prenatal diagnosis and treatment and immediate phone consultation and review of sonographic materials. A toll-free number, such as 1-800-INUTERO at the Children's Hospital of Philadelphia, should be established for consultations for families seeking information about their unborn child. A patient education video and web page detailing fetal anomalies and supporting literature can be developed, such as that available at The Center for Fetal Diagnosis and Treatment at the Children's Hospital of Philadelphia (www.fetalsurgery.chop.edu).

Many additional resources are required by a center for fetal diagnosis and treatment. For example, a Ronald McDonald House or guesthouse catering to pregnant women on bed rest is crucial to provide "a home away from home." Staff education regarding pregnant patients may be necessary. An "Adopt a Mommy-to-be" program can be developed to provide support for mothers on bed rest who have undergone fetal surgery. Assistance may be sought from numerous organizations and family agencies to fulfill additional needs.

■ Future Directions

Although beyond the scope of this chapter, the future of fetal therapy is evolving to include prenatal interventions for cardiac defects (Rychik, 2004). Cellular transplantation for such diseases as severe combined immunodeficiency (Flake et al., 1996) and hemoglobinopathies, as well as gene therapy for metabolic diseases, such as cystic fibrosis (Sylvester, Yang, Cass, Crombleholme, & Adzick, 1997), are now being performed. Further evolutions will include minimally invasive approaches to reduce the risk to the mother and the fetus and to broaden the applications for fetal surgery (Yang & Adzick, 1998).

Ongoing assessment and evaluation of all clinical experience must be reviewed, analyzed, and reported in the literature. For example, the prospective, randomized, multicenter NIH trial Management of Myelomeningocele Study (MOMS) will provide scientifically rigorous outcome information comparing prenatal myelomeningocele repair with postnatal repair (U10 HD41666). Only then will the natural history of fetal anatomic abnormalities be clarified for obstetricians, neonatologists, pediatricians, and pediatric surgeons. The mandate to the surgical nurse providing care to a fetal, neonatal, or pediatric surgery patient is to understand the natural history of the disease and the future effects on the child so that the optimal care is provided to the family.

■ Acknowledgment

The authors would like to acknowledge the contributions made by Susan K. Von Nessen, a co-author for this chapter in the first edition of this textbook.

■ Educational Materials

APSNA invites you to download the following diagnosis-related teaching tools for Chapter 11, Fetal Surgery: (1) Fetal Shunt Insertion; (2) Open Fetal Surgery. These teaching tools are available at the APSNA Web site (www.apsna.org) and the Jones and Bartlett Web site (www.jbpub.com). All teaching materials are available in English and Spanish and are free of charge. APSNA encourages their use for your patients and families.

References

Adzick, N. S., Crombleholme, T. M., Morgan, M. A., & Quinn, T. M. (1997). A rapidly growing fetal teratoma. *Lancet, 349,* 538.

Adzick, N. S., Harrison, M. R., Crombleholme, T. M., Flake, A. W., & Howell, L. J. (1998). Fetal lung lesions: Management and outcome. *American Journal of Obstetrics & Gynecology, 179,* 884–889.

Adzick, N. S., & Kitano, Y. (2003). Fetal surgery for lung lesions, congenital diaphragmatic hernia, and sacrococcygeal teratoma. *Seminars in Pediatric Surgery, 12*(3), 154–167.

Adzick, N. S. (2003). Management of fetal lung lesions. *Clinics in Perinatology, 30,* 481–492.

Adzick, N. S., Harrison, M. R., Flake, A.W., Howell, L. J., Golbus, M. S., & Filly, R. A. (1993). Fetal surgery for congenital cystic adenomatoid malformation. *Journal of Pediatric Surgery, 28,* 806–812.

Albanese, C. T., Lopoo, J., Goldstein, R. B., Filly, R. A., Feldstein, V. P., Calen, P. W., et al. (1998). Fetal liver position and perinatal outcome for congenital diaphragmatic hernia. *Prenatal Diagnosis, 18,* 1138–1142.

Altman, R. P., Randolph, J. G., & Lilly, J. R. (1974). Sacrococcygeal teratoma: American Academy of Pediatrics surgical section survey 1973. *Journal of Pediatric Surgery, 9,* 389.

Bartlett, R. H., Gazzaniga, A. B., Toomasian, J., Coran, A. G., Roloff, D., & Rucker, R. (1986). Extracorporeal membrane oxygenation (ECMO) in neonatal respiratory failure, 100 cases. *Annals of Surgery, 204,* 236–242.

Bealer, J. F., Skarsgard, E. D., Hedrick, M. H., Meuli, M., Vanderwall, K. J., Flake, A. W., et al. (1995). The PLUG odyssey: Adventures in experimental fetal tracheal occlusion. *Journal of Pediatric Surgery, 30,* 361–365.

Bergoffen, J. A., Prunett, H., & Campbell, T. J. (1993). Diaphragmatic hernia in tetrasomy 12p mosaicism. *The Journal of Pediatrics, 122,* 603–606.

Bianchi, D. W., Crombleholme, T. M., & D'Alton, M. E. (2000). Bronchopulmonary sequestration. In *Fetology* (pp. 218–288). New York: McGraw-Hill.

Bouchard, S., Johnson, M. P., Flake, A. W., Howell, L. J., Myers, L. B., Adzick, N. S., et al. (2002). The EXIT procedure: Experience and outcome in 31 cases. *Journal of Pediatric Surgery, 37,* 419–426.

Casale, D. (1990). Early urethral surgery for posterior urethral valves. *Urologic Clinics of North America, 17*(2), 361–371.

Cass, D. L., Crombleholme, T. M., Howell, L. J., Stafford, P. W., Ruchelli, E. D., & Adzick, N. S. (1997). Cystic lung lesions with systemic arterial blood supply: A hybrid of congenital cystic adenomatoid malformation and bronchopulmonary sequestration. *Journal Pediatric Surgery, 32,* 986–990.

Crombleholme, T. M., Coleman, B., Hedrick, H. L., Liechty, K., Howell, L. J., Flake, A. W., et al. (2002). Cystic adenomatoid malformation volume ratio predicts outcome in prenatally diagnosed cystic adenomatoid malformation of the lung. *Journal of Pediatric Surgery, 37*(3), 331–338.

Deprest, J., Jani, J., Van Schoubroeck, D., Cannie, M., Gallot, D., Dymarkowski, S., et al. (2006). Current consequences of prenatal diagnosis of congenital diaphragmatic hernia. *Journal of Pediatric Surgery, 41,* 423–430.

Flake, A. W. (1993). Fetal sacrococcygeal teratoma. *Seminars in Pediatric Surgery, 2,* 113.

Flake, A. W. (1997). Fetal surgery for congenital diaphragmatic hernia. *Seminars in Pediatric Surgery, 5,* 266–274.

Flake, A. W., & Howell, L. J. (1998). *Pediatric surgery and urology: Long term outcomes.* Philadelphia: W.B. Saunders.

Flake, A.W., Roncarolo, M.G., Puck, J. M., Ameida-Proada, G., Evans, M. I., Johnson, M. P., et al. (1996). Treatment of X-linked severe combined immunodeficiency (XSCID) by the in utero transplantation of paternal bone marrow. *New England Journal of Medicine, 335,* 1806–1810.

Freedman, A. L., Bukowski, T. P., Smith, C. A., Evans, M. L., Berry, S. M., Gonzalez, R., et al. (1997). Use of urinary beta 2 microglobulin to predict severe renal damage in fetal obstructive uropathy. *Fetal Diagnosis & Therapy, 12,* 1–6.

Harrison, M. R., & Adzick, N. S. (1993). Fetal surgical techniques. *Seminars in Pediatric Surgery, 2,* 136–142.

Harrison, M. R., Adzick, N. S., Estes, J. M., & Howell, L. J. (1994). A prospective study of the outcome for fetuses with diaphragmatic hernia. *Journal of the American Medical Association, 271,* 382–384.

Harrison, M. R., Adzick, N. S., Bullard, K. M., Farrell, J. A., Howell, L. J., Rosen, M. A., et al. (1997). Correction of congenital diaphragmatic hernia in utero VII: A prospective trial. *Journal of Pediatric Surgery, 32*(11), 1637–1642.

Harrison, M. R., Ross, N. A., Noall, R. A., & de Lorimier, A. A. (1983). Correction of hydronephrosis: The model: Fetal urethral obstruction produces hydronephrosis and pulmonary hypoplasia. *Journal of Pediatric Surgery, 8,* 247–256.

Hedrick, H. L. (2003). Ex utero intrapartum therapy. *Seminars in Pediatric Surgery, 10*(3), 90–195.

Hedrick, M. H., Estes, J. M., Sullivan, K. M., Adzick, N. S., & Harrison, M. R. (1994). Plug the lung until it grows (PLUG): A new method to treat congenital diaphragmatic hernia in utero. *Journal of Pediatric Surgery, 29,* 612–617.

Hedrick, M. H., Ferro, M. M., Filly, R. A., Flake, A. W., Harrison, M. R., & Adzick, N. S. (1994). Congenital high airway obstruction syndrome (CHAOS): A potential for perinatal intervention. *Journal of Pediatric Surgery, 29,* 271–274.

Howell, L. J., Burns, K. M., Lenghetti, E., Kerr, J. C., & Harkins, L. S. (2002). Management of fetal airway obstruction: An innovative strategy. *American Journal of Maternal Child Nursing, 27*(4), 238–243.

Howell, L. J., & Adzick, N. S. (2003). Establishing a fetal therapy center: Lessons learned. *Seminars in Pediatric Surgery, 12*(3), 209–217.

Holzgreve, W., Flake, A. W., & Langer, J. (1990). A fetal sacrococcygeal teratoma. In M. R. Harrison, M. S. Golbus, & R. A. Filly (Eds.), *The unborn patient: Prenatal diagnosis and treatment* (2nd ed., pp. 460–469). Philadelphia: W.B. Saunders.

Hubbard, A. M., Adzick, N. S., Crombleholme, T. M., & Haselgrove, J. C. (1997). Left-sided congenital diaphragmatic hernia: Value of prenatal MR imaging in preparation for fetal surgery. *Radiology, 203,* 636–640.

Hubbard, A. M., Crombleholme, T. M., & Adzick, N. S. (1998). Prenatal MRI evaluation of giant neck masses in preparation for the fetal EXIT procedure. *American Journal of Perinatology, 15,* 253–257.

Johnson, A. M., & Hubbard, A. M. (2004). Congenital anomalies of the fetal/neonatal chest. *Seminars in Roentgenology, 39*(2), 197–214.

Johnson, M. P., & Freedman, A. L. (1999). Fetal uropathy. *Current Opinion in Obstetrics & Gynecology, 11*(2), 185–194.

Keswani, S. G., Wilson, R. D., & Johnson, M. P. (in press). Percutaneous intrauterine fetal shunting. In J. J. Apruzzio, A. M. Vintzileos, & L. Iffy (Eds.), *Operative obstetrics* (3rd ed.). London: Taylor & Francis Books.

Lebowitz, R. L., & Griscom, N. T. (1997). Neonatal hydronephrosis: 146 cases. *Radiology Clinics of North America, 15,* 49–59.

McPherson, E. W., Ketterer, D. M., & Salsburey, D. J. (1993). Pallister Killian & Fryn's syndrome: Nosology. *American Journal of Medical Genetics, 47,* 241–245.

Metkus, A. P., Filly, R. A., Stringer, M. D., Harrison, M. R., & Adzick, N. S. (1996). Sonographic predictors of survival in fetal diaphragmatic hernia. *Journal of Pediatric Surgery, 31,* 148–152.

Pantoja, E., Llobet, R., & Gonzalez-Flores, B. (1976). Retroperitoneal teratoma: Historical review. *Journal of Urology, 115,* 52.

Quintero, R. A., Morales, W. J., Allen, M. H., Bornick, P. W., & Johnson, P. (2000). Fetal hydrolaparoscopy and endoscopic cystotomy in complicated cases of lower urinary tract obstruction. *American Journal of Obstetrics & Gynecology, 183*(2), 324–330.

Rychik, J. (2004). Frontiers in fetal cardiovascular disease. *Pediatric Clinics of North America, 51,* 1489–1502.

Skarsgard, E. D., Chitkara, L. L., Krane, A. J., Riley, E. T., Halamek, L. P., & Dedo, H. H. (1996). The OOPS procedure (operation on placental support): In-utero airway management. *Journal of Pediatric Surgery, 31*(6), 826–828.

Stolar, C., Dillon, P., & Reyes, C. (1988). Selective use of extracorporeal membrane oxygenation in the management of congenital diaphragmatic hernia. *Journal of Pediatric Surgery, 23,* 207–211.

Sylvester, K. G., Yang, E. Y., Cass, D. L., Crombleholme, T. M., & Adzick, N. S. (1997). Fetoscopic gene therapy for congenital lung disease. *Journal of Pediatric Surgery, 32,* 964–969.

Tamura, M., Tsuchida, Y., Kawano, T., Honna, T., Ishibashi, R., Iwanaka, T., et al. (1988). Piston-pump-type high frequency oscillatory ventilation for neonates with congenital diaphragmatic hernia: A new protocol. *Journal of Pediatric Surgery, 23,* 478–482.

Tsao, K., & Albanese, C. T. (2003). Prenatal therapy for obstructive uropathy. *World Journal of Surgery, 27*(1), 62–67.

Wilson, J. M., DiFiore, J. W., & Peters, C. A. (1993). Experimental fetal tracheal ligation prevents the pulmonary hypoplasia associated with fetal nephrectomy: Possible application for congenital diaphragmatic hernia. *Journal of Pediatric Surgery, 28,* 1433–1439.

Wilson, R. D., Baxter, J. K., Johnson, M. P., King, M., Kasperski, S., Crombleholme, T. M., et al. (2004). Thoracoamniotic shunts: Fetal treatment of pleural effusions and congenital cystic adenomatoid malformations. *Fetal Diagnosis and Therapy, 19,* 413–420.

Yang, E. Y., & Adzick, N. S. (1998). Fetoscopy. *Seminars in Laparoscopic Surgery, 5,* 31–39.

The Surgical Neonate

By Kim Knoerlein,
Wendy M. McKenney, Dorothy M. Mullaney,
Susan M. Quinn

Providing for the needs of the surgical neonate requires the knowledge of pathophysiology and neonatal care practices, the ability to recognize and respond to complications, and the provision of supportive care to the family. A multidisciplinary team approach toward the surgical neonate involves parents, neonatal nurses, nurse practitioners, neonatologists, pediatric surgeons, respiratory therapists, social workers, radiologists, and anesthesiologists who work together to provide high-quality care to ensure optimal outcomes.

The surgical neonate is a unique individual requiring specialized care and a distinct approach to his or her medical management during the preoperative, intraoperative, and postoperative periods. This chapter discusses specific physiologic problems experienced by the surgical neonate involving cardiorespiratory stabilization, thermoregulation, fluid and electrolyte management, drug therapy, wound care, and nutritional support. Nursing therapies are also presented and focus on the needs of the neonate and family from admission to discharge.

■ Prenatal Diagnosis, Perinatal Management, and Prenatal Family Counseling

Approximately 2% to 3% of all infants born have a major birth defect (American Academy of Pediatrics [AAP], 2002). These defects, also termed *congenital malformations*, may be due to either genetic or environmental causes. Technology is increasingly more sensitive and specific in diagnosing these malformations in utero. Many of the defects can be palliated or corrected with surgery. There are some congenital defects that may be amenable to surgery in utero, but others will require surgery in the neonatal period (see Chapter 11 for further information regarding fetal surgery). The cascade of events leading to successful neonatal surgery often begins with the prenatal diagnosis.

Several prenatal diagnostic techniques are available, not all of which are appropriate for every prenatal patient.

An assessment of risk factors should be performed prior to testing. It is important for parents to understand the difference between screening and diagnostic tests. Screening tests indicate the possibility of the infant having a problem, whereas diagnostic tests indicate whether or not the infant actually has the problem. Common screening and diagnostic tests available for prenatal diagnosis of a congenital defect or genetic abnormality include chorionic villus sampling, amniocentesis, triple-marker screen, ultrasonography, and magnetic resonance imaging (AAP, 2002; Theorell & Montrowl, 2003). Neither amniocentesis nor chorionic villus sampling assesses for structural abnormalities.

Triple-marker screening is offered to women early in pregnancy, generally around 16 to 18 weeks' gestation. It is used as a preliminary screen to identify women at high risk for having an abnormal fetus; it is not diagnostic of an abnormality. The triple marker is a blood test that screens for levels of alpha-fetoprotein, human chorionic gonadatropin, and unconjugated estriol. These three markers are often present in abnormal amounts in the face of a neural tube defect, an abdominal wall defect, or any trisomy (Zindler, 2005). If the triple-marker screen is abnormal, it is important to pursue diagnostic testing.

Prenatal ultrasonography is the most commonly used method of diagnosing a congenital defect that requires surgical intervention. This test is noninvasive and presumably safe for both the mother and the fetus. With state-of-the-art equipment and highly proficient technical skills, ultrasound is extremely accurate in detecting major abnormalities of the head, spine, heart, abdomen, kidneys, and bladder. It may also be used as a screening tool for directing further diagnostic testing, such as chromosomal analysis of fetal cells. Ultrasound is a routine screening test in many countries, although this is still a topic of controversy in the United States (Fernbach, 2003). It is possible for defects to be diagnosed by abdominal ultrasound as early as 16 to 20 weeks of gestation. Some defects may be observed even earlier in gestation if transvaginal ultrasound is used.

Magnetic resonance imaging is being used with increasing frequency to diagnosis structural abnormalities. This type of scan uses magnetic fields and radio waves to produce a high-quality structural image. Due to the quality of these images, it is possible to have a more precise image of many defects than is currently possible with ultrasonography.

Once it has been determined that a surgical procedure needs to occur in the neonatal period, decisions must be made regarding mode and place of delivery. Delivery at term gestation is preferred to minimize problems associated with transition to extrauterine life. However, this is not always feasible because of either maternal or fetal complications. Some malformations requiring surgical correction may necessitate caesarean section rather than vaginal delivery. It may be determined that it is preferable to deliver the neonate in a tertiary care facility that offers neonatal and pediatric surgical services.

Those infants who are unexpectedly delivered at a community hospital require transport to the closest tertiary center shortly after birth for further evaluation and management of the malformation. Transported infants require a warm environment, a secured airway, and adequate vascular access. Those born with gastrointestinal abnormalities also need a nasogastric tube to decompress the abdomen and to prevent aspiration of gastric contents during the transport process.

In the past few years, there have been several nursing studies performed analyzing both parents' and caregivers' response to prenatally diagnosed abnormalities, including those by Maijala, Åstedt-Kurki, Paavilainen, and Väisänen (2003) and Sandelowski and Barroso (2005). These studies describe parental need for information, including the natural history of the abnormality, the timing of the surgery, the anticipated surgical outcomes, the possible long-term sequelae, and any other foreseen problems surrounding the neonate's course.

Parents viewed their participation in the decision-making process as their first parental decision (Rempel, Cender, Lynam, Sandor, & Farquharson, 2004). Parents also expected collaboration and time among caregivers in helping them to deal with the diagnosis of an abnormal baby. Decisions in the management and treatment of the neonate require a multidisciplinary approach including parents and family, nurses, obstetricians, pediatric surgeons, nurse practitioners, neonatologists, social workers, and counselors. In addition to discussing treatment options in an open and honest manner, this team should be available to help support the parents and family in accepting and dealing with the problem of having a baby who has a malformation that will require surgery shortly after birth.

■ Neonatal Management

The key to successful management of the surgical neonate is the ability to recognize rapidly changing physiologic characteristics and provide prompt treatment. Successful preoperative stabilization of the surgical neonate enhances the infant's ability to survive the surgical intervention. After delivery and initial stabilization, all infants receive routine interventions, such as prophylactic eye ointment with erythromycin or tetracycline and vitamin K (0.5 mg for infants < 1 kg; 1 mg for infants > 1 kg). Newborns normally receive their first hepatitis B vaccine in the nursery just before discharge. However, surgical neonates who may require a lengthy hospital stay should get their scheduled series of immunizations once they are stable.

Management of the surgical neonate involves stabilization and ongoing assessment of cardiopulmonary status, thermoregulation, fluid and electrolyte balance, drug therapy, wound care, and nutritional support.

Cardiovascular and Respiratory Stabilization

The stabilization of the surgical neonate's cardiorespiratory function before surgery optimizes the ability of the neonate to survive anesthesia and surgery with fewer complications. Care providers must have a basic understanding of the unique physiology and/or pathophysiology that occurs during transition from fetal circulation to neonatal circulation. Many surgical infants require repair immediately or shortly after birth. Several disease processes put surgical infants at higher risk for mortality and morbidity, including respiratory distress syndrome, pneumonia, and congenital defects such as congenital heart disease.

A clear understanding of the process of transition from fetal circulation to neonatal circulation is important before any infant goes to surgery. Fetal cardiovascular physiology consists of four essential facts: (1) the right and left ventricles primarily perform similar tasks in the fetus and in the newborn infant, (2) only one ventricle is required for cardiovascular stability in the fetus, (3) the right ventricle is the dominant ventricle in the fetus, and (4) after embryogenesis, the size and orientation of a cardiovascular structure are determined by the flow pattern and volume of blood passing through it.

Fetal circulation ensures that the most vital organs and tissues, such as the brain and heart, receive the most highly oxygenated blood. Fetal lungs are nonfunctional, and the liver is only partially functional. Fetal circulation involves four unique anatomic features, the first being that the placenta serves as the main organ for exchange of oxygen, carbon dioxide, nutrients, and wastes. Secondly, the ductus venosus permits most blood to bypass the partially functioning liver and enter the inferior vena cava. Thirdly, the foramen ovale, an opening in the interarterial septum, allows blood to flow from the right atrium to the left atrium. The fourth anatomic difference is the patent ductus arteriosus, a tubular communication between the pulmonary artery and descending aorta that allows blood flow to bypass the lungs and go directly into the systemic circulation.

Transition from fetal to extrauterine life begins with clamping the umbilical cord and the infant's first breath, which occur almost simultaneously. Systemic vascular resistance rises when the umbilical cord is clamped, and pulmonary vascular resistance falls as the lungs expand with the infant's first breath. This enables blood to freely flow into the lungs, starting the process of oxygenation and removal of carbon dioxide necessary to sustain life. As systemic vascular resistance rises, the foramen ovale closes as the right-sided pressure in the heart increases. The ductus arteriosus normally closes within 15 to 24 hours of birth in response to increased arterial oxygen content and the effects of circulating prostaglandins. This closure of the patent ductus arteriosus is called *functional closure*. The ductus arteriosus may reopen as a result of several contributing factors, including hypoxia and acidosis. Decreased oxygen to the neonate can cause a constricted ductus to reopen and reestablish intrauterine fetal circulation, shunting blood away from the lungs. The ductus arteriosus anatomically becomes obliterated by constriction at 3 to 4 weeks of age. Hypoxia can also cause constriction of the pulmonary vascular system, causing increased pulmonary vascular resistance and, subsequently, pulmonary hypertension of the newborn.

Another disease process that may impede transitioning from fetal to newborn circulation is the presence of cyanotic congenital heart disease. Congenital heart disease occurs in approximately 1% of live births per year, making it the most commonly occurring birth defect. There are approximately 35 types of recognized heart defects occurring alone and in combination. The defects can be divided into two different categories: acyanotic, in which too much blood flows to the lungs, and cyanotic, in which there is too little blood flow to the lungs. These defects can range in severity from hemodynamically insignificant to extremely complex and life threatening. A few of the most common defects that occur within the first week of life include transposition of the great arteries, hypoplastic left ventricle, tetralogy of Fallot, coarctation of the aorta, ventricular septal defect, and pulmonary atresia. Most of these defects cause hypoxia, metabolic acidosis, and, at times, respiratory distress.

Although many infants with cyanotic heart disease present with cyanosis, they may have little to no respiratory distress. A hyperoxia test can help differentiate cyanosis caused by cardiac disease from that caused by pulmonary disease. A hyperoxia test is performed by placing the infant in 100% oxygen for 15 minutes and then obtaining an arterial blood gas. With pulmonary disease, the arterial partial pressure of oxygen (pO_2) usually rises to more than 100 mm Hg. When there is significant intracardiac right-to-left shunting, such as is seen in cyanotic heart disease, the arterial partial pressure of oxygen does not usually exceed 100 mm Hg.

Respiratory conditions that may interfere with adequate ventilation and perfusion in the surgical neonate include respiratory distress syndrome, pneumonia, transient tachypnea of the newborn, aspiration syndromes (amniotic fluid, meconium), and congenital defects such as choanal atresia. In a neonate with choanal atresia, adequate oxygenation and ventilation may require the placement of an oral airway. Other defects that involve the respiratory system include diaphragmatic hernias and tracheoesophageal fistulas. Bag-mask ventilation is contraindicated in these infants because accumulation of air within the abdomen interferes with full expansion of the lungs. Any abdominal wall defect, such as an omphalocele, gastroschisis, or bowel obstruction, may present with abdominal distention, also causing inadequate lung volumes and/or problems with lung expansion. Therefore, decompression of the stomach by placing a nasogastric tube to gentle suction is needed in these infants in the preoperative period. The establishment of adequate ventilation, oxygenation, and perfusion, and correction of acid-base status before the added stress of surgery and anesthesia optimizes the neonate's ability to sustain surgery with minimal morbidity.

A complete history, physical, and laboratory data are needed to effectively evaluate and manage the surgical neonate (Table 12-1). Assessment of the surgical neonate begins immediately after birth and includes observing the infant's ability to transition from intrauterine to extrauterine life smoothly before surgical interventions. Pharmacologic support may be necessary to improve cardiac function, which in turn improves organ perfusion. Inotropic agents, such as dopamine and dobutamine, are frequently used for this purpose. The infant is usually started on 5 µg/kg/minute, which is increased for effect to a maximum dose of 20 µg/kg/minute for both dopamine and dobutamine. The use of prostaglandins promotes dilation of the ductus arteriosus in neonates with congenital heart defects dependent on ductal shunting for oxygenation.

Use of invasive and noninvasive monitoring can be extremely helpful. Invasive monitoring includes central venous lines, such as umbilical venous catheters, to monitor pressures in the right atrium and give information on fluid status, especially if large amounts of fluid and/or blood loss are expected. Arterial catheterization, such as an umbilical artery catheter, enables monitoring of blood pressure and heart rate. It also provides easy access for blood sampling to determine oxygenation, ventilation,

and acid-base status. Monitoring during surgery allows for correction of hypoxia or metabolic acidosis immediately. Noninvasive monitoring includes the use of pulse oximetry for arterial oxygen saturation and transcutaneous end-tidal carbon dioxide (CO_2) monitoring, which provides information on ventilation. End-tidal CO_2 monitoring alerts providers should accidental extubation occur and is also useful in determining whether an infant has been successfully intubated.

Assessment of the neonate's vital signs, color, perfusion, and urine output must be performed upon return from the operating room. The clinical condition of a neonate can deteriorate more rapidly and with less warning than in any other age group. Postoperative complications seen in neonates that must be expediently corrected are respiratory distress, shock, and hemorrhage. Most infants return from the operating room on ventilatory support. Ventilatory management of the neonate is influenced by the underlying respiratory status and the primary surgical condition. The intubated neonate should be closely monitored for endotracheal tube dislodgement. Patency of the tube is maintained by suctioning as needed to prevent tube obstruction from secretions. Auscultation of breath sounds; observing for adequate chest rise, color, and perfusion; monitoring blood gases; and following oxygen saturation levels all assist in determining the surgical neonate's respiratory status. Monitoring transcutaneous end-tidal CO_2 is helpful in assessing the neonate's ventilatory status. The end-tidal CO_2 reading should correlate with arterial blood gas values. The goal is to wean any postoperative neonate off respiratory support as quickly as tolerated.

Cardiac output is assessed by observing the heart rate, blood pressure, peripheral perfusion, and urine output. An infant who is tachycardic may be in pain or may have intravascular volume depletion. The latter is especially seen in infants who undergo bowel surgery. Third spacing occurs in these infants; fluid moves into the interstitial space, causing intravascular dehydration. Significant gastric losses may also occur through decompression of the stomach by means of a Replogle tube placed to suction. Although these infants may appear grossly edematous and have poor urine output, they require significant amounts of fluid; they may require up to three times their maintenance needs for the first 24 hours after surgery. Maintenance fluids are usually ordered initially, and boluses are given as frequently as needed to avoid intravascular dehydration. Infants with tachycardia, poor peripheral perfusion, and hypotension need to be treated immediately, whether it be preoperatively, intraoperatively, or postoperatively. These parameters are reassessed

Table 12-1	Evaluation of the Surgical Neonate	
History	**Physical Examination**	**Laboratory**
• Obstetric	*Heart rate*	*Chest radiograph*
• Perinatal	• Rhythm, tachycardia, peripheral pulses, irregularities	• May identify respiratory cause for acid-base disturbance
• Labor	*Blood pressure*	*Arterial blood gases*
• Neonatal	• High or low blood pressure, wide or narrow pulse pressures	• Points to the primary acid-base derangement
• Family	*Respiratory effort*: Signs of distress	• Compensation
	• Nasal flaring, expiratory grunting, stridor, retractions, tachypnea	• Degree of hypoxemia
	General appearance: Color	
	• Cyanosis peripheral/central, pallor, mottling, gray	
	Activity	
	• Alert, lethargic, anxious, relaxed	

immediately after each intervention for the need for further volume resuscitation. Bolus fluids usually consist of normal saline and/or packed red blood cells, if blood loss is of concern, in amounts of 10 to 15 mL/kg/bolus. If after several attempts with volume replacement no improvement is noted, the use of inotropes, such as dopamine and dobutamine, may be needed. When systemic perfusion is adequate, the skin is warm, peripheral pulses are strong and easily palpated, and urine output is greater than 1 cc/kg/hour.

The use of pain medication, such as morphine and fentanyl, should be used to control moderate-to-severe pain, especially within the first 24 to 48 hours after surgery. Acetaminophen is a good alternative for procedures known to be less painful or after the first 24 to 48 hours. Evaluation tools, such as CRIES scoring (crying, requires O_2 for oxygen saturation above 95%, increased vital signs, expression, and sleeplessness) (McNair, 2004), are used to evaluate a neonate's pain level and need for pain medication. Sedation also may be necessary within the first 24 hours after surgery. It is important to remember that pain and sedation need to be treated separately because sedation does not control pain.

Thermoregulation

Neonates are uniquely vulnerable to cold stress and overheating, and the consequences of either may be devastating if not recognized early and corrected. It is imperative that the bedside nurse monitor a neonate's temperature closely and stay alert for signs of heat or cold stress. Hypothermia is common in neonates, and because of their immature skin, premature neonates are at even higher risk. More heat is lost by smaller neonates, the amount of which is inversely related to gestational age (Perlstein,

1992). Neonates are at risk for derangements in thermoregulation because of their large surface-to-mass ratio. Hyperthermia may occur, but it is more often than not caused by environmental factors. An older infant mounts a febrile response to infection, but hypothermia is more frequently seen in premature neonates who are septic. Temperature instability may be one of the first signs of sepsis the neonate exhibits. If fever is caused by an infection, the core temperature is warmer than the skin temperature, and the neonate is usually vasoconstricted (National Association of Neonatal Nurses, 1997). Evaluation for sepsis is warranted.

Neonates undergoing surgery are at high risk for hypothermia. Infants may become chilled during transfer to and from the operating room (OR), on exposure to cold surfaces and fluids, with exposure of the viscera during the surgical procedure, and secondary to the effects of sedation and anesthesia. Neonates, unlike older infants and adults, do not respond to heat loss by shivering. Instead, heat is generated through chemical thermogenesis and peripheral vasoconstriction. Upon exposure to cold, norepinephrine and thyroid hormones are released. This hormonal response induces lipolysis of brown fat stores found in the interscapular, paraspinal, and perirenal areas (Perlstein, 1992). This lipolysis and fatty acid oxidation release heat into the bloodstream. Cold stress initiates an increase in oxygen consumption, glucose use, and acid production. This further leads to depletion of glycogen stores and metabolic acidosis. Severe acidosis and hypoxia occur if steps to correct the hypothermia are not taken.

Hyperthermia is infrequent and is generally due to environmental causes. Iatrogenic causes of hyperthermia include overdressing the neonate and mechanical derangements of isolettes or radiant warmers. A temperature probe that loses contact with skin induces the temperature sensor to increase the heat output in efforts to increase the neonate's temperature. An isolette placed in direct sunlight experiences solar gain and can dramatically increase the temperature inside the isolette. This induces heat-losing mechanisms in the neonate. The skin flushes as the blood vessels dilate. The skin temperature is warmer than the core temperature. A body temperature of 42°C may cause seizures, deranged thermoregulation, and permanent brain damage (Holtzclaw, 1990). Management consists of cooling the infant and environment. It is preferable to slowly decrease the body temperature because rapid changes may induce apnea, particularly in premature neonates.

The surgical neonate requires special care to maintain euthermia. During the preoperative period, the infant is kept in a neutral thermal environment. The goal is maintenance of normal body temperature with little stress on the infant, who needs to conserve energy for the stress of surgery and recovery. Use of a transport isolette during transfer to the OR is an excellent way of maintaining optimal body temperature. If an isolette is not available for transport to the OR, the neonate should wear a cap, be placed on a radiant warmer, and be covered with warmed blankets. A layer of plastic wrap over the infant and beneath the blankets provides superior protection from heat loss. The OR should be prewarmed to a higher-than-normal temperature before the infant's arrival, and a water- or air-warming blanket heated to 40°C should be placed on the OR table under the infant.

During surgery, efforts are made to prevent heat loss. The infant should lie on the warming blanket and have only the surgical area exposed. The head covering is left on, if possible, and overhead warming lights or a servo-controlled infrared heater may be used during the procedure. Anesthetic gases are warmed and humidified. Warming skin preparation solutions, blood, and irrigating fluids plays a large role in minimizing heat loss. If the intravenous tubing is placed beneath the warming blanket, those fluids are near body temperature when infusing. Body temperature must be monitored continuously to detect alterations and may be performed by having a temperature probe placed in the esophagus, on the skin, or in the rectum.

After surgery, heat may be lost during transport from the OR to the neonatal intensive care unit (NICU). On arrival in the NICU, the surgical neonate requires a neutral thermal environment with continuous temperature monitoring. The radiant warmer or incubator is preheated to the appropriate neutral thermal temperature before the

neonate arrives to reduce heat loss to the environment. The response of the neonate's central nervous system to cold may be impaired by sedation and drugs used for anesthesia and pain control. Cardiovascular agents may cause vasodilation, further enhancing heat loss through radiation and convection. Dressings may become saturated and cool on exposure to air, further exacerbating heat losses. The surgical neonate's temperature should be continuously monitored and a neutral thermal environment should be maintained.

Fluid and Electrolytes

Fluid management of the surgical neonate compared with the older infant or adult needs to account for the physiologic and pathologic differences that are unique to this group of infants. The neonate's metabolic rate is double, water requirements are four to five times greater, and the excretion of sodium is only 10% of that in older children and adults (Adcock, Consolvo, & Berry, 1998). Fluid requirements change rapidly during the first week of life and may be higher in the premature infant. Understanding the changing water composition of the fetus and neonate enables clinicians to provide better fluid and electrolyte management.

Gestational age is a large determinant of the percentage and distribution of total body water. Both term and preterm infants are born with excess total body water, in particular, extracellular water. Newborns typically undergo a physiologic diuresis of up to 10% of their body weight over the first 4 to 5 days of life to remove this excess fluid. This is important for caregivers to understand when providing fluid and electrolytes to neonates shortly after birth, especially in managing those born extremely prematurely or growth retarded. Neonates weighing less than 1,500 g have rapidly changing fluid requirements during the first week of life and may have up to three times the fluid loss of term infants. Giving excess fluid and electrolytes during this period of natural diuresis increases the neonate's risk for patent ductus arteriosus, left ventricular failure, congestive heart failure, respiratory distress syndrome, bronchopulmonary dysplasia, and necrotizing enterocolitis (Letton & Chwals, 1997).

The kidneys play a vital role in fluid and electrolyte regulation in the neonate, although the full functional capacity of the kidney does not reach adult levels until 2 years of age. The kidney's ability to regulate fluid and electrolyte homeostasis is limited in the term and, particularly, in the preterm, infant. Neonates less than 34 weeks gestation have reduced glomerular filtration rates and tubular immaturity that alter their ability to handle filtered solutes. Accurate measurements of urine output, specific gravity, and osmolarity are especially important in the surgical neonate because of the added stress of surgery and anesthesia. Normal urine volumes are 1 to 2 mL/kg/hr with a specific gravity between 1.009 and 1.012 and urine osmolality between 250 and 290 mmol/kg (Puri & Sweed, 1996).

In the preoperative period, a complete and thorough evaluation of the fluid and electrolyte status of the surgical neonate is needed (Table 12-2). Obtaining vascular access is important to provide fluid boluses, drugs, and blood products when necessary. Stabilization of an infant's fluid and electrolyte status before surgery helps the infant endure the stress of surgery with fewer complications. Inadequate assessment of fluid intake may lead to dehydration, depletion of intravascular volume, hypotension, poor perfusion with acidosis, and hypernatremia. Administration of excess amounts of fluid, particularly in the preterm infant, may result in pulmonary edema, patent ductus arteriosus, bronchopulmonary dysplasia, and cerebral intraventricular hemorrhage.

Clinical and laboratory assessment of the neonate's fluid and electrolyte status should continue intraoperatively. Losses of fluid and blood are recorded and replaced during the procedure or shortly after surgery with packed red blood cells, normal saline, or 5% albumin. If the surgical procedure is lengthy, electrolyte and blood glucose levels are monitored, and any abnormalities are corrected. Placement of a urinary catheter provides accurate assessment of intraoperative urinary output. The environment must be kept warm to prevent further loss of heat from open peritoneal surfaces.

Careful assessment and management of fluid and electrolyte status before and during surgery often decrease complications after surgery. If the surgical neonate has not been kept well hydrated and has been hypotensive, transient renal failure with oliguria may occur and is managed with fluid restriction and correction of electrolyte imbalances such as hyperkalemia and metabolic acidosis (Gorman, 1996). Syndrome of inappropriate secretion of antidiuretic hormone (SIADH) is common in the neonatal population and results from pain, tissue injury, hypoperfusion, and ventilation. This results in fluid retention by increasing the permeability of collecting ducts and tubules of the kidney, causing increased reabsorption of water, and resulting in oliguria and hyponatremia. Antidiuretic hormone controls the concentration of sodium in the extracellular space and, when inappropriately secreted, causes water to be conserved and sodium to be excreted. Gastrointestinal drainage results in loss of additional fluids and electrolytes, such as sodium and potassium. Significant fluid losses from any drainage tube

or ostomy need to be replaced with additional fluid and electrolytes, such as half normal saline milliliter per milliliter, to keep serum levels within normal ranges.

Drug Therapy

The pharmacokinetics of a drug vary in the neonatal population and change with postconceptional age because of growth, development, and organ maturation. This presents a challenge in the neonate because of differences in absorption, distribution, metabolism, and excretion. Factors responsible for this difficulty in predicting a drug's action relate to the neonate's immature hepatic and renal function, poor perfusion that may limit absorption, delayed gastric emptying, high total body water and low body fat, illness, and decreased protein affinity for drugs. Neonatal medication doses are based on the infant's weight. Thus, doses can vary tremendously in this population. Caregivers need to be knowledgeable about the drug, dosage, and delivery route to ensure that the correct medication is given to the neonate. All drug dosage calculations should be double-checked by two nurses before administration.

Absorption of a drug depends on the site of administration and how effectively it transfers into the circulation. The most reliable route of drug administration in the neonate is the intravenous route. Drugs are delivered directly into the bloodstream, bypassing the absorption phase and rapidly reaching serum drug concentrations for an immediate drug response. Although intravenous drug therapy is ideal, several problems with the use of this route of drug administration in neonates must be recognized. Rapid serum drug concentrations may lead to undesired and toxic reactions because adequate and equal distribution to all organs does not always occur. Peak serum concentrations may be less than trough concentrations because of inadequate infusion of the entire drug.

In the neonate, absorption from the gastrointestinal tract is delayed and depends on gastrointestinal pH, gastric emptying time, enzyme activity, microbial colonization, and clinical status. Neonates have a gastric pH ranging from 6 to 8, with decreased gastric acid production during the first 30 days of life. Delayed gastric emptying time in the neonate slows passage of a drug into the intestines, resulting in a prolonged absorption phase (Ward, 1994).

Drugs given by the intramuscular route rely on adequate perfusion and muscle mass for greater absorption. In a sick or hypothermic neonate, perfusion may not be adequate, causing delayed drug action. With limited amounts of muscle mass, injections may enter the subcutaneous tissue, where absorption is slow and unpredictable. Multiple intramuscular injections should be

Table 12-2 **Assessment of Fluid and Electrolyte Status in the Neonate**

Physical Assessment	Fluid Intake and Output	Monitor Laboratory Data	Hemodynamic Monitoring
Mucous membranes	*Measurement of losses*	*Hematocrit*	*Central venous pressures*
	Urine, stool/stoma, vomitus,	Drops with overload	Indicated for monitoring right
Skin	drainage	Elevated with dehydration	heart pressures to assess ve-
Poor turgor with hypovolemia	Weight of dressings		nous return and blood volume
Dependent or pitting edema	Urinary catheter for meticulous	*Serum and urine electrolytes*	May be helpful in the infant
with overload	monitoring		with myocardial insufficiency,
	External urine collection device	*Serum osmolality*	SIADH, renal tubular necrosis, or
Eyes	or diaper weights	Normal, 280–295 mOsm/L	rapid fluid shifts
Sunken in dehydration	Strict measurement		Normal range, 4–8 mm Hg
Periorbital edema with over-		*BUN and creatinine*	
load	*Determine adequacy of urine*	Not very helpful in first 24 hours	
	output	of life	
Fontanelle	Average 1–2 mL/kg/hr	Provides indirect data about	
Depressed with dehydration		ECF and GFR	
Bulging with overload	*Monitor specific gravity and/or*		
	urine osmolarity	CO_2 and HCO_2	
Peripheral perfusion	Neonates cannot concentrate	Indirect measures of intravascu-	
Capillary refill time slowed	urine above 1.015–1.020	lar volume depletion	
with hypovolemia			
	Monitor weight	*Total protein*	
Liver size	Daily or bid weights using same	May indicate intravascular	
Increased with overload CHF	scale	albumin depletion	
	Determine appropriate weight		
Neurologic changes	gain or loss		
Tachycardia may indicate hy-			
povolemia			
Hypotension is a late sign of			
hypovolemia			
Alterations in ECG may denote			
acid-base or electrolyte			
imbalance			

Abbreviations: bid-twice daily; BUN-blood urea nitrogen; CHF-congestive heart failure; CO_2-carbon dioxide; ECF-extracellular fluid; ECG-electrocardiogram; GFR-glomerular filtration rate; HCO_2-bicardonate; SIADH-syndrome of inappropriate antidiuretic hormone.

avoided because of ineffective drug concentrations and potential damage to the neonate's tissues that may lead to abscesses.

Distribution is the movement of the absorbed drug to and through body fluids, organs, and tissues. An increase in total body water of the neonate, often seen after surgery, may require a larger per kilogram drug dose to achieve the desired concentration and effect (Kenner, Amlung, & Flandermeyer, 1998a). Because fluid status changes rapidly, drug monitoring is needed to ensure adequate serum levels for effective treatment in compromised neonates.

The primary site of drug metabolism is in the liver. Other organs, such as the kidneys, intestines, lungs, adrenal glands, and skin, have a more limited capacity to perform this function. Many drugs require biotransformation before they can be eliminated from the body. Biotransformation may frequently be accelerated or slowed in the sick neonate because of organ damage, drug interactions, poor nutrition, or disease state. The first-pass effect occurs when a drug moves directly from the intestinal absorption site to the liver and gets metabolized and excreted before reaching target organ sites (Martin, 1993). This may alter drug availability, and with the poor gastrointestinal motility often seen in the premature neonate, accentuated and unpredictable circulating concentrations of the drug may take place.

The elimination of both metabolized and unchanged drug from the body is called *excretion*. The kidneys provide this function through glomerular filtration, tubular excretion, and tubular reabsorption. Other important organs of excretion are the lungs, gastrointestinal tract, and liver. Glomerular function increases steadily after birth, whereas tubular function matures more slowly, causing a glomerular and tubular imbalance. Renal function of neonates may be changed by hypoxemia, decreased perfusion, and nephrotoxic drugs, such as gentamicin, indomethacin, and amphotericin B, all of which alter drug elimination. Increased glomerular function normally reflects improved cardiac output, decreased renal vascular resistance, redistribution of intrarenal blood flow, and changes in basement membrane permeability. This may be impaired in neonates after surgical procedures or illness, which makes dosing requirements unpredictable. Carefully individualized titration and blood level monitoring is necessary to ensure safe serum levels of renally excreted medications.

Risks of anesthesia are greater in the neonate than in the older infant and adult because of multiple factors related to prematurity, underlying disease processes, and limited physiologic reserves. Problems that may present with anesthetic administration in the neonatal population include the inability to maintain a patent airway and poor ventilation and oxygenation, leading to respiratory arrest, hypothermia, hypotension, and fluid overload. Adequate preoperative assessment of cardiovascular and respiratory status is necessary to ensure stability during the surgical procedure. Continuous monitoring is essential during the operation to prevent complications.

The difficulty in pain management of neonates is in the interpretation of physiologic and behavioral indicators, the neonate's only means of communication. Physiologic parameters that may indicate pain include increased heart and respiratory rates, elevated blood pressure, desaturation, pallor, dilated pupils, apnea, cyanosis, muscle tremors, and palmar sweating. In addition, behavioral parameters include localized motor activity, such as facial grimacing, brow bulge, eye squeeze, nasolabial furrow, open or pursed lips, stretched mouth, taut tongue, chin quiver, crying, agitation, and alteration of sleep state. It may be difficult to distinguish pain from agitation. Pain assessment measures are unreliable in neonates with low birth weights, who receive mechanical ventilation and who are neurologically impaired or sedated. These infants may have a delay or lack of response to painful stimuli because of depletion of physiologic reserves that affect their response capability, thus making it difficult for caregivers to assess pain (Stevens & Franck, 1995).

Agitation may be caused by numerous factors, such as environmental overstimulation, respiratory insufficiency, neurologic irritability, and a need to change position. Many problems lead to agitation in the neonate and must be distinguished from pain. Environmental stimulation, such as loud noises, bright lights, or certain stimuli associated with unpleasant events, may trigger the neonate to exhibit agitation. Nursery staff are able to minimize noxious stimuli by elimination of unnecessary noise, limiting the number of people at the bedside, and protecting the neonate's environment. Nurses caring for these infants must use their expertise in assessment to distinguish these factors from actual pain and discomfort. A goal of neonatal nurses is to provide comfort and relief of pain by effectively communicating the infant's needs to the health care team. Two approaches to pain management in neonates are nonpharmacologic and pharmacologic (Table 12-3).

Postoperative pain is anticipated in the surgical neonate; therefore, pharmacologic agents are instituted. Continuous-drip infusions of morphine or fentanyl are frequently used in neonates postoperatively. Morphine provides better sedative effects and there is less tolerance and physical dependence when it is used for long periods of time. Monitor for adverse effects, which include decreased intestinal motility, abdominal distention, respiratory depression, urine retention, and tolerance. Fentanyl is short acting and more potent than morphine. One major problem with continuous long-term fentanyl administration is the development of tolerance and physical dependence within 3 to 5 days. Wean neonates off fentanyl over several days to prevent the effects of drug withdrawal. Further information regarding pain management may be found in Chapter 5 of this text.

Wound Care

The surgical neonate is vulnerable to infection during hospitalization. Thus, the nurse must provide careful wound care in an attempt to prevent infection. Wound healing follows a pattern and is consistent for humans of any age. What is unique in the neonatal population is how rapidly they heal and how much less scar hypertrophy occurs. However, wound healing may be compromised for many reasons. Infection, poor nutrition, impaired circulation, hematomas, and seromas can all contribute to wound dehiscence. Wound dehiscence is managed with wet-to-dry dressings to allow the wound to granulate and contract. Further information regarding wound management may be found in Chapter 34 of this text.

Wound infection may occur during or after the surgical procedure and is a complicating factor. Neonates are at an immunologic disadvantage because immunoglobulins A and M do not transfer from the mother to the fetus in utero. However, immunoglobulin G transfers across the placenta beginning at 32 weeks' gestational age; thus near-term neonates receive passive immunization from their mothers. Although the neonate can mount an immune response with granulocytes, there is impaired neutrophil migration and a relative lack of complement factor, which makes this response less effective. Neonates have minimal-to-no antigen exposure, and overwhelming sepsis may develop from bacterial proliferation and overgrowth. Postoperative wound infections in the newborn may require treatment with antibiotics. Infection occurs more frequently after a "contaminated" surgery, such as an intestinal perforation, versus a "clean" surgery, such as ligation of a patent ductus arteriosus.

The first dressing change is typically performed by the surgeons. Gentle restraints or analgesia may be required if the dressing change is painful or the infant is vigorous. Nursing assessment of the surgical site is ongoing. These observations may provide the first indication of wound infection or poor healing. If any suspicion of infection exists, blood cultures are drawn before broad-spectrum antibiotics are initiated that target aerobes and anaerobes, and gram-positive and gram-negative organisms. Obtaining urine and cerebrospinal fluid needs to be considered because neonates are vulnerable to overwhelming sepsis with infection from any site.

Nutritional Support

At birth, the neonate has substantial nutritional demands because of a high metabolic rate and rapid growth and development. Compared with older infants, the neonate has limited caloric stores. Surgical neonates are at a much higher risk for malnutrition as a result of increased metabolic demands from surgery, nutrient losses, and sepsis. In the neonate, the gastrointestinal tract is structurally and functionally mature enough by 33 to 34 weeks' gestation to adequately absorb nutrients to support growth. However, several anatomic and physiologic characteristics exist that may compromise the neonate's nutrition, such as poor suck-swallow coordination, absent or weak gag reflexes, and an incompetent gastroesophageal sphincter, which put the neonate at risk for aspiration.

Another characteristic of neonates that limits adequate intake is their small stomach size, with an average capacity of 30 mL. They also have delayed gastric emptying time and decreased intestinal motility, both of which become more pronounced after surgical interventions. Intestinal

enzymes needed for protein digestion and carbohydrate and fat absorption are decreased because of immaturity or compromise of the gastrointestinal system, which affects growth and development of all organ systems.

Early identification of the surgical neonate at risk for nutritional deficiency is the first step toward proper nutritional management. Daily caloric requirements in healthy neonates average 100 to 120 kcal/kg/day but may be as high as 180 kcal/kg/day for premature or medically compromised neonates. This intake may be achieved with total parenteral nutrition, 20 kcal per ounce formulas, or breast milk, which is the preferred formula because it contains immunoglobulins and digestive enzymes and enhances gut growth. Expected weight gain for preterm neonates is approximately 20 to 30 g/kg/day, and term neonates average 10 to 15 g/kg/day. Daily weight changes may reflect fluctuations in body water, but the average over several days indicates growth trends.

Approximately 20% to 30% of surgically stressed neonates have increased nutritional requirements because of their need to promote wound healing, maintain adequate respiratory function, and resist infection (Taylor, 1997). Daily caloric requirements should be assessed on an individual basis and reassessed as the neonate's condition changes. An appropriate distribution of calories for adequate nutrition in healthy or compromised neonates should contain 8% to 12% of total caloric intake as protein, 35% to 55% as carbohydrates, and 35% to 55% as fat. Carbohydrates, especially glucose, are one of the neonate's main energy nutrients and are essential to the brain for normal metabolism. Premature neonates need approximately 4 to 6 mg/kg/min of glucose, and term neonates need 8 to 10 mg/kg/min to use and to maintain glucose stores. Protein is needed for adequate growth, synthesis of enzymes and hormones, wound healing, and increased energy. Neonates undergoing surgery need 2.5 to 3.5 g/kg/day of protein to maintain positive nitrogen balance and for sufficient weight gain. Fats are a major source for growth, metabolism, and muscle activity, with total daily needs of 3 to 4 g/kg/day. As a rule, no more than 60% of calories should be given as fat to allow for metabolic clearing and to prevent complications of fat malabsorption (Fletcher, 1994). Surgical neonates require optimal nutritional intake before surgery to promote successful recovery during the postoperative healing phase.

The development of total parenteral nutrition has increased the quality and length of survival in surgically compromised neonates who would otherwise be malnourished or die. Total parenteral nutrition may be infused by peripheral intravenous line, percutaneously inserted central catheter, or central venous line access. It

Table 12-3	Pharmacologic and Nonpharmacologic Interventions for Pain Management in Neonates
Pharmacologic	**Nonpharmacologic**
Mild pain	*Environmental interventions*
Acetaminophen (Tylenol)	Dim lights; decrease or minimize noise; time out periods; turning off
Moderate-to-severe pain	radios and unnecessary alarms; speak softly; conduct rounds away
Opioids	from bedside; use acoustical tile and spot lighting
Morphine	*Infant interventions*
Fentanyl	Provide boundaries for infants; group together invasive proce-
Systemic analgesia	dures; pacifier-nonnutritive sucking; hand-to-mouth sucking;
Epidural (bupivacaine with an opioid fentanyl or morphine)	holding during painful procedure; gentle handling; rest periods
Local anesthetics	between procedures; minimal handling protocol initiated;
Lidocaine	swaddling/containment/nesting; positioning on side or prone
EMLA (eutectic mixture of local anesthetics)	(stomach)
Agitation control	Kinesthetic motion (rhythmic, repetitive, cyclic stimulation)
Sedative/hypnotic	(i.e., waterbed, rocking); tactile stimulation (i.e., massage, stroking)
Lorazepam (Ativan)	
Midazolam (Versed)	
Chloral hydrate	

is initiated in neonates who are without enteral intake for more than 3 days or have delayed intestinal function. Further explanation of total parenteral nutrition may be found in Chapter 3 of this text.

Nurses have an important task in the initiation of enteral feedings to premature or compromised neonates. Close monitoring during the advancement of feedings can provide clues to intolerance. Nursing assessment for signs of feeding difficulties include bilious aspirates, vomiting, diarrhea, and abdominal distention. Stool consistency and color should also be noted and the stool checked for reducing substances, indicative of carbohydrate malabsorption, and blood in the stool, an early sign of necrotizing enterocolitis and a common occurrence in premature infants. Any of these signs warrant further investigation and should be reported immediately to the surgical team.

To facilitate tolerance of enteral feedings, nurses should provide neonates the opportunity for nonnutritive sucking during gavage feedings, which accelerates maturation of the sucking reflex, decreases oxygen consumption, and improves weight gain (Kenner, Amlung, & Flandermeyer, 1998b). Prone or right-side-down position during or after feedings may also be initiated to improve gastric emptying time and prevent regurgitation and aspiration. Reducing stress and stimulation before and during feedings decreases fluctuations in oxygenation that may interfere with gut perfusion and function.

Plotting anthropometric measurements of daily weight, weekly head circumference, length, fluid, and caloric in-

take on the bedside growth chart allows nurses and clinicians to evaluate for adequate growth and nutrition of individual neonates. The most sensitive indicator of good nutrition in neonates is the head circumference, with average increases between 0.5 cm and 1.0 cm per week. If problems are seen, adjustments are made in the nutritional plan to ensure optimal growth.

Family Focus, Discharge, and Follow-up

Parenting the surgical neonate is unlike parenting the normal newborn. Different approaches must be initiated by the health care team for successful parental attachment, newborn care, and discharge planning. Nurses need to focus their educational efforts on family adaptation to stresses that accompany the surgical neonate, in addition to the stresses parents experience in having a newborn. Parents of surgical neonates often do not immediately experience normal newborn events, such as holding and feeding their infant. This is due to early stabilization of the critically ill neonate requiring immediate surgical interventions or transport to a local tertiary care facility for further evaluation and management. In some cases, parents have no preparation for their infant's surgical interventions until immediately after delivery. This may interfere with parent-infant attachment and may continue for some period of time.

Parents of the surgical neonate are often unable to complete the three final steps of attachment: (1) hearing and seeing the infant, (2) touching and holding the infant, and (3) caretaking, as identified by Klaus and Kennell

(1979), for days to, sometimes, weeks after the birth of their infant. Parents often show hesitancy in accepting care responsibilities because of this delayed parent-infant attachment, which may lead to interaction deprivation. This may affect the mother's commitment to her infant, her maternal self-confidence in her ability to mother the infant, and altered behavior toward the infant in such areas as infant stimulation and skilled care giving (Barnett, Leiderman, Grobstein, & Klaus, 1970). Parent-infant bonding may be strengthened if parents are allowed to feed, bathe, and change their newborn. Mothers who are breastfeeding should be encouraged to provide breast milk for the infant despite their feeding status. Mothers can store their expressed milk in sterile plastic bags or containers and freeze them for later use. This gives mothers the sense that they are providing something that is beneficial for their infants.

Moehn and Rossetti (1996) looked at the effects of neonatal intensive care on parental emotions and attachment. The study has provided nurses with insights on how to empower parents as caregivers. It concluded that nurses must be sensitive listeners and must acknowledge parental feelings and provide for their needs, knowing that parents experience stressors based on their infant's condition and their personal experiences. Additionally, nurses should identify parental stressors through interaction and communication with parents rather than by assumptions, and they should include parents in the everyday care of their infants to allow parents the opportunity to assume the caregiver role. Nurses must also help prepare parents throughout the hospital course for the neonate's discharge home. Maintaining daily communication with parents to keep them informed of their infant's progress is a top priority of the health care team members. Providing parents with a consistent nurturing environment eases the transition into successful parenting and facilitates the process of acceptance of their surgical neonate.

In the prenatal period, a tour of the NICU allows parents the opportunity to meet the members of the health care team and familiarize themselves with the unique NICU environment. During the tour, nurses describe what parents should expect in the immediate preoperative period and throughout the neonate's stay in the hospital. This affords parents the opportunity to prepare for the birth of their child and the surgery. Initial nursing responsibilities include helping parents become familiar with intrusive medical equipment and helping parents understand the need for stabilization of their infant before surgery. Once their baby is born, allowing parents to perform simple care for their infant strengthens parent-infant attachments and eases the feeling of helplessness during the initial preoperative period.

Parents should be helped to cope with the stress of uncertainty. During pregnancy, they fantasize their newborn to be healthy and perfect. With the diagnosis of a surgical anomaly, those perceptions are shattered for the whole family, leaving them in a psychologically disorganized state in which their normal coping skills become inadequate. Encouraging parents to verbalize their feelings and concerns is most helpful during this stressful time. Nurses are able to share with parents ways in which they may personalize their infant's bedside with pictures of their family, stuffed animals, and colorful name cards. This gives the parents an opportunity to feel as if they are able to do something for their infant.

Most critically ill neonates are sensitive to environmental stimuli and gentle touching because of their limited energy reserves. Parents are initially unable to determine when to soothe, when to touch, and when not to touch. Parents may see their infant respond to their touch by turning away, grimacing, and crying inconsolably. Parents view this type of infant behavior as negative, making it difficult for them to cope and understand. Nurses must guide parents in understanding their infant's cues for overstimulation, pain, and contentment.

"Going home" are two words that elicit joy, disbelief, anxiety, and ambivalence in the parents of the surgical neonate. While in the hospital, parents come to depend on the supportive environment of the NICU to understand and cope with the behavior and care of their infant. The transition from hospital to home begins on admission. For most parents, taking home their newborn infant is one of the most stressful times. When their infant has had surgery and has been hospitalized since birth, the stress is even greater. Nurses need to help parents become the primary caregivers for their neonate and instill in them the confidence and skills necessary to care for their infant on their own (Moehn & Rossetti, 1996). The surgical neonate may often go home needing more than just normal newborn care. Parents are instructed in medication administration, formula preparation, use of special equipment, and emergencies that require health care provider input. Many resources are available to families to smooth the transition home. Educational pamphlets given to parents are an excellent way to educate them regarding such things as signs of infection, how to care for a gastrostomy tube, and wound care.

Before discharge, a systematic assessment to collect information about the needs of each surgical neonate and his or her family is warranted. This information identifies concerns in the home environment and with the parent-infant interaction and is used to evaluate areas for further interventions or referrals to other services. Nurses familiar with the infant and family play a vital role in this assessment process. Their input determines the types of services that may be needed to provide a smooth transition to the home environment for parents and their infant.

Most parents return for a postoperative surgical visit within 2 weeks of discharge. This follow-up visit provides an opportunity to assess wound healing, monitor weight gain, and reinforce discharge teaching. Encourage parents to ask questions and begin to discuss additional surgical interventions that may be necessary. Further follow-up appointments with their primary care provider are needed to initiate the infant's immunizations and monitor the neonate's developmental progress.

■ Conclusion

Nurses and clinicians who provide care to surgical neonates must have a thorough working knowledge and understanding of neonatal physiology and care practices that set them apart from other infants. Initiation of routine prenatal screening has allowed early detection of fetal problems that will necessitate surgical evaluation immediately after delivery. Prenatal counseling and referral to the closest high-risk perinatal center that offers pediatric surgical services provide the neonate with the best possible chance for survival.

Considerable challenges exist in the neonate's medical and surgical management, some of which may require immediate interventions. Stabilization of the neonate before surgery must take place to optimize the neonate's ability to withstand anesthesia and the surgical procedure with minimal complications. Neonates are at increased risk for problems with thermoregulation, fluid and electrolyte disturbances, cardiorespiratory compromise, pain, inadequate nutrition, and infection.

Family support throughout the hospital stay is the responsibility of all health care team members. Parental participation in their infant's care from admission to discharge builds confidence and provides the skills needed to care for their infant at home. Neonates require expert care from a multidisciplinary team whose members have a thorough knowledge of the principles of management during the preoperative, intraoperative, and postoperative phases to ensure the best possible outcomes.

■ Acknowledgment

The authors would like to acknowledge the important contributions made by Katherine E. Keener and Linda Miranda McNamara to this chapter in the first edition of this textbook.

References

Adcock, E. W., Consolvo, C. A., & Berry, D. D. (1998). Fluid and electrolyte management. In G. G. Merenstein & S. L. Garner (Eds.), *Handbook of neonatal intensive care* (4th ed., pp. 243–258). St. Louis, MO: Mosby.

American Academy of Pediatrics. (2002). *Guidelines for perinatal care* (5th ed.). Elk Grove Village, IL: The Academy.

Barnett, C. R., Leiderman, P. H., Grobstein, R., & Klaus, M. H. (1970). Neonatal separation: The maternal side of interactional deprivation. *Pediatrics, 45,* 197–205.

Fernbach, S. (2003). Hereditary influences on health promotion of the child and family. In M. J. Hockenberry, D. Wilson, M. L. Winkelstein, & N. E. Kline (Eds.), *Wong's nursing care of infants and children* (7th ed., pp. 110–138). St. Louis, MO: Mosby.

Fletcher, A. (1994). Nutrition. In G. Avery, M. Fletcher, & M. MacDonald (Eds.), *Neonatology: Pathophysiology and management of the newborn* (4th ed., pp. 330–356). Philadelphia: Lippincott-Raven.

Gorman, W. A. (1996). Fluid and electrolyte balance in the newborn. In P. Puri (Ed.), *Newborn surgery* (pp. 72–81). Oxford, England: Butterworth-Heinemann.

Holtzclaw, B. (1990). Temperature problems in the post-operative period. *Critical Care Nursing Clinics of North America, 2,* 589–598.

Kenner, C., Amlung, S., & Flandermeyer, A. (1998a). Principles of neonatal drug therapy. In C. Kenner, S. Amlung, & A. Flandermeyer (Eds.), *Protocols in neonatal nursing* (pp. 604–615). Philadelphia: Saunders.

Kenner, C., Amlung, S., & Flandermeyer, A. (1998b). Neonatal development. In C. Kenner, S. Amlung, & A. Flandermeyer (Eds.), *Protocols in neonatal nursing* (pp. 660–678). Philadelphia: Saunders.

Klaus, M., & Kennell, J. (1979). Care of the parents. In M. Klaus & A. Fanaroff (Eds.), *Care of the high risk neonate* (pp. 146–172). Philadelphia: Saunders.

Letton, R., & Chwals, W. (1997). Fluid and electrolyte management. In K. Oldham, P. Colombani, & R. Foglia (Eds.), *Surgery of infants and children: Scientific principles and practice* (pp. 83–96). Philadelphia: Lippincott-Raven.

Maijala, H., Åstedt-Kurki, P., Paavilainen, E., & Väisänen, L. (2003). Interaction between caregivers and families expecting a malformed child. *Journal of Advanced Nursing, 42,* 37–46.

Martin, R. (1993). Pharmacology in neonatal care. In P. Beachy & J. Deacon (Eds.), *Core curriculum for neonatal intensive care nursing* (pp. 501–519). Philadelphia: Saunders.

McNair, C. (2004). Postoperative pain assessment in the neonatal intensive care unit. *Archives of Disease in Childhood, Fetal and Neonatal Edition, 89,* F537–F541.

Moehn, D., & Rossetti, L. (1996). The effects of neonatal care on parental emotions and attachment. *Infant-Toddler Intervention, 6,* 229–246.

National Association of Neonatal Nurses. (1997). *Neonatal thermoregulation: Guidelines for practice.* Petaluma, CA: The Association.

Perlstein, P. (1992). Physical environment. In A. Fanaroff & R. Martin (Eds.), *Neonatal-perinatal medicine: Diseases of the fetus and infant* (pp. 401–419). St. Louis, MO: Mosby.

Puri, P., & Sweed, Y. (1996). Preoperative assessment. In P. Puri (Ed.), *Newborn surgery* (pp. 41–51). Oxford, England: Butterworth-Heinemann.

Rempel, G. R., Cender, L. M., Lynam, M. J., Sandor, G. G., & Farquharson, D. (2004). Parents' perspectives on decision making after antenatal diagnosis of congenital heart disease. *Journal of Obstetric, Gynecologic and Neonatal Nursing, 33,* 64–70.

Sandelowski, M., & Barroso, J. (2005). The travesty of choosing after positive prenatal diagnosis. *Journal of Obstetric, Gynecologic and Neonatal Nursing, 34,* 307–318.

Stevens, B., & Franck, L. (1995). Special needs of pre term infants in the management of pain and discomfort. *Journal of Obstetric and Gynecologic Neonatal Nursing, 24,* 856–862.

Taylor, L. (1997). Nutrition and central venous access. In D. Nakayama, C. Bose, N. Chescheir, & R. Valley (Eds.), *Critical care of the surgical newborn* (pp. 125–153). New York: Futura.

Theorell, C., & Montrowl, S. (2003). Diagnostic processes. In C. Kenner & J. Wright Lott (Eds.), *Comprehensive neonatal nursing* (3rd ed., pp. 810–843). Philadelphia: Saunders.

Ward, R. (1994). The use of therapeutic drugs. In G. Avery, M. Fletcher, & M. MacDonald (Eds.), *Neonatology: Pathophysiology and management of the newborn* (4th ed., pp. 1271–1299). Philadelphia: Lippincott-Raven.

Zindler, L. (2005). Ethical decision making in first trimester pregnancy screening. *Journal of Perinatal and Neonatal Nursing, 19,* 122–131.

Necrotizing Enterocolitis

By Betty R. Kasson

Necrotizing enterocolitis (NEC) is a baffling disease that is the source of the most common surgical emergency in the neonate (Kosloske & Musemeche, 1989). It is primarily a disease of prematurity, but it can also affect the term neonate (Andrews, Sawin, Ledbetter, Schaller, & Hatch, 1990). The overall mortality rate for infants with NEC is 25%, with the rate of mortality for more premature babies approaching 66% (Foglia, 1995). NEC has been attributed to perinatal factors, such as hypoxia and ischemia (Nowicki, 1990), and postnatal factors, including exchange transfusions through umbilical vein catheters, placement of umbilical arterial catheters, cardiovascular abnormalities, hyperviscosity, ischemia of the intestinal mucosa, feeding of hyperosmolar formulas and medicines, and cleanliness of the neonatal intensive care unit (Rowe, 1986; Lawrence, Bates, & Gaul, 1982). Infectious agents have also been implicated, including the clostridias, *Escherichia coli*, and *Klebsiella* (Han, Sayed, Chance, Brabyn, & Shaheed, 1983). After many careful studies over 25 years, no single factor has been demonstrated as the sole cause of NEC. It is now believed that NEC is the common final pathway resulting from a variety of factors (Kleigman & Walsh, 1987). Current studies indicate that both developmental and inflammation regulation mechanisms are involved (Nanthakumar, Fusunyan, Sanderson,

& Walker, 2000; Claud et al., 2004; Caplan, Simon, & Jilling, 2005; Neu, Chen, & Beierle, 2005).

■ Epidemiology

NEC is primarily a disease of premature infants who have been fed. NEC occurs in 1% to 2.4% of live births (Rowe, 1986) and accounts for 10% of deaths in very-low-birth-weight infants (Foglia, 1995). In the premature infant, NEC usually occurs within a week to 10 days after the initiation of feedings. In the term neonate (5%–25% of cases), NEC occurs within 1 to 4 days of life if feeding starts on day 1 (Andrews et al., 1990). Udall (1990) described a decrease in the risk of NEC at 34 to 35 weeks gestational age. He believes that this is due to intestinal maturation and the development of an intact intestinal mucosal barrier. Goldman (1980) reported that NEC is a rare phenomenon in the unfed infant; feeding clearly plays a role in the development of NEC. In one study, NEC was equally distributed between males and females and showed no racial or seasonal distribution (Wilson et al., 1981).

NEC can present as individual or "cluster" cases, and the cause appears to be different for the two types. There are several reports of sudden clusters of cases occurring in neonatal intensive care units in which an infectious viral or bacterial organism was isolated, and appropriate infection control enforcement resolved the epidemic (Han et al., 1983; Moomjian, Peckham, Fox, Pereira, & Schaberg, 1978). Several of the organisms isolated were normal colonic flora, and there was no clear explanation for why they suddenly caused disease.

Pathogenesis

There is general agreement that NEC is the result of a cluster of factors. Rowe (1986) classified these factors as indirect (e.g., perinatal hypoxia or low flow states due to cardiac disease) and direct (e.g., bacterial overgrowth in the intestine by a particular organism, or feeding). A brief discussion of some factors believed to contribute to NEC follows.

Ischemia

Ischemia is the major indirect factor implicated in NEC. Low flow states in the bowel vascular system lead to necrosis of the bowel. These observations were made in babies with cardiac defects, umbilical arterial and venous catheters, and hyperviscosity. All of these factors can cause decreased blood flow to the intestine. Hypoperfusion leads to oxygen deprivation and the build-up of metabolic waste products, resulting in mucosal damage. The evidence for this mechanism is not conclusive. Rowe (1986) matched "at risk" NEC babies with similar babies without risk factors and found no difference in the incidence of NEC. A study on ischemia and reperfusion noted that it may be the return of blood flow after a period of low flow that causes NEC. During the high-flow (hyperemic) recovery period following an ischemic event, endothelial cells swell and cell membranes are disrupted. Inflammatory cellular mediators, such as platelet-activating factor (PAF) and oxygen-free radicals are released from the cells. In animal studies, these compounds have caused NEC-like injury (Foglia, 1995; Ford, Watkins, Reblock, & Rowe, 1997; MacKendrick & Caplan, 1993). A 2005 review by Nowicki favored a disruption in the relationship of a vasoconstrictor protein (ET-1) and a vasodilator free radical (NO). It appears the usual balance toward NO and vasodilation can be changed to vasoconstriction by the presence of inflammation.

Direct Factors

Immature Infant Immunologic Defenses

The neonatal gastrointestinal tract is immunologically immature (Udall, 1990). Premature infants have a limited capacity to defend against bacterial toxins because the intestine in the neonate is actually adapted to absorb whole macromolecules in order to get passive immunity from breast milk. The maternal immune system is part of the neonatal host defense because under normal circumstances, neonates rely on breast milk to provide phagocytes, B cells, T cells, and immunoglobulin A (IgA). The lymphatic tissue in the neonatal intestine is not able to produce B and T lymphocytes at a level that can effectively control bacterial overgrowth without this maternal "boost." Neonatal and premature intestine is also deficient in IgA, which is thought to suppress bacterial growth and keep bacteria from adhering to the intestinal mucosa.

The distal ileum and the cecum have increased lymph tissue, decreased secretory function, and immature mucus production in the premature infant. There is little mucus to protect the bowel mucosa, and the protective lymphoid tissue is not yet functional. This means that premature infants have a decreased ability to defend against bacterial toxins that can damage the ileal and cecal mucosa and helps explain why these regions of the bowel are those most commonly affected by NEC.

Neonates may develop abnormal bacterial flora because normal gut colonization is delayed or absent. Most babies establish bacterial colonization from contact with and feeding by their mothers. This mechanism provides a large variety of organisms that colonize the gut in a balanced and competitive fashion. Nanthakumar et al. (2000) cited studies showing that the organisms found in the gut of breast-fed neonates are mostly lactobacilli and bifidobacteria. In formula-fed infants, enterobacteria and gram-negative organisms predominate (Hoy, Wood, Hawkey, & Puntis, 2000). Lawrence et al. (1982) proposed that the physical isolation, the cleanliness of neonatal intensive care unit procedures, and the use of antibiotics conspired to produce a situation in which one or two dominant bacterial species might proliferate and produce a large amount of toxin damaging to the neonatal gut. They noted that in germ-free animal models, the bacteria that proliferated in a similar situation were all toxin-producers. It is not yet known whether premature babies undergoing "kangaroo therapy," in which there is skin-to-skin contact between the premature infant and the parent, colonize their intestinal tracts in a balanced way despite not being fed.

Claud et al. (2004) exposed human fetal intestinal cells and adult intestinal cells to *Salmonella* organisms. The immature intestinal cells demonstrated an exaggerated inflammatory response. The authors hypothesized that the immature human intestine is not able to cope with large numbers and types of new bacteria and responds with an outpouring of inflammatory factors that can damage the intestine itself. A 2005 review by Neu et al. identified intestinal and immune function immaturity challenged by bacterial colonization as the complex of factors associated with NEC.

Nonimmunologic Defense Mechanisms

Neonates have decreased gastric acid production for the first month of life. Gastric acid is the first line of defense against the introduction of bacteria into the enteric system and is an effective killer of swallowed organisms. Without a high acid environment, large numbers of bacteria travel from the stomach into the bowel (Hyman et al., 1985).

Neonates also produce a lower level of pancreatic enzymes that can attack and break down proteins. Because bacterial toxins are proteins, the secretion of pancreatic enzymes into the duodenum inactivates these toxins. Without an effective pancreatic enzyme system, the neonate is more vulnerable to the effects of these toxins (Lebenthal & Leung, 1988).

Udall (1990) observed that the mucous membrane of the neonate is not "closed." The neonatal gut is able to absorb large macromolecules in order to achieve passive immunity through breast milk. The premature gut is even more permeable, and the translocation of bacterial and viral particles and toxins across the mucous membrane has been demonstrated histologically (Ballance, Dahms, Shenker, & Kliegman, 1990). The closure of this membrane is thought to be a maturational event, and the decrease in the risk of NEC at 35 weeks gestation is consistent with this timing. In one study, mothers who had been treated with steroids in the antenatal period had infants with a lower incidence of NEC than a matched control group. The difference was thought to be due to earlier maturation of the bowel because of the steroid treatment (Bauer, Morrison, Poole, & Korones, 1984).

Factors characteristic of the premature gastrointestinal tract that have been implicated in NEC include poor motility, lack of mucus production, and decreased function of lymphoid tissue. MacKendrick and Caplan (1993) described a condition in which these factors interact. Poor motility for moving bacteria through the bowel, poor mucus production for entrapping bacteria, and lack of phagocytes and mucosa-protecting IgA combine to make the bowel vulnerable to bacterial toxins and inflammatory compounds.

Feeding

Very few unfed infants develop NEC. One theory that connects feeding to mucosal damage involves the over-growth of intestinal bacteria when it is provided with a carbohydrate source. This is supported by the evidence that hydrogen gas, a product of carbohydrate fermentation, is found in the bowel. Primary digestion of formula in infants takes place in the enzyme-rich environment of the small bowel and is not characterized by hydrogen-producing fermentation. Studies on the digestion of formula by premature infants show that all lactose is not digested by enzymes, and that the residual undergoes fermentation in the ileum and colon (Kien, Liechty, & Mullett, 1990). This provides an important second source of nutrition for the infant but also creates a situation that encourages the overgrowth of bowel-damaging bacteria (Cheu, Brown, & Rowe, 1989).

A study of 926 preterm infants by Lucas and Cole (1990) showed that NEC was six to 10 times more common in formula-fed than in breast-fed babies, and that babies fed a combination of breast milk and formula had three times more NEC than those that were breast fed only. They concluded that breast milk significantly decreased the incidence of NEC in preterm infants. However, some infants fed only breast milk have developed NEC. As cited earlier, evidence for a different pattern of bacterial intestinal colonization in breast and formula-fed infants may explain this difference. These studies, Lucas and Cole's evidence, and the presence of phagocytes, B and T cells, and IgA in breast milk support the important role that breast milk plays in the health of the neonatal gastrointestinal system.

Having a premature infant with NEC is a very stressful event for parents who frequently feel helpless and exhausted. The nurse plays a vital role in encouraging the mother of an infant with NEC to keep pumping and keep producing milk. Parents of acutely ill, ventilated infants sometimes feel that there is nothing they can do for their child. The evidence presented by Lucas and Cole shows the importance of producing breast milk for later feedings.

Vasoactive and Inflammatory Cellular Mediators

In animal models, cell mediators, such as platelet activating factor, inflammatory cytokines, interleukins, and tumor necrosis factor alpha have all produced a clinical and histologic picture that looks like NEC. Ischemia-reperfusion injuries and metabolism of carbohydrates by gas-producing organisms also release a burst of these vasoactive compounds. The action of these compounds seems to lead to vasoconstriction and bowel necrosis (Foglia, 1995). In their 2004 study, Claud et al. demonstrated the decreased expression of a regulatory gene in an immature human intestinal cell line. This regulatory suppression resulted in the increased release of cellular inflammatory cytokines discussed earlier.

Compounds that block the production of PAF, such as nitric oxide, reduce bowel injury in animal models (MacKendrick, Caplan, & Hsueh, 1993; Nowicki, 2005). Increasing evidence suggests that PAF and toll-like receptors are mediators in the inflammatory pathway that creates the clinical picture of NEC, no matter what the causative factors are (Caplan & Hsueh, 1990; Caplan et al., 2005). The work by Claud et al. (2004) also implicates the cytokine interleukin-8. Warner and Warner (2005) reviewed the role of epidermal growth factor, a compound known to be active in normal intestinal repair and development. They suggest that deficiency of epidermal growth factor may contribute to NEC. The experimental work of Feng, El-Assal, & Besner (2005) on epidermal growth factor has demonstrated this protective effect in vitro.

The Presentation of NEC

Because NEC is the result of many interacting factors, the presentation is also variable. NEC can range from a mild illness that responds to a few days of antibiotics and gastric decompression to a life-threatening condition characterized by thrombocytopenia, respiratory failure, and cardiovascular collapse.

Clinical Signs

Early clinical signs may be nonspecific, including lethargy, poor feeding, bilious emesis, and temperature instability. Abdominal distention, an increase in prefeeding gastric residual volumes, and gross or occult blood in the stools are other frequent findings. This picture has factors in common with the presentation of sepsis, feeding intolerance, and hypomotility of prematurity. Often, a nasogastric tube can cause gastric bleeding resulting in stools that are positive for occult blood, complicating the picture. Careful observation for abdominal distention and tenderness, increasing gastric residuals, and fecal blood is the key to early diagnosis (Foglia, 1995; Kleigman & Walsh, 1987; Rowe, 1986).

Physical Findings

Physical findings in later NEC may include a green or bluish hue to the abdominal wall, labia, or scrotum. The neonatal abdominal wall is thin, and meconium spilled into the peritoneal cavity can sometimes be seen as dark coloration under the skin (Fig. 13-1). Abdominal wall

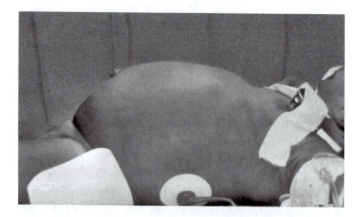

Figure 13-1 The abdomen of an infant with abdominal distention and meconium staining of the lower quadrants. (Courtesy of Sam Alaish, M.D., 2005, Baltimore, Maryland.)

erythema is frequently an indicator of the underlying inflammation of peritonitis. Abdominal wall edema, tenderness, and rigidity usually accompany it. Increasing abdominal girth or a palpable fixed loop of bowel is another physical finding (Rowe, 1986).

Laboratory Findings

Laboratory findings are frequently nonspecific and indicative of generalized sepsis. There may be either an increase or a decrease in the white blood cell count. The decrease is more ominous because it indicates that the infant is unable to generate a systemic immune response. A continuing fall in platelets below 100,000/mm³ is also ominous and is frequently associated with intestinal perforation and sepsis. Electrolyte abnormalities are indicative of fluid shifts and the capillary leakage associated with infection. An increase in the C-reactive protein is also a good nonspecific indicator of sepsis (Foglia, 1995).

Radiologic Evaluation

Radiographs are important for noting a change from the normal bowel gas pattern. They can detect free gas in the abdomen, in the venous system of the liver (portal venous gas), and in the wall of the bowel (pneumatosis intestinalis). Radiographs may be obtained as often as every 6 hours if NEC is suspected. Plain abdominal films may show a change from the normal "honeycomb" gas pattern to distended loops of bowel with thickened, edematous walls. "Fixed" loops, large gas-filled loops that are in the same position from film to film, may indicate segmental necrosis (Fig. 13-2). Pneumatosis intestinalis is seen early in NEC and can change over a matter of hours as gas pockets in the bowel wall fill and empty (Fig. 13-3). There are two forms of pneumatosis: a cystic form, which appears early and is characterized by pockets of gas in the inner-

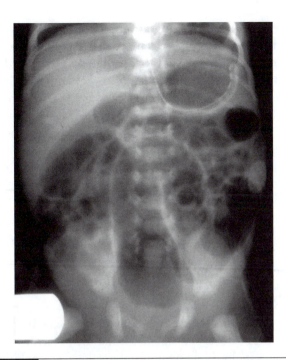

Figure 13-2 An anteroposterior radiograph of an infant with dilated loops of bowel and abdominal distention.
(Courtesy of Sam Alaish, M.D., 2005, Baltimore, Maryland.)

most mucosal layer of the bowel, and a linear form indicative of gas in the muscular or outermost (serosal) layer. Cysts and blebs may appear in the serosa as well (Foglia, 1995).

Portal venous gas is seen as a dark, treelike pattern over the light shadow of the liver in the right upper quadrant and indicates that bowel gas has moved into the capillary system of the mesentery and has traveled into the portal vein. Pneumoperitoneum, free gas in the abdomen, is always an indication for surgery, because it shows that the bowel wall has been perforated. In mechanically ventilated infants, however, it is important to be sure that the abdominal free gas is not the result of the migration of gases from the thoracic or mediastinal spaces caused by overventilation. Free gas is more difficult to see on a supine film, because air rises, and the film is taken through the gas with the bowel loops as background. When it is detected on this radiographic view, it forms a round or oval shadow overlying the abdominal contents (football sign). The free gas can also outline the falciform ligament lying just to the right of the vertebral column. Free gas is best seen on a cross-table lateral or left lateral decubitus film. In a cross-table lateral, the film is taken supine from the side so that the free gas that has risen to the anterior abdominal wall appears as a dark shadow above the bowel. The left lateral decubitus film, taken with the baby's left side down and shot from the side, allows the free gas to rise to the right side, where the air is outlined against the shadow of the liver (Fig. 13-4). Small amounts of gas can best be seen on this film because there is no interference from the gas within the bowel.

■ Management

Medical Management of NEC

More than half of babies with the clinical picture of NEC are managed without surgical intervention. Treatment and surveillance consist of the elements listed in Table 13-1. The goals of medical management are to detect and fight infection, to support ventilation and oxygenation, to provide adequate intravascular volume, and to decrease

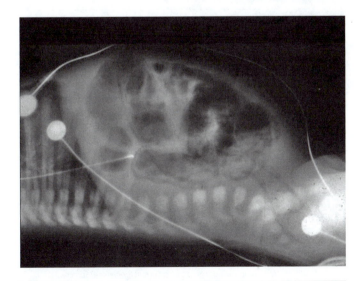

Figure 13-3 A cross-table lateral radiograph of an infant with pneumatosis throughout the bowel.
(Courtesy of Sam Alaish, M.D., 2005, Baltimore, Maryland.)

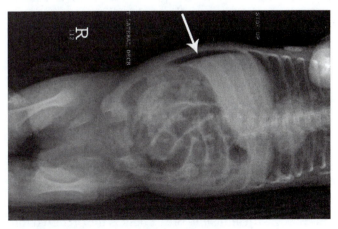

Figure 13-4 A left lateral decubitus radiograph with dilated bowel loops and free gas rising to the right side and outlining the liver.
(Courtesy of Sam Alaish, M.D., 2005, Baltimore, Maryland.)

Table 13-1	Medical Management of Necrotizing Enterocolitis

Aggressive fluid resuscitation

Gastrointestinal rest with nasogastric drainage to suction

Peripheral and central blood cultures

Antibiotic coverage for aerobes and anaerobes

Close monitoring of abdominal girth

Correction of volume and electrolyte abnormalities

Mechanical ventilation to correct blood gas abnormalities

Correction of coagulopathies

Total parenteral nutrition

Serial physical examinations

Serial radiographs

the work of the bowel and its metabolic needs to a minimum. Physiologic management goals support the baby's metabolism and equilibrium. Bowel rest allows the damaged organ to heal.

When the bowel is full of food, its work is increased. It has to meet both its tissue metabolic needs and the needs of digestion and absorption. It requires greater amounts of oxygen and more blood flow to supply nutrients and remove metabolic wastes. Feeding also provides fermentable material to fuel the growth of bacteria and the production of bacterial toxins. Bowel rest, decompression, and nasogastric suction remove the substrate for bacterial overgrowth, decrease the work of the bowel, and allow the oxygen and nutrients to be used for metabolism and healing.

Without the enteral route, achieving an adequate level of nutrition is a challenge. Babies with NEC require 120 to 150 Kcal/kilogram/day, depending on their gestational age and weight. This level of parenteral nutrition requires central venous access, and peripherally inserted central catheters have supported a major advance in providing nutrition for these babies (Ryder, 1993).

Infants with NEC may be critically ill, requiring aggressive fluid resuscitation, ventilation, inotropes, diagnostic procedures, and antibiotic therapy. NEC is superimposed on the special needs and problems of prematurity, and this can be a devastating combination, even without a frank bowel perforation.

When feedings are restarted, the initial volumes are very small (1 mL/hour or less), and they are advanced slowly (1–2 mL/hr). The feedings are given by continuous nasogastric infusion. Breast milk is the preferred formula because of the presence of its immunologically active components. If breast milk is not available, elemental formulas with predigested proteins and fats may be used.

There is close monitoring for abdominal girth changes, blood in the stools, increasing gastric residuals, and behavioral changes during the feeding advances. Feedings are stopped if there is any sign of recurrence of NEC. Achieving full enteral feedings can be a lengthy process with many interruptions. This is a difficult time for parents. When feedings are begun, they believe that there is real progress. When feedings have to be stopped, parents may become despondent. It is important to let parents know that many increases, decreases, and stops in the feeding regimen are not unusual in a baby who has had NEC, and that these changes are not indicative of final outcome. It is not easy for parents to "ride the feeding roller coaster" with NEC. Reminding them that this is an expected part of the disease helps allay unnecessary anxiety.

Indications for Surgery

Surgery is indicated when medical management fails, or when the bowel is perforated. The failure of medical management includes many of the signs listed in Table 13-2. An infant with a clear intestinal perforation or a significant number of other clinical signs will require operation. Bell, Ternberg, and Feigin (1978) developed clinical staging criteria for NEC that define stages of severity and the therapeutic interventions appropriate for each. The Bell criteria are still useful and have been modified by other clinicians (Kleigman & Walsh, 1987).

If the infant is unstable and transport to the operating room would be hazardous, the operation is performed in the neonatal intensive care unit. Anesthesia, scrub, and circulating nurses, sterile operating packs, and all neces-

Table 13-2	Signs of the Failure of Medical Management

Hypothermia

Apnea

Hyperbilirubinemia

[a]Uncorrectable metabolic acidosis

[a]Falling platelet counts requiring repeated transfusions

[a]Unexplained coagulopathies

[a]Increasing rigidity of the abdominal wall

[a]Free gas or portal venous gas on radiograph

Oliguria

Bleeding

[a]Indications for immediate operation.

From Foglia, R. (1995). Necrotizing enterocolitis. *Current Problems in Surgery, 32*, 759–823; Rowe, M. I. (1986). Necrotizing enterocolitis. In K. J. Welch, J. G. Randolph, M. M. Ravitch, I. A. O'Neill, and M. I. Rowe (Eds.), *Pediatric surgery* (4th ed., pp. 944–958). Chicago: Yearbook Medical Publishers.

sary equipment are brought to the infant's bedside. Foglia (1995) found that about 50% of infants with intraoperative findings of NEC had diagnosed intestinal perforation before surgery. This leads to the conclusion that in about half of the cases, a multifactorial picture is as diagnostic for NEC as a radiograph showing free gas.

On opening the abdomen, the surgeon may find a swollen, purple bowel with areas of full- or partial-thickness necrosis (white, green, or gray patches), or a skip pattern in which normal bowel is present between areas of pneumatosis, edema, and necrosis. There may be visible blisters (pneumatosis) on the serosal surface of the bowel. The bowel wall may be thin and friable and is usually hemorrhagic (Fig. 13-5). The peritoneal fluid may be bloody with necrosis, or turbid and brown with perforation. There may be fibrinous exudate over the serosa, and areas of mucosal slough (Rowe, 1986; Foglia, 1995). The most common areas of involvement are the terminal ileum, cecum, and right colon, but any portion of the bowel may be involved. The goal of surgery is to remove only the bowel that is fully necrotic, and to leave any marginal areas in the hope that they will survive. This can be a difficult decision because studies of the microscopic changes during NEC show that there can be active development of necrosis right next to areas that are healing and building new mucosa (Ballance et al., 1990).

The marginal bowel is brought to the abdominal skin surface (exteriorized) so that leaky internal anastomoses

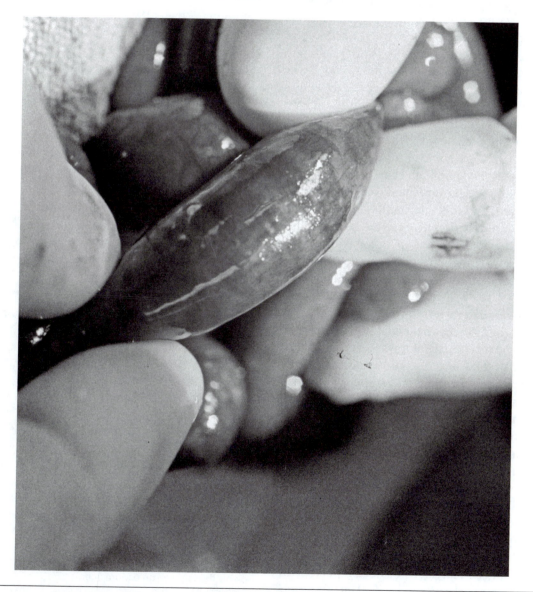

Figure 13-5 A segment of necrotic bowel showing hemorrhage and gray patches.

(From Rowe, M. I. [1986]. Necrotizing enterocolitis. In K. J. Welch, J. G. Randolph, M. M. Ravitch, J. A. O'Neill, & M. I. Rowe [Eds.], *Pediatric surgery* [4th ed., pp. 944–958]. Chicago: Yearbook Medical Publishers.)

do not contaminate the peritoneal cavity with stool. Fully resected areas may undergo primary anastomosis with good results (Tan, Kiely, Agrawal, Brereton, & Spitz, 1989). Multiple ostomy formation is preferred over the excision of normal bowel that lies between involved areas so as to retain as much bowel as possible. This means that a baby may have several stomas on the abdomen, although stool is only produced by the proximal stoma. The other stomas are called mucous fistulas. These are sections of bowel not connected to the fecal stream. It is also important to save the ileocecal valve, if possible. This valve both slows the transit time of nutrients through the small bowel to give time for adequate absorption and prevents the reflux of bacteria-laden colon contents into the small bowel. The remaining bowel adapts by increasing its surface area until maximum enteral absorption is achieved. How much small bowel is necessary to avoid lifelong dependence on TPN is still debated. Sondheimer, Cadnapaphornchai, Sontag, and Zerbe (1998) found an inverse relationship between the length of small bowel remaining and the duration of time on parenteral nutrition. There is also current discussion among pediatric specialists as to whether the ileocecal valve is as vital to the outcome of the short gut patient as is currently believed (Kaufman et al., 1997).

At the end of the operation, the viable and marginal bowel is measured, and this information is used to formulate a long-term nutrition plan for the infant. Sometimes, the plan includes a repeat operation within 24 to 36 hours to reevaluate marginal bowel.

After the operation, the surgeon describes the findings to the family. Usually, the family does not understand the implications for enteral feeding of removing of a portion of the bowel and is overwhelmed if stoma formation was required. The full impact of the surgeon's information is processed over the next days and weeks, and nurses' explanations and interpretations are an important part of this process. Assessing the parents' understanding of the current information and readiness to learn more helps the family adapt to the situation. Using diagrams, drawings, and articles, as well as providing access to resources on the Internet and parent support groups, further supports their intellectual and emotional well-being.

In some instances, a peritoneal drain is placed instead of using a more conventional surgical approach. This is more frequently performed in very-low-birth-weight and in unstable infants who may not tolerate an operation. Morgan, Shochat, & Hartman, (1994) reported the drainage procedure as definitive in 18 of 29 infants weighing less than 1,500 grams. No further operation was required, and the infants did well. Because very-low-birth-

weight infants have a 66% mortality rate from more conventional management of NEC, this procedure is a reasonable alternative in these infants. If there is no improvement after 24 hours of drainage, an open procedure is frequently performed.

Long-Term Consequences

The long-term consequences of necrotizing enterocolitis include short bowel syndrome, strictures, adhesions, and malabsorption (Foglia, 1995), with short bowel syndrome as the major complication. Stevenson, Kerner, Malachowski, & Sunshine (1980) studied late morbidity in prematurely born infants and found that 81% of children had no problems related to the gastrointestinal tract. They concluded that the long-term prognosis in NEC is encouraging. Rowe (1986) reviewed several authors who matched very-low-birth-weight infants with and without NEC and reported no increased problems in developmental, neurologic, growth, or nutritional status or gastrointestinal function 1 to 2 years after NEC. Schwartz, Richardson, Hayden, Swischuk, and Tyson (1980) reviewed 62 patients and found post-NEC strictures in 25% of them. Not all of these strictures were symptomatic, and more recent data would be valuable in evaluating outcomes (Fig. 13-6). Strictures in the bowel beyond the

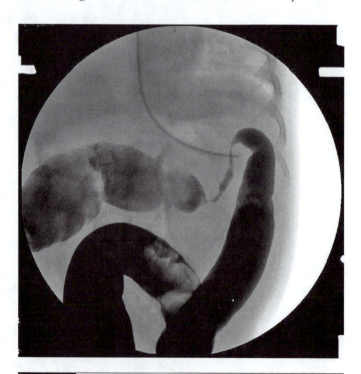

Figure 13-6 A stricture of the transverse colon proximal to the splenic flexure seen on barium enema.
(From Foglia, R. [1995]. Necrotizing enterocolitis. *Current Problems in Surgery, 32,* 759–823; Rowe, M. I. [1986]. Necrotizing enterocolitis. In K. J. Welch, J. G. Randolph, M. M. Ravitch, J. A. O'Neill, & M. I. Rowe [Eds.], *Pediatric surgery* [4th ed., pp. 944–958]. Chicago: Yearbook Medical Publishers.)

ostomy are not usually symptomatic, because they do not impede stool flow. Before the ostomy is closed, a contrast study of this isolated bowel is performed to identify strictures that may cause obstruction and bleeding when the continuity of the bowel is restored.

Short-Bowel Syndrome

The most serious consequence of necrotizing enterocolitis is short-bowel syndrome (SBS). SBS is defined as an inability to meet the nutritional needs of normal growth and development through the enteral route. The definition is functional, rather than being either the percentage of bowel resected or the length of bowel remaining. In North America, over one third of SBS cases result from NEC (Georgeson, 1998; Georgeson & Brown, 1998). Normal bowel absorbs nutrients, vitamins, and fluids; produces enzymes and hormones; and recirculates bile. The complications of SBS are the result of disruptions of these functions. The segment of the bowel resected determines what kinds of problems will result, because different parts of the bowel have different functions. In NEC, the jejunum, ileum, and cecum are affected most often.

The jejunum has the greatest surface area, with long villi, deep crypts between them, and loose junctions between cells. It receives hyperosmotic boluses of food mixed with pancreatic enzymes and bile that cause influxes of fluid into the intestine through the spaces between cells. Most nutrients are also absorbed here. Resection of the jejunum causes malnutrition until the ileum adapts to take over the absorptive function.

The ileum reabsorbs fluids secreted into the jejunum; absorbs fat-soluble vitamins, vitamin B_{12}, and bile acids; and secretes the hormones controlling gastric emptying and intestinal transit time. Except for fluid reabsorption, these functions cannot be taken over by other segments of the bowel. If the ileum is resected, fat soluble and vitamin B_{12} deficiencies result, and gastric emptying and transit time are disordered (Vanderhoof & Langnas, 1997). The ileum also terminates in the ileocecal valve, which controls emptying from the small bowel into the colon and prevents the reflux of bacteria-laden large bowel contents into the ileum. The resection of the ileocecal valve seems to lengthen dependence on parenteral nutrition (Kaufman et al., 1997). Overall, resection of the jejunum is better tolerated than ileal resection. The ileum adapts to increase absorption, although its site-specific functions are not replicable in other bowel segments (Vanderhoof & Langnas). Resection of the cecum affects water reabsorption and may lead to chronic diarrhea.

Bowel adaptation begins immediately after resection, but it may be months before the enteral route can provide full calories. Survival for infants with SBS increased from 50% to 85% with the advent of total parenteral nutrition (TPN) (Georgeson & Brown, 1998). Prognostic factors for how long a child will remain on TPN and whether he or she will achieve full enteral feeding are difficult to determine. In a small group of patients with SBS, Sondheimer et al. (1998) found that both small-bowel length after surgery and the percentage of calories taken enterally at 52 weeks postgestational age were predictive of how long the infants were dependent on TPN.

In bowel adaptation, villi lengthen and crypts deepen to increase surface area, the bowel dilates and lengthens, and transit time of intestinal contents decreases (Georgeson, 1998). Improvement in nutrient absorption lags behind the increase of surface area (Vanderhoof, 1996). The adaptation process is dependent on enteral nutrition, and increase of mucosal surface area does not proceed without nutritional support. Complex nutrients and long-chain fatty acids appear to be a more powerful stimulant for these adaptive changes than simple sugars and short-chain fats. Formulas high in fats and proteins are preferred because they have a lower osmotic load and cause less diarrhea than those high in carbohydrates. Gastric, pancreatic, and biliary secretions acting directly on the bowel mucosa also stimulate adaptation (Vanderhoof & Langnas, 1998). Therefore, early closure of ostomies and restoration of bowel continuity promote adaptation by providing an uninterrupted route to the bowel mucosa (Georgeson). Continuous feeding is also beneficial because it keeps the bowel in constant contact with the stimulating nutrients (Vanderhoof & Langnas). Hormonal secretions, such as enteroglucagon, insulin-like growth factor I, and epidermal growth factor, are among those being studied to determine their role in adaptation (Georgeson).

The small intestine is short in the premature infant and nearly doubles its length in the third trimester (Touloukian & Walker-Smith, 1983). Because bowel elongation is also proportional to increase in body length, the capacity for bowel elongation after resection is greatest in the premature infant. Premature infants experience less time dependent upon parenteral nutrition than affected term neonates (Kaufman et al., 1997).

There are several surgical interventions that may be beneficial in SBS. After resection, the small bowel dilates as its surface area increases during adaptation. This dilatation can result in dysmotility, malabsorption, bacterial overgrowth, and sepsis. Children with dilated dysmotile bowel benefit from a tapering enteroplasty, in which the bowel is streamlined to increase its functional motility. The intestinal plication achieves the same goal while preserving maximal intestinal surface area. In this procedure, a longitudinal fold is made that tapers the bowel by folding the extra tissue inwards and stitching the fold along the area where there are no blood vessels (the antimesenteric surface) (Georgeson & Brown, 1998).

Stricture resection for partial small-bowel obstruction is important for releasing tight anastomoses, promoting flow of bowel contents, and preventing bacterial overgrowth. Strictures are a common complication of NEC, and the stricturoplasty can improve bowel function substantially (Vanderhoof, 1996).

Bowel dilatation also creates extra tissue when it can be used in an intestinal doubling (Bianchi) procedure by dividing the dilated bowel longitudinally into two segments and attaching them end to end. This improves motility similar to that achieved by the enteroplasty and increases mucosal surface area over the next 6 to 9 months. Kimura's doubling technique encourages new blood supply for the bowel from the abdominal wall or liver before division of the dilated bowel (Georgeson & Brown, 1998). The serial transverse enteroplasty (STEP) procedure (Kim et al., 2003) uses the GIA stapler to lengthen dilated bowel by staple firings into the antimesenteric border of the bowel every 2 cm, alternating directions. This produces a zig-zag track through the bowel that doubles the functional length. The serial transverse enteroplasty procedure can be performed after a previous Bianchi procedure.

There are also surgical procedures to decrease intestinal transit time and encourage bowel dilatation. In these procedures, intestinal valves are created to slow the progress of enteric contents from one segment to the next. Success requires the right balance of slowing the transit of bowel contents without developing the symptoms of obstruction (Georgeson & Brown, 1998). A review of operative strategies by Petty and Ziegler (2005) discusses these approaches.

Chapter 30 provides a comprehensive discussion of small-intestinal transplantation. Outcomes have greatly improved since the development of the immunosuppressive drug tacrolimus. Fluid and electrolyte problems and osmotic and secretory diarrhea characterize the postoperative course. Lymphoproliferative disease, sepsis, cytomegalovirus infections, and rejection are also common. Small-bowel transplantation and liver transplantation are performed in conjunction when TPN-induced cholestatic disease results in liver failure. Success has been limited in small-bowel transplantation alone (Vanderhoof, 1996; Georgeson, 1998).

There are many complications of SBS beyond malabsorption. Parenteral nutrition–induced liver disease is the most common cause of death from SBS (Vanderhoof, 1996). Liver disease from long-term TPN is frequent, with some degree of cholestasis present in all children receiving parenteral nutrition. Vanderhoof (1996) reported that an enteral intake of 20% to 30% of calories is effective in preventing liver disease. Gallstones (cholelithiasis) are also common in children receiving parenteral nutrition. They result from the disordered pathway for bile salt reabsorption and altered bilirubin metabolism. Because biliary tract disease may be silent, some authors are now recommending cholecystectomy when stones are discovered. Renal stone formation from disordered calcium absorption may also occur (Georgeson & Brown, 1998).

Excess secretion of gastric acid caused by overproduction of the hormone gastrin (hypergastrinemia) is the result of a disrupted feedback loop from the small bowel to the stomach. If the condition is untreated, gastritis and gastric and duodenal ulcer disease result. Gastric acid production can be managed medically with hydrogen ion and proton pump blocking agents (Vanderhoof, 1996).

Trace mineral and vitamin deficiencies are common once parenteral nutrition is discontinued. Ileal resection predisposes the child to fat-soluble vitamin deficiencies from disordered bile transport and poor fat absorption. Vitamin B_{12} deficiencies also occur because the ileum is the only place where B_{12} is absorbed. Many trace minerals are absorbed poorly, and zinc, copper, calcium, magnesium, and iron serum levels should be checked routinely in patients with SBS. Unexplained skin rashes and hair loss should include trace mineral malabsorption in the differential diagnosis (Vanderhoof, 1996).

Bacterial overgrowth is a major complication in SBS. The motility of the normal small bowel rapidly moves bacteria into the colon. The dilatation, dysmotility, and enteral stasis that accompany SBS provide an optimal environment for the growth of bacteria. Feeding regimens that leave undigested nutrients in the bowel provide the nourishment for rapid bacterial growth. Bacterial overgrowth results in enteritis, diarrhea, bacterial translocation with bacteremia, and colonization with unusual organisms, such as lactobacilli. Lactobacilli ferment carbohydrate to a product that cannot be metabolized by human cells, and which causes acidosis and coma (Georgeson & Brown, 1998; Georgeson, 1998). Kaufman et al. (1997) found that bacterial overgrowth and associated inflammation of the enteric tract contribute to prolonged dependence on parenteral nutrition. The treatment of bacterial overgrowth is both medical and surgical. Antibiotics, prokinetic agents that improve bowel motility, adjustment of feeding regimens to decrease the amount of undigested nutrients, and the surgical enteroplasties discussed previously all may play a role (Vanderhoof & Langnas, 1997; Georgeson & Brown). Long-term TPN has been implicated in a suppression of intestinal mucosal immunity and other pathology in children with SBS. Duran's 2005 literature review of 414 children with SBS showed no direct evidence between TPN and bacterial overgrowth, impaired neutrophil function, decreased immune function, or villous atrophy.

Parenteral nutrition requires central venous access, and long-term indwelling catheters have significant management problems. Even with scrupulous care, sepsis and bacteremia are constant threats in children who translocate bacteria across the bowel wall into the bloodstream. Children who are dependent on central catheters for TPN have crises when their catheters occlude, break, become colonized with bacteria, or malfunction. Emboli from clots proximal to the catheter tip may be thrown into the central circulation, and thromboses may result from partial occlusion of vessels by the catheter itself. Long-term maintenance and care of these catheters is of primary importance to the health of these children (Ryder, 1993).

The nursing care of the SBS child requires expert assessment and intervention. Feeding a baby with diminished absorptive surface requires constant vigilance for evidence of malabsorption as the feedings are advanced. Increasing frequency and volume of stool or a more watery consistency indicates an overload of the bowel's absorptive capacity and the potential for dehydration and electrolyte loss. Evaluation of the reducing substances in the stool, a method of monitoring for undigested carbohydrates, is a good objective measure of the degree of carbohydrate malabsorption. If feeding advances are continued in the face of increasing evidence of malabsorption, the intestinal mucosa may slough—a setback of days or weeks. However, the short bowel increases its surface area substantially over time, and it is important to take advantage of the opportunity to increase enteral feeding. Achieving the balance between malabsorption and adaptation is the art of managing these babies. Practical concerns for parents include protecting intravenous access from contamination and traumatic removal. The nurse's observations, documentation, and teaching are vital parts of advancing the enteral feedings as safely and rapidly as possible. Helping parents understand how all these factors interact is an important part of the nursing care of these babies.

■ Developmental Issues

NEC is primarily a disease of the premature infant. An appropriate developmental plan, such as the Neonatal Individualized Developmental Care and Assessment Plan (NIDCAP) (Als & Gilkerson, 1995), is important in achieving optimal neurodevelopmental outcomes while enteric problems are being addressed medically and surgically. Appropriate positioning, consistent caregivers, premature skin care, sensitivity to cues for overstimulation, and examination skills using neurodevelopmental guidelines for soothing and calming are important to achieving developmental milestones. Developmental specialists provide the expertise necessary for developing and individualizing plans of care. Neurodevelopmental evaluation should continue at regular intervals through the preschool years to ensure the best outcomes for these children.

Very-low-birth-weight and premature infants who are small for gestational age demonstrate stunted growth at 10 years of age under the best of circumstances (Knops et al., 2005). This is good information for parents who may otherwise blame themselves for a child's growth failure after NEC.

Babies who have been intubated and unable to eat for long periods of time develop an aversion to oral feedings. They lack the practice in coordinating the breathe-suck-swallow sequence that infants need to nipple successfully. The early intervention of a feeding specialist is an important component in the care of these infants.

■ Planning for Home

Many babies with NEC go home with some combination of ostomy care, central venous catheter care, complex feeding regimens, and home parenteral nutrition. While the infant is in the hospital, individualized teaching plans for the parents are crucial. Learning ostomy management, central line care, gavage feeding, or gastrostomy care takes time and commitment on the part of parents and nurses. Other important issues include planning for a back-up caregiver, helping siblings respond to a compromised infant, and modifying the home to accommodate equipment and new routines. Intervention by case managers, social workers, primary nurses, and home nurses before discharge is valuable in smoothing the transition from hospital to home.

Having a baby with necrotizing enterocolitis is a confusing and frightening event for parents. Feeding a child is one of the most basic bonding experiences for a parent, and many parents of a child who cannot be fed feel inadequate. The multifactorial etiology of NEC may engender a parental soul-searching session looking for "what we did wrong." The sense that you cannot do anything but wait and see what happens once NEC develops also contributes to the feelings of frustration and helplessness. The nurse is a key part of the team providing information and comfort to the parents through this difficult period. A knowledge of what factors are thought to be involved in the development of NEC, an understanding of the diagnostic and therapeutic interventions likely to be used, and a grasp of the actual long-term morbidity from NEC are invaluable in soothing parental fears and helping them understand the realities of their baby's situation.

■ Future Research

The cause of necrotizing enterocolitis is still not known, but the outcome may be a lifetime of chronic bowel, nutrition, and behavior problems. Further research is needed in many areas. The direction of current medical research is to identify the biochemical pathways that lead to NEC in animal models. In the meantime, many issues of interest to nurses and families remain unstudied. The modification of diet to maximize nutrition, minimize bowel upset, and support normal growth and development in children with NEC has not been fully investigated. The effect of kangaroo therapy on neonatal bacterial colonization is still unknown. Feeding development in babies with NEC who are not fed orally for long periods of time needs further evaluation. Studies of self-image in children with short-bowel syndrome and ostomies would be a valuable addition to the literature. Studies of the coping behaviors of parents raising a child with a chronic bowel problem would also add information that would be useful in assisting these families. There are many opportunities for research in physiological, developmental, and psychosocial areas.

■ Educational Materials

APSNA invites you to download the following diagnosis-related teaching tool for Chapter 13, Necrotizing Enterocolitis: Necrotizing Enterocolitis. This teaching tool is available at the APSNA Web site (www.apsna.org) and the Jones and Bartlett Web site (www.jbpub.com). All teaching materials are available in English and Spanish and are free of charge. APSNA encourages their use for your patients and families.

References

Als, H., & Gilkerson, L. (1995). Developmentally supportive care in the neonatal intensive care unit. *Zero to Three, 15*(6), 2–10.

Andrews, D. A., Sawin, R. S., Ledbetter, D. J., Schaller, R. T., & Hatch, E. I. (1990). Necrotizing enterocolitis in term neonates. *The American Journal of Surgery, 159,* 507–509.

Ballance, W. A., Dahms, B. B., Shenker, N., & Kliegman, R. M. (1990). Pathology of necrotizing enterocolitis: A ten-year experience. *The Journal of Pediatrics, 117*(1), S6–S13.

Bauer, C. R., Morrison, J. D., Poole, W. K., & Korones, S. B. (1984). A decreased incidence of necrotizing enterocolitis after prenatal glucocorticoid therapy. *Pediatrics, 73,* 682–688.

Bell, M. J., Ternberg, J. L., & Feigin, R. D. (1978). Neonatal necrotizing enterocolitis: Therapeutic decisions based upon clinical staging. *Annals of Surgery, 187,* 1–7.

Caplan, M. S., & Hsueh, W. (1990). Necrotizing enterocolitis: Role of platelet activating factor, endotoxin, and tumor necrosis factor. *Journal of Pediatrics, 117*(1 Part 2), S47–S51.

Caplan, M. S., Simon, D., & Jilling, T. (2005). The role of PAF, TLR and the inflammatory response in neonatal necrotizing enterocolitis. *Seminars in Pediatric Surgery, 14*(3), 145–151.

Cheu, H. W., Brown, D. R., & Rowe, M. I. (1989). Breath hydrogen excretion as a screening test for the early diagnosis of necrotizing enterocolitis. *American Journal of the Diseases of Childhood, 143,* 156–159.

Claud, E. C., Lu, L., Anton, P. M., Savidge, T., Walker, W. A., & Cherayil, B. J. (2004). Developmentally regulated IkB expression in intestinal epithelium and susceptibility to flagellin-induced inflammation. *Proceedings of the National Academy of Science, U S A, 101*(19), 7404–7408.

Duran, B. (2005). The effects of long-term parenteral nutrition on gut mucosal immunity in children with short bowel syndrome: A systematic review. *BioMed Central Nursing, 4,* 2.

Feng, J., El-Assal, O. N., & Besner, G. G. (2005). Heparin-binding EGF-like growth factor (HB-EGF) and necrotizing enterocolitis. *Seminars in Pediatric Surgery, 14*(3), 167–174.

Foglia, R. (1995). Necrotizing enterocolitis. *Current Problems in Surgery, 32*(9), 759–823.

Ford, H., Watkins, S., Reblock, K., & Rowe, M. (1997). The role of inflammatory cytokines and nitric oxide in the pathogenesis of necrotizing enterocolitis. *Journal of Pediatric Surgery, 32*(2), 275–282.

Georgeson, K. (1998). Short-bowel syndrome. In J. A. O'Neill, M. I. Rowe, J. L. Grosfeld, E. W. Fonkalsrud, & A. G. Coran (Eds.), *Pediatric surgery* (Vol. 2, 5th ed., pp. 1223–1232). St. Louis, MO: Mosby.

Georgeson, K., & Brown, P. (1998). Short bowel syndrome. In M. D. Stringer, K. D. Oldham, P. D. Mouriquand, & E. R. Howard (Eds.), *Pediatric surgery and urology: Long term outcomes* (pp. 237–242). London: W.B. Saunders.

Goldman, H. I. (1980). Feeding and necrotizing enterocolitis. *American Journal of the Diseases of Childhood, 134,* 553–555.

Han, V. K. M., Sayed, H., Chance, G. W., Brabyn, D. G., & Shaheed, W. A. (1983). An outbreak of *Clostridium difficile* necrotizing enterocolitis: A case for oral vancomycin therapy? *Pediatrics, 71*(6), 935–941.

Hoy, C. M., Wood, C. M., Hawkey, P. M., & Puntis, J. W. L. (2000). Duodenal microflora in very low birth weight neonates and relation to necrotizing enterocolitis. *Journal of Clinical Microbiology, 38*(12), 4539–4547.

Hyman, P. E., Clarke, D. D., Everett, S. L., Sonne, B., Stewart, D., Harada, T., et al. (1985). Gastric acid secretory function in preterm infants. *Journal of Pediatrics, 106*(3), 467–471.

Kaufman, S. S., Loseke, C. A., Lupo, J. V., Young, R. J., Murray, N. D., Pinch, L. W., et al. (1997). Influence of bacterial overgrowth and intestinal inflammation on duration of parenteral nutrition in children with short bowel syndrome. *The Journal of Pediatrics, 131,* 356–361.

Kien, C. L., Liechty, E. A., & Mullett, M. D. (1990). Effects of lactose intake on nutritional status in premature infants. *The Journal of Pediatrics, 116*, 446–449.

Kim, H. B., Lee, P. W., Garza, J., Duggan, C., Fauza, D., & Jaksic, T. (2003). Serial transverse enteroplasty for short bowel syndrome: A case report. *Journal of Pediatric Surgery, 38*(6), 881–885.

Kliegman, R. M., & Walsh, M. C. (1987). Neonatal necrotizing enterocolitis: Pathogenesis, classification and spectrum of illness. *Current Problems in Pediatrics, 27*, 219–287.

Knops, N. B. B., Sneeuw, K. C. A., Brand, R., Hille, E. T. M., denOuden, A. L., Wit, J. M., et al. (2005). Catch-up growth up to ten years of age in children born very pre-term or with very low birth weight. *BioMed Central Pediatrics, 5*, 26.

Kosloske, A. M., & Musemeche, C. (1989). Necrotizing enterocolitis of the neonate. *Clinical Perinatology, 16*, 97–111.

Lawrence, G., Bates, J., & Gaul, A. (1982). Pathogenesis of necrotizing enterocolitis. *The Lancet, i*, 137–142.

Lebenthal, E., & Leung, Y. K. (1988). Feeding the premature and compromised infant: Gastrointestinal considerations. *Pediatric Clinics of North America, 35*(2), 215–238.

Lucas, A., & Cole, T. J. (1990). Breast milk and neonatal necrotizing enterocolitis. *Lancet, 336*, 1519–1523.

MacKendrick, W., & Caplan, M. (1993). Necrotizing enterocolitis: New thoughts about pathogenesis and potential treatments. *Pediatric Clinics of North America, 40*(5), 1047–1059.

MacKendrick, W., Caplan, M., & Hsueh, W. (1993). Endogenous nitric oxide protects against platelet-activating factor-induced bowel injury in the rat. *Pediatric Research, 34*(2), 222–228.

Moomjian, A. S., Peckham, G. J., Fox, W. W., Pereira, G. R., & Schaberg, D. A. (1978). Necrotizing enterocolitis: Endemic versus epidemic form [Abstract]. *Pediatric Research, 12*, 530.

Morgan, L. J., Shochat, S. J., & Hartman, G. E. (1994). Peritoneal drainage as primary management of perforated NEC in the very low birth-weight infant. *Journal of Pediatric Surgery, 29*, 310–315.

Nanthakumar, N. N., Fusunyan, R. D., Sanderson, S., & Walker, W. A. (2000). Inflammation in the developing human intestine: A possible pathophysiologic contribution to necrotizing enterocolitis. *Proceedings of the National Academy of Science, U S A, 97*(11), 6043–6048.

Neu, J., Chen, M., & Beierle, E. (2005). Intestinal innate immunity: How does it relate to the pathogenesis of necrotizing enterocolitis. *Seminars in Pediatric Surgery, 14*(3), 137–144.

Nowicki, P. (1990). Intestinal ischemia and necrotizing enterocolitis. *The Journal of Pediatrics, 117*(1), S14–S19.

Nowicki, P. T. (2005). Ischemia and necrotizing enterocolitis: Where, when and how. *Seminars in Pediatric Surgery, 14*(3), 152–158.

Petty, J. K., & Ziegler, M. M. (2005). Operative strategies for necrotizing enterocolitis: The prevention and treatment of short bowel syndrome. *Seminars in Pediatric Surgery, 14*(3), 191–198.

Rowe, M. I. (1986). Necrotizing enterocolitis. In K. J. Welch, J. G. Randolph, M. M. Ravitch, J. A. O'Neill, & M. I. Rowe (Eds.), *Pediatric surgery* (4th ed., pp. 944–958). Chicago: Yearbook Medical Publishers.

Ryder, M. A. (1993). Peripherally inserted central venous catheters. *Nursing Clinics of North America, 28*(4), 937–971.

Schwartz, M. Z., Richardson, J., Hayden, C. K., Swischuk, L. E., & Tyson, K. R. T. (1980). Intestinal stenosis following successful medical management of necrotizing enterocolitis. *Journal of Pediatric Surgery, 15*(6), 890–899.

Sondheimer, J. M., Cadnapaphornchai, M., Sontag, M., & Zerbe, G. O. (1998). Predicting the duration of dependence on parenteral nutrition after neonatal intestinal resection. *The Journal of Pediatrics, 132*(1), 80–84.

Stevenson, D. K., Kerner, J. A., Malachowski, N., & Sunshine, P. (1980). Late morbidity among survivors of necrotizing enterocolitis. *Pediatrics, 66*(6), 925–927.

Tan, C. E. L., Kiely, E. M., Agrawal, M., Brereton, R. J., & Spitz, L. (1989). Neonatal gastrointestinal perforation. *Journal of Pediatric Surgery, 24*(9), 888–892.

Touloukian, R. J., & Walker-Smith, G. J. (1983). Normal intestinal length in preterm infants. *Journal of Pediatric Surgery, 18*, 720–722.

Udall, J. N. (1990). Gastrointestinal host defense and necrotizing enterocolitis. *The Journal of Pediatrics, 117*(1), S33–S43.

Vanderhoof, J. A. (1996). Short bowel syndrome in children and small intestinal transplantation. *Pediatric Clinics of North America, 43*(2), 533–550.

Vanderhoof, J. A., & Langnas, A. N. (1997). Short bowel syndrome in children and adults. *Gastroenterology, 113*, 1767–1778.

Warner, B. W., & Warner, B. B. (2005). Role of epidermal growth factor in the pathogenesis of neonatal necrotizing enterocolitis. *Seminars in Pediatric Surgery, 14*(3), 175–180.

Wilson, R., Kanto, W. P., McCarthy, B. J., Burton, T., Lewin, P., Terry, J., et al. (1981). Epidemiologic characteristics of necrotizing enterocolitis: A population-based study. *American Journal of Epidemiology, 114*(6), 880–887.

Nursing Care of Children with Surgical Lesions of the Head, Neck, and Thoracic Cavity

CHAPTER 14

Common Cysts

By M. Elizabeth Foster

Discovery of a lump or bump on a child initiates a cascade of parental anxiety and action that prompts a visit to the pediatrician. Despite parental fears, most unexplained superficial lumps carry a low risk of malignancy in the pediatric population. Many lumps and bumps are seen and carefully observed or treated by primary care physicians. Those that classically present as specific lesions or fail to respond to various salts and salves, antibiotics, steroids, and reassurance are often referred to a pediatric surgeon. Embryologic accidents result in numerous reparable conditions that may present as lumps or bumps. This chapter focuses on common cysts and superficial lumps: branchial cleft remnants, thyroglossal duct cysts, lymphangiomas, vascular anomalies, lymphadenitis, dermoid cysts, ganglion cysts, and pilonidal cysts. Excluded are torticollis, teratomas, dermatologic lesions, tumors, and cystic lesions of internal organs. Table 14-1 summarizes the standard surgical approach to common cysts in childhood.

■ Branchial Cleft Remnants

During the fifth week of embryologic development, major head and neck structures are formed from a series of four internal pharyngeal pouches and external clefts separated by five pharyngeal arches. The external and middle ear, mandible, larynx, laryngeal muscles, nerves and vessels, thyroid gland, parathyroid glands, and thymus gland are among these structures. Pharyngeal arches contain mesenchymal tissue that becomes cartilage, bone, muscle, and blood vessels. Arches are covered externally with squamous epithelium (ectoderm) and internally with cuboidal epithelium (endoderm). Ectodermal tissues become skin over the lower face and neck, ear, thyroid, and cricoid cartilages and bone. Endoderm forms blood vessels and mucous membranes of the pharynx. Mesoderm forms facial and laryngeal muscle and cranial nerves V, VII, IX, and X (trigeminal, facial, glossopharyngeal, and vagus, respectively). The pharyngeal arches, pouches, and clefts are known as branchial (gill-like) arches, pouches, and clefts, although human embryos do not develop gills (Skandalakis, Gray, & Todd, 1994; Soper & Pringle, 1986).

Incomplete, failed, or persistent embryologic development of the branchial arches results in several anomalies or defects in the neck. Two common branchial cleft remnants are branchial cleft sinuses and cysts. As the arch structures finish forming, the branchial pouches and clefts obliterate. If obliteration is incomplete, a sinus tract, fistula, or cyst is the result. Sinuses and cysts are more

Table 14-1   **Summary of Common Cysts and the Straightforward Surgical Approaches[a]**

Cyst	Location	Surgical Indications	Incision	Wound Closure	Complications
First branchial cleft	In front, behind, or below earlobe	Risk of infection	Curved, vertical incision in front of ear to jaw	Subcutaneous with topical collodion or wound closure strips	Facial nerve paralysis, damage to parotid gland, infection, recurrence
Second branchial cleft	Sternocleido mastoid; lower ⅓ & anterior	Risk of infection	Elliptical around opening of sinus or cyst	Subcutaneous with topical collodion or wound closure strips	Hypoglossal & glossopharyngeal nerve damage, bleeding, infection, recurrence
Thyroglossal duct cyst	Midline on or above hyoid bone; movement with swallow	Risk of infection	Transverse just above cyst	Subcutaneous with topical collodion or wound closure strips	Respiratory distress, dysphagia, infection, bleeding, recurrence
Cystic hygroma	Posterior triangle of neck, axilla, cheek, chest, buttocks	Risk of infection, airway obstruction, disfigurement, extreme size, or recurrent infections	Transverse to accommodate removal	Subcutaneous or sutured with drain(s)	Airway obstruction, edema, bleeding, infection, facial nerve damage, recurrence
Hemangioma	Anywhere	Rare; threat to facial or vital structures; extreme size; cosmetic	Transverse to accommodate removal	Subcutaneous or sutured with or without drain(s)	Bleeding, infection, recurrence
Capillary malformation	Anywhere	Cosmetic	None; laser	None	Failure, bleeding, infection
Arteriovenous malformation	Anywhere	Severe bleeding	Depends on location	Subcutaneous with nonabsorbable skin sutures	Bleeding, pain, infection, recurrence
Venous malformation	Anywhere	Decrease bulk of lesion; cosmetic	Depends on location	Subcutaneous with nonabsorbable skin sutures	Bleeding, pain, infection, recurrence
Dermoid cyst	Palpebral ridge of eye, head	Risk of infection; cosmetic	Transverse to accommodate removal	Subcutaneous with topical collodion or wound closure strips	Infection
Ganglion cyst	Dorsal or volar surface of wrist, foot	Risk of infection; pain; interference with joint function	Transverse to accommodate removal	Subcutaneous with topical collodion or wound closure strips	Recurrence, infection
Pilonidal cyst	Sacrococcygeal region	Infection/abscess; pain	Midline; lateral to midline; oblique to midline; flap	Primary closure or secondary intention	Recurrence, infection, wound failure

[a]Complexity, clinical data, cyst physiology, and complications potentially alter the surgical approach and outcome and are excluded from this listing.

common than true fistulas. Branchial cleft remnants originating from the second arch are the most common (90%), followed by those of the first arch (8%). Third and fourth arch anomalies are rare (2%) (Friedberg, 1989; Roback & Telander, 1994; Soper & Pringle, 1986; Smith, 1998).

Preauricular sinuses are tracts that remain after formation of the external ear from the first and second arches. It is believed these are not true branchial cleft remnants but are the result of abnormal infolding and entrapment of epithelium during external ear formation. These sinuses are autosomal dominant with incomplete penetrance and usually present as a preauricular or helical pit. Bilateral presentation occurs in 25% of affected individuals (Friedberg, 1989). The pits may fill with debris and become infected. Surgical excision is indicated for cosmetic reasons or to prevent recurrent infections.

True first branchial cleft anomalies are rare but do occur as cysts that lie in front, behind, or below the earlobe or in the submandibular area (Fig. 14-1). A first branchial sinus has an external opening below the mandible and above the hyoid bone. Some sinus tracts have internal openings to the external ear canal and are true fistulas (Soper & Pringle, 1986). In close proximity to these tracts are the facial nerve (cranial nerve VII) and the parotid gland, which increase the risk and difficulty of surgical excision. Lymphadenitis is the differential diagnosis with first branchial remnants. Complete surgical excision of first branchial remnants is indicated to prevent infection and is performed in the absence of inflammation and infection.

The operation requires general anesthesia, nerve stimulators and probes, and adequate exposure of the facial nerve and parotid gland by means of a curved, vertical incision in front of the ear carried down to just below the jaw. A drain may be placed if fluid or pus is encountered during excision. Wound closure is performed in layers with absorbable sutures, and the skin is closed subcutaneously. Topical collodion or wound closure strips may be applied. Mild paresis of the facial nerve frequently occurs and should resolve within 6 weeks of the procedure. Complications include persistent facial nerve paralysis, wound infection, or recurrence caused by incomplete excision (Soper & Pringle, 1986; Smith, 1998).

Second branchial cleft remnants present as sinus tracts during the first decade of life and as cysts during the second decade. A skin tag or ectopic cartilage (Fig. 14-2) is often present at the opening, and, occasionally, the tract may be palpated deep in the neck. The sinus or cyst is usually located on the lower third and anterior border of the sternocleidomastoid muscle. Differential diagnoses include cystic hygroma and lymphadenitis. Complete sur-

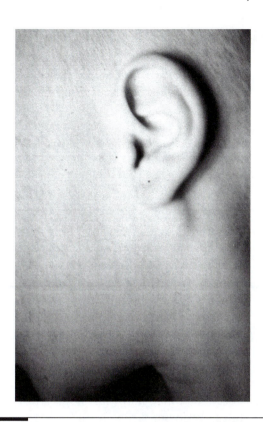

Figure 14-1 First branchial cleft cyst located below the earlobe.

gical excision is indicated for second branchial sinuses and cysts to prevent infection and is performed in the absence of inflammation and infection.

General anesthesia, good airway control, and slight hyperextension of the neck are required throughout the procedure. An external sinus is approached by means of an elliptical incision around the opening, preferably in a skin crease (Fig. 14-3); cysts are approached similarly, and the incision is made around the cyst. If bilateral cysts are present, both may be removed during the same operation. A second (stepladder) incision may be required in an older child when the sinus is low on the sternocleidomastoid to facilitate complete removal of the tract. This allows adequate exposure of the carotid artery branches and the hypoglossal and glossopharyngeal nerves (cranial nerves XII and IX, respectively). Wound closure is performed in layers, without a drain, and the skin is closed with subcutaneous sutures. Complications include infection, recurrence because of incomplete excision, bleeding, and damage to cranial nerves IX and XII (Friedberg, 1989; Roback & Telander, 1994; Soper & Pringle, 1986; Smith, 1998). First and second branchial sinuses and cysts are lined with stratified squamous epithelium and may contain skin appendages, such as sweat glands, hair follicles, and sebaceous glands. Cartilage and muscle tissue

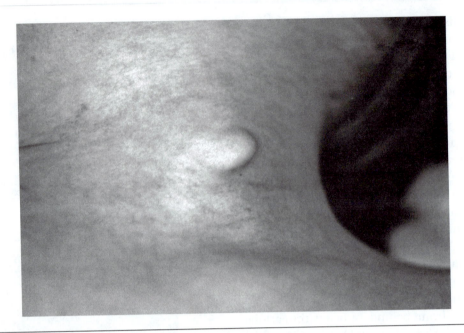

Figure 14-2 Second branchial cleft remnant with skin tag marking the site of the lesion.

have also been identified in the histologic study of these lesions (Bill & Vadheim, 1955).

Third branchial cleft remnants are rare and are often located near the thyroid and along the anterior border of the sternocleidomastoid muscle at the clavicular insertion. Differential diagnoses of third and fourth branchial cleft remnants include thymic cyst, cystic hygroma, acute suppurative thyroiditis, ectopic bronchogenic cyst, pyriform sinus fistula, and congenital lateral cervical cyst of infancy. Fourth branchial cleft remnants are also rare and

are located low in the neck similar to third cleft remnants (Soper & Pringle, 1986; Smith, 1998; Mahomed & Youngson, 1998).

Infection and drainage are common presenting signs of branchial cleft remnants. Preoperative nursing care of children with branchial cleft cysts includes monitoring compliance with the medical regimen and education related to hospital-specific ambulatory surgery procedures and process. Most children are discharged several hours after the procedure with the exception of those with res-

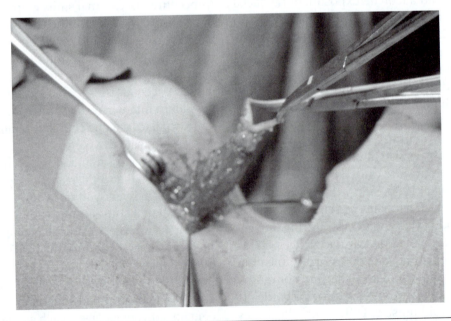

Figure 14-3 Excision of a second branchial cyst and sinus tract.

piratory or anesthesia complications. Nursing care includes instructions to the parent(s) about wound care, activity, pain control, bathing, diet, and complications. Discharge instructions for parents should include information about complications, such as late stridor, dysphagia, and cranial nerve injury. Table 14-2 (Bates, 1983) may be used as a guide for cranial nerve function assessment. A regular diet is resumed when the child is fully alert and able to swallow liquids without aspiration. Normal activity is resumed on postoperative day (POD) 2, with instruction to avoid strenuous activity for 5 to 7 days as well as trauma to the operative area. Sponge bathing is recommended until POD 3. A follow-up visit is planned to assess wound healing, nerve damage, and any signs of recurrence. Topical antibiotic ointments and creams are not recommended for incision care, but oral antibiotics may be prescribed for several days for patients with a previous infection. Pain control is achieved with narcotic agents on PODs 1 and 2 and nonnarcotic agents thereafter as needed. Collodion or wound closure strips applied to the incision are left to peel off spontaneously, usually by POD 5 to 7.

■ Thyroglossal Duct Cyst

Development of the thyroid gland occurs between the third and 10th week of embryologic development, with the beginning marked by an endodermal thickening in the primitive pharynx. The thickening becomes a diverticulum at the posterior third of the tongue (foramen caecum) and then develops a bilobed shape as it projects downward on its tract. By the 10th week, the thyroid is in its normal adult position, and the tract remains connected to the tongue, but the tract's channel obliterates. The tract is behind, in front of, or, rarely, through the hyoid bone. Persistence of the tract permits the accumulation of a colloid-like material secreted by the epithelial lining of the tract. A thyroglossal duct cyst is the result of this accumulation and usually appears between the second and 10th year of life (Skandalakis, Gray, & Todd, 1994; Solomon & Rangecroft, 1984). Distribution between sexes is equal, and the cyst is seen as an asymptomatic midline neck mass over the hyoid bone (Fig. 14-4). Classically, the cyst is round and firm with no external opening and moves up with tongue thrust or swallowing. The cyst may be seen just lateral to the midline, usually to the left, and is rarely seen in the foramen caecum or suprasternally. Differential diagnoses include ectopic thyroid, thyroid nodule, cervical lymphadenopathy, hemangioma, lipoma, and midline dermoid cyst. Oral flora may infect the thyroglossal duct cyst through the thyroglossal duct, causing an eruption through the skin, erythema, and tenderness over the cyst (Solomon & Rangecroft; Soper & Pringle, 1986).

Surgical excision is indicated at diagnosis unless infection is present. The Sistrunk procedure (Sistrunk, 1928)

Table 14-2 Cranial Nerve Assessment Guidelines for Postoperative Care of the Child Undergoing Excision of a Cystic Lesion of the Head or Neck

Cranial Nerve	Name	Function	Assessment
5	Trigeminal	Motor: jaw movement Sensory: sensation on face	Clench teeth; sharp/dull pain sensation on face; hot or cold sensation on face; corneal reflex; infants < 4 mo: rooting reflex
7	Facial	Motor: facial muscle movement Sensory: taste on anterior ⅔ of tongue	Facial symmetry; raise eyebrows; frown; close eyes tight; show teeth; smile; puff out cheeks; infants: observe facial symmetry while crying
9	Glossopharyngeal	Motor: swallowing Sensory: sensation—tongue, pharynx, & eardrum; taste	Listen for hoarseness or speech changes; watch movement of uvula when patient says "ah"; gag reflex
10	Vagus	Motor: movement of palate, pharynx, larynx Sensory: sensation—pharynx & larynx	Same as for glossopharyngeal
12	Hypoglossal	Motor: tongue movement	Stick out tongue; look for asymmetry or deviation from midline tongue strength; infants: pinch nostrils and look for baby to open mouth and raise the tip of the tongue

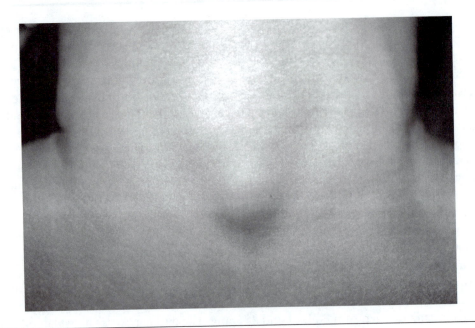

Figure 14-4 Thyroglossal duct cyst presents as a midline mass over the hyoid bone.

involves excising the cyst and its tract upward to the base of the tongue, including dividing and removing part of the hyoid bone adjacent to the tract (Fig. 14-5). General anesthesia, good airway control, and midline positioning of the head are required, and the cyst is approached through a transverse incision at or just above the cyst. The cyst and tract are dissected, and the tract is ligated at the foramen caecum. Wound closure is performed in layers, and the skin is closed subcutaneously. Collodion and/or wound closure strips are placed over the incision,

and a drain is not necessary unless fluid or pus is encountered during excision (Soper & Pringle, 1986).

Histologic examination usually reveals that the cyst is lined with ciliated columnar respiratory epithelium or stratified squamous epithelium (Sade & Rosen, 1968). Complications include infection, recurrence as a result of incomplete excision, bleeding, and airway obstruction resulting from edema or bleeding. Perioperative nursing care of children with thyroglossal duct cysts is similar to that of children with branchial cleft cysts. Uncomplicated

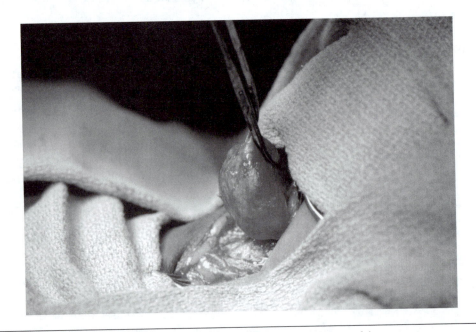

Figure 14-5 Excision of thyroglossal duct cyst. The tract is excised up to the foramen caecum of the tongue.

excisions and postoperative courses permit discharging the child several hours after the procedure. A 23-hour observance is indicated after excision of a thyroglossal duct cyst if any possibility of airway problems is suspected or noted after surgery or if a drain is in place.

■ Lymphangioma (Cystic Hygroma)

Lymphangiomas are characterized by the presence of fluid-filled, endothelium-lined spaces derived from lymphatic vessels. Three types of lymphangiomas are described as: (1) simple: capillary-sized, thin-walled lymph channels; (2) cavernous: dilated lymph channels; and (3) cystic: cysts of varying sizes with thick fibrous walls. When the cystic type of lymphangioma is located in the primitive jugular lymph sac, it is called a *cystic hygroma*. Lymphatic tissue and fluid are unable to drain in normal channels and become sequestered in a loculated mass (Skandalakis, Gray, & Ricketts, 1994). Although most cystic hygromas are located in the neck and axilla, some clinicians describe cystic lymphangiomas anywhere on the body as cystic hygromas (Figs. 14-6 and 14-7). Ninety percent of cystic hygromas are seen before 2 years of age. Diagnosis of fetal cystic hygroma by sonography before 30 weeks gestation is strongly associated with chromosomal and structural anomalies that often result in fetal death. Chromosomal anomalies include Turner's syndrome (45X)

and Down syndrome (trisomy 21). Structural defects are cardiac, renal, neural tube, eye, skeletal, anorectal, or genital in origin (Chervenak et al., 1983; Langer et al., 1990).

Enlargement of the cystic hygroma progresses with the child's growth and is hastened by bacterial or viral infection. Spontaneous regression is rare; surgical excision offers the best hope of a cure. The common presentation is a soft, painless mass in the posterior triangle of the neck. The mass is loculated, fluctuant, not attached to skin, and not movable on deep palpation, and it transilluminates. Cystic hygromas are benign and have no symptoms of their own, but their growth may cause disfigurement, dysphagia due to esophageal compression, and dyspnea due to airway obstruction. Extensive radiologic studies are not necessary to diagnose cystic hygroma because of its uniqueness; however, a computed tomographic scan or magnetic resonance imaging is helpful in defining the boundaries of the lesion and its invasion of surrounding structures. Differential diagnoses include branchial cleft cyst, hemangioma, dermoid cyst, and lipoma (Filston, 1994; Ravitch & Rush, 1986).

Surgical excision is indicated at diagnosis unless inflammation or infection is present. The cystic hygroma is approached through a transverse cervical incision large enough to accommodate removal (Fig. 14-8). General anesthesia, good airway control, and positioning of the head away from the affected side are required for the procedure. Some lesions are excised simply, others require

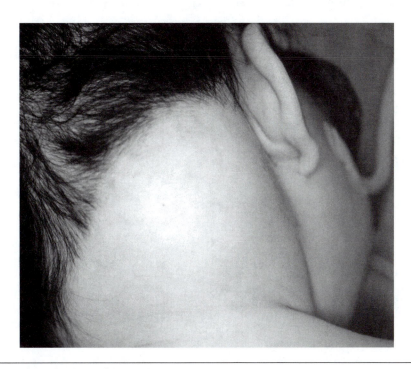

Figure 14-6 Cystic hygroma in the posterior neck.

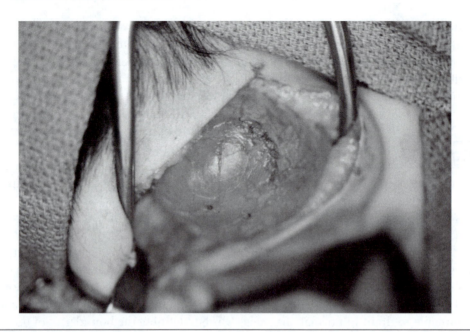

Figure 14-7 Operative view of cystic hygroma in Figure 14-6. The mass is clear and loculated.

extensive dissection, and a few are unresectable. Sclerotherapy has been shown to aid with regression for cystic hygromas that are unresectable. Axillary hygromas are approached by means of an incision in an axillary skin crease with the arm raised during the procedure. Mediastinal extension is approached from the cervical incision alone or by extending the incision down the anterior midline. Splitting the sternum may be necessary to remove the cyst wholly. A drain or drains are placed to capture any residual fluid or blood after extensive resection (Filston, 1994; Ravitch & Rush, 1986). Complications include recurrence requiring reoperation, injury to the mandibular branch of the facial nerve, lingual edema, bleeding, infection, and airway obstruction (Filston; Ninh & Ninh, 1974).

Nursing care of the child undergoing resection of a cystic hygroma includes airway management and monitoring, fluid balance, cranial nerve function assessment

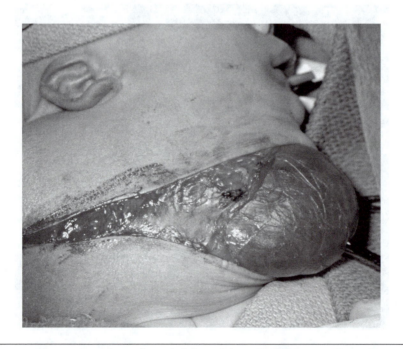

Figure 14-8 Large cystic hygroma of posterior and anterior neck delivered through a large transverse incision.

(see Table 14-2), pain control, and nutrition for wound healing. Supporting the family's adjustment to a potentially disfiguring lesion and/or scar on the child is important. Intensive care monitoring is required after an extensive resection, and nurses should inform the parent(s) of the presence of tubes, drains, lines, and equipment before visiting. The intensive care unit environment is frightening, and an explanation of sights, sounds, and scenarios is imperative and indicated for managing parental anxiety and fear. Edema and bleeding are usually responsible for airway complications and require careful assessment and attention for the first 48 hours after surgical excision. The facial and hypoglossal cranial nerves (VII and XII, respectively) are assessed for motor and sensory function (see Table 14-2). Pain control is initially achieved with narcotic agents that require monitoring oxygen saturation levels and cardiac and respiratory rates. The drain or drains are removed when output is minimal. Wound closure is performed in layers with subcutaneous skin closure. Activity is permitted as tolerated, with attention being paid to avoiding trauma to the operative site.

Shock, anger, guilt, fear, depression, rejection, and a sense of loss of a healthy infant are the most common emotions expressed by parents when the infant has a birth defect or requires a major operation (Mercer, 1990). Nurses are in a position to support and validate the family's emotions while encouraging bonding and adaptation to the infant with an illness.

Hemangiomas and Vascular Malformations

Hemangiomas and arteriovenous malformations (AVMs) are the most common head and neck masses in children. Venous malformations and capillary malformations are other common vascular malformations in children. They are all the result of faulty embryologic development of peripheral blood vessels. The process is described as unopposed angiogenesis.

Hemangiomas appear in the first few weeks of life, are more common in females, and are seen as soft, compressible masses (Fig. 14-9). A bluish hue to the skin over the lesion is common. Hemangiomas progress through two phases: proliferation and involution. Proliferation is characterized by enlargement of the lesion during the first 6 to 8 months of life, followed by growth of the lesion commensurate with the child until the end of the first year. Involution takes place over several years and is characterized by shrinking and color changes from red to bluish purple. Most hemangiomas spontaneously and completely regress by 5 to 10 years of age without intervention. Lesions that threaten facial features or vital structures or those that are extremely large may be treated with steroids to hasten regression. Indications for steroid therapy include bleeding, ulceration, visual obstruction, nasal obstruction, rapid lesion growth, or parental concern about facial deformity.

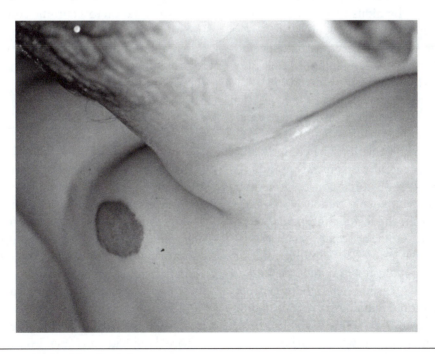

Figure 14-9 Hemangioma on the shoulder of an infant.

Steroid therapy is most effective in superficial lesions and may halt the growth of both superficial and deep lesions. However, steroids do not shorten the natural course of hemangiomas. Triamcinolone acetonide is injected via a small-bore needle in an outpatient setting. Treatment intervals and drug doses vary by institution, and successful therapy is indicated by a 50% or greater reduction in lesion size. Failure to respond to steroids is the rare indication to excise the lesion or treat it with sclerotherapy, laser therapy, or interferon (Filston, 1994; Mulliken & Fishman, 1998; Chen, Yeong, & Horng, 2000). Aggressive reassurance and tincture of time are the primary modes of therapy for most hemangiomas because they are benign and spontaneously resolve. The nurse's role is to support and validate the parents' feelings and promote bonding and attachment to an infant with a disfiguring lesion.

AVMs are less common than hemangiomas and may be evident shortly after birth. These lesions are characterized by a patch of warm, purple skin, a palpable mass, and a bruit or thrill when superficial. Trauma and puberty contribute to enlargement of the malformation. Long term, these lesions produce ischemic skin changes, pain, and intermittent bleeding within the lesion. The most severe effects of AVM are congestive heart failure because of shunting of blood through the AVM and limb hypertrophy when they occur in an extremity. Excision is usually performed in late childhood or adolescence or if the lesion causes life-threatening bleeding, but complete surgical excision is seldom possible. Selective embolization is useful as the first line of palliative therapy during bleeding or painful episodes. Embolization to occlude the nidus is not recommended mainstay therapy, because collateral vessels contribute to the reformation of the lesion; however, partially occluding the nidus before surgical excision minimizes bleeding during the procedure (Mulliken & Fishman, 1998).

Venous malformations usually appear as a blue patch anywhere on the body, superficially or deep. They may be local or extensive, nondescript or disfiguring, and grow with the child. Venous malformations are compressible, expand when dependent, and worsen during puberty. Compression garments are required conservative therapy to minimize dependent edema, venous congestion, sequestration of blood in the lesion, and pain. Sclerotherapy with 1% sodium tetradecyl sulfate (small lesions) or absolute ethanol (large lesions) is helpful before surgical resection, which is indicated to reduce the bulk of the lesion or for cosmetic reasons. Sclerotherapy is performed by an interventional radiologist. Venous malformations tend to recur (Mulliken & Fishman, 1998).

Capillary malformation (port wine stain) is a macular, vascular lesion that occurs on the face, trunk, or limbs. During adolescence, it produces skin darkening, soft tissue nodules, and hypertrophy. Capillary malformations in the limbs are associated with Klippel-Trenaunay and Parkes-Weber vascular anomaly syndromes. Klippel-Trenaunay syndrome features a vascular anomaly (usually capillary malformation, varicose veins, or hypoplastic or aplastic deep veins) and pronounced limb hypertrophy. Parkes-Weber syndrome features the same limb hypertrophy, but the vascular anomaly is an arteriovenous fistula. Problems encountered in both syndromes include joint pain, skin ulcerations, and the need for a prosthetic shoe or heel lift for the unaffected leg when the lower extremities are involved. Capillary malformations of the face are sometimes associated with Sturge-Weber sequence, which also features hemangiomata of eye structures and meninges, seizures, paresis, and mental deficiency (Jones, 1988). Flashlamp pulsed-dye laser is the treatment for capillary malformations, and 70% to 80% are significantly lightened with this therapy (Mulliken & Fishman, 1998).

Vascular anomalies are chronic and have an impact on the physical, emotional, and social aspects of the affected child's and family's life. Grotesque and disfiguring lesions affect the child's body image development and self-esteem and cause a sense of being different. Social isolation, rejection, and feelings of abandonment may dominate the child's behaviors as a result of ridicule and rejection from other children and adults. Limited mobility, pain, and risk for trauma interfere with physical activities for the child with a vascular malformation. The nursing role is largely supportive and should facilitate the child's adaptation to a chronic condition through validation of feelings and reinforcement of positive attributes. Parental bonding and acceptance of the child are crucial to providing a nurturing and supportive environment for the child (Mercer, 1990).

■ Lymphadenopathy

Lymphadenopathy is enlargement of a lymph node(s), and lymphadenitis is a form of lymphadenopathy with additional symptoms of local pain, tenderness, and fever. Enlarged nodes are a common and normal finding during puberty, and cervical nodes up to 1 cm in diameter are normal in children less than 12 years of age. Nonspecific reactive cervical lymphadenopathy is self-limiting and usually the result of an upper respiratory viral infection or other systemic viral illnesses, such as Epstein-Barr virus. Bacterial infections may also cause cervical lymphadenitis (Fig. 14-10). These infections typically respond to a course of antibiotics unless the nodes

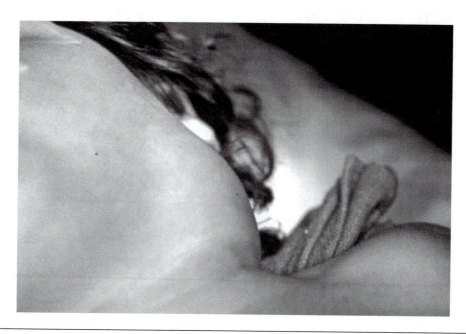

Figure 14-10 Cervical lymphadenitis caused by bacterial infection of the node.

develop an abscess within them. An abscess requires incision and drainage for treatment. Granulomatous diseases produce chronic lymphadenopathy and may involve several nodes (Fig. 14-11) (Bodenstein & Altman, 1994; Friedberg, 1989).

Treatment of lymphadenopathy involves several approaches that are based on the history, chronicity, presentation, and differential diagnoses. A summary of common surgical lymphadenopathies is listed in Table 14-3 for brevity and is not intended as an exhaustive list of all lymphadenopathy seen in childhood. Suppurative lymphadenitis is usually benign, self-limiting, and a clinical finding or symptom of a systemic disease rather than a singular disease entity. Suppurative lymphadenopathy may be approached surgically by incision and drainage, whereas nonsuppurative lymphadenopathy requires excision, biopsy, or fine-needle aspiration when indicated. Surgical therapy is intended as diagnostic,

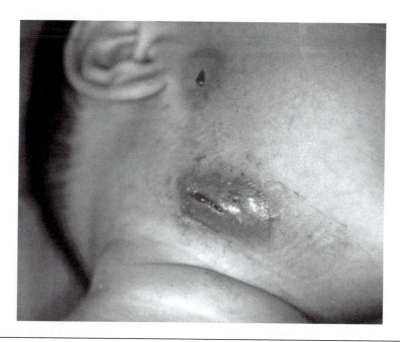

Figure 14-11 Spontaneous drainage of lymphadenitis caused by atypical mycobacterium.

Table 14-3 **Summary of Surgical Indications and Approaches to Lymphadenitis**

Classification of Node Inflammation	Most Common Causative Agent[a]	Medical Management	Indications for Surgery[b]	Surgical Approach[b]	Surgical Outcomes[b]
Reactive lymphadenopathy	Upper respiratory virus; Epstein-Barr virus; Kawasaki syndrome	Observation	None	None	None
Bacterial lymphadenitis	*Staphylococcus; Streptococcus; Haemophilus influenzae*	Penicillin Cephalosporin	Fluctuance Induration	Incision and drainage	Diagnostic and curative
Fungal lymphadenitis (usually in immuno-compromised patient)	*Candida albicans*	Amphotericin B	Fluctuance Induration May defer surgery until medical therapy ended	Incision and drainage	Diagnostic and palliative
Granulomatous infection: tuberculous lymphadenitis	*Mycobacterium tuberculosis*	Isoniazid Rifampin Pyrazinamide	Chronicity Diagnosis	Fine-needle aspirate Excisional biopsy	Diagnostic and palliative
Granulomatous infection: atypical mycobacterium	*Mycobacterium scrofulaceum Mycobacterium avium Mycobacterium kansasii*	Rifampin Clarithromycin Anti-tuberculosis meds	Draining tracts with skin involvement	Excision	Diagnostic and curative
Granulomatous infection: cat scratch fever	*Bartonella henselae*	Observation	Discomfort because of size	Aspiration	Palliative
Toxoplasmosis	*Toxoplasma gondii*	Pyrimethamine	Diagnosis	Excisional biopsy	Diagnostic

[a]American Academy of Pediatrics. (2000). *2000 red book: Report of the Committee on Infectious Diseases* (25th ed.). Elk Grove Village, IL: American Academy of Pediatrics.
[b]Bodenstein, L., & Altman, R. P. (1994). Cervical lymphadenitis in infants and children. *Seminars in Pediatric Surgery, 3*, 134–141.

curative, palliative, or any combination of these outcomes. The nursing role with surgical treatment of lymphadenitis is educational with regard to hospital-specific ambulatory surgery procedures and process. Instructions for wound care, bathing, activity, complications, and appropriate medical and surgical follow-up should be given before discharge. After incision and drainage, the wound often requires cleaning and packing of the cavity on a daily or twice-daily basis. Packing prevents early skin closure as the wound heals by secondary intention. The nurse explains the rationale and demonstrates the wound care regimen to the parent(s) and determines whether the parent(s) can safely perform the procedure. Bathing is permitted if the wound needs to be washed out. Clean excisions are closed primarily with subcutaneous skin closure and topical collodion and/or wound closure strips. Normal activity is resumed with instruction to avoid strenuous activity for 5 to 7 days and trauma to the operative site. Medical follow-up for lymphadenitis includes compliance with the antibiotic regimen and referral or follow-up with the primary care physician or an infectious disease specialist. Surgical follow-up allows assessment of wound healing and assessment for complications.

Dermoid Cyst

Dermoids are a type of sebaceous cyst that contain ectodermal elements, such as sebaceous glands, hair follicles, and connective tissue. They are most commonly located along the supraorbital palpebral ridge, are attached to the bony fascia, are movable, and are nontender (Fig. 14-12). Other locations include scalp, forehead, nose, neck, jaw, and suprasternal area. Epidermoid cysts have a similar presentation and differ only by their contents, which is sebaceous without skin appendages. Dermoids and epidermoids in the midline of the skull are studied on plain films for penetration to the epidural space; no other diagnostic studies are indicated for dermoids. If the cyst penetrates to the epidural space, a computed tomographic scan and neurosurgery consult are appropriate management. Differential diagnoses include lipoma, lymphangioma, thyroglossal duct cyst, and pilomatrixoma. Calcified epithelioma of Malherbe (pilomatrixoma) is a hamartoma of hair follicle origin and a common type of sebaceous cyst. Pilomatrixoma may occur anywhere except the palms and soles (no hair follicles). Indications for surgical excision are cosmetic, risk for infection, and to establish pathologic diagnosis. Dermoids and other sebaceous cysts are benign, are cured with surgical excision, and usually do not recur (Guarisco, 1991; Knight & Reiner, 1983; Pryor, Lewis, Weaver, & Orvidas, 2005).

The nursing role is educational with regard to hospital specific ambulatory surgery procedures and process. Instructions about incision care, bathing, activity, complications, and follow-up are given. Excision of a sebaceous cyst is often perceived as trivial; however, it is important to approach the family with sincerity and allay their anxiety about the surgical procedure. The incision is closed subcutaneously and covered topically with collodion and/or wound closure strips. Most dermoid cysts are 1 to 1.5 cm in diameter, and the incision is commensurate with the size of the lesion. Bathing is permitted on the first postoperative day, but soaking the incision should be avoided. Normal activity is resumed, with instruction to avoid trauma to the operative site. Regular diet is resumed when the child is fully alert and able to tolerate liquids without aspiration. Pain control is achieved with nonnarcotic agents.

■ Ganglion Cyst

Ganglion cysts originate from the capsule of a joint or from a tendon sheath. They are most commonly seen on the dorsal surface of the wrist (70%), occasionally on the volar surface of the wrist (20%), and rarely on the foot or other locations. Most ganglions are 1 to 2 cm in diameter; are round, nontender, or slightly tender; and may interfere with function of the wrist or foot (Fig. 14-13). Differential diagnoses include giant cell tumor of the tendor sheath, lipoma, true synovial cyst, or tenosynovitis of the extensor tendons. Ganglion cysts contain a thick, clear fluid that may be aspirated or injected with steroids as means of treatment. Surgical excision is the best method of treatment and one that offers the lowest rate of recurrence (Smith & Yandow, 1996). The oldest method for treating a ganglion cyst is to hit it with the family Bible; this bursts the cyst, permitting the capsule to scar. Aspiration, injection, and traumatic methods of treatment

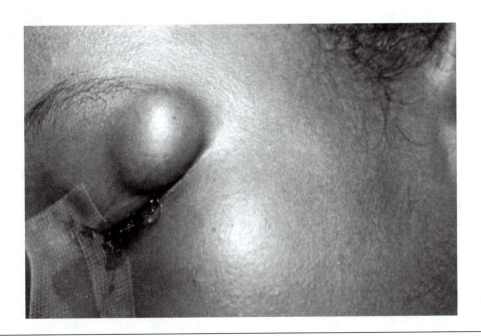

Figure 14-12 Dermoid cyst on the palpebral ridge of the eye.

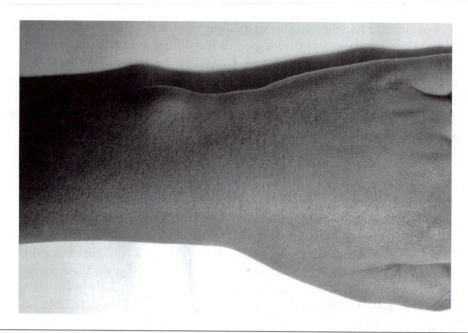

Figure 14-13 Ganglion cyst on the dorsal surface of the wrist.

have a significant recurrence rate between 70% and 90% and are often abandoned in favor of surgical excision (Nahra & Bucchieri, 2004).

Ganglion cysts are excised in the operating room under general or regional anesthesia. A transverse incision is made, and blunt dissection to the cyst stalk is performed. The cyst is excised at the base of the stalk, the wound is irrigated and injected with local anesthetic, and the skin is closed with sutures (may be subcutaneous or nonabsorbable).

The nursing role is educational with regard to hospital-specific ambulatory surgery procedures and process. Instructions about incision care, bathing, activity, complications, and follow-up are given. The affected wrist is immobilized in a soft splint for 7 to 10 days after surgery. The family is instructed on removal and replacement of the splint for bathing and wrist movement. Bathing is permitted on POD 2, but soaking the incision should be avoided. If the skin was closed with nonabsorbable sutures, they are removed on POD 7. Normal activity is resumed, with instruction to avoid trauma to the operative site. Regular diet is resumed when the child is fully alert and able to tolerate liquids without aspiration. Pain control is achieved with narcotic agents on PODs 1 and 2 and nonnarcotic agents thereafter as needed.

■ Pilonidal Sinus

Once believed to be congenital in origin, it is now widely accepted that pilonidal sinus is an acquired condition due

to rates of recurrence following wide excision, age at onset, and gender distribution. The term is from Latin "pilus" meaning hair, and "nidus" meaning nest. Pilonidal disease peaks in the second decade of life (range, 15–45 years) and occurs predominantly in hirsute Caucasian males (80%) (Chamberlain & Vawter, 1974; Hull & Wu, 2002; da Silva, 2000). It is rare in African-American individuals and almost nonexistent in Asians. In pediatrics, the disease appears most often in adolescence after the onset of puberty. The disease process occurs primarily in the sacrococcygeal region and natal cleft, but interdigital pilonidal disease has been reported in the hands of hairdressers, barbers, dog groomers, sheep shearers, and cow milkers from the intrusion of hair into the skin. A sacral pit containing hair is commonly the source of the problem. Friction in the natal cleft causes hair shafts to penetrate the skin and initiate an inflammatory response. The result is a painful erythematous abscess over the sacrococcygeal region, typically in line with the natal cleft. The abscess may spontaneously drain and heal, or drain and form a secondary tract. Numerous hair follicles may be involved, causing several sinus tracts and cysts below the skin. Recurrence rates are strongly correlated with the persistence and/or recurrence of hair in the wound.

The goals of treatment are to minimize pain and debilitation after the procedure, reduce the rate of recurrence, and facilitate complete healing. This is achieved in several widely accepted methods of treatment. The simplest technique is incision and curettage of all sinus tracts, creating one large wound that is left open to heal by secondary intention. Using general or local anesthesia, the patient is placed in a prone jack-knife position or lateral position. Daily cleansing and packing of the wound are initiated until the wound heals completely. This may take 2 to 6 weeks, depending on wound size, wound environment, compliance, and complications. Systemic antibiotics are optional. Shaving or use of depilatory cream is imperative while the wound heals to prevent inclusion of hair in the wound. The advantage of this procedure is its simplicity. The disadvantages are prolonged wound care, higher risk of infection, and pain. One step further in this procedure is marsupialization, in which the skin edges are sewn to the base of the curettaged wound in an effort to minimize wound size, prevent premature wound closure, and speed recovery. In Bascom's operation, the pilonidal follicles are excised individually, and a small incision is made lateral to the natal cleft and excised follicle(s). A piece of gauze is run through the excised follicle(s) and the incision to scrub away hair and granulation tissue. The follicle(s) and incision are left unsutured to heal. Again, systemic antibiotics are optional. All of the open procedures take considerable time to heal and still pose the threat of recurrence. Time away from work or school is also an important consideration in the decision regarding the use of an open technique (Hull & Wu, 2002; Petersen, Kock, Stelzner, Wendlandt, & Ludwig, 2002; da Silva, 2000).

Primary closure techniques involve excising the infected sinus tracts and closing the incision (1) along the midline, (2) oblique or lateral to the midline, or (3) with the creation of a flap over the wound. Midline closures have the highest incidence of early wound failure and recurrence, most likely due to suture line tension, contamination, and continued penetration of hair from friction in the natal cleft. Oblique and lateral closures have better outcomes but are still affected by wound failure and recurrence. Several flap techniques are described in the literature: the Karydakis flap, the Dufourmentel rhomboid flap, the Limberg rhomboid flap, V-Y plasty, and Z-plasty. Detailed discussion of each flap is beyond the scope of this chapter, but each technique flattens the natal cleft in the area of the cyst and reduces suture line tension by avoiding the cleft. Oblique, lateral, and flap closures offer the quickest recovery time in the absence of complications (Petersen et al., 2002; Spivak, Brooks, Nussbaum, & Friedman, 1996; Hull & Wu, 2002). Many patients experience recurrence of pilonidal disease even after an uncomplicated postoperative course. The use of antibiotics is not universally agreed upon; consideration of the entire clinical picture guides the choice for or against antibiotics. Wound drains are another variable factor in management of the disease process. Complete drainage and evacuation of hair and devitalized tissue are crucial for successful healing, regardless of the chosen treatment method.

Nursing care of pilonidal disease focuses on wound care and pain relief. Treatment takes weeks, and nurses must be diligent in providing wound care and teaching the patient and family how to care for the wound at home. Frequent assessment of the wound environment and communication with the physician are key to early detection and intervention for complications. A long-term wound care plan is initiated in the immediate postoperative period and is altered as needed during the course of healing. Draining the abscess offers great pain relief that is quickly offset when dressing changes begin (open procedure). Nurses must also be diligent with pain assessment and treatment according to institutional protocol. Analgesic agents should be administered as needed for dressing changes (open procedure) and as needed during the postoperative phase (open and closed procedures). A regular diet is initiated in the usual fashion after the effects of anesthesia dissipate. Activity level is tailored to the wound type to avoid tension on the suture line and pressure to the area. Prolonged sitting is discouraged in both open and closed procedures. Hygiene is also specific to the surgical procedure used. Open procedures require wound cleansing and dressing on a daily basis; moisture on the sutures should be avoided with closed procedures. All aspects of postoperative care must be tailored to the individual, the family, and the surgical procedure.

■ Conclusion

A simple and straightforward surgical approach is curative for most of the common cysts of childhood. These cases are often clean and straightforward, and they carry a low risk and incidence of complications and problems. The safety and efficacy of pediatric anesthesia have also contributed to minimal hospital stays and low complication rates after superficial cyst removal.

■ Educational Materials

APSNA invites you to download the following diagnosis-related teaching tools for Chapter 14, Common Cysts: Lymphadenopathy, branchial cleft cyst, cystic hygroma, dermoid cyst, ganglion cyst, pilonidal cyst, and thyroglossal duct cyst. These teaching tools are available at the APSNA Web site (www.apsna.org) and the Jones and Bartlett Web site (www.jbpub.com). All teaching materials are available in English and Spanish and are free of charge. APSNA encourages their use for your patients and families.

References

American Academy of Pediatrics. (2000). *2000 red book: Report of the Committee on Infectious Diseases* (25th ed.). Elk Grove Village, IL: American Academy of Pediatrics.

Bates, B. M. (1983). *A guide to physical examination* (3rd ed.). Philadelphia: Lippincott.

Bill, A. H., & Vadheim, J. L. (1955). Cysts, sinuses and fistulas of the neck arising from the first and second branchial clefts. *Annals of Surgery, 142*, 904–908.

Bodenstein, L., & Altman, R. P. (1994). Cervical lymphadenitis in infants and children. *Seminars in Pediatric Surgery, 3*(3), 134–141.

Chamberlain, J. W., & Vawter, G. F. (1974). The congenital origin of pilonidal sinus. *Journal of Pediatric Surgery, 9*(4), 441–444.

Chen, M. T., Yeong, E. K., & Horng, S. Y. (2000). Intralesional corticosteroid therapy in proliferating head and neck hemangiomas: A review of 155 cases. *Journal of Pediatric Surgery, 35*(3), 420–423.

Chervenak, F. A., Isaacson, G., Blakemore, K. J., Breg, W. R., Hobbins, J. C., Berkowitz, R. L., et al. (1983). Fetal cystic hygroma: Cause and natural history. *New England Journal of Medicine, 309*(14), 822–825.

Filston, H. C. (1994). Hemangiomas, cystic hygromas, and teratomas of the head and neck. *Seminars in Pediatric Surgery, 3*(3), 147–159.

Friedberg, J. (1989). Pharyngeal cleft sinuses and cysts, and other benign neck lesions. *Pediatric Clinics of North America, 36*(6), 1451–1469.

Guarisco, J. L. (1991). Congenital head and neck masses in infants and children. *Ear, Nose, and Throat Journal, 70*(2), 75–82.

Hull, T. L., & Wu, J. (2002). Pilonidal disease. *Surgical Clinics of North America, 82*(6), 1169–1185.

Jones, K. L. (Ed.). (1988). *Smith's recognizable patterns of human malformations* (4th ed.). Philadelphia: W.B. Saunders.

Knight, P. J., & Reiner, C. B. (1983). Superficial lumps in children: What, when, and why? *Pediatrics, 72*(2), 147–153.

Langer, J. C., Fitzgerald, P. G., Desa, D., Filly, R. A., Golbus, M. S., Adzick, N. S., et al. (1990). Cervical cystic hygroma in the fetus: Clinical spectrum and outcome. *Journal of Pediatric Surgery, 25*(1), 58–62.

Mahomed, A., & Youngson, G. (1998). Congenital lateral cervical cysts of infancy. *Journal of Pediatric Surgery, 33*(9), 1413–1415.

Mercer, R. T. (1990). *Parents at risk*. New York: Springer.

Mulliken, J. B., & Fishman, S. J. (1998). Vascular anomalies: Hemangiomas and malformations. In J. A. O'Neill, M. I. Rowe, J. L. Grosfeld, E. W. Folkalsrud, & A. G. Coran (Eds.), *Pediatric surgery* (Vol. 2, 5th ed., pp. 1939–1952). St. Louis, MO: Mosby.

Nahra, M. E., & Bucchieri, J. S. (2004). Ganglion cysts and other tumor related conditions of the hand and wrist. *Hand Clinics, 20*(3), 249–260.

Ninh, T. N., & Ninh, T. X. (1974). Cystic hygroma in children: A report of 126 cases. *Journal of Pediatric Surgery, 9*(2), 191–195.

Petersen, S., Kock, R., Stelzner, S., Wendlandt, T. P., & Ludwig, K. (2002). Primary closure techniques in chronic pilonidal sinus: A survey of the results of different surgical approaches. *Diseases of the Colon and Rectum, 45*(11), 1458–1467.

Pryor, S. G., Lewis, J. E., Weaver, A. L., & Orvidas, L. J. (2005). Pediatric dermoid cysts of the head and neck. *Otolaryngology–Head and Neck Surgery, 132*(6), 938–942.

Ravitch, M. M., & Rush, B. F. (1986). Cystic hygroma. In K. J. Welch, J. G. Randolph, M. M. Ravitch, J. A. O'Neill, & M. I. Rowe (Eds.), *Pediatric surgery* (Vol. 1, 4th ed., pp. 533–539). Chicago: Year Book Medical.

Roback, S. A., & Telander, R. L. (1994). Thyroglossal duct cysts and branchial cleft anomalies. *Seminars in Pediatric Surgery, 3*(3), 142–146.

Sade, J., & Rosen, G. (1968). Thyroglossal cysts and tracts: A histological and histochemical study. *Annals of Otology, Rhinology, and Laryngology, 77*, 139–145.

da Silva, J. H. (2000). Pilonidal cyst: Cause and treatment. *Diseases of the Colon and Rectum, 45*(8), 1146–1156.

Sistrunk, W. E. (1928). Technique of removal of cysts and sinuses of the thyroglossal duct. *Surgery, Gynecology and Obstetrics, 46*, 109–112.

Skandalakis, J. E., Gray, S. W., & Ricketts, R. R. (1994). The lymphatic system. In J. E. Skandalakis & S. W. Gray (Eds.), *Embryology for surgeons* (2nd ed., pp. 877–897). Baltimore: Williams and Wilkins.

Skandalakis, J. E., Gray, S. W., & Todd, N. W. (1994). The pharynx and its derivatives. In J. E. Skandalakis & S. W. Gray (Eds.), *Embryology for surgeons* (2nd ed., pp. 17–64). Baltimore: Williams and Wilkins.

Smith, C. D. (1998). Cysts and sinuses of the neck. In J. A. O'Neill, M. I. Rowe, J. L. Grosfeld, E. W. Fonkalsrud, & A. G. Coran (Eds.), *Pediatric surgery* (Vol. 1, 5th ed., pp. 757–771). St. Louis, MO: Mosby.

Smith, J. T., & Yandow, S. M. (1996). Benign soft–tissue lesions in children. *Orthopedic Clinics of North America, 27*(3), 645–654.

Solomon, J. R., & Rangecroft, L. (1984). Thyroglossal–duct lesions in childhood. *Journal of Pediatric Surgery, 19*(5), 555–561.

Soper, R. T., & Pringle, K. C. (1986). Cysts and sinuses of the neck. In K. J. Welch, J. G. Randolph, M. M. Ravitch, J. A. O'Neill, & M. I. Rowe (Eds.), *Pediatric surgery* (Vol. 1, 4th ed., pp. 539–552). Chicago: Year Book Medical.

Spivak, H., Brooks, V. L., Nussbaum, M., & Friedman, I. (1996). Treatment of chronic pilonidal disease. *Diseases of the Colon and Rectum, 39*(10), 1136–1139.

Esophageal Defects

By Danuta E. Nowicki

Defects of the esophagus, whether congenital, acquired, or functional, are among the most common anomalies in children. Congenital defects include esophageal atresia (EA), tracheoesophageal fistula (TEF), laryngotracheo-esophageal clefts, congenital esophageal stenosis, and esophageal duplication. Corrosive injuries to the esophagus, esophageal strictures, and foreign bodies in the esophagus are among the acquired esophageal defects. Achalasia and gastroesophageal reflux (GER) are examples of functional disorders of the esophagus. Prompt identification of the disorder is necessary for appropriate management. This chapter focuses on EA, TEF, corrosive injuries to the esophagus, esophageal stricture, and esophageal replacement.

■ Congenital Defects

Esophageal Atresia and Tracheoesophageal Fistula

Of all the potential anomalies involving the esophagus and trachea, EA and the associated TEF are the most common and the most fatal if not promptly diagnosed and treated surgically. Before 1939, there was 100% mortal-

ity in infants born with EA/TEF (Raffensperger, 1990). Advances in medical and surgical care in the past 40 years have led to a survival rate of near 100% in otherwise healthy infants born with the disorder (Randolph, Newman, & Anderson, 1989). The cause of death in the ill infants is attributed to extreme prematurity and associated anomalies.

Often referred to as one condition, EA/TEF is in reality two entities, which may present separately or, more commonly, occur together. EA refers to the condition wherein there has been a disruption in the development of the esophagus, preventing it from becoming a continuous tube. This results in the formation of a proximal and distal pouch. TEF is an abnormal connection, by way of the fistula, between the esophagus and the trachea. Most common is a combination of the two, in which the esophagus has failed to fuse as a continuous tube, and a fistula connects the proximal, distal, or both pouches to the trachea.

Incidence and Etiology

EA/TEF occurs in approximately 1:3000–4500 births, with a slight male predominance (Bankier, Brady, & Myers, 1991; Filston & Shorter, 2000; Raffensperger, 1990). Prematurity is common with EA or EA with an associated TEF; 34% of these infants weigh less than 2,500 g (Holder,

1993). In general, infants with pure TEF are not born prematurely; their average gestational age is 37 weeks.

The origin of these anomalies is not known. They usually occur sporadically, although there are reports of several family members having EA/TEF. The anomaly is found in twins, siblings, and offspring of adults who themselves had the disorder (Bankier et al., 1991; Filston & Shorter, 2000; Harmon & Coran, 1998; Raffensperger, 1990).

Embryology

The foregut of the embryo is seen as a single-cell-layer tube at 19 to 23 days of gestation. This tube gives rise to the esophagus and the pharynx. The dorsal foregut, or primitive esophagus, begins to divide from the ventral trachea at the level of the carina by a union between two proliferating ridges of cells composing the epithelial lining. This division progresses in a cephalad direction and is completed to the level of the larynx by approximately the 26th day. A disruption in this process is thought to result in a TEF (Beasley, 1991a; Raffensperger, 1990).

EA is thought to occur as a result of the unavailability of tissue caused by the rapid growth and elongation of the primitive esophagus. An interruption of the vascular supply to the area during development may also play a role in the cause (Beasley, 1991a; Harmon & Coran, 1998; Filston & Shorter, 2000; Raffensperger, 1990).

Classification

Although EA and TEF occur as isolated entities, a combination is more common. The classification of these defects has marked clinical significance in the treatment, management, and eventual outcome of these children. Following are the most commonly recorded classifications based on the pathological condition they represent and rate of occurrence. Their alphabetical ranking is based on Gross' (1953) method of classification (Fig. 15-1).

Associated Anomalies

Approximately 50% of infants born with EA/TEF have other anomalies that vary in severity and associated mortality (Table 15-1). In addition to surgical correction for EA/TEF, the infant may require corrective repairs of the associated anomalies. Associated cardiac anomalies are the most common and the most lethal. The incidence of cardiovascular anomalies ranges from 14.7% to 28% (David & O'Callaghan, 1974; Greenwood & Rosenthal, 1976; Mee, 1991). EA/TEF is also a component of the VATER or VACTERL association (Quan & Smith, 1973). This association of anomalies includes defects of the vertebrae, anorectal malformations, cardiac defects, renal defects, and defects of the radius and/or limbs. Although most patients do not exhibit all the associated defects, if one defect is present, others should be suspected. The most common associated gastrointestinal defect found in this grouping is imperforate anus.

Pathophysiology

Swallowing by the fetus begins at about 14 weeks' gestation. By the end of pregnancy, the fetus swallows several hundred milliliters or half the amniotic fluid volume daily (Stokes, 1991). It is estimated that the fetus may get as much as 10% to 14% of its nutrition from the amniotic fluid (Mulvihill, Stone, Debas, & Fonkalsrud, 1985). Infants with EA have a small stomach because it has not been dilated through swallowing. The size of the stomach may be problematic in the creation of a gastrostomy or gastric fundoplication and may limit the ability to advance feedings. EA prevents saliva and oral intake from reaching the stomach. Strenuous attempts at swallowing by the fetus cause hypertrophy and distention of the upper pouch. The pooling of liquid or food in the blind upper pouch compresses the trachea, interfering with the development of the tracheal cartilage. This may lead to tracheomalacia, a condition in which the tracheal wall is especially soft and pliable (Filler & Forte, 1998). If there is an associated proximal TEF, the pooled liquid in the upper pouch crosses the fistula, causing respiratory distress.

The presence of a TEF allows the passage of food and gas between the trachea and the esophagus in either direction. Thus, air forced across the fistula as an infant cries may elicit a belch. If the child has the more common distal fistula between the lower esophageal pouch and trachea, the stomach may become massively dilated and the diaphragms elevated, causing respiratory compromise. A distal fistula also allows gastric contents to pass along the fistula to the trachea, causing respiratory complications, such as tracheobronchitis, pneumonia, and atelectasis.

Clinical Presentation

Often, the first sign of EA is polyhydramnios on the prenatal maternal ultrasonographic scan (Filston & Shorter, 2000; Harmon & Coran, 1998; Stringer et al., 1995). The failure to identify the fetal stomach and/or the presence of a dilated proximal pouch is strongly suggestive of EA. If this anomaly is suspected, the presence of associated anomalies should be investigated. After birth, the pooling of secretions in the upper pouch or inability to tolerate oral feeding with coughing and choking is suspicious. After effective oral/pharyngeal suctioning, the infant appears normal until he or she is fed again. If an associated

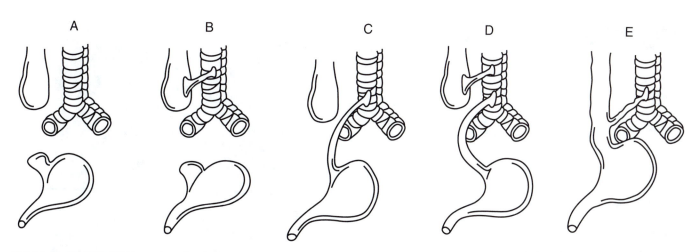

Type A, Isolated EA (3.7%–7%). Almost always found with a long gap between the proximal and distal pouches. Type B, EA with proximal TEF (0.8%). The proximal esophageal pouch is usually short because of tethering by the fistula to the trachea. This results in a long esophageal gap. Type C, EA with distal TEF (86%). This combination is the most common presentation of the anomaly. The upper esophagus usually ends blindly between the seventh cervical and fifth thoracic vertebra. There is usually a short esophageal gap. The upper pouch is larger then the distal esophageal segment because of dilation and hypertrophy, which occur by efforts of the fetus to swallow amniotic fluid. There may be muscular continuity between the esophageal pouches. The distal esophagus, which has its origins from trachea, connects by way of the fistula to a membranous portion of the lower trachea. Type D, EA with proximal and distal TEF (0.7%–6%). Type E, Isolated TEF (4.4%–7%). Not an esophageal atresia but included in the grouping. The continuity of the esophagus is intact. One or multiple fistulas may occur between the esophagus and trachea at any level from the carina to the cricoid but usually occur around the lower cervical to upper thoracic area. The fistula inserts higher on the trachea than on the esophagus. The defect is often referred to as an H-type fistula.

Figure 15-1 Classification of esophageal atresia (EA)/tracheoesophageal fistula (TEF).
From Filston, H. C. & Shorter, N. A. (2000). Esophageal atresia and tracheoesophageal fistula. In K. W. Ashcraft, J. P. Murphy, R. J. Sharp, D. J. Sigalet, & C. L. Snyder (Eds.), *Pediatric surgery* (3rd ed., pp. 438–369). Philadelphia: W.B. Saunders Company.

distal TEF is present, the infant may have a distended abdomen from air being forced through the fistula into the stomach.

TEF, without the presence of EA, may not be recognized for several months (Andrassy et al., 1980; Crabbe, Kiely, Drake, & Spitz, 1996). The severity of respiratory symptoms depends on the size and the number of fistulas present. Abdominal distention, especially after feedings, is common. Often, these infants are discharged home. Only after multiple visits to the primary health provider's office for choking episodes is aspiration resulting from a TEF suspected.

Diagnosis

A quick diagnostic test to evaluate for EA/TEF is to attempt to pass a No. 10 to 12 French feeding/Replogle tube down the esophagus. A smaller tube is too flexible and folds on itself. If resistance is met when the tube is advanced, usually at about 10 to 12 cm, a radiographic film should be obtained with the tube in position. The presence of EA/TEF can be confirmed with a simple chest/abdominal radiographic film (Myers & Beasley, 1991; Raffensperger, 1990). The tip of the feeding tube indicates the length of the proximal pouch. The presence of air in the stomach indicates a distal TEF. Air in the stomach but not in the small intestine is suggestive of associ-

ated duodenal atresia. A gasless stomach is diagnostic of pure EA (Fig. 15-2), although a distal fistula so small as to not allow the passage of air may rarely be present. This initial radiographic film also reveals information about the child's pulmonary status, cardiac size and contour, and possibly vertebral anomalies.

A contrast study of the upper pouch may be obtained to evaluate whether a proximal fistula is present. With care to avoid aspiration, 0.5 cc of oral contrast is placed in the upper pouch with a small feeding tube (Harmon & Coran, 1998). Under fluoroscopic guidance, this may accurately locate the level of the pouch and the presence of a fistula. Contrast in the trachea suggests a proximal TEF, although this may also indicate spillover from the pouch. Because of the risk of aspiration during this test, bronchoscopy can be performed at the time of esophageal repair and replaces the need for these upper pouch studies (Harmon & Coran) (Fig. 15-3).

The isolated TEF may be diagnosed with a limited upper gastrointestinal study or esophagram. A small nasogastric tube is passed into the distal esophagus and contrast media is slowly injected while the tube is gradually withdrawn. The esophagram may show abnormal peristalsis. Failure to identify a fistula radiologically indicates the need for bronchoscopy/esophagoscopy for diagnosis (Andrassy et al., 1980).

Table 15-1	Common Associated Anomalies
Cardiac	
ASD	
VSD	
Tetralogy of Fallot	
Truncus arteriosus	
PDA	
Coarctation of the aorta	
Arch anomalies	
Vascular ring	
Gastrointestinal	
Anorectal (imperforate anus/cloaca)	
Duodenal (atresia/stenosis)	
Pyloric (atresia/stenosis)	
Esophagus (congenital stenosis)	
Hirschsprung's disease	
Others	
Urinary Tract	
Renal defects	
Hypospadias	
Orthopedic	
Vertebral	
Limb	
Chromosomal	
Trisomy 21	
Trisomy 18	

Abbreviations: ASD, atrial septal defect; PDA, patent ductus arteriosus; VSD, ventricular septal defect.

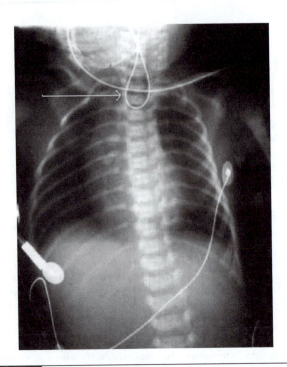

Figure 15-2 Radiographic film of infant with pure esophageal atresia.

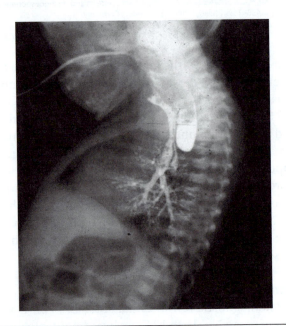

Figure 15-3 Note spillover of contrast from upper pouch study outlining bronchial tree.

Associated anomalies can be excluded with echocardiography, renal ultrasonography, and radiographic films/ultrasonography of the spine. Because repair of the esophagus is usually performed through a right thoracotomy, the side of the aortic arch must be identified. Approximately 5% of children have an aberrant right aortic arch, which may require the surgeon to approach the esophagus from a left thoracotomy in order to facilitate exposure during the repair (Harrison, Hanson, Mahour, Takahashi, & Weitzman, 1977).

Preoperative Management

If the diagnosis of EA/TEF is suspected, the infant should be transferred to a tertiary care center where pediatric surgeons are available. Once EA/TEF is diagnosed, the goals of preoperative care include prevention of aspiration pneumonia, provision of respiratory support, and evaluation of associated anomalies. Broad-spectrum antibiotics covering respiratory flora should be started as soon as possible. If respiratory support is needed, the team member with

the most experience should intubate the infant. Bag/mask ventilation should be avoided because it may cause massive abdominal distention if a TEF is large.

Infants with EA awaiting primary repair must have their proximal esophageal pouch drained with a small single- or double-lumen tube on continuous or intermittent low suction (Fig. 15-4). The patency of the suc-

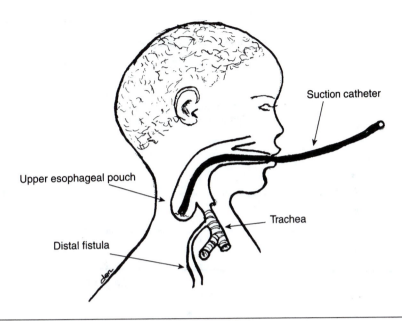

Figure 15-4 Infant with esophageal atresia and distal tracheoesophageal fistula.

tion catheter should be frequently assessed. These infants do better when placed prone or on their sides with the head of the bed slightly elevated. The esophageal pouch has a 1–2 mL capacity, and malfunction of the drainage tube can lead to aspiration, desaturation, and bradycardia. Some surgeons advocate irrigating these tubes with 0.5 mL sterile normal saline every 2 hours, although this may increase the risk of aspiration (Roy, 1991).

A decision must be made whether any surgery is indicated for associated anomalies before the repair of the esophagus. The severity of a cardiac anomaly may supersede the need to repair the esophagus (Filston & Shorter, 2000). A definitive repair of the esophagus may be deferred in the severely ill infant who requires ventilatory support (Raffensperger, 1990). Since 1982, physiologic status has been used as the sole basis for repair without regard to weight, gestation, or pulmonary condition (Randolph et al., 1989).

A gastrostomy tube may be placed at the time of cardiac repair to decompress the stomach. The infant with an associated imperforate anus or intestinal atresia will need to have a repair or stoma within the first day of life. If clinically stable, this surgery can be paired with the esophageal repair (Raffensperger, 1990).

Operative Repair

Repair of EA or EA/TEF can fall into three scenarios: primary repair, delayed repair, and staged repair (Figs. 15-5 and 15-6). Primary repair includes the ability to get the two ends of the esophagus together and ligate and divide any fistula in one surgical procedure. Preservation of na-

tive esophageal tissue is superior to anything used to replace it. If a long gap exists between the two segments of the esophagus, then primary repair may not be possible. Assessing gap length between the esophageal ends provides easily measurable criteria that can be used to predict long-term outcome (Brown & Tam, 1996). Several techniques have been used to stretch both blind ends of the esophagus to gain length. Some surgeons favor frequent stretching of the proximal esophageal pouch at the bedside with a bougie or a similar catheter to gain length for closure (Raffensperger, 1990). Elongation of the proximal pouch occurs over several months. Others have developed a technique that consists of multistaged extrathoracic elongation of the proximal esophagus (Kimura et al., 2001). With this technique, traction sutures anchor the end of the proximal esophagus that is brought out as a stoma to the anterior chest wall. In approximately 2 months, the child returns to the operating room where the stoma is taken down and placed in a lower position on the chest. This process is continued until there is adequate length for anastomosis of the esophageal ends. The distal pouch may also be stretched in a retrograde manner through the gastrostomy, provided that a TEF is not present. Others believe that the pouch gains length through growth and does not need stretching (Beasley, 1991b). Infants usually remain in the hospital while awaiting the delayed repair.

Depending on his or her clinical condition, the infant may wait several weeks to months before repair is attempted. During this time, he or she is managed on gastrostomy feedings and suction drainage of the upper

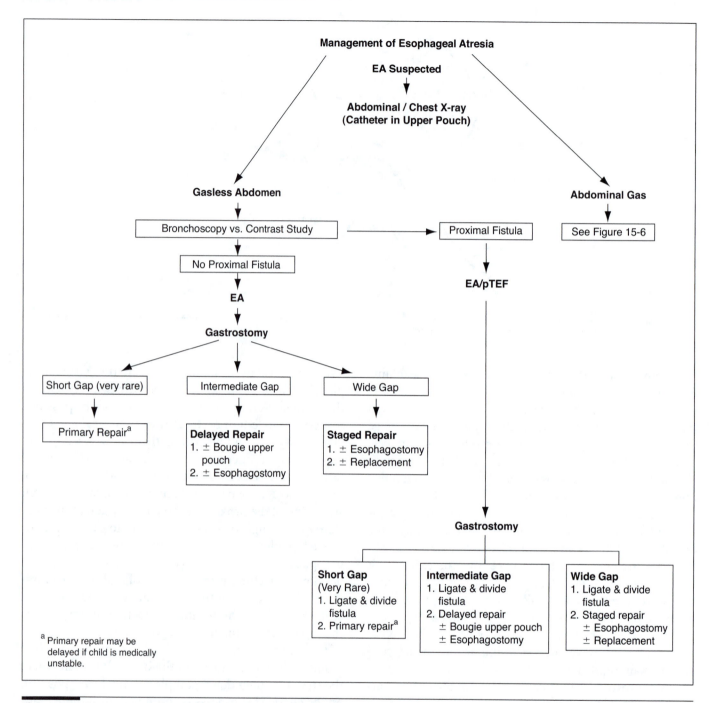

Figure 15-5 Management of esophageal atresia: gasless abdomen. EA: esophageal atresia. pTEF: proximal tracheoesophageal fistula.

pouch to prevent aspiration of secretions. Few references to home care of these infants have been found in literature; however, in selected situations, this can be a safe and successful option (Aziz, Schiller, Gerstle, Ein, & Langer, 2003; Hollands, Lankau, & Burnweit, 2000). Improved survival is found in the poor-risk infant if the esophageal repair is delayed, and delaying primary repair has been found to have a better outcome than a staged repair (Raffensperger, 1990).

Although now seldom performed, some surgeons create an esophagostomy to drain the proximal pouch while awaiting delayed repair. Indications for cervical esophagostomy include little or no distal esophagus, ultralong gap between the pouches, life-threatening anastomotic complications, and long gap without appropriate facility for prolonged upper pouch care (Myers, Beasley, & Auldist, 1991b). An esophagostomy allows the infant to be discharged home. However, creation of an esophagostomy may sacrifice much-

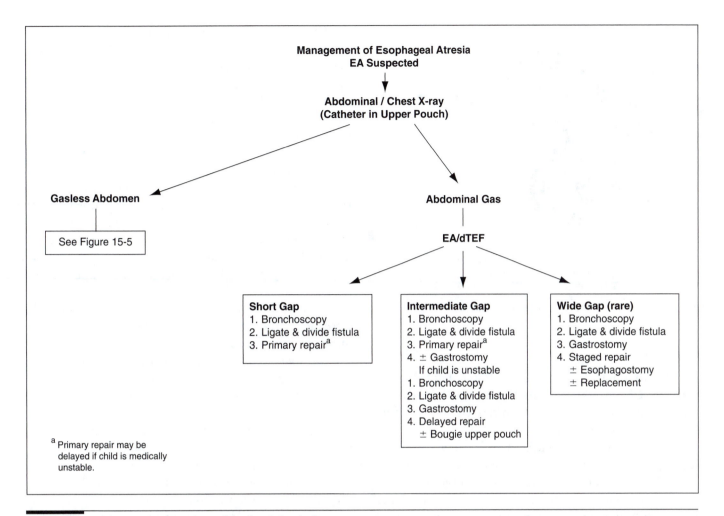

Figure 15-6 Management of esophageal fistula: abdominal gas.
EA, esophageal atresia; dTEF, distal tracheoesophageal fistula.

needed esophageal length and commit the surgeon to performing an esophageal substitution (Spitz, 1995).

Primary repair is the preferred operative plan (Fig. 15-7). Ideally, the gap between the pouches should be no wider then two to three vertebral bodies to avoid postoperative tension on the anastomosis (Beasley, 1991b; Raffensperger, 1990). Traditionally, this repair has been accomplished by means of a posterolateral thoracotomy on the side opposite the aortic arch (Harrison et al., 1977). The tips of the pouches are excised and brought together by end-to-end (Beasley & Auldist, 1991) or end-to-side anastomosis (Poenaru, Laberge, Neilson, Nguyen, & Guttman, 1991; Touloukian & Seashore, 2004). The anastomosis may be difficult because the proximal pouch may be two to four times larger in diameter then the distal pouch. The esophagus, having no serosal lining, does not hold sutures well. If a considerable gap is present between the two pouches, a circular myotomy may be performed on the proximal pouch to gain esophageal length (Raffensperger). A chest tube or soft drain is usually placed

in the retropleural space next to the anastomosis to allow any drainage from the surgical site to be recognized. Some surgeons favor not leaving a drain at the site and identify anastomotic complications by clinical deterioration and radiologic changes. In one review, only 47% of patients with anastomotic complications were noted to have drainage from the surgical drains. Of these, 80% required the placement of additional drains (McCallion, Hannon, & Boston, 1992). The success of the anastomosis depends on the gentle handling of tissue, the blood supply, and lack of tension on the suture line rather than any particular technique. A gastrostomy tube is occasionally placed to assist with feedings and/or decompression, although the trend is to avoid gastrostomies whenever possible (Santos, Thompson, Johnson, & Foker, 1983; Shaul, Schwartz, Marr, & Tyson, 1989). If it is impossible to bring the two ends of the esophagus together, the infant undergoes a staged repair.

The first successful thoracoscopic repair of EA was performed in 1998 as an effort to avoid morbidity asso-

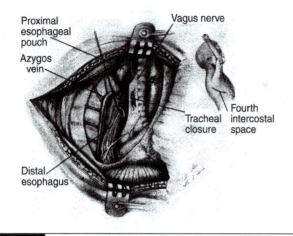

Figure 15-7 Operative approach for exposure of tracheoesophageal fistula and repair of esophageal atresia.

Reprinted with permission. Randolph, J. G. (1986). Esophageal atresia and congenital stenosis. In K. J. Welch, J. G. Randolph, M. M. Ravitch, J. A. O'Neill, Jr., & M. I. Rowe (Eds.), *Pediatric surgery* (4th ed., pp. 682–696). New York: Year Book Medical.

ciated with thoracotomy in infants (Rothenberg, Patrick, Bealer, & Chang, 2001; Holcomb et al., 2005). In the past few years, the technique has been refined and is widely performed with favorable results.

The infant with isolated EA has placement of a feeding gastrostomy. Usually, the ends of the pouches are too far apart to be brought together safely. Surgery to anastomose the pouches is delayed, with the hope of gaining length with time, or is planned for eventual esophageal replacement. Staged repair is reserved for those infants with severe respiratory distress, very high proximal pouches, or severe associated anomalies (Raffensperger, 1990; Randolph et al., 1989).

The operative repair of an isolated TEF involves division of the fistula and repair of the esophageal and tracheal defects. Most of these fistulas are above or at the level of the clavicle and can be reached by the cervical approach (Raffensperger, 1990).

Postoperative Management

Care of the infant after repair of EA/TEF includes effective pain management, evaluation, and support of all organ systems, with focus on the respiratory and gastrointestinal systems, and care of surgical wounds and drains.

Pain Management: The level of the infant's pain is assessed by means of physiologic indicators. The infant may be kept on continuous intravenous analgesics or intermittent boluses. In addition to effective pain relief, pain control is important as the infant risks disruption of the anastomosis due to excessive movement and crying from inadequate pain relief.

Respiratory: The healthy infant who has undergone primary repair of an EA/TEF, isolated TEF, or pure EA may be extubated soon after surgery, whereas a smaller, ill infant may require prolonged ventilation. Frequent suctioning of the pharynx is needed until the infant is able to swallow his or her own saliva. The suction catheter is often measured from the upper dental ridge to the anastomosis by the surgeon and is marked. An approximate measure can be taken from the tip of the nose to the earlobe. Deep suctioning should be avoided to prevent disruption of the anastomosis (Beasley & Auldist, 1991; Raffensperger, 1990). The infant should be positioned to reduce strain on the esophageal anastomosis; if the infant is placed supine, care must be taken to prevent extension of the neck (Raffensperger). Post-operatively, gentle chest physiotherapy is provided three to four times daily. Infants with isolated TEF repairs have considerable dissection of the trachea and may be hoarse and stridorous during the postoperative period.

Gastrointestinal: Traditionally, a contrast esophagram is obtained 5 to 10 days after repair to assess for anastomotic leaks (Raffensperger, 1990; Santos et al., 1983). If no leak is demonstrated on radiologic examination, oral feedings are initiated. The chest drains are removed after the infant begins oral feedings without signs of anastomotic leak. Signs indicative of leak include fluid from chest drains resembling saliva or formula/breast milk, respiratory distress, and sepsis. Some surgeons forego the contrast esophagram and feed the infants orally as early as the third day after surgery (Brown, Eyres, & Myers, 1991). Others do not place drains or chest tubes at the time of repair (McCallion et al., 1992). Those infants are watched for respiratory distress and sepsis before being fed.

If a gastrostomy tube is present, feedings are started as soon as bowel function returns. Because of the possibility of gastric reflux, many elect to delay feeds until the anastomosis is well healed in order to protect the surgical site (Raffensperger, 1990). A jejunal tube may be passed through the gastrostomy for feeding the gut downstream. Patency of enteral tubes should be maintained by irrigating them with 1 to 2 mL of sterile normal saline every 3 to 4 hours or per the surgeons' preference. Delay in enteral feedings necessitates the administration of parenteral nutrition. Infants with isolated TEF repair can start oral feeding 4 to 7 days after surgical repair (Raffensperger).

Esophagostomies: Infants that have undergone an esophagostomy need frequent assessment of the patency of the stoma. If the esophagostomy becomes occluded, the infant is at risk of aspiration pneumonia and respiratory compromise. These children may begin gastrostomy feedings as soon as bowel function returns, provided that no surgery has been performed on the distal pouch and no fistula ligation has been performed. Oral sham feedings (feedings given when there is esophageal discontinuity) should be started as soon as the esophagostomy has healed, usually within a few days. Although messy because the feedings come out the esophagostomy, sham feedings enable the infant to develop and maintain oral skills, such as sucking and swallowing. The skills of an enterostomal therapist in fitting a pouch over the stoma are invaluable. The infant who is not sham fed may refuse oral feeding once the esophageal repair is completed.

Dressings/Tube Care: In general, surgical dressings over incisional sites are removed within 24 hours. Wounds are kept clean and dry. Chest tubes should be well secured and dressed. The surgeon should be notified of leakage at the incision or around chest tube insertion sites because this may indicate disruption or leakage at the anastomosis. The patency of the chest tube should be checked, and the physician should be informed if blockage is suspected. The gastrostomy tube should be dressed and secured well. Because these infants may have very small stomachs, the maximum capacity in the reservoir balloon should be clarified with the surgeon if this type of device has been placed. The reservoir balloon should be checked every 4 to 5 days, or per institutional protocol.

Complications

The most common and dangerous early postoperative complication after repair of EA/TEF is anastomotic leak (Harmon & Coran, 1998; Touloukian & Seashore, 2004). Small leaks often close spontaneously. Larger leaks, especially those occurring within the first few days after repair, may necessitate re-exploration. The area of anastomosis may need to be resutured. However, if complete disruption occurs at the anastomotic site, the proximal esophagus may need to be brought out as an esophagostomy. Some surgeons have reported good results in saving the native esophagus by resuturing the primary repair with or without a pleural patch (Chavin, Field, Chandler, Tagge, & Otherson, 1996). Complications of a leak may include sepsis, mediastinitis, and recurrent fistulas.

Recurrent TEFs may not be recognized for months or years. Diagnosis is made by contrast esophagram or bronchoscopy. Surgical repair is necessary. There have been reports on the successful use of fibrin glue, a biologic product, injected into the fistula through a bronchoscope as an alternate to tying and dividing the fistula (Gutierrez et al., 1994).

Esophageal anastomotic strictures occur frequently. They primarily cause difficulty in swallowing and may lead to choking and respiratory difficulty. Diagnosis is made by barium swallow or esophagoscopy (Raffensperger, 1990). The treatment is esophageal dilation. Opinion varies regarding whether children need routine dilation after repair. Some surgeons elect to perform dilation in infants as early as 2 weeks after surgery, especially if the anastomosis was performed under tension (Raffensperger; Santos et al., 1983). These dilations may continue monthly for some time. Others may follow the progress of their patients with scheduled esophagrams.

GER is a frequent occurrence in children with EA/TEF repair. It is exacerbated by poor peristaltic clearance of the esophagus caused by intrinsic motor dysfunction (Jolly et al., 1980; Tovar et al., 1995). The incidence of GER is documented in over 50% of these patients (Holder, 1993; Wheatley, Coran, & Wesley, 1993). Anastomotic tension may cause shortening of the intraabdominal esophagus, deform the gastroesophageal junction, and cause reflux. Treatment, medical or surgical, is generally the same as for GER not associated with EA/TEF. Many surgeons favor not doing a fundoplication because of the poor pumping action of the esophagus (Curci & Dibbins, 1988; Wheatley et al.); however, GER may be severe enough to require fundoplication in 6% to 45% of patients (Snyder et al., 1997). A partial wrap fundoplication (Thal/Toupet) may be performed or the reflux managed through use of jejunal rather then gastric feedings. Esophageal mucosal pathology as a result of reflux is a concern for children with a history of EA. In one report of long-term follow-up, esophageal metaplasia has been reported in 18% of children who have a history of EA (Schalamon, Lindahl, Saarikoski, & Rintala, 2003). In this study, the patient's symptoms had poor correlation with the histologic findings. Most esophageal pathology was identified before the age of 3 years. Children with repeated normal biopsy findings on upper endoscopy within 2 years after repair are unlikely to progress to having histologic changes from esophagitis. It is suggested that those with mild esophagitis be followed up with upper endoscopy and biopsy until 6 years of age. Another study showed the declining incidence of GER as the child matured; GER was found in one fourth of these children followed up into the late teen and early adult years (Little et al., 2003).

Children with esophagostomies need frequent evaluation for esophagostomy stenosis or obstruction of the tract that may lead to respiratory distress. The child may need gentle dilatation of the esophagostomy tract on a daily or twice-daily basis by the caregiver. Obstruction of the tract may require removal of a foreign body. Skin around the esophagostomy may become macerated, preventing the fit of an appliance device over the site in infants who sham feed.

Tracheal obstruction caused by tracheomalacia and/or pressure of the innominate artery or aorta is not uncommon. Tracheomalacia affects 10% to 20% of children after repair of EA (Harmon & Coran, 1998). These infants are predisposed to anterior-posterior collapse of the trachea. The onset occurs at approximately 2 to 3 months of age and resolves within 1 to 2 years as the cartilage becomes firmer. Those with severe obstruction may exhibit "dying" (apneic) spells (Filler & Forte, 1998). These spells are most common during or immediately after eating and are thought to be caused by obstruction of the trachea by the food-filled esophagus. Surgical correction by aortopexy is reserved for children with life-threatening attacks.

At various stages throughout their management, children with EA/TEF may present a nutritional challenge. Severely ill infants require total parenteral nutrition by means of a central venous catheter. Others may be dependent on gastrostomy or jejunostomy feeds. Weight gain should be carefully monitored in all infants. The transition to oral feedings may be slow and difficult for some infants, who may expend excessive energy in the effort to feed. Some infants with EA/TEF require a higher caloric intake to grow well. Once table foods are introduced, children should be encouraged to eat slowly and wash their food down with substantial liquid. Lifelong esophageal dysmotility is present in many of these children (Tomaselli et al., 2003). Food debris is the most common cause of foreign body obstruction in the esophagus (Schier, Kom, & Michel, 2001; Zigman & Yazbeck, 2002). Parents should be advised to cut table foods into small pieces and to avoid hot dogs, ends of French fries, and other sharp foods. All children should adhere to GER precautions. Many times, consultation with a speech or occupational therapist is indicated if the infant shows difficulty in coordinating sucking and swallowing. Nutritional management should be continued on an outpatient basis, especially with those infants who are waiting for delayed or staged repair.

Discharge Criteria

Discharge planning is initiated at the time of the infant's arrival at the hospital but facilitated when the surgical plan has been established. Discharge criteria include an extensive list of potential needs (Table 15-2). The child's primary caregiver should begin to learn the care of the child as early as possible. The home environment should be assessed to identify specific infant and caregiver needs. Home nursing visits should be arranged after dis-

Table 15-2 Discharge Criteria
• CPR training
• Oxygen
• Pulse oximeter
• Cardiac monitor
• Apnea monitor
• Suction machine and accessories
• Enteral pump and accessories
• IV infusion pump and accessories
• Enteral formula
• Total parenteral nutrition
• Medications
• Gastrostomy/jejunostomy supplies
• Home nursing
• Respite care
• Resource phone numbers
• Referral to support groups

charge to assess growth and respiratory progress of the infant.

Infants with primary repair may be discharged within 2 weeks of surgery. Infants who require staged repair may be sent home between surgical procedures (Aziz et al., 2003; Hollands et al., 2000). Criteria for discharge include tolerating feedings and appropriate weight gain. The plan for discharge includes scheduled appointments, radiologic tests, scheduled dilatations, and future surgical procedures. Chronically ill children are at risk for developmental delay, and all attempts should be made to frequently assess skills and milestones.

Long-Term Evaluation

Limited data are available regarding long-term status of children who have undergone EA repair. The available data have primarily focused on complications such as esophageal motility, pulmonary function (Spitz, 1996), and GER. Concern for esophageal mucosal changes because of GER necessitates long-term surveillance by way of upper endoscopy with biopsy (Schalamon et al., 2003). In 1984, a parent support group for children with EA was established in Germany; it soon became the largest of its kind worldwide (Schier et al., 2001). A report of a study from this group summarized the long-term experience of the parents and children with EA, rather than the surgeons. Results of a comprehensive questionnaire reveal a fascinating insight into the day-to-day life of these children. Topics covered in the questionnaire include associated anomalies, types of surgeries, complications of surgeries, methods of esophageal pouch stretching, feeding difficulties, dietary restrictions, management of reflux, frequency of pulmonary infections, and performance in school and social activities. These parents stressed the importance of a support group in the exchange of information on current treatment, as well as monitoring the progress of their children. Despite life-long complications, children with EA/TEF generally have good long-term quality of life.

Laryngotracheoesophageal Cleft

A rare anomaly, laryngotracheoesophageal cleft is related to and may be associated with EA/TEF. With this defect, closure of the tracheoesophageal septum is completely lacking. A cleft exists in the midline, between the posterior aspect of the trachea/larynx and the anterior portion of the esophagus. In its more severe presentations, it is highly lethal (Ryan, Muehrcke, Doody, Kim, & Donahoe, 1991). Repairs are tenuous and tracheostomy is left in place for months, sometimes years.

Congenital Esophageal Stenosis

Rossi first described isolated congenital esophageal stenosis in 1826 (Murphy, Yazbeck, & Russo, 1995). In 1987, Nihoul-Fekete et al., defined the entity as "... an intrinsic stenosis of the esophagus present although not necessarily symptomatic at birth, which is caused by congenital malformation of the esophageal wall architecture" (Murphy et al.). Diagnosis includes evaluation with a contrast esophagram and esophagoscopy. The stenotic area is usually short and amenable to repeated dilations. Resection is the best treatment for severe cases in which there is circumferential involvement of the esophagus (Murphy et al.; Ohkawa, Takahashi, Hoshino, & Sato, 1975).

■ Acquired Defects

Corrosive Injury to the Esophagus

Children are by nature curious creatures and do not hesitate to put various substances in their mouths. Parental negligence, ignorance, or child abuse are also potential causes of ingestion (Raffensperger, 1990). In the older child, suicidal intent must be considered. A high degree of family stress, such as the loss of a family member, physical illness, or mental illness, is associated with corrosive ingestion (Raffensperger).

Corrosive substances come in various liquid, gel, and crystal forms. Liquids tend to be gulped rapidly by children and primarily cause injury to the mouth, hy-

popharynx, esophagus, stomach, and occasionally the small intestine. Little evidence of oral injury may exist because the substance may have been swallowed too rapidly. Solid substances tend to stick to the oral mucosa and are spit out by the child as they begin to cause pain. These agents primarily cause injury to oral structures and surrounding skin. However, they may cause damage to the esophagus as well (Shikowitz, Levy, Villano, Graver, & Pochaczevsky, 1996). Alkaline chemicals are the most damaging. They cause liquefaction necrosis of the esophagus, which can involve mucosa, submucosa, and muscular wall (Shikowitz et al.). Liquefaction continues until dilution is sufficient to alter the caustic agent to a near neutral pH. Acid injuries most often involve the antrum of the stomach.

The effect of caustic injury depends on the extent of damage to the wall of the esophagus (Fig. 15-8). The depth of injury predicts the amount of stricture formation. Mucosal erythema alone is usually without significant sequelae. Full-thickness injury may lead to perforation of the esophagus, mediastinitis, and injury to mediastinal structures.

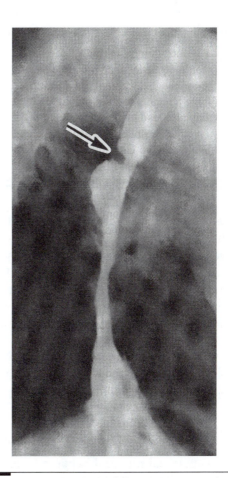

Figure 15-8 Injury to esophagus following ingestion of oven cleaner.

Clinical Presentation

Ingestion of a caustic substance should be suspected if the child is found drooling and refusing foods. The child may have a hoarse cry or respiratory distress (Millar & Cywes, 1998; Raffensperger, 1990).

Diagnosis

Diagnosis and treatment are contingent on identification of the ingested substance. Caregivers are encouraged to bring the container of the suspected substance to the hospital with the child. The child remains NPO during the evaluation phase. The oral cavity should be carefully examined under strong lighting, and suction equipment should be available. The amount of damage to the oral mucosa does not predict the extent of injury to the esophagus. Injury to the esophagus after ingestion is immediate. What passes into the stomach is most often in such a dose that it is buffered with gastric acid to neutrality, thereby halting further injury.

With the exception of household bleach, a mild irritant that does not require extensive evaluation (Anderson, Rouse, & Randolph, 1990), ingestion of most substances, particularly those containing either sodium or potassium hydroxide, calls for endoscopic evaluation. Esophagoscopy to evaluate the extent of injury should be carried out within 24 hours of ingestion.

Treatment

Initial treatment involves supportive care with intravenous fluids before determination of the extent of injury. Vomiting should not be induced, because this returns the substance to the esophagus, where it can do further damage. Ingestion of large amounts of fluid should also be avoided because this may also lead to vomiting.

Admission to the hospital is based on the child's clinical condition. An intensive care unit admission should be arranged for the child who has had a massive ingestion of an alkaline substance. Radiologic studies of the chest and neck help determine extent of tracheal edema, mediastinal widening, and signs of perforation. Esophagoscopy is usually performed with the child under general anesthesia. The rigid esophagoscope is passed up to but not through the most proximal observed injury. Flexible endoscopy has the added advantage of allowing the stomach and duodenum to be evaluated (Anderson, Rouse, et al., 1990).

Depth of injury is graded as first, second, and third degree as with skin burns. First-degree injury is characterized by superficial mucosal hyperemia, edema, and sloughing. Second-degree injury involves transmucosal injury; the entire wall of the esophagus has exudate, and ulceration is present. The injury extends into muscle. Third-degree injury involves erosion through the esophagus into the periesophageal tissues, including the mediastinum, or perforation into the pleural or peritoneal cavities (Raffensperger, 1990).

Linear burns are of less clinical significance than circumferential burns, which cause stricture. Tracheostomy placement is indicated for extensive injuries that cause increasing stridor (Raffensperger, 1990). Shock and signs of peritonitis are indicative of necrosis and possible stomach perforation. Early esophageal perforation indicates almost total destruction of the esophagus. In this case, an esophagostomy and gastrostomy should be placed. Plans should begin for eventual esophageal substitution. Some surgeons advocate immediate esophagectomy and gastrectomy in the event of massive ingestion to prevent liquefaction necrosis of the mediastinal structures. Minimally invasive esophagectomy with a combined thoracoscopic and laparoscopic approach is being performed in many institutions and has been associated with a decreased hospital stay and a more rapid return to normal activities (Nwomeh, Luketich, & Kane, 2004).

The first 4 days after the ingestion constitute the acute inflammatory phase. Children with first-degree injuries are given fluids and allowed to resume a regular diet within 24 to 48 hours (Anderson, Rouse, et al., 1990). These children do not stricture. The subacute phase lasts up to 15 days. At the end of this phase, the necrotic tissue sloughs and leaves a denuded ulcerated surface. Swelling decreases, and swallowing may return to normal function. The child may be re-endoscoped during the subacute phase to evaluate extent of injury and healing. The third phase takes place during the 3rd to 4th weeks following ingestion; the inflammatory reaction subsides and tissue contraction begins. Normal tissue is replaced by dense fibrous scar tissue. Re-epithelialization is usually complete by the sixth week (Shikowitz et al., 1996).

Steroid therapy to decrease inflammatory response and thus prevent stricture formation has been in use since the 1950s. Dexamethasone, 0.3 mg/kg/day in four divided doses, is begun within the first 2 days of injury (Raffensperger, 1990). Steroids are continued until there is evidence that the mucosa has healed. More recent information has strongly suggested that the use of steroids in the treatment of esophageal injury is ineffective (Anderson, Rouse, et al., 1990; Millar & Cywes, 1998; Shikowitz et al., 1996). Antibiotics are usually begun immediately after the injury to prevent infection and are continued while the child is receiving steroids.

Some surgeons advocate early esophageal dilatation before strictures develop. Others may use esophageal stents or nasogastric tubes to prevent stricture formation. If evidence of stricture formation is present, a gastrostomy may be placed to assist with feedings, as well as retrograde dilatations (Millar & Cywes, 1998).

Complications

Complications can be divided into three phases (Shikowitz et al., 1996). The acute phase occurs during the first 72 hours. This is when there is a high risk of circulatory collapse and pulmonary necrosis secondary to aspiration. The latent phase occurs during the first and second week, when infection, perforation, and abscess can occur. The third phase, or delayed complications, result when esophageal stricture occurs. Strictures are the most common sequela of corrosive injury to the esophagus. These are treated with scheduled dilations and in severe cases may require resection. In severe cases of esophageal stricture, esophageal replacement may be indicated. Severe damage to the hypopharynx, larynx, and cervical esophagus make eventual esophageal substitution challenging (Raffensperger, 1990; Shikowitz et al.).

Other, more serious, complications include TEF and aortoesophageal fistula resulting from erosion and damage to the mediastinal structures (Millar & Cywes, 1998).

Follow-Up Care

In cases of mild damage to the esophagus, the child may be discharged from the hospital if he or she is asymptomatic and has a normal esophagram. The child should be closely followed up clinically and re-evaluated with an esophagram as needed.

Suicide attempt should be included in the differential diagnosis in the older child who has ingested a large quantity of caustic substance. After stabilization of the child's condition, psychiatric evaluation and intervention share an equal role in the ongoing medical management. Even those who have not made a suicide attempt may need such intervention because injuries caused by ingestion may adversely affect the emotional outcome as well as physical well-being of the child.

Esophageal Stricture

Acquired esophageal strictures in childhood are most likely a result of reflux esophagitis, corrosive injury, or anastomotic scarring (Allmendinger et al., 1996). The scarring across an anastomosis is made worse by the presence of GER. The management of this situation includes treatment of the stricture and the identification, correction, and prevention of reflux.

Clinical Presentation

Presenting signs and symptoms of stricture include drooling, inability to swallow saliva or fluids, ability to take liquids but not solids, and regurgitation of undigested food. Stricture should be suspected if the preceding signs are accompanied by a positive history of esophageal surgery, injury, or reflux disease.

Diagnosis

The diagnosis is established with an esophagram (Holder, 1993). Esophagoscopy is used to evaluate the character and length of stricture, the ability to dilate the defect, and the condition of the mucosa (Miller & Cywes, 1998). Passing a barium-filled Penrose tube down the esophagus at the time of esophagoscopy yields an accurate fluoroscopic view of the length and character of the stricture (K.D. Anderson, personal communication, June 1998).

Treatment

Universal treatment of esophageal strictures involves dilation with various types of dilators. Sedation for dilation varies but may include oral and intravenous sedation or general anesthesia. Methods of dilation vary among surgeons. Antegrade methods of dilation include the passing of rubber/silicone or balloon dilators through the mouth. Proponents of balloon dilation report that it produces a uniform radial force, causing decreased trauma on the esophagus than bougie dilators that exert a shearing axial force (Allmendinger et al., 1996; Ashcraft, 1993). Retrograde dilation with Tucker dilators through an existing gastrostomy is considered one of the safest methods of dilating. The disadvantage of retrograde dilation is that a guide string is left in the esophagus between dilations. This string, which exits the mouth or nostril, often causes much distress to the older child. Potential complications of dilation include perforation and septicemia. After routine dilation, the child is awakened, allowed to drink, and discharged home. Recent description of placement of a self-expanding biocompatible stent across the strictured area after dilation shows promising results in preventing further stenosis (Broto, Asensio, & Vernet, 2003).

The number of dilations needed before abandoning the esophagus and committing to the replacement of the organ varies among surgeons. Short strictures may be treatable by resection with end-to-end esophageal anastomosis, or stricturotomy (Anderson, Acosta, Meyer, & Sherman, 2002). The child's quality of life should be considered in the evaluation of the response to dilations. Frequency of dilations depends on the child's clinical condition. The child who is able to take modified oral feedings and goes months between dilations may not need to have the esophagus replaced. In contrast, the child who is fed by gastrostomy and needs to undergo dilation every few weeks because of the inability to swallow oral secretions should have the esophagus replaced in an effort to normalize life as much as possible. The timing of substitution depends on failure of dilation as a primary method of treatment (Pederson, Klein, & Andrews, 1996).

Follow-Up

Subsequent dilations are performed at scheduled intervals as required by the patient's symptoms. Esophagrams may not be indicated if the esophagus is routinely visualized during dilation. Occasionally, the stricture persists radiographically, but the child can compensate by more forceful swallowing and thorough mastication of food.

Foreign Body in the Esophagus

Congenital or acquired esophageal strictures may halt the passage of an object that may have otherwise been swallowed without difficulty. Common culprits are fibrous foods, such as meats and stringy vegetables; foods with sharp edges, such as french fries and corn chips; and bulky foods, such as breads and tortillas. In children with normal esophageal anatomy, the areas of physiologic narrowing, such as the cricopharyngeus, aortic arch, and cardioesophageal sphincter, are often the sites where objects lodge. In this case, the foreign body is usually something in the child's immediate environment, such as a small toy, coin, safety pin, or other sharp item (Gans & Austin, 1993). Swallowed batteries from toys or calculators are problematic because they may cause corrosive injury as well.

Clinical Presentation

The child may be initially seen with dysphagia, drooling, choking, or pain. If the swallowed object is large, coughing and respiratory distress may be present as the object distends the esophagus and compresses the trachea. Oftentimes, the caregiver may have witnessed the ingestion or has evidence of the ingestion from other items found in the environment. Aspiration pneumonia, fever, cough, signs of perforation, or TEF may develop if the presence of a foreign body has been missed or neglected (Gans & Austin, 1993).

Diagnosis

Diagnostic tests include plain films of the chest and neck. If the item is radiopaque, the size and location of the object will be evident. If the object is difficult to visualize, a barium swallow may be needed (Raffensperger, 1990).

Treatment

Removal of foreign bodies is best accomplished with the child under general anesthesia. Endotracheal intubation is used to prevent respiratory obstruction by pressure of the foreign body or endoscope. Retrieval of the foreign body is usually successful with the use of the endoscope and forceps (Gans & Austin, 1993; Raffensperger, 1990).

Follow-Up

Although difficult to remove all potential objects for aspiration from the environment, parents should be counseled or given written information on how to childproof their environment. Particular emphasis should be placed on the provision of age-appropriate toys for their children.

■ Functional Defects of the Esophagus

Functional disorders of the esophagus are few but severely limit the ability to eat and thrive when present. They may affect the capacity to attain normal developmental milestones. The most common functional disorder is GER. Chapter 23 is devoted to the management of this condition. Other functional disorders include diffuse esophageal spasm, as seen in achalasia; lack of normal peristalsis, as evidenced in scleroderma; and impaired function, as seen when esophageal diverticula are present. The latter are so rare that they are rarely seen in clinical practice in children.

Achalasia

Achalasia is a condition in which there is diffuse spasm in the distal portion of the esophagus, causing failure to relax with swallowing. The etiology of the condition is unknown. It is primarily a disease of older people, with symptoms not occurring until adulthood. When it occurs in childhood, the mean onset is 8.5 years, although it has been diagnosed in infants.

At one time, it was thought that achalasia was caused by a defect of the ganglion cells in Auerbach's plexus. This has not been proved in children. Histopathology of several muscle specimens has revealed absence of neural plexus and ganglion cells in some but not all patients.

Clinical Presentation

The presenting complaint is difficulty in swallowing. Some children are able to swallow liquids or pureed foods but have difficulty with solids. In time, the proximal esophagus becomes distended, and the child vomits retained food and fluid. Infants and younger children may fail to gain weight and may be labeled as having failure to thrive. Teenagers lose weight over several months. There may be episodes of nocturnal aspiration of esophageal contents leading to pneumonia. The differential diagnosis includes GER due to similarity of symptoms.

Diagnosis

In achalasia, a dilated esophagus with an air-fluid level may be seen on chest x-ray study. A barium swallow is diagnostic and demonstrates a dilated proximal esophagus with a narrowing, or bird-beak deformity, in the distal portion (Fig. 15-9). Little of the contrast material may be seen passing into the stomach. Dysmotility is noted in the proximal esophagus. Manometric studies in the older child demonstrate lack of peristalsis of the esophagus with little or no relaxation of the lower esophageal sphincter. Often, the child may undergo esophagoscopy that reveals concentric narrowing of the distal portion of the esophagus. The area easily accommodates an esophagoscope or dilators, because no true stricture is present.

Operative Repair

Dilation of the narrowed portion provides only temporary relief. Surgery is the only definitive treatment for achalasia. The esophageal myotomy, or Heller myotomy, has been the accepted surgical procedure for over 80 years (Ashcraft, 2000). Through a left thoracotomy or midline upper abdominal approach, the distal esophagus is located and mobilized. A longitudinal incision is made through the muscle layers over the dilated esophagus down to the mucosa. The division is carried out until the mucosa pouches out of the incision. The technique is similar to the pyloromyotomy. Some surgeons carry this incision onto the stomach and then do a partial fundoplication to prevent GER. Others elect not to extend the incision in this manner, and avoid doing a fundoplica-

tion. Laparoscopic or thoracoscopic myotomy may also be performed with success equivalent to that of the open procedure (Lelli, Drongowski, & Coran, 1997; Rothenberg et al., 2001). When re-operation is required, it is because of reflux or recurrent obstruction.

Postoperative Care

As with other types of esophageal surgeries, the child receives supportive postoperative care. The child is kept well hydrated via the intravenous route. Antibiotics are continued for 48 to 72 hours. Approximately 5 to 6 days after surgery, a contrast esophagram is obtained to exclude leakage of esophageal contents from the surgical site. If a leak is not demonstrated, then oral feeds may be started. The child is quickly advanced to a regular diet for age. Discharge from the hospital occurs when the child tolerates regular foods.

Complications and Follow-Up Care

Complications are rare but include perforation of the stomach or esophagus at the time of surgery. The perforation is immediately identified and repaired. There is a possibility of GER developing that would require fundoplication at a later date if it is not able to be managed medically. The child is at risk for metaplasia developing in the distal esophagus in untreated GER. Because of this increased risk, regular endoscopic surveillance of these children is warranted. The child might also experience recurrent obstructive symptoms that may require esophageal dilatation or reoperation.

■ Esophageal Replacement

Although pediatric surgeons generally agree that the native esophagus is superior to anything used to replace it, there may be a time when substitution is necessary (Stone, Fonkalsrud, Mahour, Weitzman, & Takiff, 1985). Age of replacement varies with condition, but it can be performed in early infancy if the child is clinically stable (Vargas-Gomez, 1994). Pederson et al. (1996) reported replacement as early as 36 days after birth in premature infants.

Indications for Replacement

The most common reason for substitution is long-gap EA followed by severe caustic injury and benign strictures that are too long for resection and primary anastomosis (Campbell, Weber, Harrison, & Campbell, 1982; Stone et al., 1985). These strictures are caused by reflux esophagitis, corrosive injury, or anastomotic scarring. Barrett's epithelium in the distal esophagus may also warrant full

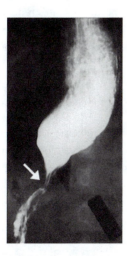

Figure 15-9 Note massive dilation of proximal esophagus.

replacement. Major disruption of an anastomosis may also lead to esophageal replacement.

Preoperative Care

Children with esophageal disease are a nutritional challenge. Many children with an esophageal defect have a gastrostomy tube in place to provide adequate calories. The child's pulmonary status should be assessed, particularly if aspiration has been a part of the clinical picture. Although these children require aggressive pulmonary care, usually they do not improve until the esophageal defect is repaired.

Postoperative Care

Properties of the ideal esophageal substitute are as follows: it should closely mimic, in size and function, the native esophagus, particularly in reference to peristaltic activity; it should not occupy a large space in the thorax; and it should have a good blood supply (Table 15-3). In addition, the operative procedure should be relatively straightforward with a low complication rate (Spitz, 1992).

Regardless of technique, the intestinal tract must be thoroughly cleansed before surgery. Various methods of cleansing include elemental diet, laxatives, and rectal irrigations. This preparation may begin several days before surgery, and much of it can be done at home. Older children may begin a liquid diet as early as 3 days before surgery, switching to clear liquids the day before. Most are admitted to the hospital the day before to ensure that the bowel is adequately cleansed before surgery. Intravenous antibiotics are given on call to the operating room to prevent postoperative infection. Many surgeons advocate the use of oral antibiotics before surgery to decrease the bacterial flora in the intestine.

■ Operative Repair

Colon Interposition

The colon remains the most frequently used organ for replacing the esophagus (Campbell et al., 1982; Lindahl, Louhimo, & Virkola, 1983; Spitz, 1992) (Fig. 15-10). Right, left, or transverse colon is used per surgeon preference (Fig. 15-11). The colon may be placed in the retrosternal position posterior to the left lung by means of a left thoracotomy or by way of the trans-hiatal route eliminating the need for thoracotomy. The arguments against retrosternal replacement include increased incidence of leakage at anastomosis, higher rate of cervical stricture, dysphagia, and cervical bulge on swallowing (Ahmad et al., 1995). Those who favor this method claim better function with fewer complications (Stone et al., 1985). It is imperative to identify that no cardiac anomaly is present that would require correction by means of a median sternotomy because this approach would be difficult with a retrosternal colon in place. The colon is anastomosed to the cervical esophagus through a separate neck incision. The transposed colon may be placed in an isoperistaltic or antiperistaltic manner. In early studies, the colon was

---

Table 15-3   Types of Esophageal Replacements: Advantages and Disadvantages

Procedure	Advantages	Disadvantages
Colon interposition	Readily available; good blood supply; easy to mobilize; adequate length usually attained	Leaks/strictures at anastomotic sites; redundancy of graft over time; slow transit time/stasis of food; GER; may have difficulty swallowing; may have cervical bulge on swallowing; transient diarrhea
Reversed gastric tube	Ease of procedure; good blood supply; adequate length usually attained; rapid transit of food; readily available	Leaks/strictures at cervical anastomosis; may not be long enough to reach proximal esophagus high in neck; GER
Gastric transposition ("pull-up")	Ease of procedure; adequate length usually attained; good blood supply; readily available	Bulk in chest may cause respiratory problems; GER; may have delayed gastric emptying; poor blood supply if needed high in neck; transient dysphagia; may have transient dumping syndrome
Jejunal interposition	Adequate length readily available; caliber of substitution similar to esophagus; peristaltic activity	Precarious blood supply making needed length difficult to attain

Abbreviation: GER, gastroesophageal reflux.

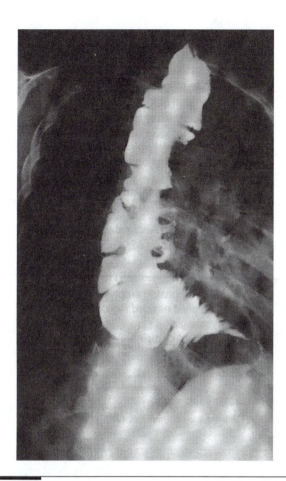

Figure 15-10 Esophagram of esophageal replacement with colonic interposition.

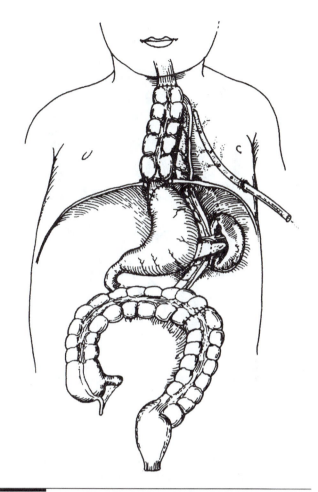

Figure 15-11 Diagram of esophageal substitution with transverse colonic segment.

Reprinted with permission. Ashcraft K. W. (1993). The esophagus. In K. W. Ashcraft & T. M. Holder (Eds.), *Pediatric surgery*, (2nd ed., pp. 228–248). Philadelphia: W.B. Saunders.

described as merely a conduit dependent on gravity to propel food; later research claims that sequential propulsive waves might be present with isoperistaltic placement (Kelly, Shackelford, & Roper, 1983). Additional procedures may include appendectomy, gastrostomy, gastric fundoplication, and pyloroplasty or pyloromyotomy.

Reversed Gastric Tube

A relatively straightforward procedure, the reversed gastric tube has become the favored method of replacement in several major pediatric centers around the world (Anderson, Noblett, Belsey, & Randolph, 1990; Lindahl et al., 1983). After determining that the stomach is large enough with a preoperative contrast study, the abdominal cavity is entered by means of a midline or left subcostal incision. A tube is fashioned from the greater curvature of the stomach based on a pedicle of the left gastroepiploic artery. This tube is then tunneled through the native esophageal bed, retrosternally or transthoracically (Fig. 15-12). The child should be prepared for a colon interposition if the stomach is found to be un-

suitable during surgery. Pyloroplasty is not usually necessary. A small, intussuscepted portion of the distal gastric tube at its junction with the stomach can be sutured to prevent reflux (Buras, Jacir, & Anderson, 1986).

Gastric Transposition

A gastric pull-up is technically the simplest replacement procedure. Anatomic variants, such as a small stomach, unsuitable colon, or previous failed interpositions, may make this the only available option. In this procedure, the stomach is exposed by means of a midline abdominal incision, and the previous gastrostomy site is closed. The stomach is then brought up into the chest through the hiatus and anastomosed to the proximal stump of the healthy esophagus (Fig. 15-13). A pyloroplasty usually accompanies the procedure (Spitz, 1992). Early problems reported include gastric reflux, dumping syndrome, and dysphagia. These usually resolve in time.

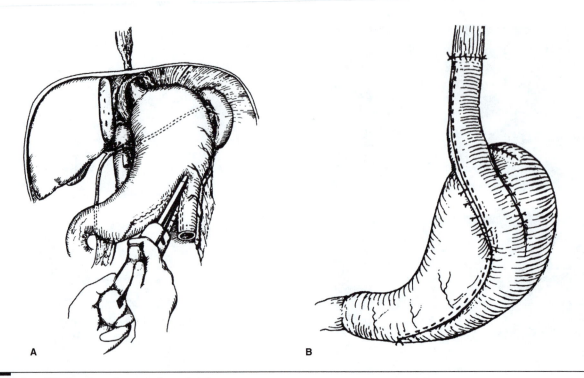

A

B

Figure 15-12 A and B Creation of reversed gastric tube.
Reprinted with permission. Ashcraft, K. W. (1993). The esophagus. In K. W. Ashcraft & T. M. Holder, (Eds.), *Pediatric surgery* (2nd ed., pp. 228–248). Philadelphia: W.B. Saunders.

Because many of these children are born with a tenuous respiratory system, there is concern of having a potential distendable organ in the chest. However, it appears that the stomach tubularizes with time and functions more like a conduit than a reservoir in this position (Davenport et al., 1996). Recently, it has been reported that the denervated stomach as an esophageal substitute is not merely a conduit but a contractile organ that demonstrates increasing motor activity with time (Collard, Romangnoli, Otte, & Kestens, 1998). This activity may aid in the propulsion of food. The presence of a single surgical anastomosis, an excellent blood supply to the transposed organ, and the fact that adequate length is almost always obtained ensure good results with this procedure (Spitz, 1992). Long-term outcome of this procedure has shown favorable results with no deterioration in function of the transposed stomach (Spitz, Kiely, & Pierro, 2004).

Jejunal Transposition

Theoretically, the use of the jejunum as a substitute is ideal because it has the appropriate diameter and peristaltic action (Fig. 15-14). There is technical difficulty in attaining length without sacrificing adequate vascularity (Cusick, Batchelor, & Spicer, 1993). Despite extensive reports of Russian experience with the procedure, there is no detailed information on the ages of the children,

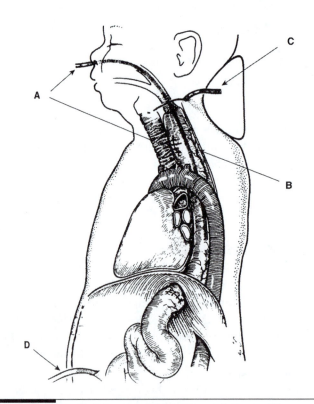

Figure 15-13 Lateral diagram of child with gastric transposition. A, nasogastric decompression tube; B, pulled-up gastric segment; C, drain at cervical anastomosis; and D, jejunal feeding tube.
Source: Reprinted with permission. Spitz, L. (1995). Gastric replacement of the esophagus. In L. Spitz & A. G. Coran (Eds.), *Rob & Smith's operative surgery: Pediatric surgery,* (5th ed., pp. 152–158). New York: Chapman & Hall Medical.

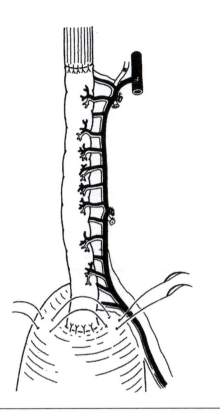

Figure 15-14 Esophageal substitution using piece of jejunum.
Reprinted with permission. Cusick, E. L., Batchelor, A. A. G., & Spicer, R. D. (1993). Development of technique for jejunal interposition in long-gap esophageal atresia. *Journal of Pediatric Surgery, 28*, 990–994.

complications, or long-term functional results (Ring, Varco, L'Heureux, & Foker, 1982). Ring et al. (1982) reported minimal complications in the early and late postoperative periods in 16 children who underwent jejunal replacement surgery. Free jejunal grafts with microvascular surgery are routinely performed to augment and attain length in colonic and gastric tube interpositions that do not reach a short proximal esophageal pouch.

Postoperative Care

Close monitoring is required in the early postoperative period. The child may remain intubated for several days, depending on the postoperative respiratory status. The head should be slightly elevated to decrease the amount of stress on the cervical anastomosis. A Penrose drain is usually left in the neck at the site of the cervical anastomosis to drain any fluid collection. A gastrostomy tube is present in those children who have undergone a colon interposition, reversed gastric tube, or jejunal transposition. A jejunal tube is placed in those who have undergone a gastric pull-up. It is imperative that these enteral tubes are left to gravity drainage until peristalsis commences. Clamping these tubes prematurely may cause reflux into the transposed segment

and lead to disruption or stricture formation at the anastomotic sites (Raffensperger, 1990).

If there is no drainage from the neck wound, a contrast study is obtained approximately 1 week later. The cervical drain is removed if there are no radiologically demonstrated leaks at the time of the study. The child is then allowed to eat orally (Ahmad et al., 1995). Commencement of an oral diet as early as 4 days after surgery has been reported, provided that there is no leakage from the cervical drain and no indication of disruption of the anastomosis (Marujo, Tannuri, & Maksoud, 1991). The diet is advanced slowly. Soft food cut into small pieces is offered until the child is old enough to understand the principle of thorough mastication. The child should eat upright and remain in this position for at least 1 hour after eating. If there is a demonstrated leak at the cervical anastomosis, the child is kept NPO until there is resolution of this leak.

Enteral feedings are resumed after intestinal function returns. The feeding tubes are not removed until it is proved that there are no delayed surgical complications and the child is able to eat orally and sustain weight.

Parenteral antibiotics are administered for approximately 7 days to avoid postoperative infections at the anastomotic and incisional sites. As with any major abdominal and thoracic surgery, pain is to be expected. Children should be kept pain free by the use of epidural catheters to deliver analgesia in addition to intravenous agents.

Complications

Low complication rates and good functional results depend on experience with the operative technique rather than on which substitute is used (Campbell et al., 1982). Complications can be grouped as immediate, intermediate, and long term.

Necrosis of the transposed segment is most often seen with colon interpositions and is considered an immediate complication because it is seen mostly in the early postoperative period (Stone et al., 1985). The occurrence is reported to be as high as 18%. When this occurs, the transposed segment is removed, a cervical esophagostomy is placed, and the child is allowed to recover before attempting another interposition.

Anastomotic leak at the cervical esophagocolic/gastric anastomosis is another immediate complication and has been described in 2.8% to 70% of cases (Campbell et al., 1982; Ring et al., 1982; Stone et al., 1985). Most of these leaks close spontaneously. A rare and unfortunate complication is perforation through the cervical anastomosis by a suction catheter. Catheters should be measured from the upper dental ridge before each intervention.

Other early and less common complications include wound infections, pneumonia, pneumothorax, pericarditis, and Horner's syndrome (Stone et al., 1985).

The list of long-term complications is extensive. Strictures may develop at the anastomotic areas and are the most common (Borgnon et al., 2004). Anastomosis to a scarred proximal esophagus, as in corrosive injury, predisposes to stricture formation (Bassiouny & Bahnassy, 1992). Persistent strictures may need to be surgically revised.

Food obstruction in the neoesophagus can be a result of narrowing at the site of stricture and/or ingestion of large amounts or pieces of food without adequate fluid intake (Lindahl et al., 1983). Fibrous foods, such as meats and certain vegetables, can be particularly troublesome and may need to be removed endoscopically.

Over time, these colons may become very boggy and redundant (Lindahl et al., 1983). Food can sit for long periods of time in a patulous colon interposition. Fetid breath can be a social problem. Ingestion of substantial liquid aids in the propulsion of food. Graft redundancy may need revision or replacement if causing severe dysphagia (Bassiouny & Bahnassy, 1992).

Dumping syndrome is due to rapid gastric emptying and is usually seen in children who eat a hypertonic meal. It is more common in children who have undergone a gastric pull-up. This is usually a transient problem. It does not appear to be associated with the presence or absence of pyloroplasty (Ravelli, Spitz, & Milla, 1994).

Transient diarrhea may be observed after colon transposition. On average, two to three loose stools daily are reported but with only occasional social inconvenience. Stool incontinence is common in children who have also undergone repair of high imperforate anus. It is possible that resecting colon for replacement causes decreased water absorption in the shortened colon, thus aggravating the condition in these children (Anderson, Noblett, et al., 1990).

Children with a gastric pull-up have been identified as having problems with *anemia*, as documented by low serum ferritin levels. Iron absorption is facilitated by presence of acid in the stomach. It is thought that poor absorption is caused by atrophic gastritis and hypochlorhydria. It is suggested that these children receive iron supplementation (Davenport et al., 1996).

GER is present in 60% of children who have undergone colonic interposition. Antireflux procedures can be performed at the time of surgery; however, this may cause problems in a colon that depends mostly on gravity to empty. Some surgeons believe that GER is better controlled when the replacement surgery is delayed until the infant is able to sit up for feedings. The colon is thought to be resistant to peptic ulceration because of its mucus production. Alkaline secretions of the colon neutralize the refluxed gastric acid. However, ulceration with bleeding may occur in the interposed segment and is more common in colon substitution. Food stasis within the colon segment causing ulceration has been reported. These children should be followed up for possible dysplastic changes that may lead to cancer. Reflux is also present in children who have undergone a gastric pull-up or reversed gastric tube procedure. These children should also adhere to reflux precautions. A modified plication at the lower end of the gastric tube is often successful in minimizing reflux (Buras et al., 1986). A comparative study between children who underwent a colon interposition in the United Kingdom and those who underwent a reversed gastric tube in the United States did not identify GER as a major problem in either population (Anderson, Noblett, et al., 1990). Feeding through an enteral tube in the early postoperative period and continuous or small frequent feeds instead of feeding large boluses minimizes the risk of reflux into the replaced segment. Postoperative pneumonia is almost always due to aspiration.

A transient early growth delay is present in those who have had EA. This appears to resolve in the early adolescent period. No evidence of growth delay exists in children who have undergone esophageal replacement for other conditions (Campbell et al., 1982; Stone et al., 1985). Other long-term complications include small-bowel obstruction from adhesions and dysphagia (Borgnon et al., 2004). Death is rare with this surgery and is usually attributable to pulmonary complications (Ahmad et al., 1995).

Discharge Planning

As with any medically fragile child, considerable effort should be devoted to planning for discharge from the hospital. Patients with complications usually have an extensive list of needs. Most of these children do well. Follow-up care should focus on nutritional status. A consultation with a dietician may be obtained to assist the family and medical team in choosing appropriate foods and recommending supplementation via an enteral tube when indicated.

These children should be observed for any signs of anastomotic stricture, especially if there was an anastomotic leak in the postoperative period. The surgeon may elect to place the child on a schedule for dilation or decide to follow up the child with dilation on an as-needed basis. The family is instructed to call the office if the child is experiencing increased difficulty swallowing or regurgitating food.

If these children are school age, they may find themselves behind in their studies because of missed school days. Effort should be made to commence studies as soon as possible during hospitalization and convalescence at home. Involving the school nurse is beneficial because he or she can function as the child's advocate once the child returns to school. Copies of discharge instructions as well as telephone numbers of the primary health team should accompany the child back to school.

■ Acknowledgments

The author wishes to thank Drs. Donald Shaul, Kasper Wang, Juan Acosta, and Dean Anselmo for their technical support in this endeavor.

■ Educational Materials

APSNA invites you to download the following diagnosis-related teaching tool for Chapter 15, Esophageal Defects: Esophageal atresia and tracheoesophageal fistula. This teaching tool is available at the APSNA Web site (www.apsna.org) and the Jones and Bartlett Web site (www.jbpub.com). All teaching materials are available in English and Spanish and are free of charge. APSNA encourages their use for your patients and families.

References

Ahmad, S. A., Sylvester, K. G., Hebra, A., Davidoff, A. M., McClane, S., Stafford, P. W., et al. (1995). Esophageal replacement using the colon: Is it a good choice? *Journal of Pediatric Surgery, 31*(8), 1026–1031.

Allmendinger, N., Hallisey, M. J., Markowitz, S. K., Hight, D., Weiss, R., & McGowan, G. (1996). Balloon dilatation of esophageal strictures in children. *Journal of Pediatric Surgery, 31*(3), 334–336.

Anderson, K. D., Noblett, H., Belsey, R., & Randolph, J. G. (1990). Long-term follow-up of children with colon and gastric tube interposition for esophageal atresia. *Surgery, 111*(2), 131–136.

Anderson, K. D., Rouse, T. M., & Randolph, J. G. (1990). A controlled trial of corticosteroids in children with corrosive injury of the esophagus. *New England Journal of Medicine, 323*, 637–640.

Anderson, K. D., Acosta, J. M., Meyer, M. S., & Sherman, N. J. (2002). Application of the principles of myotomy and stricturoplasty for treatment of esophageal stricture. *Journal of Pediatric Surgery, 37*(3), 403–406.

Andrassy, R. J., Ko, P., Hanson, B. A., Kubota, E., Hays, D. M., & Mahour, G. H. (1980). Congenital esophageal fistula without esophageal atresia. *American Journal of Surgery, 140*, 731–733.

Ashcraft, K. W. (1993). The esophagus. In K. W. Ashcraft & T. M. Holder (Eds.), *Pediatric surgery* (2nd ed., pp. 228–248). Philadelphia: W.B. Saunders.

Ashcraft, K. W. (2000). The esophagus. In K. W. Ashcraft, J. P. Murphy, R. J. Sharp, D. L. Sigalet, & C. L. Snyder (Eds.), *Pediatric surgery* (3rd ed., pp. 325–347). Philadelphia: W.B. Saunders.

Aziz, D., Schiller, D., Gerstle, J. T., Ein, S. H., & Langer, J. (2003). Can "long-gap" esophageal atresia be safely managed at home while awaiting anastomosis? *Journal of Pediatric Surgery, 38*(5), 705–708.

Bankier, A., Brady J., & Myers, N. A. (1991). Epidemiology and genetics. In S. W. Beasley, N. A. Myers, & A. W. Auldist (Eds.), *Oesophageal atresia* (pp. 19–27). New York: Chapman & Hall.

Bassiouny, I. E., & Bahnassy, A. F. (1992). Transhiatal esophagectomy and colonic interposition for caustic esophageal stricture. *Journal of Pediatric Surgery, 27*(8), 1091–1096.

Beasley, S. W. (1991a). Embryology. In S. W. Beasley, N. A. Myers, & A. W. Auldist (Eds.), *Oesophageal atresia* (pp. 31–42). New York: Chapman & Hall.

Beasley, S. W. (1991b). Oesophageal atresia without fistula. In S. W. Beasley, N. A. Myers, & A. W. Auldist (Eds.), *Oesophageal atresia* (pp. 137–158). New York: Chapman & Hall.

Beasley, S. W., & Auldist, A. W. (1991). Oesophageal atresia with distal tracheo-esophageal fistula. In S. W. Beasley, N. A. Myers, & A. W. Auldist (Eds.), *Oesophageal atresia* (pp. 119–134). New York: Chapman & Hall.

Broto, J., Asensio, M., & Vernet, J. M. (2003). Results of a new technique in the treatment of severe esophageal stenosis in children: Poliflex stents. *Journal of Pediatric Gastroenterology and Nutrition, 37*(2), 203–206.

Brown, A. K., & Tam, P. K. (1996). Measurement of gap length in esophageal atresia: A simple predictor of outcome. *Journal of the American College of Surgeons, 182*(1), 41–45.

Brown, T. C. K., Eyres, R., & N. A. Myers. (1991). Anaesthesia and perioperative care. In S. W. Beasley, N. A. Myers, & A. W. Auldist (Eds.), *Oesophageal atresia* (pp. 103–115). New York: Chapman & Hall.

Borgnon, J., Tounian, P., Auber, F., Larroquet, M., Boeris Clemen, F., Girardet, J. P., et al. (2004). Esophageal replacement on children by an isoperistaltic gastric tube: A 12-year experience. *Pediatric Surgery International, 20*, 11–12.

Buras, R. R., Jacir, N. N., & Anderson, K. D. (1986). An antireflux procedure for use with the reversed gastric tube. *Journal of Pediatric Surgery, 21*(6), 545–547.

Campbell, J. R., Webber, B. R., Harrison, M. W., & Campbell, T. J. (1982). Esophageal replacement in infants and children by colon interposition. *The American Journal of Surgery, 144*, 29–34.

Chavin, K., Field, G., Chandler, J., Tagge, E., & Otherson, H. B. (1996). Save the child's esophagus: Management of major disruption after repair of esophageal atresia. *Journal of Pediatric Surgery, 131*(1), 48–52.

Collard, J. M., Romangnoli, R., Otte, J. B., & Kestens, P. J. (1998). The denervated stomach as an esophageal substitute is a contractile organ. *Annals of Surgery, 227*(1), 33–39.

Crabbe, D. C. G., Kiely, E. M., Drake D. P., & Spitz, L. (1996). Management of the isolated tracheoesophageal fistula. *European Journal of Pediatric Surgery, 6*, 67–69.

Curci, M. R., & Dibbins, A. W. (1988). Problems associated with a Nissen fundoplication following tracheoesophageal fistula and esophageal atresia repair. *Archives of Surgery, 123*, 618–620.

Cusick, E. L., Batchelor, A. A. G., & Spicer, R. D. (1993). Development of a technique for jejunal interposition in long-gap esophageal atresia. *Journal of Pediatric Surgery, 28*(8), 990–994.

Davenport, M., Hosie, G. P., Tasker, R. C., Gordon, I., Kiely, E. M., & Spitz, L. (1996). Long-term effects of gastric transposition in children: A physiological study. *Journal of Pediatric Surgery, 31*(4), 588–593.

David, T. J., & O'Callaghan, S. E. (1974). Cardiovascular malformation and oesophageal atresia. *British Heart Journal, 36*, 559.

Filler, R. M., & Forte, V. (1998). Lesions of the larynx and trachea. In J. A. O'Neill, Jr., M. I. Rowe, J. L. Grosfeld, E. W. Fonkalsrud, & A. G.

Coran (Eds.), *Pediatric surgery* (5th ed., pp. 863–872). St. Louis, MO: Mosby.

Filston, H. C., & Shorter, N. A. (2000). Esophageal atresia and tracheoesophageal fistula. In K. W. Ashcraft, J. P. Murphy, R. J. Sharp, D. J. Sigalet, & C. L. Snyder (Eds.), *Pediatric surgery* (3rd ed., pp. 438–369). Philadelphia: W.B. Saunders.

Gans, S. L., & Austin, E. (1993). Foreign bodies. In K. W. Ashcraft & T. M. Holder (Eds.), *Pediatric surgery* (2nd ed., pp. 82–88). Philadelphia: W.B. Saunders.

Greenwood, R. D., & Rosenthal, A. (1976). Cardiovascular malformations with tracheoesophageal fistula and esophageal atresia. *Pediatrics, 57,* 87.

Gross, R. E. (1953). *The surgery of infancy and childhood.* Philadelphia: W.B. Saunders.

Gutierrez, C., Barrios, J. E., Lluna, J., Vila, J. J., Garcia-Sala, C., Roca, A., et al. (1994). Recurrent tracheoesophageal fistula treated with fibrin glue. *Journal of Pediatric Surgery, 29*(12), 1567–1569.

Harmon, C. M., & Coran, A. G. (1998). Congenital anomalies of the esophagus. In J. A. O'Neill, Jr., M. I. Rowe, J. L. Grosfeld, E. W. Fonkalsrud, & A. G. Coran (Eds.), *Pediatric surgery* (5th ed., pp. 941–967). St. Louis, MO: Mosby.

Harrison, M. R., Hanson, B. A., Mahour, G. H., Takahashi, M., & Weitzman, J. J. (1977). The significance of right aortic arch in repair of esophageal atresia and tracheoesophageal fistula. *Journal of Pediatric Surgery, 12,* 861–869.

Holder, T. M. (1993). Esophageal atresia and tracheoesophageal malformations. In K. W. Ashcraft & T. M. Holder (Eds.), *Pediatric surgery* (2nd ed., pp. 249–269). Philadelphia: W.B. Saunders.

Holcomb, G. W., 3rd, Rothenberg, S. S., Bax, K. M., Martinez-Ferro, M., Albanese, C. T., Ostlie, D. J., et al., (2005). Thoracoscopic repair of esophageal atresia and tracheoesophageal fistula: A multi-institutional analysis. *Annals of Surgery, 242*(3), 422–428.

Hollands, C. M., Lankau, C. A., & Burnweit, C. A. (2000). Preoperative home care for esophageal atresia—A survey. *Journal of Pediatric Surgery, 35*(2), 279–282.

Jolly, S. G., Johnson, D. G., Roberts, C. C., Herbst, J. J., Matlak, M. E., McCombs, A., et al. (1980). Patterns of gastroesophageal reflux in children following repair of esophageal atresia and distal tracheoesophageal fistula. *Journal of Pediatric Surgery, 15,* 857–867.

Kelly, J. P., Shackelford, M. D., & Roper, C. L. (1983). Esophageal replacement with colon in children: Functional results and long-term growth. *The Annals of Thoracic Surgery, 36*(6), 634–640.

Kimura, K., Nishijima, E., Tsugawa, C., Collins, D. L., Lazar, E. L., Stylianos, S., et al. (2001). Multistaged extrathoracic esophageal elongation procedure for long gap esophageal atresia: Experience with 12 patients. *Journal of Pediatric Surgery, 36*(11), 1725–1727.

Lelli, J. L., Drongowski, R. A., & Coran, A. G. (1997). Efficacy of the transthoracic modified Heller myotomy in children with achalasia: A 21-year experience. *Journal of Pediatric Surgery, 32*(2), 338–341.

Lindahl, H., Louhimo, I., & Virkola, K. (1983). Colon interposition or gastric tube? Follow-up study of colon-esophagus and gastric tube-esophagus patients. *Journal of Pediatric Surgery, 18*(1), 58–63.

Little, D. C., Rescorla, F. J., Grosfeld, J. L., West, K. W., Scherer, L. R., & Engum, S. A. (2003). Long-term analysis of children with esophageal atresia and tracheoesophageal fistula. *Journal of Pediatric Surgery, 38*(6), 852–856.

Marujo, W. C., Tannuri, U., & Maksoud, J. G. (1991). Total gastric transposition: An alternative to esophageal replacement in children. *Journal of Pediatric Surgery, 26*(6), 676–681.

McCallion, W. A., Hannon, R. J., & Boston, V. E. (1992). Prophylactic extrapleural chest drainage following repair of esophageal atresia: Is it necessary? *Journal of Pediatric Surgery, 27*(5), 561.

Mee, R. B. B. (1991). Congenital heart disease. In S. W. Beasley, N. A. Myers, & A.W. Auldist (Eds.), *Oesophageal atresia* (pp. 229–239). New York: Chapman & Hall.

Millar, J. W., & Cywes, S. (1998). Caustic strictures of the esophagus. In J. A. O'Neill, Jr., M. I. Rowe, J. L. Grosfeld, E. W. Fonkalsrud, & A. G. Coran (Eds.), *Pediatric surgery* (5th ed., pp. 969–979). St. Louis, MO: Mosby.

Mulvihill, S. J., Stone, M. M., Debas, H. T., & Fonkalsrud, E. (1985). The role of amniotic fluid in fetal nutrition. *Journal of Pediatric Surgery, 20*(6), 668–672.

Murphy, S. G., Yazbeck, S., & Russo, P. (1995). Isolated congenital esophageal stenosis. *Journal of Pediatric Surgery, 30*(8), 1238–1241.

Myers, N. A., Beasley, S. W., & Auldist, A. W. (1991a). Associated anomalies. In S. W. Beasley, N. A. Myers, & A. W. Auldist (Eds.), *Oesophageal atresia* (pp. 211–226). New York: Chapman & Hall.

Myers, N. A., Beasley, S. W., & Auldist, A. W. (1991b). Oesophageal replacement. In S. W. Beasley, N. A. Myers, & A. W. Auldist (Eds.), *Oesophageal atresia* (pp. 171–190). New York: Chapman & Hall.

Myers, N. A., & Beasley, S. W. (1991). Diagnosis. In S. W. Beasley, N. A. Myers, & A. W. Auldist (Eds.), *Oesophageal atresia* (pp. 77–91). New York: Chapman & Hall.

Nwomeh, B. C., Luketich, J. D., & Kane, T. D. (2004). Minimally invasive esophagectomy for caustic esophageal stricture in children. *Journal of Pediatric Surgery, 39*(7), e1–e6.

Ohkawa, H., Takahashi, H., Hoshino, Y., & Sato, H. (1975). Lower esophageal stenosis in association with tracheobronchial remnants. *Journal of Pediatric Surgery, 10*(4), 453–457.

Pederson, J. C., Klein, R. L., & Andrews, D. A. (1996). Gastric tube as the primary procedure for pure esophageal atresia. *Journal of Pediatric Surgery, 31*(9), 1233–1235.

Poenaru, D., Laberge, J. M., Neilson, I. R., Nguyen, L. T., & Guttman, F. M. (1991). A more than 25-year experience with end-to-end versus end-to-side repair for esophageal atresia. *Journal of Pediatric Surgery, 26*(4), 472–477.

Quan, L., & Smith, D. W. (1973). The VATER association—vertebral defects, anal atresia, T-E fistula with esophageal atresia, radial and renal dysplasia: A spectrum of associated defects. *Journal of Pediatrics, 82,* 104.

Raffensperger, J. D. (Ed.). (1990). *Swenson's pediatric surgery* (5th ed.). Norwalk, CT: Appelton & Lange.

Randolph, J. G., Newman, K. D., & Anderson, K. D. (1989). Current results in repair of esophageal atresia with tracheoesophageal fistula using physiologic status as a guide to therapy. *Annals of Surgery, 209*(5), 526–531.

Ravelli, A. M., Spitz, L., & Milla, P. J. (1994). Gastric emptying in children with gastric transposition. *Journal of Pediatric Gastroenterology and Nutrition, 19*(4), 403–409.

Ring, W. S., Varco, R. L., L'Heureux, P. R., & Foker, J. E. (1982). Esophageal replacement with jejunum in children. *Journal of Thoracic Cardiovascular Surgery, 83,* 918–927.

Rothenberg, S. S., Patrick, D. A., Bealer, J. F., & Chang, J. H. (2001). Evaluation of minimally invasive approaches to achalasia in children. *Journal of Pediatric Surgery, 36*(5), 808–810.

Roy, R. N. D. (1991). Transport of the neonate with oesophageal atresia. In S. W. Beasley, N. A. Myers, & A. W. Auldist (Eds.), *Oesophageal atresia* (pp. 93–102). New York: Chapman & Hall.

Ryan, D. P., Muehrcke, D. D., Doody, D. P., Kim, S. H., & Donahoe, P. K. (1991). Laryngotracheoesophageal cleft (Type IV): Management and repair of lesions beyond the carina. *Journal of Pediatric Surgery, 26*(8), 962–970.

Santos, A. D., Thompson, T. R., Johnson, D. E., & Foker, J. E. (1983). Correction of esophageal atresia with distal tracheoesophageal fistula. *Journal of Thoracic Cardiovascular Surgery, 85,* 229–236.

Schalamon, J., Lindahl, H., Saarikoski, H., & Rintala, R. J. (2003). Endoscopic follow-up in esophageal atresia—For how long is it necessary? *Journal of Pediatric Surgery, 38*(5), 702–704.

Schier, F., Korn, S., & Michel, E. (2001). Experiences of a parent support group with the long-term consequences of esophageal atresia. *Journal of Pediatric Surgery, 36*(4), 605–611.

Shaul, D. B., Schwartz, M. Z., Marr, C. C., & Tyson, K. R. T. (1989). Primary repair without routine gastrostomy is the treatment of choice for neonates with esophageal atresia and tracheoesophageal fistula. *Archives of Surgery, 124,* 1188–1191.

Shikowitz, M. J., Levy, J., Villano, D., Graver, L. M., & Pochaczevsky, R. (1996). Speech and swallowing rehabilitation following devastating caustic ingestion: Techniques and indicators for success. *Laryngoscope, 106,* 1–12.

Snyder, C. L., Ramachandran, V., Kennedy, A. P., Gittes, G. K., Ashcraft, K. W., & Holder, T. M. (1997). Efficacy of partial wrap fundoplication for gastroesophageal reflux after repair of esophageal atresia. *Journal of Pediatric Surgery, 32*(7), 1089–1092.

Spitz, L. (1992). Gastric transposition for esophageal substitution in children. *Journal of Pediatric Surgery, 27*(2), 252–259.

Spitz, L. (1995). Cervical esophagostomy. In L. Spitz & A. G. Coran (Eds.), *Rob & Smith's operative surgery: Pediatric surgery* (5th ed., pp. 121–123). New York: Chapman & Hall.

Spitz, L. (1996). Esophageal atresia: Past, present, and future. *Journal of Pediatric Surgery, 31*(1), 19–25.

Spitz, L., Kiely, E., & Pierro, A. (2004). Gastric transposition in children-a 21-year experience. *Journal of Pediatric Surgery, 39*(3), 276–281.

Stokes, K. B. (1991). Pathophysiology. In S. W. Beasley, N. A. Myers, & A. W. Auldist (Eds.), *Oesophageal atresia* (pp. 59–71). New York: Chapman & Hall.

Stone, M. M., Fonkalsrud, E. W., Mahour, G. H., Weitzman, J. J., & Takiff, H. (1985). Esophageal replacement with colon interposition in children. *Annals of Surgery, 203*(4), 346–351.

Stringer, M. D., McKenna, K. M., Goldstein, R. B., Filly, R. A., Adzick, N. S., & Harrison, M. R. (1995). Prenatal diagnosis of esophageal atresia. *Journal of Pediatric Surgery, 30*(9), 1258–1263.

Touloukian, R. J., & Seashore, J. H. (2004). Thirty-five year institutional experience with end-to side repair for esophageal atresia. *Archives of Surgery, 139*(4), 371–374.

Tomaselli, V., Volpi, M. L., Dell'Agnola, C. A., Bini, M., Rossi, A., & Indriolo, A. (2003). Long-term evaluation of esophageal function in patients treated at birth for esophageal atresia. *Pediatric Surgery International, 19*(1-2), 40–43.

Tovar, J. A., Diez-Pardo, J. A., Murcia, J., Prieto, G., Molina, M., & Polanco, I. (1995). Ambulatory 24-hour manometric and pH metric evidence of clearance capacity in patients with esophageal atresia. *Journal of Pediatric Surgery, 30*(8), 1224–1231.

Vargas-Gomez, M. (1994). Esophageal replacement in patients under 3 months of age. *Journal of Pediatric Surgery, 29*(4), 487–491.

Wheatley, M. J., Coran, A. G., & Wesley, J. R. (1993). Efficacy of the Nissen fundoplication in the management of gastroesophageal reflux following esophageal atresia repair. *Journal of Pediatric Surgery, 28*(1), 53–55.

Zigman, A., & Yazbeck, S. (2002). Esophageal foreign body obstruction after esophageal atresia repair. *Journal of Pediatric Surgery, 37*(5), 776–778.

Congenital Lung Malformations

By Teri Coha

Congenital cystic lesions of the lung are uncommon, making up only a small percentage of the pediatric surgical population. The most common are congenital cystic adenomatoid malformation (CCAM), pulmonary sequestration, bronchogenic cyst, and congenital lobar emphysema (CLE). These abnormal cystic lesions are pathologically distinct but share similar clinical and embryologic characteristics (dell' Agnola, Tadini, Mosca, Colnaghi, & Wesley, 1996). Their origins remain poorly understood. They may be diagnosed antenatally, in early life, or later. The significant increase in the use of prenatal ultrasound of the fetus has improved the likelihood of an early diagnosis and has contributed a wealth of information about these malformations. All mothers carrying a fetus with a prenatally diagnosed lung lesion should be referred to a tertiary care center, with a neonatal intensivist, perinatologists, and pediatric surgeons available for delivery.

Overall, congenital lung malformations occur at a 1.3 to 1 ratio of males to females. No ethnic or racial predominance has been found, and the malformations are rarely familial. Both the right and the left lung are equally affected, bilateral involvement is rare, and usually, only one lobe on the affected side is diseased (Buntain, Isaacs, Payne, Lindesmith, & Rosenkrantz, 1974). Because other congenital defects may be associated with congenital lung malformations, a thorough assessment is indicated on all patients (Shanmugam, MacArthur, & Pollock, 2005).

Congenital diaphragmatic hernia (CDH) is also discussed in this chapter because it significantly affects lung development. However, CDH is a more complex lesion with many possible treatments and is discussed separately.

■ Congenital Cystic Adenomatoid Malformation

CCAM is characterized by solid, cystic, or mixed masses that communicate with the normal tracheobronchial tree and derive their vascular supply from the pulmonary circulation. CCAMs result from failure of normal bronchoalveolar development and the formation of cysts of varying sizes. The cysts range in size from less than 1 mm to more than 10 cm (Horak et al., 2003; McLean et al., 2004). They are generally confined to one lobe of the lung, and bilateral lung involvement is uncommon (Adzick, Harrison, Crombleholme, Flake, & Howell, 1998). Most CCAMs are diagnosed prenatally, with a small percentage of patients diagnosed after the newborn period and a few reports of CCAM diagnosed in adults

(MacDonald, Forte, Cutz, & Crysdale, 1996; Lackner, Thompson, Rikkers, & Galbraith, 1996).

Stocker, Madewell, and Drake (1977) developed a classification of CCAMs by dividing them into three distinct pathological types based on the size of the cyst and its microscopic appearance. Type 1 refers to single or multiple cysts (between one and four) greater than 2 cm in diameter, lined by ciliated pseudostratified columnar epithelium, type 2 is described as multiple small cysts less than 1 cm in diameter lined by ciliated cuboidal epithelium, and type 3 is described as a large bulky, noncystic lesion, lined by ciliated cuboidal epithelium involving the entire lobe or lobes with no normal lung tissue visible (Fig. 16-1). Seeds and Azizkhan (1990) defined type 1 as the replacement of normal lung tissue by multiple large cysts in a lobar distribution that varies in size and is anechoic and type 2 as a diffuse lesion that results in replacement of the entire lung with microscopic cysts that enlarge the lung and are echodense. Adzick, Flake, and Crombleholme (2003) classified prenatally diagnosed CCAM into two groups based on gross anatomy and ultrasound. Macrocystic disease consists of single or multiple cysts 5 mm or larger on prenatal ultrasound, and microcystic lesions appear as a solid and bulky mass.

The clinical spectrum of prenatally diagnosed CCAM is quite variable. In some fetuses, the cysts grow rapidly, causing nonimmune hydrops and fetal demise, whereas in others, the mass may spontaneously regress and disappear (Adzick et al., 1998; MacGillivray, Harrison, Goldstein, & Adzick, 1993). Ultrasonography can provide ongoing information about the CCAM, including lobe of involvement, Stocker class, macrocystic versus microcystic appearance, degree of mediastinal shift, and the degree of hydrops (Crombleholme et al., 2002).

Prognosis depends primarily on the size, not the lesion type (Adzick et al., 2003). Prognosis is poor for neonates with bilobar lesions, bilateral lesions, and pulmonary hypoplasia (Shanmugam et al., 2005) and in the presence of polyhydramnios and fetal hydrops (Usui et al., 2004). Prenatal counseling, especially related to elective termination of the pregnancy, should acknowledge that these children have a positive outcome in the absence of fetal hydrops. In the absence of hydrops, the survival rate for infants with CCAM is 100% (Crombleholme et al., 2002).

The recommended treatment for CCAM is pulmonary resection. Infants who are symptomatic at birth usually need early excisional surgery. Elective surgery is recommended for infants and children who are symptomatic, have evidence of mediastinal shift, or have involvement of a significant part of the lung (Ayed & Owayed, 2003; Usui et al., 2004). Shanmugam, MacArthur, and Pollock (2005) prefer lobectomy in patients with extensive unilobar involvement and in patients who require emergent resections.

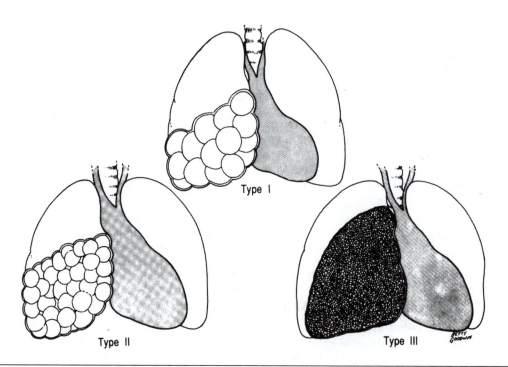

Figure 16-1 Congenital cystic adenomatoid malformations.

■ Pulmonary Sequestration

Pulmonary sequestration is an isolated lobe of lung tissue without bronchial connection to the tracheobronchial system. The arterial blood supply is often provided by an aberrant artery arising from the aorta or one of its branches (Savic, Birtel, Tholen, Funke, & Knoche, 1979; Adzick et al., 2003). The anomaly originates from the embryonic foregut, making it one of the bronchopulmonary foregut malformations that include enteric cysts, bronchogenic cysts, esophageal duplication, and tracheoesophageal fistulas. It occurs

> *"when there is separation of a segment of the lung or a separate out pouching from the foregut anlage. The timing of the separation is important in that if the sequestered lung tissue arises before pleura formation, the sequestration will be intralobar and surrounded by normal lung tissue. When the sequestration arises after pleural development, it will be invested by its own pleura and will be extralobar and separate from the remaining pulmonary parenchyma"*

(Seeds & Azizkhan, 1990, p. 233) (Fig. 16-2).

Intralobar sequestrations are commonly located in the posterior basilar region of the lower lobe. Extralobar sequestration is generally found in the left posterior costophrenic angle (Shanmugam et al., 2005). The isolated area can interfere with the growth and development of adjacent structures.

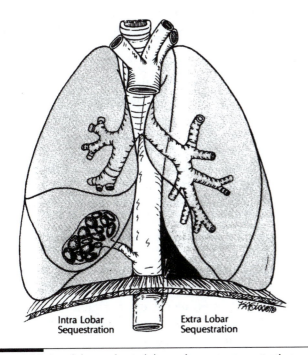

Figure 16-2 Intralobar and extralobar pulmonary sequestration.

Associated congenital malformations, such as diaphragmatic hernia, pectus excavatum, foregut duplications, and congenital heart defects, have been described (Shanmugam et al., 2005). The diagnosis of pulmonary sequestration is made in the newborn period as a result of the effect on respiratory function, in older children with chronic respiratory infections, and more commonly in the antenatal period with ultrasonography (Evans, 1996). Doppler ultrasonography may identify the anomalous systemic artery from the aorta to the fetal lung lesion, confirming the diagnosis of pulmonary sequestration (King, Pilling, & Walkinshaw, 1995; MacGillivray et al., 1993).

Seeds and Azizkhan (1990) recommended resection in the neonatal period, projecting a good prognosis for those without severe pulmonary hypoplasia. Early resection is also recommended based on reports of serious complications occurring in patients with unresected pulmonary sequestrations (Takeda et al., 1999; Shanmugam et al., 2005). An extralobar sequestration is separate from the normal lung by its own plural envelope, making excision relatively straightforward. Patients with intralobar sequestration may require lobectomy because of inflammatory changes from infections and vascular adhesions (Shanmugam et al.).

Adzick, Harrison, Crombleholme, Flake, and Howell (1998) reported on a series of 39 cases of extralobar sequestration diagnosed between 18 and 36 weeks gestation that were monitored with the use of ultrasound. In 28 of the fetuses, the lesion completely or nearly completely disappeared. At birth, the infants were asymptomatic and the lesions were detectable only with computed tomography or magnetic resonance imaging but not on chest x-ray study. This group was followed up without resection. Most of the remaining infants in this study had larger extralobar sequestrations and underwent postnatal resection for respiratory symptoms. Three fetuses developed hydrops and underwent weekly fetal thoracenteses; one had a thoracoamniotic shunt placed, and all survived.

■ Bronchogenic Cyst

Bronchogenic cysts are "solitary unilocular cystic structures that are filled with fluid or mucus" (Langston, 2003). They are remnants of the primitive foregut containing tissue that is normally found in the trachea or bronchi, and they are frequently attached to, but do not communicate with, the trachea or bronchi. The stage of embryonic development determines location of the lesion: the paratracheal or bronchial versus intraparenchymal. Cysts located in the mediastinum near the trachea, esophagus, carina, or main bronchi probably form early during separation of the embryonic foregut. Those that occur later in development, during budding and branching, grow within the lung parenchyma (Nobuhara, Gorski, LaQuaglia, & Shamberger, 1997; St-Georges et al., 1991). Hyaline cartilage plates are necessary for a diagnosis of bronchogenic cysts. The most common location is in the mediastinum just above the tracheal bifurcation (Langston). Extrathoracic cysts have presented as soft masses over the border of the sternum (Rodgers, Harman, & Johnson, 1986), over the scapula (Jona, 1995), or as neck masses (Nobuhara et al.).

Bronchogenic cysts are frequently diagnosed during childhood. There is no gender predominance, and rarely is there an associated malformation (Nobuhara et al., 1997; Ribet, Copin, & Gosselin, 1996). Infants and children present with respiratory distress or other symptoms resulting from compression of the lesion on surrounding structures, or with gastrointestinal complaints of vomiting or poor feeding. Mediastinal bronchogenic cysts produce symptoms by causing airway obstruction, whereas pulmonary cysts produce symptoms of infection or compression, including cough and hemoptysis (Nobuhara et al.; Ribet et al.).

Diagnosis is confirmed with chest radiograph examination, barium esophagram, or chest computed tomographic scans (Nobuhara et al., 1997; Rodgers et al., 1986).

The literature supports surgical excision at the time of diagnoses even in asymptomatic patients. Left untreated, prognosis is unpredictable and late complications are frequent, including the threat of bacterial or fungal infection and malignancy (Nobuhara et al., 1997; Ribet et al., 1996; St-Georges et al., 1991). Segmentectomy is an option for small cysts (Ribet et al.).

■ Congenital Lobar Emphysema

CLE is a marked hyperinflation state occurring in one or more lobes of the lung (Shanmugam et al., 2005; Langston, 2003). The etiology of CLE is unclear. In most cases, no airway anomaly is identified (Olutoye, Coleman, Hubbard, & Adzick, 2000). In approximately half of the cases, there is an intraluminal bronchial obstruction caused by abnormal mucosal folds, bronchial stenosis, bronchial kinking, or bronchomalacia from a cartilage deficiency (Horak et al., 2003). The congenital deficiency of bronchial cartilage allows air to enter the affected area on inspiration, where it is trapped when the abnormally flaccid bronchial walls collapse on expiration. Massive air trapping and overdistention leave the lobe physiologically useless and

causes compression atelectasis of the ipsilateral lobe or lobes. The overdistended lobe may also push the mediastinum toward the opposite side, causing compression atelectasis of the other lung and interfering with venous return to the heart (Hendren & McKee, 1966) and cardiac output. Another theory is that a lesion, such as a redundant bronchial fold or mucus plug, acts as an intraluminal obstruction or "one way valve," again allowing air to enter but not to leave (Kravitz, 1994).

CLE is primarily a condition of early infancy, usually presenting at birth and rarely seen after 6 months of age. Symptoms may be mild to severe, ranging from slight wheezing and increased respiratory rate to respiratory distress (Wansaicheong & Ong, 1999; Hendren & McKee, 1966). Cardiac defects are the most common congenital anomaly associated with lobar emphysema (Buntain et al., 1974; Hendren & McKee). In infants old enough to crawl and put objects in their mouth, foreign body aspiration is considered in the differential diagnosis.

Olutoye, Coleman, Hubbard, and Adzick (2000) reported on two cases of CLE identified on prenatal ultrasound and fetal magnetic resonance imaging. The mass in both fetuses regressed in utero and became indistinguishable from adjacent normal lung tissue. Both infants developed respiratory distress with significant air trapping in the neonatal period, requiring lobectomy.

CLE has been diagnosed on prenatal ultrasound (Olutoye et al., 2000; Wansaicheong & Ong, 1999). It may appear on a plain chest film as a hyperexpanded and hyperlucent area in the lung (Hendren & McKee, 1966) or as a radiopaque mass due to delayed clearance of lung fluid from the affected lobe (Olutoye et al.). Bronchoscopy is necessary in older children to exclude endobronchial masses (Shanmugam et al., 2005).

Controversy exists about the timing and necessity of surgery. Even though a CLE may decrease in size over the course of the pregnancy, prominent air trapping postnatally can occur. The definitive treatment for CLE is lobectomy. Excision of the affected lobes allows normal expansion and ventilation of adjacent lobes previously compressed (Hendren & McKee, 1966; Othersen, 1993). For patients with mild symptoms and those who are asymptomatic, observation is an option the surgeon and patient may choose (Wansaicheong & Ong, 1999; Takeda et al., 1999).

Diagnosis of Congenital Lung Malformations

The increase in routine use of prenatal ultrasonography has resulted in earlier detection of congenital cystic malformations. Once detected, serial monitoring prenatally and continuing postnatally is recommended. Regular monitoring has provided valuable information on the natural history of these lesions and the pathophysiologic features that affect the neonate's outcome. It gives the physician and family information with which they can form a course of management. Large lesions may regress in size. Those that do not regress can lead to a variety of secondary problems, including mediastinal shift, hypoplasia of normal lung tissue, polyhydramnios, cardiovascular compromise, and the development of nonimmune hydrops (Adzick et al., 2003). Adzick, Flake, and Crombleholme (2003) found that prognosis depended primarily on the size of the lung mass and the physiologic changes in the neonate as a result of the mass such as the development of hydrops fetalis (refer to Chapter 11).

Congenital lung malformations not diagnosed antenatally are generally recognized in the first 6 months of life. Neonates present with symptoms of respiratory distress, tachypnea, cyanosis, and dyspnea, from a space-occupying lesion. In children, the common symptoms include fever, cough, stridor, recurrent pulmonary infections, or persistent radiographic abnormalities (Horak et al., 2003). Bronchogenic cysts and intralobar pulmonary sequestrations are more common diagnoses of late presentation. Diagnosis in infants and children can generally be made on the basis of symptoms and chest radiography. Computed tomography, magnetic resonance imaging, or Doppler ultrasonography may also be used to evaluate the lesion (Aktogu, Yunca, Halilcolar, Ermete, & Buduneli, 1996; Hemanz-Schulman, 1993; Schwartz & Ramachandran, 1997). A definitive diagnosis of the lesion may not occur in some cases until after excision. An accurate diagnosis may be of lesser importance for surgical treatment than for anatomic definition (dell' Agnola et al., 1996).

Hydrops Fetalis

Hydrops fetalis is generally defined as "the presence of fetal subcutaneous tissue edema accompanied by serous effusion(s) in one or more body cavities" (Cassady, 2005). The edema is generalized, not dependent, as in adults, because the fetus is essentially weightless. Fetal hydrops was once believed to be the consequence of maternal isoimmunization of fetal blood group antigens foreign to the mother, such as those in the Rhesus (Rh) family. Later, factors other than isoimmune hemolytic disease were identified as causes of hydrops. Nonimmune hydrops fetalis refers to the occurrence of hydrops without hematologic evidence of fetomaternal blood group incompatibility. The nonimmune type has been recognized in the presence of cardiac anomalies, renal disease, gastrointestinal disorders, and chromosomal anomalies. It also occurs when there is compression of venous return and cardiac output by a mass as in CCAM, pulmonary sequestration, and CDH (Rodriguez et al., 2005).

When hydrops is present in conjunction with a congenital lung malformation, the probability of in utero or neonatal death is great and fetal intervention may be indicated (Adzick et al., 1993; Brown, Lewis, Brouillette, Hilman, & Brown, 1995; Bullard & Harrison, 1995). In the absence of fetal hydrops, many of these infants can easily be carried to term and ultimately do well.

Treatment

In the presence of nonimmune hydrops associated with a congenital lung lesion, fetal death often occurs. If the fetus is less than 32 weeks, an intrauterine intervention may be an option. Interventions with some reported success include fetal thoracentesis, thoracoamniotic shunting, or surgical resection of the enlarged pulmonary lobe. Thoracentesis has demonstrated some success, but the fluid may reaccumulate (Brown et al., 1995). In centers where thoracoamniotic catheters were used, some were successful, whereas others found the catheters difficult to place and reported limited long-term decompression. Resection of the mass in utero is also occasionally successful with resolution of hydrops, return of the mediastinum to the midline, and impressive in utero growth of the lung (Adzick et al., 1993; Bullard & Harrison, 1995).

After confirmation of the diagnosis, additional evaluation includes amniocentesis or percutaneous umbilical blood sampling to exclude chromosomal anomalies and a fetal echocardiogram to assess for fetal heart disease. If the fetus is greater than 32 weeks, early delivery and ex utero resection is advised (Bullard & Harrison, 1995).

In congenital lung malformations diagnosed after the neonatal period, treatment varies. In general, patients who initially present with symptoms undergo surgical excision. However, the treatment for asymptomatic patients is controversial (Shanmugam et al., 2005).

Many authors express concern over the potential for complications when surgical excision is postponed, including compression of adjacent tissue and organs, infection with risk of rupture and hemorrhage, recurrence in the case of segmental resection, and development of malignancy (Shanmugam et al., 2005; Aktogu et al., 1996; dell' Agnola et al., 1996; Gharagozloo, Dausmann, McReynolds, Sanderson, & Helmers, 1995; Nobuhara et al., 1997; Schwartz & Ramachandran, 1997). Other authors state that monitoring asymptomatic patients is acceptable, citing cases of infants and children who remain asymptomatic (Bromley, Parad, Estroff, & Benacerraf, 1995). However, because congenital malformations are rare and most are removed early, the true natural history of unresected malformations is unclear.

Congenital Diaphragmatic Hernia

Anatomy and Physiology

The diaphragm is a dome-shaped fibromuscular sheet that separates the thoracic and abdominal cavities. Development of the diaphragm begins in the 4th week of gestation.

> *"The normal diaphragm is composed of several components, including the septum transversum, which forms the central tendon; the pleuroperitoneal membrane, which forms the dorsolateral portion; the intercostal muscle group which forms the posterior lateral muscle; and the dorsal crura, which is formed from the esophageal mesentery. By week 7, these peritoneal folds extend medially to fuse centrally, with further muscularization occurring over time"*

> (Katz, Wiswell, & Baumgart, 1998).

CDHs occur when the diaphragm develops abnormally, resulting in an opening or defect between the thorax and the abdomen. The factors that contribute to the abnormal development remain unclear. The defect may be a small slit or a total absence of the diaphragm (de Lorimier, 1993). Stomach, liver, and/or intestines are able to enter the chest through the defect during early stages of lung development. The compression of the abdominal organs on the developing lung buds is believed to be the reason for abnormal lung growth or pulmonary hypoplasia (Gosche, Islam, & Boulanger, 2005). The lungs have fewer bronchial divisions than normal, and there is a deficiency in the alveolar number. Because the pulmonary arterial tree develops at the same time as the airways, the growth of the arterial tree is also affected by the mass in the chest. There is a decrease in the pulmonary vasculature, and the pulmonary arteries have an abnormally thick muscularis (de Lorimier). Although the vascular and bronchial abnormalities are more severe on the side of the defect, lung development on the contralateral side is affected by pressure from a shift of the mediastinum (Katz et al., 1998). These features are the cause of hypoxemia and persistent pulmonary hypertension postnatally. They are the primary reason for the high morbidity and mortality associated with CDH (Gosche et al.).

Incidence and Diagnosis

CDH occurs in 1 in 3,300 live births (Katz et al., 1998) and 1 in 2,200 births when stillbirths are included (de Lorimier, 1993). It is more common in males and accounts for 8% of all major congenital anomalies (Hekmatnia, 2003). The left-sided posterolateral hernia or Bochdalek hernia occurs in approximately 90% of the cases. Less common is the Morgagni hernia, occurring in 5% to 10% of the cases. This is an anterior midline hernia through the sternocostal hiatus of the diaphragm. Most of these occur on the right side (Hekmatnia).

The diagnosis of CDH is often made using prenatal ultrasound when loops of bowel are identified in the thoracic cavity (Doyle & Lally, 2004). Additional evaluation to identify associated malformations and chromosomal abnormalities can then take place. Prenatal diagnosis allows for early consultation with the family regarding therapeutic options and expectations. Delivery should be planned at a center experienced in the use of inhaled nitric oxide, high-frequency ventilation, and extracorporeal membrane oxygenation (ECMO) (Moya & Lally, 2005).

Associated Anomalies

The number of infants with coexisting major anomalies ranges between 37% and 47% (Colvin, Bower, Dickinson, & Sokol, 2005). The Bagolan et al.'s (2004) study found cardiac anomalies, including patent ductus arteriosus and ventricular septal defects, to be the most common defect associated with CDH. Musculoskeletal anomalies were the second most common association. Anomalies of the genitourinary, gastrointestinal, and central nervous system are also found in infants with CDH (Fauza & Wilson, 1994).

Presentation

Infants with CDH generally develop symptoms of respiratory distress in the first 24 hours of life. High-risk infants are those diagnosed prenatally and those presenting with respiratory distress within 2 hours of birth (Bagolan et al., 2004). Infants in respiratory distress swallow air, which distends the bowel, compressing functioning lung (de Lorimier, 1993). It is important to avoid bag and mask ventilation in the delivery room because it results in additional distention of the stomach and bowel with air, which further compromises pulmonary function (Moya & Lally, 2005). Those with extreme pulmonary hypoplasia and atelectasis from surfactant deficiency develop hypoxemia, hypercarbia, and acidosis, leading to a cycle of pulmonary vasospasm, pulmonary hypertension, right-to-left shunting of blood, and worsening hypoxemia, hypercarbia, and acidosis. This cycle results in pulmonary hypertension of the newborn and death if it is not quickly interrupted (Breaux et al., 1995). The abdomen, devoid of abdominal viscera, is often flat or scaphoid; bowel sounds may be heard in the chest; and the heart sounds may be displaced.

The clinical picture of CDH in children who present later in life is a combination of respiratory and gastrointestinal symptoms. Because of its rarity and the great variability of symptoms, late diagnosis CDH can be difficult. Chest x-ray study supplemented by upper gastrointestinal series to confirm the presence of abdominal viscera in the chest is the most common study used to make a diagnosis.

Baglaj and Dorobisz (2005) reviewed 349 cases of CDH presenting after the neonatal period, reported in the literature before 2003. Before the diagnosis of CDH, 56 (16%) of the children had radiologic studies relevant to the diagnosis of CDH that were interpreted as normal. The studies include chest x-ray, barium enema, abdominal radiography, and upper gastrointestinal study. In 16 asymptomatic children, the diagnosis was made on chest x-ray study performed for another reason, and in four children, it was found incidentally during an operation. Fourteen children in the series died of complications related to CDH.

Treatment

CDH is a complex problem of pulmonary hypoplasia and pulmonary hypertension. Infants with CDH often have persistent pulmonary hypertension of the newborn (PPHN). A variety of respiratory therapies are used to manage PPHN and pulmonary hypoplasia associated with CDH, including conventional ventilation, nitric oxide, high-frequency oscillation ventilation, and ECMO.

Nitric oxide is a vasodilator that is highly selective to the pulmonary vasculature. It has been effective in infants with pulmonary hypertension and respiratory failure but has not proved helpful in infants with CDH (Smith, Jesudason, Featherstone, Corbett, & Losty, 2005; Elbourne, Field, & Mugford, 2005).

High-frequency oscillation ventilation is another mode of treatment for infants with respiratory distress. Although infants with respiratory distress syndrome or pneumonia respond favorably, the benefit of high-frequency oscillation ventilation in the treatment of infants with CDH is unclear (Bohn, Pearl, Irish, & Glick, 1996; Smith et al., 2005).

The traditional treatment for PPHN in all infants, including those with CDH, was hyperventilation. This treatment often resulted in significant pulmonary barotrauma (Bohn et al., 1996). Although the best mode of ventilation has not yet been proved, avoiding iatrogenic barotrauma as a treatment strategy has resulted in an improved survival rate (Bagolan et al., 2004). In 1985, Wung, James, Kilchevsky, and James published a study that demonstrated successful treatment of persistent pulmonary hypertension of the newborn with pressure-limited venti-

lation and permissive hypercapnia. The goal is to maintain preductal oxygen saturation at greater than 90%, ignoring postductal saturations and hypercarbia (Katz et al., 1998). Bagolan and colleagues (2004) found gentle ventilation and permissive hypercarbia increased the survival and decreased the morbidity in infants with high-risk CDH.

ECMO is a form of cardiopulmonary bypass that allows rest for the heart and lungs by allowing oxygen and carbon dioxide exchange to occur mechanically outside the body. It is effective for infants in severe but reversible hypoxemic respiratory distress that occurs from persistent pulmonary hypertension, meconium aspiration, and sepsis (Khan & Lally, 2005). In CDH, the hypoxemic respiratory distress is the result of pulmonary hypertension and pulmonary hypoplasia. Although hypertension is potentially reversible, the hypoplasia may not be, depending on its severity.

In the 1980s, infants with CDH underwent emergent surgical repair, and ECMO was used for those who developed severe hypoxemia after surgery. With the understanding that surgery could be delayed, the use of ECMO changed to a component of preoperative stabilization. ECMO is generally reserved for infants who have failed to respond to maximal medical management. However, with the recognition of the significance of ventilator-induced lung injury in CDH, some centers now institute ECMO earlier than in the past to avoid barotrauma (Khan & Lally, 2005). There are so many variables among centers in patient selection, criteria for use, and patient management before and after ECMO, however, that it is difficult to determine the true affect of ECMO. A combined review of five ECMO centers of infants who were stabilized with ECMO and repaired on ECMO showed a 43% survival rate (Doyle & Lally, 2004). The Extracorporeal Life Support Organization reports a 58% survival rate in infants with CDH treated with ECMO.

Surgical repair of the defect immediately after birth was one of the first approaches used for the treatment of CDH. It seemed logical that adequate ventilation required removal of the abdominal viscera from the thoracic cavity. However, not all centers found a significant difference in survival between infants who underwent early repair within the first 24 hours after birth and those whose surgery was delayed more than 24 hours after birth (Rozmairek, Qureshi, Cassidy, Ford, & Hackam, 2004). The hypoplastic lungs and associated pulmonary hypertension are the cause of respiratory distress more so than the defect and pressure from the visceral organs. Therefore, optimizing the physiologic status of the neonate is more important than the timing of the surgical repair (Rozmiarek et al.).

Operative repair through a subcostal incision allows access to the diaphragm for a primary repair or patch closure after visceral reduction. A primary repair is performed when possible, and a muscle flap or synthetic patch is used when the defect is too large for primary repair. The repair is influenced by the size of the infant, the size of the defect, and the size of the abdominal cavity (Bohn et al., 1996).

In some situations, CDH is amenable to fetal surgery (refer to Chapter 11 for more information).

Outcome

The reported mortality rate associated with CDH varies widely. Published reports often detail specific patient populations, such as neonates referred to a tertiary pediatric surgical center, and may not include the infants who died before arrival at the center. These reports also do not include terminated pregnancies or cases of in-utero fetal demise (Colvin et al., 2005). The mortality rate in comprehensive, population-based studies remains high, 62% to 68% (Stege, Fenton, & Jaffray, 2003; Colvin et al.). A significant number of cases succumb either prenatally or in the first few hours of life. Rozmiarek, Qureshi, Cassidy, Ford, and Hackam (2004) report a 64% survival of live born infants. Generally, the survival rate is highest for those infants born with an isolated diaphragmatic lesion, lower for those with CDH and other nonchromosomal anomalies, and approaching zero in infants with chromosomal defects (Langham et al., 1996). The presence of cardiac and renal dysfunction has a significant negative affect on outcome (Rozmairek et al.). Wilson, Fauza, Lund, Benacerraf, & Hendren (1994) reviewed 183 cases of CDH and found no correlation between prenatal diagnoses of isolated CDH and outcome, even when the diagnosis occurred before 25 weeks' gestation. Infants with CDH and an associated congenital anomaly, especially a cardiac anomaly, fared poorly. The authors believe that infants with an associated anomaly are more likely to be diagnosed early because of the accompanying congenital malformation and that these additional risk factors lead to a poor outcome (Colvin et al., 2005).

Long-Term Consequences

Survivors of CDH have a significant morbidity, often resulting in prolonged hospitalization and the need for gastrostomy tubes and oxygen therapy. The follow-up studies on infants with CDH reveal a multitude of issues that vary in severity and frequency. The most common problems associated with CDH are gastroesophageal reflux, chronic lung disease necessitating oxygen therapy, and failure to thrive requiring gastrostomy placement (Katz et al., 1998;

Downard et al., 2003). Other complications include adhesive bowel obstruction, recurrence of the hernia particularly in patients with patch repairs, and neurodevelopmental delays (Katz et al.).

Gastroesophageal reflux is evident in 62% to 80% of infants at the time of discharge (D'Agostino et al., 1995; Kieffer et al., 1995). The etiology of gastroesophageal reflux in children with CDH is multifactorial, including esophageal dilation, malposition of the stomach with a widened angle of His, a shorter intraabdominal portion of the esophagus, and increased intraabdominal pressure resulting from reintroduction of the herniated viscera into the infant's abdominal cavity (Kieffer et al.). Persistent feeding problems are also common. These infants tire easily, have inefficient suck, and may completely refuse oral feedings. Chronic lung disease, chest deformity, gastroesophageal reflux, esophagitis, and hypotonia all play a role in prolonged feeding difficulties (D'Agostino, 1997).

Chronic lung disease has been described in approximately one third of children with CDH. Prolonged artificial ventilation and residual lung hypoplasia are the cause of persistent lung problems (D'Agostino, 1997; Ijsselstijn, Tibboels, Hop, Molenaar, & de Jongste, 1997).

Routine developmental assessments are necessary to identify developmental delays early, and primary care physicians should refer these children for treatment. Delays in gross motor skills are more common than problems with cognitive skills (D'Agostino, 1997).

■ Conclusion

Congenital lung malformations are an uncommon but interesting finding in the pediatric population. Significant acute and chronic issues related to the disease and its treatment, in particular, affect infants with CDH. The outcome for the family is based on the surgical care and the treatment, teaching, and support the family receives from the nursing staff.

■ Acknowledgments

I would like to thank Dr. C. Stolar, Dr. T. Weiner, and Kerri Keller, APN, for their assistance with editing this chapter.

■ Educational Materials

APSNA invites you to download the following diagnosis-related teaching tool for Chapter 16, Congenital Lung Malformations: Thoracotomy. This teaching tool is available at the APSNA Web site (www.apsna.org) and the Jones and Bartlett Web site (www.jbpub.com). All teaching materials are available in English and Spanish and are free of charge. APSNA encourages their use for your patients and families.

References

Adzick, S., Flake, A., & Crombleholme, T. (2003). Management of congenital lung lesions. *Seminars in Pediatric Surgery, 12*, 10–16.

Adzick, N., Harrison, M., Crombleholme, T., Flake, A., & Howell, L. (1998). Fetal lung lesions: Management and outcome. *American Journal of Obstetrics and Gynecology, 179*, 884–889.

Adzick, S., Harrison, M., Flake, A., Howell, L., Golbus, M., Filly, R., et al. (1993). Fetal surgery for cystic adenomatoid malformation of the lung. *Journal of Pediatric Surgery, 28*, 806–812.

Aktogu, S., Yunca, G., Halilcolar, H., Ermete, S., & Buduneli, T. (1996). Bronchogenic cysts: Clinicopathological presentation and treatment. *European Respiratory Journal, 9*, 2017–2021.

Ayed, A., & Owayed, A. (2003). Pulmonary resection in infants for congenital pulmonary malformation. *Chest, 124*, 98–101.

Baglaj, M., & Dorobisz, U. (2005). Late-presenting congenital diaphragmatic hernia in children: A literature review. *Pediatric Radiology, 35*, 478–488.

Bagolan, G., Casaccia, G., Crescenzi, F., Nahom, A., Trucchi, A., & Giorlandino, C. (2004). Impact of a current treatment protocol on outcome of high-risk congenital diaphragmatic hernia. *Journal of Pediatric Surgery, 39*, 313–318.

Bohn, D., Pearl, R., Irish, M., & Glick, P. (1996). Postnatal management of congenital diaphragmatic hernia. *Clinics in Perinatology, 23*, 843–872.

Breaux, C., Simmons, M., & Georgeson, K. (1995). Management of infants with congenital diaphragmatic hernia with ECMO. In J. Zwischenberger & R. Bartlett (Eds.), *Extracorporeal cardiopulmonary support in critical care.* Ann Arbor, MI: Extracorporeal Life Support Organization.

Bromley, B., Parad, R., Estroff, J., & Benacerraf, B. (1995). Fetal lung masses: Prenatal course and outcome. *Journal of Ultrasound in Medicine, 14*, 927–936.

Brown, M., Lewis, D., Brouillette, R., Hilman, B., & Brown, E. (1995). Successful prenatal management of hydrops, caused by congenital cystic adenomatoid malformation, using serial aspirations. *Journal of Pediatric Surgery, 30*, 1098–1099.

Bullard, K., & Harrison, M. (1995). Before the horse is out of the barn: Fetal surgery for hydrops. *Seminars in Perinatology, 19*, 462–473.

Buntain, W. L., Isaacs, H., Payne, V. C., Lindesmith, G. G., & Rosenkrantz, J. G. (1974). Lobar emphysema, cystic adenomatoid malformation, pulmonary sequestration, and bronchogenic cyst in infancy and childhood: A clinical group. *Journal of Pediatric Surgery, 9*, 85–93.

Cassady, G. (2005). Hydrops fetalis. Retrieved January 5, 2006, from http://www.emedicine.com/ped/topic1042.htm

Colvin, J., Bower, C., Dickinson, J., & Sokol, J. (2005). Outcomes of congenital diaphragmatic hernia: A population-based study in western Australia. *Pediatrics, 116*(3), 356–363.

Crombleholme, T., Coleman, B., Hedrick, H., Liechty, K., Howell, L., Flake, A., et al. (2002). Cystic adenomatoid malformation volume ratio predicts outcome in prenatally diagnosed cystic adenomatoid malformation of the lung. *Journal of Pediatric Surgery, 37*, 331–338.

D'Agostino, J. (1997). Congenital diaphragmatic hernia: What happens after discharge? *Maternal Child Nursing, 22*, 263–266.

D'Agostino, J., Bembaum, J., Gerdes, M., Schwartz, I., Coburn, C., Hirschi, R., et al. (1995). Outcome for infants with congenital diaphragmatic hernia requiring extracorporeal membrane oxygenation: The first year. *Journal of Pediatric Surgery, 30*, 10–15.

dell' Agnola, C., Tadini, B., Mosca, F., Colnaghi, M., & Wesley, J. (1996). Advantages of prenatal diagnosis and early surgery for congenital cystic disease of the lung. *Journal of Perinatal Medicine, 24*, 621–631.

de Lorimier, A. (1993). Diaphragmatic hernia. In K. Ashcraft & T. Holder (Eds.), *Pediatric surgery* (2nd ed., p. 230). Philadelphia: W.B. Saunders.

Downard, C., Jaksic, T., Garza, A. D., Nemes, L., Jennings, R., & Wilson, J. (2003). Analysis of an improved survival rate for congenital diaphragmatic hernia. *Journal of Pediatric Surgery, 38*, 729–732.

Doyle, N., & Lally, K. (2004). The CDH study group and advances in the clinical care of the patient with congenital diaphragmatic hernia. *Seminars in Perinatology, 28*, 174–184.

Elbourne, D., Field, D., & Mugford, M. (2005). Extracorporeal membrane oxygenation for severe respiratory failure in newborn infants. Cochrane Library. Retrieved January 22, 2006, from http://www.cochrane.org/reviews/en/ab001340.html

Evans, M. (1996). Hydrops fetalis and pulmonary sequestration. *Journal of Pediatric Surgery, 31*, 761–764.

Fauza, D., & Wilson, J. M. (1994). Congenital diaphragmatic hernia and associated anomalies. *Journal of Pediatric Surgery, 29*, 1113–1117.

Gharagozloo, F., Dausmann, M., McReynolds, S., Sanderson, D., & Helmers, R. (1995). Recurrent bronchogenic pseudocyst 24 years after incomplete excision. *Chest, 108*, 880–883.

Gosche, J. R., Islam, S., & Boulanger, S. C. (2005). Congenital diaphragmatic hernia: Searching for answers. *American Journal of Surgery, 190*, 324–332.

Hekmatnia, A. (2003). Congenital diaphragmatic hernia. Retrieved January 20, 2006, from www.emedicine.com/radio/topic187.htm

Hemanz-Schulman, M. (1993). Cysts and cystlike lesions of the lung. *Radiologic Clinics of North America, 31*, 631–649.

Hendren, H., & McKee, D. (1966). Lobar emphysema of infancy. *Journal of Pediatric Surgery, 1*, 24–39.

Horak, E., Bodner, J., Gassner, I., Schmid, T., Simma, B., Grassl, G., et al. (2003). Congenital cystic lung disease: Diagnostic and therapeutic considerations. *Clinical Pediatrics, 42*, 251–261.

Ijsselstijn, H., Tibboels, D., Hop, W., Molenaar, J., & de Jongste, J. (1997). Long-term pulmonary sequelae in children with congenital diaphragmatic hernia. *American Journal of Respiratory Critical Care Medicine, 155*, 174–180.

Jona, J. (1995). Extramediastinal bronchogenic cysts in children. *Pediatric Dermatology, 12*, 304–306.

Katz, A., Wiswell, T., & Baumgart, S. (1998). Contemporary controversies in the management of congenital diaphragmatic hernia. *Clinics in Perinatology, 25*, 219–248.

Khan, A., & Lally, K. (2005). The role of extracorporeal membrane oxygenation in the management of infants with congenital diaphragmatic hernia. *Seminars in Perinatology, 29*, 118–122.

Kieffer, J., Sapin, E., Berg, A., Beaudoin, S., Bargy, F., & Helardot, P. (1995). Gastroesophageal reflux after repair of congenital diaphragmatic hernia. *Journal of Pediatric Surgery, 30*, 1330–1333.

King, S. J., Pilling, D. W., & Walkinshaw, S. (1995). Fetal echogenic lung lesions: Prenatal ultrasound diagnosis and outcome. *Pediatric Radiology, 25*, 208–210.

Kravitz, R. (1994). Congenital malformations of the lung. *Pediatric Clinics of North America, 41*, 453–472.

Lackner, R., Thompson, A., Rikkers, L., & Galbraith, A. (1996). Cystic adenomatoid malformation involving an entire lung in a 22-year-old woman. *Annals of Thoracic Surgery, 61*, 1827–1829.

Langham, M., Kays, D., Ledbetter, D., Frentzen, B., Sanford, L., & Richards, D. (1996). Congenital diaphragmatic hernia: Epidemiology and outcome. *Clinics in Perinatology, 23*, 671–688.

Langston, C. (2003). New concepts in the pathology of congenital lung malformations. *Seminars in Pediatric Surgery, 12,* 17–37.

MacDonald, M., Forte, V., Cutz, E., & Crysdale, W. (1996). Congenital cystic adenomatoid malformation of the lung referred as "Airway Foreign Body." *Archives of Otolaryngology and Head and Neck Surgery, 122,* 333–336.

MacGillivray, R., Harrison, M., Goldstein, R., & Adzick, S. (1993). Disappearing fetal lung lesions. *Journal of Pediatric Surgery, 28,* 1321–1325.

McLean, S., Pfeifer, J., Siegel, M., Jensen, E., Schuler, P., Hirsch, R., et al. (2004). Congenital cystic adenomatoid malformation connected to an extralobar pulmonary sequestration in the contralateral chest: Common origin? *Journal of Pediatric Surgery, 39,* 313–317.

Moya, F., & Lally, K. (2005). Evidence-based management of infants with congenital diaphragmatic hernia. *Seminars in Perinatology, 29,* 112–117.

Nobuhara, K., Gorski, Y., LaQuaglia, M., & Shamberger, R. (1997). Bronchogenic cysts and esophageal duplications: Common origins and treatment. *Journal of Pediatric Surgery, 32,* 1408–1413.

Olutoye, O., Coleman, B., Hubbard, A., & Adzick, S. (2000). Prenatal diagnosis and management of congenital lobar emphysema. *Journal of Pediatric Surgery, 35,* 792–795.

Othersen, B. (1993). Pulmonary and bronchial malformations. In K. Ashcraft & T. Holder (Eds.), *Pediatric surgery* (2nd ed., pp. 176–187). Philadelphia: W.B. Saunders.

Ribet, M., Copin, M., & Gosselin, B. (1996). Bronchogenic cysts of the lung. *Annals of Thoracic Surgery, 61,* 1636–1640.

Rodgers, B., Harman, K., & Johnson, A. (1986). Bronchopulmonary foregut malformations: The spectrum of anomalies. *Annals of Surgery, 5,* 517–524.

Rodriguez, M., Bruce, J., Jimenez, X., Romaguera, R., Bancalari, E., Garcia, O., et al. (2005). Nonimmune hydrops fetalis in the liveborn: Series of 32 autopsies. *Pediatric and Developmental Pathology, 8,* 369–378.

Rozmiarek, A., Qureshi, F., Cassidy, L., Ford, H., & Hackam, D. (2004). Factors influencing survival in newborns with congenital diaphragmatic hernia: The relative role of timing of surgery. *Journal of Pediatric Surgery, 39*(6), 821–824.

Savic, B., Birtel, F., Tholen, W., Funke, H., & Knoche, R. (1979). Lung sequestration: Report of seven cases and review of 540 published cases. *Thorax, 34,* 96–101.

Schwartz, M., & Ramachandran, R. (1997). Congenital malformations of the lung and mediastinum: A quarter century of experience from a single institution. *Journal of Pediatric Surgery, 32,* 44–47.

Seeds, J., & Azizkhan, R. (1990). *Congenital malformations: Antenatal diagnosis, perinatal management, and counseling.* Rockville, MD: Aspen.

Shanmugam, G., MacArthur, K., & Pollock, J. (2005). Congenital lung malformation—antenatal and postnatal evaluation and management. *European Journal of Cardio-Thoracic Surgery, 27,* 45–52.

Smith, N., Jesudason, E., Featherstone, N., Corbett, H., & Losty, P. (2005). Recent advances in congenital diaphragmatic hernia. *Archives of Diseases in Children, 90,* 426–428.

Stege, G., Fenton, A., & Jaffray, B. (2003). Nihilism in the 1990's: The true mortality of congenital diaphragmatic hernia. *Pediatrics, 112,* 532–535.

St-Georges, R., Deslauriers, J., Duranceau, A., Vaillancourt, R., Deschamps, C., Beauchamp, G., et al. (1991). Clinical spectrum of bronchogenic cysts of the mediastinum and lung in the adult. *Annals of Thoracic Surgery, 52,* 6–13.

Stocker, J. T., Madewell, J. E., & Drake, R. M. (1977). Congenital cystic adenomatoid malformation of the lung. *Human Pathology, 8,* 155–171.

Takeda, S., Miyoshi, S., Inoue, M., Omori, K., Okumura, M., Yoon, H., et al. (1999). Clinical spectrum of congenital cystic disease of the lung in children. *European Journal Cardiothoracic Surgery, 15,* 11–17.

Usui, N., Kamata, S., Sawai, T., Kamiyama, M., Okuyama, H., Kubota, A., et al. (2004). Outcome predictors for infants with cystic lung disease. *Journal of Pediatric Surgery, 39,* 603–606.

Wansaicheong, G. K., & Ong, C. L. (1999). Congenital lobar emphysema: Antenatal diagnosis and follow up. *Australasian Radiology, 43,* 243–245.

Wilson, J., Fauza, D., Lund, D., Benacerraf, B., & Hendren, H. (1994). Antenatal diagnosis of isolated congenital diaphragmatic hernia is not an indicator of outcome. *Journal of Pediatric Surgery, 29,* 815–819.

Wung, J., James, S., Kilchevsky, E., & James, E. (1985). Management of infants with severe respiratory failure and persistence of the fetal circulation, without hyperventilation. *Pediatrics, 76,* 488–494.

Common Thoracic Problems

By Frances T. Gill

Diseases of the thorax in children pose diagnostic and interventional challenges for pediatric surgical teams. Although the etiology of these diseases may be congenital, traumatic, or infectious, the proposed treatment plan must be individualized to meet the clinical needs of each patient.

■ Empyema

The pleural cavity is composed of two membranes that maintain close contact with each other: the visceral pleura, covering the lung, and the parietal pleura, lining the thoracic wall. Five to 15 mL of pleural fluid is present that reduces the surface tension and allows for easy expansion and recoil of the lungs. Although fluid collections greater than 25 cc are defined as effusions, patients may accumulate up to 300 cc in the pleural space before symptoms become evident. If the fluid becomes infected, it is known as *empyema*. Pneumonia is the most frequent cause of empyema in children, although chest trauma, neoplastic processes, immunodeficiency, or infection in the retroesophageal or mediastinal space may also predispose the child to the formation of empyema (Gates, Caniano, Hayes, & Arca, 2004).

Pneumonia is a common childhood disease, with an incidence of between 1.0 and 4.5 cases per 100 children annually. Most cases are viral, but bacterial infection is responsible in 20% to 30% of patients (Schultz et al., 2004). Parapneumonic effusions occur in at least 40% of bacterial pneumonias, with up to 60% of these effusions resulting in the formation of empyema (Schultz et al.). During the early course of the disease, the pleura becomes inflamed and the leakage of protein, fluid, and white blood cells ensues. As this inflammatory response continues, bacteria invade the fluid, and a purulent exudate or empyema forms.

The incidence of empyema complicating community-acquired pneumonia is increasing and is causing significant childhood morbidity (Jaffe & Balfour-Lynn, 2005). The most common causative agent of complicated pneumonia in children has been *Streptococcus pneumoniae*. With the advent of the pneumococcal conjugate vaccine (Prevnar©; Wyeth-Lederle) in 2000, this incidence has been declining. Instead, group A *streptococcus*, *Staphylococcus aureus*, *Pseudomonas aeruginosa* and methicillin-resistant *S. aureus* (MRSA) as the common agents of complicated parapneumonic effusion in children have emerged (Schultz et al., 2004; Alfaro, Fergie, & Purcell, 2005; Barbato et al., 2003).

There are three defined stages in the development of empyema: (1) the acute or exudative stage is characterized by thin serous fluid with minimal debris; (2) the fibrinopurulent stage is associated with thicker fluid and thick fibrin strands; (3) the organizing stage is characterized by a thick fibrous peel and ultimately, scar formation (Gates, Caniano, et al., 2004).

Children with complicated pneumonias usually present with a history of fever, cough, pleuritic chest pain, general malaise, loss of appetite, emesis, and abdominal discomfort. Upon initial assessment, the patient "appears sick," often sitting quietly in the bed with pale skin, extreme lethargy, and variable degrees of respiratory distress. Physical findings can also include fever, tachypnea with nasal flaring and substernal retractions, tachycardia, dry mucus membranes, decreased or absent breath sounds, and a distended abdomen. Dehydration due to poor intake and increased insensible fluid losses from tachypnea and fever is common. Mild-to-moderate nutritional deficiency may be evidenced by a low serum albumin level (Gates, Hogan, Weinstein, & Arca, 2004).

The child should be placed in a position of comfort while interventions are performed efficiently. Parents need to be actively involved with the care team from the start, lending reassurance and support to their child. Management begins with vital signs, including pulse oximetry; intravenous access; blood testing for complete blood count, electrolyte panel, albumin, and possible blood gases; blood/urine culture; and posteroanterior/lateral chest x-ray study. This film may highlight an infiltrate in the area of the pneumonia, a fluid collection, or even a complete "white out." Tracheal deviation is less common (Fig. 17-1). An abdominal film often demonstrates dilated loops of bowel consistent with ileus.

Although there are varied opinions related to the management of empyema, the goals of treatment are to treat the pneumonia with broad-spectrum antibiotics (e.g., Augmentin, cefotaxime) and chest physiotherapy, drain the fluid, and optimize the expansion of the lung. Initially, the patient is given broad-spectrum antibiotics, maintenance intravenous fluids, and supplemental oxygen as needed. Vancomycin is the gold standard therapy for treating serious infections caused by MRSA, whereas clindamycin is a valuable agent for empyema caused by less severe MRSA isolates (Schultz et al., 2004). Currently, there are no clear guidelines that determine the duration of antibiotic therapy for empyema (Gates, Caniano, et al., 2004).

General pediatric surgery, pulmonary, infectious disease, and nutrition consultations may be warranted. Supportive care includes antipyretics and analgesics. Sedatives should be avoided to prevent central nervous system depression with a concomitant decrease in respiratory effort. Fluid and electrolyte balance must be mon-

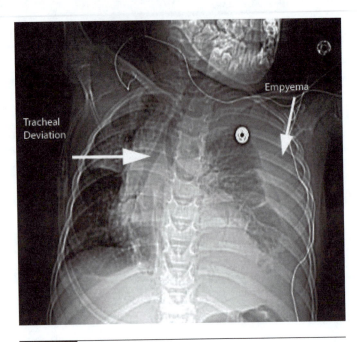

Figure 17-1 Chest x-ray study with tracheal deviation.
(Reprinted with permission by Stephen Dunn, MD.)

itored closely to ensure proper hydration. Bronchodilator therapy does not have a role in the treatment of effusions in children and may potentially worsen their V/Q mismatch, exacerbating hypoxemia (Balfour-Lynn et al., 2005). Serial chest x-ray studies allow the care providers to gauge the progress of the disease. Ultrasound or computed tomographic (CT) scan can provide more definitive information related to the lung and pleural fluid and assist in guiding appropriate treatment (Fig. 17-2).

If there is no improvement or there is worsening of pulmonary function within 48 to 72 hours, then more

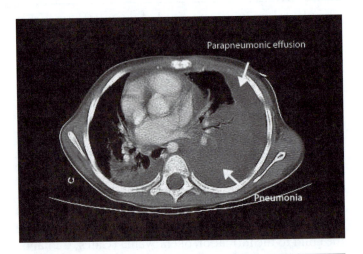

Figure 17-2 Computed tomogram of the chest demonstrating empyema.
(Reprinted with permission by Stephen Dunn, MD.)

aggressive treatment is warranted. Four commonly used strategies are (1) chest tube drainage, (2) chest tube drainage with instillation of fibrinolytics into the pleural cavity, (3) open thoracotomy with decortication, and (4) video-assisted thoracoscopic surgery (VATS).

Chest tube drainage is often used for patients with large pleural effusions and worsening clinical symptoms. Adequate sedation is needed before placement of the tube, and this can be accomplished with ketamine or midazolam and fentanyl in a monitored setting. This should include cardiopulmonary monitoring, pulse oximetry, suction and readily available resuscitative equipment.

The size of the catheter used depends on the characteristics of the fluid to be drained. Pigtail catheters can be used for thin, free-flowing fluid to minimize discomfort for the patient. Thicker fluid needs a larger-bore tube to facilitate adequate drainage. Placement at the 4th or 5th intercostal space at the midaxillary line is common. The tube should be directed posteriorly and superiorly toward the apex of the lung. In severe cases, a second tube may also be inserted in the dependent portion of the pleural cavity to increase drainage. At the time of insertion, a sample of pleural fluid should be collected for cytology, culture, and sensitivity. This helps guide the appropriate antibiotic therapy. A confounding point is that up to 45% of these cultures prove negative because of previous outpatient treatment with antibiotics (Gates, Caniano, et al., 2004).

Securing the chest tube with appropriate suturing, petroleum gauze, and an occlusive dressing is imperative to preventing tube migration and air leakage. A chest x-ray study after insertion confirms whether the tube is in the proper position and that no pneumothorax is present.

The chest tube is attached to a system with three chambers: collection, water seal, and suction control. The collection chamber collects air, fluid, and debris drained from the chest. The water seal chamber acts as a one-way valve to allow air out while preventing it from entering the pleural space. The water level is usually filled to provide for a suction of 20 cm of water. This chamber also allows for the ability to monitor for an air leak. Air leakage is usually a sign of parenchymal injury and usually resolves. Persistent air leak can be due to a bronchopulmonary fistula, disruption of a surgical staple line, perforation of the bronchus or esophagus, or often a leak in the system. To test for an air leak, one first assesses the patency of the tube and the integrity of the occlusive dressing. The suction is turned off. Bubbling in the water seal chamber indicates either a true air leak or a leakage from the collection system. The chest tube is then clamped, and if the leak persists, there is a leak in the collection system; if the leak disappears, then a true anatomic leak exists. During the course of treatment with chest tube drainage, the patient may experience a lower volume of output than is expected, even when the chest x-ray study demonstrates significant fluid retention. Troubleshooting the drainage system should include assessment of the patency of the tube. Kinking of the tubing at the entrance site can occur, thus impeding the free flow of drainage. Obstruction of drainage may also be due to clot or debris clogging the tubing. In this case, gentle milking of the tube may move the substance into the collection chamber.

Removal of the chest tube dressings before tube removal should be avoided. An occlusive dressing at the tube insertion site should always be kept intact and reinforced as needed. Clamps and extra occlusive dressings should be kept at the bedside in the event that the chest tube should inadvertently be dislodged or disconnected. Chest tubes are usually removed when the 24-hour drainage total is below 100 to 200 cc. Before discontinuation of the tube, the child should be given IV pain medication. When possible, the child should be encouraged to perform a Valsalva maneuver, or inhale and hold the breath. In younger or uncooperative patients, coordination with the respiratory patterns at the time of removal is attempted. As the tube is removed, an occlusive dressing is immediately applied to provide a seal. This dressing should be left in place for 72 hours before changing to prevent transfer of air into the pleural space.

Continuation of intravenous antibiotic therapy is a controversial subject. Many clinicians continue until the child is afebrile for at least 48 hours and the chest tube is removed. Others believe that a full 2-week course of antibiotic is warranted. Many patients continue oral antibiotics for 2 to 3 weeks thereafter (Balfour-Lynn et al., 2005).

Increased fibrin deposits with gelatinous fluid can impede drainage and decrease lung expansion, thus leading to a prolonged clinical course (Wells & Havens, 2003). In these cases, direct instillation of fibrinolytics with temporary clamping of the chest tube has proved to be a valuable adjunct to pleural drainage. These drugs should not be used in children with suspected bronchopulmonary fistula or chest tube air leakage because clamping the tube after instillation may lead to tension pneumothorax. The main risk of the use of fibrinolytics is bleeding because there are not standardized dosages for use in children (Gates, Hogan, et al., 2004).

Recently, the agent alteplase (tissue plasminogen activator [tPA]; Genentech, San Francisco, CA) has been widely used for fibrinolysis. Two milligrams in 50 mL of normal saline is instilled into the chest tube and left in place for 1 hour before reconnection to the drainage system with water seal suction. This dose can be repeated every 12 hours based on clinical symptoms. Previously, urokinase was used, but this medication is now unavailable due to manufacturing issues. Streptokinase, once commonly used for fibrinolysis, has limited indication because repeated dosage is contraindicated.

After the administration of alteplase, chest tube output and serial chest x-ray studies are followed up closely (Gates, Hogan, et al., 2004). The child is assessed for improvement of respiratory symptoms, fever, and oxygen utilization. If no improvement is noted within 48 to 72 hours, surgical intervention is an appropriate option.

Surgical intervention is planned for children who have had a lack of clinical or radiologic response to medical management with antibiotics, chest tube drainage, and fibrinolytic therapy (Balfour-Lynne et al., 2005). Open thoracotomy with decortication is an invasive procedure that is reserved for children who present late in their disease process and have complex or chronic empyema with a thick pleural rind (Balfour-Lynn et al.). This approach requires an open chest incision for removal of the pleural collection.

Most commonly today, VATS is performed to remove thick fibrinous material that impedes pleural drainage (Fig. 17-3). A small incision is made in the chest for insertion of the scope, whereas one or two additional instruments are introduced to assist with removal of debris from the pleural cavity (Gates, Caniano, et al., 2004).

Patients who have undergone VATS procedure need careful attention to their respiratory status and their need for supplemental oxygen postoperatively. Vital signs, including pulse oximetry, should be monitored frequently. Encouraging the frequent use of an incentive spirometer will facilitate pulmonary toilet. Positioning the child in semi- to high-Fowler's position provides for comfort and optimal expansion of the lungs.

Attention to the child's nutritional status is important at this stage of illness. Collaboration with the clinical nutritionist is beneficial for determining appropriate feedings to increase the caloric intake for healing purposes.

Chest x-ray studies are obtained to follow the progress of the disease. It is important to acknowledge that the appearance of the film often lags behind the clinical progress of the patient. Marked pleural opacity is usually present on films at discharge from the hospital, which progressively resolves without further intervention within 2 to 16 months (Satish, Bunker, & Seddon, 2003).

The optimal approach in the management of a given patient with an empyema is not well standardized because of a lack of well-controlled clinical trials. However, numerous studies have demonstrated that use of early VATS in appropriate patients results in a significant decrease in hospital length of stay (Gates, Hogan, et al., 2004; Schultz et al., 2004; Gates, Caniano, et al., 2004).

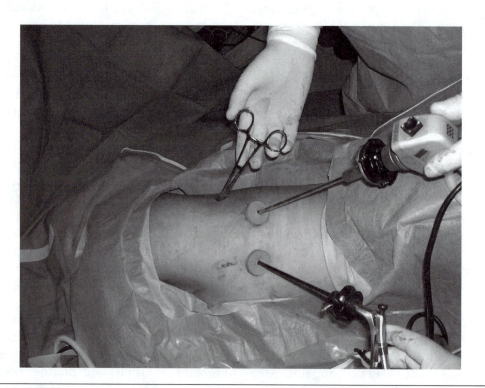

Figure 17-3 Video-assisted thoracic surgery.
(Reprinted with permission by Stephen Dunn, MD.)

Pneumothorax

Pneumothorax is the accumulation of air in the pleural cavity, with secondary lung collapse (Fig. 17-4) (Ozcan, McGahren, & Rodgers, 2003). This condition can occur from a disruption in the surface of the pleura that can be primary or secondary. Patients who sustain primary spontaneous pneumothorax have no history of past lung disease. Often, at the time of diagnosis, a CT scan reveals blebs in the apical portion of the lung. Frequently, patients are tall, lean males, particularly those who smoke (Chan, Clarke, Daniel, Knight, & Seevanayagam, 2001). Secondary spontaneous pneumothorax often occurs in those patients with a history of underlying lung disease. Traumatic pneumothorax can be caused by blunt or penetrating injury. Iatrogenic injury can occur from hospital procedures (e.g., central line placement, mechanical ventilation).

Presenting symptoms vary. A small pneumothorax may not cause significant symptoms. Patients with a larger pneumothorax complain of the sudden onset of stabbing chest pain, often radiating to the shoulder. Complaints of shortness of breath, tachypnea, cyanosis, and inability to inhale deeply are common. On examination, the patient may be apprehensive and have absent or decreased breath sounds on auscultation. A diagnostic chest x-ray study reveals increased lucency and intrapleural air outlining the collapsed lung. Abdominal films may show dilated loops of bowel due to the volume of swallowed air associated with increased respiratory rate or, rarely, pneumoperitoneum. Escape of air into the mediastinal space may reveal palpable crepitus along the chest or neck surfaces and can also be seen on chest x-ray study.

Treatment of pneumothorax depends on the source and the severity of the air leak. The primary goals of treatment are re-expansion of the lung and prevention of recurrences (Ozcan et al., 2003). The use of supplemental humidified oxygen increases the time of resorption of air in the pleural space. Monitoring vital signs closely, including pulse oximetry, is needed. Providing maintenance intravenous fluid prevents dehydration due to insensible losses from an increased respiratory rate. Analgesia to alleviate pleural pain and fever should be offered on a scheduled basis. Serial x-ray studies are often obtained to help guide the treatment plan. A CT scan may be helpful in identifying existing lung disease or the number of apical blebs present.

Small, minimally symptomatic pneumothoraces may resolve without the need for aspiration. Emergent percutaneous needle aspiration of air may be used for patients in significant distress with pain, dyspnea, and hypoxemia. This may be accomplished with insertion of a large-bore intravenous catheter into the second intercostal space and then attached to a stopcock and syringe. If the pneumothorax is clinically significant and associated with hypoxia and tachypnea, a chest tube is necessary. The advent of a percutaneous chest drainage catheter (Thal Quik, Cook Critical Care, Bloomington, IN) uses the Seldinger entry technique, thus avoiding the larger incision needed in standard thoracotomy chest tube placement. This technique is performed by inserting the needle into the 4th or 5th intercostal space while pulling back on the syringe provided. When air or fluid returns, entrance into the thoracic cavity has been accomplished. The syringe is then removed from the needle, and a guidewire is inserted into the chest cavity through the needle. The needle is then removed, a nick is made in the skin with a small blade, and a dilator is passed over the wire until the desired tube size tract is reached. The dilator is then removed over the wire, and the appropriate-sized chest tube is placed. The wire is then removed, and the chest tube is secured and placed to suction. This has proved to be beneficial for the drainage of air and nonloculated fluid collections. Other techniques include placement of a Heimlich valve or pigtail catheter.

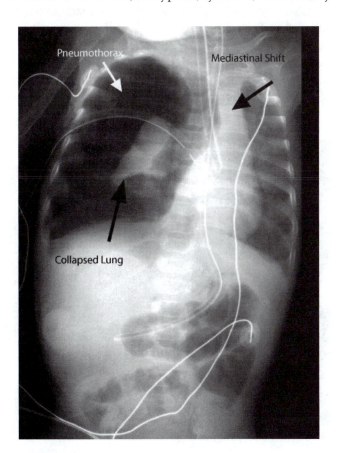

Figure 17-4 Chest x-ray study: pneumothorax.
(Reprinted with permission by Stephen Dunn, MD.)

After a spontaneous pneumothorax, there is a 30% to 75% chance of experiencing a recurrence and a 50% chance of a contralateral occurrence (Rodgers, 2003). There has been controversy related to the timing of surgery for spontaneous pneumothorax. Although VATS with blebectomy and pleurodesis for the first episode of pneumothorax has been recommended by some, more commonly, this procedure is often reserved for patients with recurrence. Early surgery should be considered for patients who have bilateral pneumothoraces, persistent air leak greater than 7 days, severe symptoms, or underlying pulmonary disease (i.e., cystic fibrosis) or blebs on CT scan (Rodgers). The VATS approach enables the surgeon to use a staple to remove the abnormal tissue, followed by mechanical pleurodesis to adhere the lung to the chest wall (Qureshi et al., 2005). Mechanical pleurodesis can be accomplished with a Bovie scratch pad or gauze. These treatment options have significantly decreased the incidence of recurrence in the affected lung, although pneumothorax of the contralateral side may be seen.

■ Pectus Deformities

Pectus deformities include two types of abnormalities of the chest wall: pectus excavatum and the much less common pectus carinatum. In up to 20% of cases, a concomitant musculoskeletal abnormality, such as scoliosis, kyphosis, neurofibromatosis, or myopathy, may be seen. Associated syndromes include Marfan's, Poland's, Pierre Robin, Ehlers-Danlos, or prune-belly (Hebra, 2003).

Pectus Excavatum

Pectus excavatum is due to abnormal growth of the costal cartilage of the chest wall resulting in a sunken appearance of the sternum (Figs. 17-5A and B). This is the most common chest wall deformity, affecting 1 in 1,000 children, with a male to female ratio of 5:1 (Goretsky, Kelly, Croitoru, & Nuss, 2004). Because 46% of patients have a family history of pectus excavatum, there is current research examining the probability of an inherited disorder of connective tissue (Goretsky, 2005). This abnormality is usually evident at birth and increases in severity during the period of rapid bone growth associated with puberty. At this point, the once malleable chest wall becomes more rigid. Subjective symptoms often include variations in exercise tolerance, chest pain, or shortness of breath, presumably caused by altered cardiopulmonary function due to cardiac displacement and reduction in lung volume (Wu, Knauer, McGowan, & Hight, 2001; Lawson et al., 2005). Significant psychosocial impairment due to a negative body image is very common. Conditions that may be associated with pectus excavatum include Marfan's syndrome, marfanoid habitus, Ehlers-Danlos syndrome, and cardiac irregularities.

During the initial patient evaluation, the degree of deformity is evaluated. A complete history and physical begin the work-up. There may be significant asymmetry of the chest wall as well as costal margin flaring and kypho-

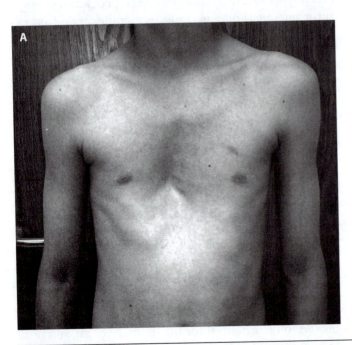
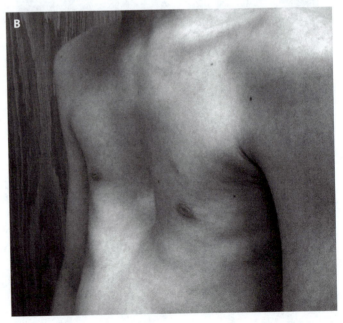

Figure 17-5A and B A, Preoperative anterior view of pectus excavatum. B, Preoperative lateral view of pectus excavatum.
(Reprinted with permission by Stephen Dunn, MD.)

sis. Scoliosis and asthma are common associations. Photographs are obtained for documentation of the defect. A CT scan may be ordered to determine the degree of cardiac and pulmonary compression, sternal torsion, or asymmetry of the chest (Fig. 17-6). It is also used to measure the Haller index at the deepest aspect of the pectus. This is completed by measuring from side to side inside the rib cage and dividing that measurement by the distance from the sternum to the vertebral body (Swoveland, Medvick, Kirsh, Thompson, & Nuss, 2001). A normal chest has a ratio of less than two. Severe pectus is often defined as Haller index greater than 3.25. In some centers, CT is no longer used due to the inherent risks of radiation exposure in children (Zallen & Glick, 2004).

Pulmonary function tests are performed to determine changes in vital capacity and air flow, which may indicate restrictive and/or obstructive airway disease in these patients (Lawson et al., 2005). Exercise pulmonary function tests may reveal significant impairment in maximum exercise tolerance, even if the static measurements are normal. Cardiac evaluation is needed as well. A cardiologist is consulted, and an electrocardiogram and echocardiogram are obtained. Decreased cardiac output, mitral valve prolapse, and arrhythmias have been documented in this population (Goretsky et al., 2004). This evaluation is especially important in patients with marfanoid habitus or Marfan's syndrome, in which cardiac abnormalities are particularly common.

After testing is completed, the decision regarding appropriate treatment is made. In mild cases, the child is referred to a nonoperative program of posture and exercise components in an attempt to stop the progression of

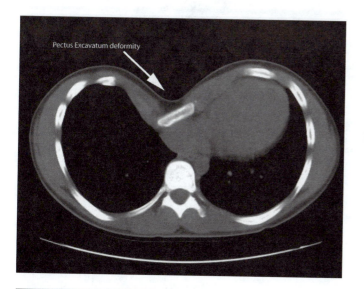

Pectus Excavatum deformity

Figure 17-6 Computed tomographic scan in pectus excavatum. (Reprinted with permission by Stephen Dunn, MD.)

the defect. Reexamination 6 months later is planned. In moderate-to-severe cases, a surgical option is discussed with the patient and family. Selection criteria may include a Haller index greater than 3.25, compromise of the cardiopulmonary system, or documented progression of the deformity. Any recurrence following either an open or minimally invasive operative procedure may warrant a repeated surgical correction. Although body image concerns are often paramount in the patient's presentation, it is the physical symptoms that usually warrant surgical intervention. Often, surgical care providers are placed in a position of justifying the child's case for pectus repair to third party payers. Documentation of specific physiologic criteria assists in the insurance certification process. Acting in the role of patient advocate is often needed, and perseverance on the child's behalf is key.

Ravitch (1949) described the early technique of pectus repair. This open procedure, once seen as the standard approach to pectus repair, required a transverse or longitudinal incision in the midchest, usually followed by cartilage removal from four to five ribs on each side. Remodeling the chest with the use of a sternal osteotomy was followed by bar placement. This bar was then sutured to the ribs for stabilization. Jackson-Pratt drains were left in place until postsurgical drainage had ceased. Hospital time was usually 5 to 6 days. Patients experienced a moderate degree of postoperative pain treated with narcotic analgesia. The cosmetic result of the surgery was well accepted by most patients.

Different modifications of the classic Ravitch approach have been described. It is imperative that this procedure not be attempted until the child has begun the pubertal growth spurt to avoid complications and recurrence (Hebra, 2003). One modification uses a smaller incision, with the creation of a subcutaneous flap over the muscle fascia. A small wedge osteotomy is performed laterally for stabilization. This is held in place by two heavy nonabsorbable sutures. Proponents of this approach describe excellent results with low morbidity and comparatively shorter lengths of hospital stay than with the traditional Ravitch procedure (Davis & Weinstein, 2004). Another method, described by Funkalsrud (2004) described exposing the deformed costal cartilages and resecting a short chip medially adjacent to the sternum and laterally at the level of the chest that has a more normal contour. A transverse anterior sternal osteotomy is performed, followed by placement of a stainless steel bar (Adkins strut) behind the sternum for support. Rib sutures are placed to avoid migration of the bar. Most struts were removed within 6 months. The results of each have been described as good to excellent, but each method involves destruction of the flexible cartilage with replacement with a fibrous scar.

A minimally invasive approach to remodel the chest in patients with pectus excavatum was first described in 1998 by Donald Nuss (Nuss, Kelly, Croitoru, & Katz, 1998). Also known as the minimally invasive repair of pectus excavatum, the Nuss procedure requires no cartilage incision, no resection, and no sternal osteotomy. Dissection near the growth plate of the bone is not performed with this approach. The optimal age at operation is between 7 and 14 years, but it has been successfully performed into adulthood.

An internal brace is used to recontour the chest. This brace, known as the *Lorenz bar* (Walter Lorenz Surgical, Inc., Jacksonville, FL), has rounded ends and blunt edges and is made of stainless steel.

A team approach is needed to achieve optimal outcomes for the pectus patient. The surgeon, nurse practitioner, staff nurse, respiratory therapist, anesthesiologist/pain management team, physical therapist, child life specialist, and social worker all play an important role in the success of the surgery. Before surgery, parents and children should be clearly educated about expectations regarding pain and the need for aggressive pulmonary therapy after surgery. Explaining the use of pain scales and medications helps the child prepare for important communication related to his

or her comfort while giving the child a sense of control in the hospital environment. Time should be spent to build trust and encourage the child and the family to ask questions. Nursing responsibilities require checking identification, vital signs, weight, allergies, pertinent past medical history, and appropriate consents. Ensuring that a preoperative broad-spectrum antibiotic has been given before the first incision is necessary to prevent infection.

The first steps in the operating room are devoted to positioning. The patient is placed supine, and the shoulders are well padded with attention to the brachial plexus to prevent injury. General anesthesia is administered, and the thoracic epidural catheter is inserted between T4 and T12 for postoperative pain management. A Foley catheter is inserted. A nasogastric tube is placed for the duration of the procedure. The area of the chest directly over the deepest segment of the deformity is measured. The bar is then bent to this custom size (Fig. 17-7). Intercostal spaces are measured until the center of the pectus is identified. Incisions are made on each lateral chest wall. Direct visualization of the bar passing behind the sternum is accomplished by use of a thoracoscope. The Lorenz bar introducer is advanced slowly through the left incision, making a substernal tunnel (Fig. 17-8). The introducer is then used to elevate the sternum. With this completed, umbilical tape is tied onto the introducer that is then re-

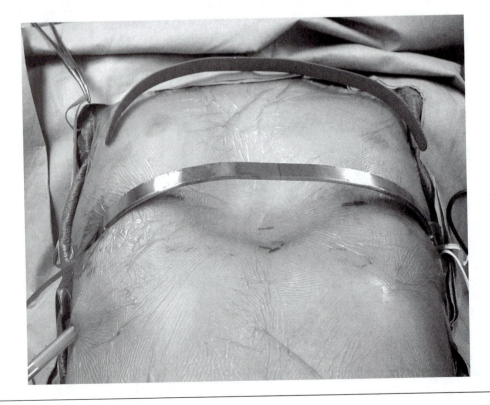

Figure 17-7 Sizing the bar.
(Reprinted with permission by Stephen Dunn, MD.)

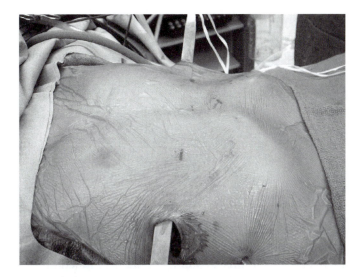

Figure 17-8 Introducer.
(Reprinted with permission by Stephen Dunn, MD.)

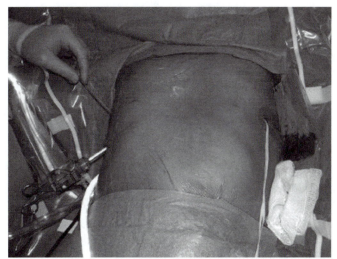

Figure 17-9 Umbilical tape.
(Reprinted with permission by Stephen Dunn, MD.)

moved slowly (Fig. 17-9). This tape within the substernal tunnel provides traction for guiding the convex pectus bar into place. The bar is then passed through the tunnel from the right side of the chest. At this point, the rotational instrument is used to flip the bar 180 degrees (Fig. 17-10). A bar stabilizer is placed on the left side and wired to the bar (Fig. 17-11). Heavy absorbable sutures are used around the bar and the rib on the right side. In some patients, a second stabilizer may be needed. (Nuss, 2005).

Nursing vigilance is paramount in the postoperative period. Upon return from the operating room, the patient must remain in the supine position with only a small pil-

low under the head for comfort. Pulmonary toilet is instituted with the consistent use of hourly incentive spirometry that should be continued every 2 hours during sleeping times. Assessment of vital signs, including pulse oximetry and auscultation of breath sounds, should be documented every 4 hours. Supplemental oxygen may be needed initially. An increased heart rate and/or blood pressure may indicate inadequate pain control. Standardized pain scales provide objective data related to the degree of discomfort. Thoracic epidural analgesia is provided with a mixture of hydromorphone or fentanyl and bupivacaine. The epidural catheter should be assessed hourly for patency and effectiveness. Often, a patient-controlled

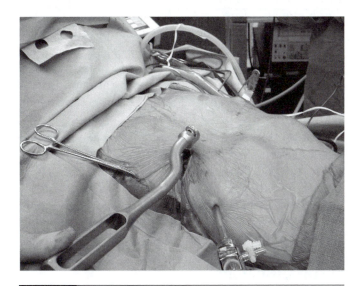

Figure 17-10 Flipping the bar.
(Reprinted with permission by Stephen Dunn, MD.)

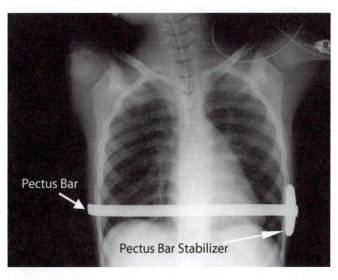

Figure 17-11 Chest x-ray study with Lorenz bar in place.
(Reprinted with permission by Stephen Dunn, MD.)

analgesia pump is used for delivery of the medication. Breakthrough pain is controlled by narcotic analgesia as well as intravenous or oral nonsteroidal anti-inflammatory medications. An H2 blocker (e.g., ranitidine [Zantac]) and muscle relaxants (e.g., diazepam [Valium] or methocarbamol [Robaxin]) are added. An antiemetic medication (e.g., ondansetron [Zofran]) is provided, as needed, for nausea. A Foley catheter remains in place until the first postoperative day. Fluid and electrolyte balance must be monitored closely. Normal saline bolus fluid at 20 mL/kg should be given if the urine output decreases. Constipation, common with the use of narcotic analgesia, should be prevented. The use of stool softeners and stimulant laxatives should be started as soon as the patient is tolerating liquids by mouth.

Patient positioning is challenging during the early postoperative days. The patient is not permitted to roll in the bed, lie on the side, rotate or flex the spine, or slouch. A sign posted over the bed should alert staff not to pull on the patient's arms during repositioning. On the second postoperative day, the patient gets out of bed to a chair by pivoting to sitting from the supine position. Sitting on the side of the bed should be discouraged because bending of the thorax may occur. The patient should also be cautioned not to ambulate without assistance in the early postoperative period.

The epidural catheter is removed between the second and fourth postoperative day. Before removal, the patient should be premedicated with narcotics and muscle relaxants. Immediately after removal, a schedule of medications by mouth is begun. Scheduled medications may include Percocet or loracarbef (Lorabid), diazepam or methocarbamol, ketorolac (Toradol), and ranitidine. Morphine and lorazepam (Ativan) are used, as needed, for breakthrough pain. Within 24 hours, the medication regimen that will be used at home is introduced. These may include nonsteroidal anti-inflammatory medications (e.g., ibuprofen, naproxen), methocarbamol or diazepam, Percocet, ranitidine, docusate sodium (Colace), and lorazepam as needed. Ibuprofen should be continued around the clock for several weeks, whereas the diazepam or methocarbamol can be weaned to twice daily after several days. The Percocet doses should be tapered from every 4 hours to longer periods after the first week at home.

Typically, length of hospital stay is between 3 to 5 days. Each child should wear a Medic Alert bracelet to signify the pectus bar placement. The company producing this bracelet can be reached by calling 1-888-633-4298 or visiting on line at www.medicalert.org. After discharge, the patient can anticipate being home for 2 to 3 weeks. Daily walking and continued breathing exer-

cises are prescribed. A postoperative examination is planned within 3 weeks. Return to school occurs when the patient has discontinued use of all narcotic analgesia. Heavy lifting and use of backpacks must be avoided for 2 months. Attendance at gym class is not permitted for 6 weeks. After 2 months, practice with sport teams may begin, but actual contact must wait for 3 months. Clear communication with the school nurse and faculty is an important part of follow-up care. Documentation is often needed to ensure that specific restrictions will be honored. In some cases, a request for a second set of books to avoid carrying a heavy load is helpful. Other children may need to leave the classroom 5 minutes before the bell rings to avoid being jostled in the hallways. Follow-up is planned for 6 months, including pulmonary function testing. A chest ray study is obtained only if the patient is experiencing pain, or if the appearance of the chest changes. A full history and physical, including photographs, allow the practitioner to evaluate the results of the repair.

Complications related to minimally invasive pectus repair include pneumothorax, shifting of the bar, ongoing pain, wound infection, cracked stabilizer, or trauma. Parents need an established contact person with whom to communicate concerns. Children should be readily evaluated if concern exists.

Outpatient bar removal is planned between 2 to 3 years after surgery. After removal, patients are strongly encouraged to continue an exercise program. A certified physical therapist can use a progressive weight-lifting program that focuses on the development of healthy muscle mass supporting the remodeling of the chest.

Medical concerns can arise for the future. Patients who have undergone pectus repair may receive cardiopulmonary resuscitation, but increased force would be needed. Defibrillation is permitted, but the paddles would have to be placed in an anterior-posterior position to be most effective. Magnetic resonance imaging can be performed, but the bar may increase the artifact effect. A CT scan is the preferred test for these patients (Swoveland et al., 2001).

Currently, the Nuss procedure has become the preferred method for pectus excavatum repair in many centers worldwide. Repeated studies have shown that it is an effective and successful method of surgical repair with low morbidity, shorter length of hospital stay, and high patient satisfaction. Figures 17-12A and B show the postoperative results of an adolescent with pectus excavatum repair.

Pectus Carinatum

Pectus carinatum is an abnormal protrusion of the anterior chest wall. This is a rare deformity occurring in 1 in

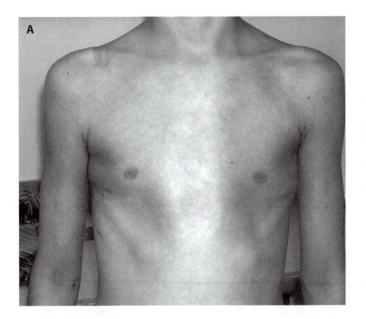

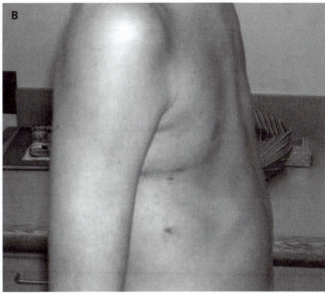

Figure 17-12A and B A, Postoperative anterior view of pectus excavatum. B, Postoperative lateral view of pectus excavatum. (Reprinted with permission by Stephen Dunn, MD.)

1,500 children, predominantly in males (4:1). Although the etiology is unknown, a genetic component is suggested by the approximately 25% of patients with a family history of chest wall defects (Goretsky et al., 2004). The protrusion is first noted in childhood, usually after a significant growth spurt (Fig. 17-13). These children do not usually complain of symptoms.

Treatment options include a custom-fitting brace that provides compression of the anterior and posterior chest cavity. This has been shown to be safe and effective for early pectus carinatum. In a study by Frey et al. (2005), the orthotic brace was used for 14 to 16 hours per day for 2 to 2½ years. In more severe defects, a modified Ravitch procedure may be performed. In this approach, sternal osteotomies are performed, and the bone is bent down until the desired correction is made. Suture fixation is usually adequate to keep the sternum in the new position (Hebra, 2003).

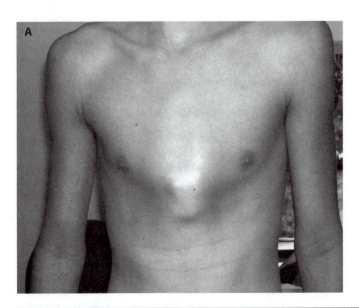

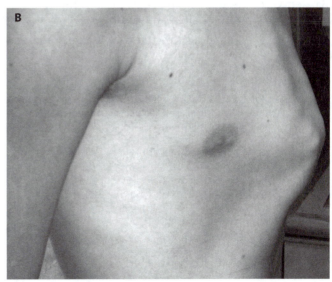

Figure 17-13A and B A, Anterior view of pectus carinatum. B, Lateral view of pectus carinatum. (Reprinted with permission by Stephen Dunn, MD.)

Conclusion

This chapter has presented an overview of the more common chest wall defects as well as the surgical interventions for these diagnoses. Advances in the field of pediatric thoracic surgery have been made with the development of innovative laparoscopic techniques and equipment. Pain management techniques have improved the quality of the postoperative experience. Pediatric surgical nurses caring for children with thoracic procedures possess a thorough understanding of the physiology of the defect and pathological condition as well as the basic principles of the corrective surgical techniques. Pediatric surgical nurses improve the quality of the child's and family's experience by providing education, reassurance, and nurturing care before, during, and after thoracic procedures.

Acknowledgments

I would like to thank Philip J. Wolfson, MD, Kirk Reichard, MD, and Christopher Giaquintos, PA-C, for their unwavering friendship and patient assistance with this chapter. I would also like to recognize the work of Louise Flynn, author of this chapter in the first edition of this textbook.

Educational Materials

APSNA invites you to download the following diagnosis-related teaching tool for Chapter 17, Common Thoracic Procedures: Minimally invasive repair of pectus excavatum (Nuss procedure). This teaching tool is available at the APSNA Web site (www.apsna.org) and the Jones and Bartlett Web site (www.jbpub.com). All teaching materials are available in English and Spanish and are free of charge. APSNA encourages their use for your patients and families.

References

Alfaro, C., Fergie, J., & Purcell, K. (2005). Emergence of community-acquired methicillin-resistant staphylococcus aureus in complicated parapneumonic effusions. *Pediatric Infectious Disease Journal*, 24(3), 274–275.

Balfour-Lynn, I. M., Abrahamson, E., Cohen, G., Hartley, J., King, S., Parikh, D., et al. (2005). BTS guidelines for the management of pleural infection in children. *Thorax*, 60(Suppl. 1), i1–i21.

Barbato, A., Panizzolo, C., Monciotti, C., Marcucci, F., Stefanutti, G., & Gamba, P. G. (2003). Use of urokinase in childhood pleural empyema. *Pediatric Pulmonology*, 35P, L50–L55.

Chan, P., Clarke, P., Daniel, F., Knight, S., & Seevanayagam, S. (2001). Efficacy study of video-assisted thoracoscopic surgery pleurodesis for spontaneous pneumothorax. *Annals of Thoracic Surgery, 71*, 452–454.

Davis, J. T., & Weinstein, S. (2004). Repair of the pectus deformity: Results of the Ravitch approach in the current era. *The Annals of Thoracic Surgery*, 78(2), 421–426.

Frey, A., Durrent, G., Garcia, V., Brown, R., Inge, T., Ryckman, F., et al. (2005). Non-operative management of pectus carinatum. In the American Pediatric Surgical Association Meeting (p. A110). Phoenix, AZ, May 2005.

Funkalsrud, E. (2004). Open repair of pectus excavatum with minimal cartilage resection. *Annals of Surgery*, 240(2), 231–235.

Gates, R. L., Caniano, D. A., Hayes, J. R., & Arca, M. J. (2004). Does VATS provide optimal treatment of empyema in children? A systematic review. *Journal of Pediatric Surgery*, 39(3), 381–386.

Gates, R. L., Hogan, M., Weinstein, S., & Arca, M. J. (2004). Drainage, fibrinolytics, or surgery: A comparison of treatment options in pediatric empyema. *Journal of Pediatric Surgery*, 39(11), 1638–1642.

Goretsky, M. (2005). Evaluation of the patient with chest wall deformities. In *Minimally Invasive Correction of Pectus Excavatum: The Nuss Procedure Workshop and Training Manual*. Norfolk, VA: Children's Hospital of the King's Daughters.

Goretsky, M., Kelly, R., Croitoru, D., & Nuss, D. (2004). Chest wall anomalies; pectus excavatum and pectus carinatum. *Adolescent Medical Clinics*, 15, 455–471.

Hebra, A. (2003). Pectus deformities. In P. Mattei (Ed.), *Surgical directives* (pp. 485–492). Philadelphia: Lippincott Williams & Wilkins.

Jaffe, A., & Balfour-Lynn, I. M. (2005). Management of empyema in children. *Pediatric Pulmonology*, 40(2), 148–156.

Lawson, M., Mellins, R., Tabangin, M., Kelly, R., Croitoru, D., Goretsky, M., et al. (2005). Impact of pectus excavatum on pulmonary function before and after repair with the Nuss procedure. *Journal of Pediatric Surgery*, 40, 174–180.

Nuss, D. (2005). Minimally invasive correction of pectus excavatum. In *Minimally Invasive Correction of Pectus Excavatum: The Nuss Procedure Workshop and Training Manual*. Norfolk, VA: Children's Hospital of the King's Daughters.

Nuss, D., Kelly, R. E., Croitoru, D. P., & Katz, M. E. (1998). A 10-year review of a minimally invasive technique for the correction of pectus excavatum. *Journal of Pediatric Surgery, 33*(4), 545–552.

Ozcan, C., McGahren, E. D., & Rodgers, B. M. (2003). Thoracoscopic treatment of spontaneous pneumothorax in children. *Journal of Pediatric Surgery*, 38(10), 1459–1464.

Qureshi, F. G., Sandulache, V. C., Richardson, W., Ergun, O., Ford, H. R., & Hackman, D. J. (2005). Primary vs. delayed surgery for spontaneous pneumothroax in children; which is better? *Journal of Pediatric Surgery*, 40, 166–169.

Ravitch, M. M. (1949). The operative treatment of pectus excavatum. *Annals of Surgery*, 129(4), 429–444.

Rodgers, B. M. (2003). Pneumothorax. In P. Mattei (Ed.), *Surgical directives* (pp. 493–495). Philadelphia: Lippincott Williams & Wilkins.

Satish, B., Bunker, M., & Seddon, P. (2003). Management of thoracic empyema in childhood: Does the pleural thickening matter? *Archive of Disease in Childhood*, 88, 918–921.

Schultz, K. D., Fan, L. L., Pinsky, J., Ochoa, L., O'Brian-Smith, E., Kaplan, S. L., et al. (2004). The changing face of pleural empyemas in children: Epidemiology and management. *Pediatrics*, 113(6), 113:1735.

Swoveland, B., Medvick, C., Kirsh, M., Thompson, K., & Nuss, D. (2001). The Nuss procedure for pectus excavatum correction. *AORN Journal*, 74(6), 828–841.

Wells, R. G., & Havens, P. L. (2003). Intrapleural fibrinolysis for parapneumonic effusion and empyema in children. *Radiology*, 228(2), 370–377.

Wu, P. C., Knauer, E. M., McGowan, G. E., & Hight, D. W. (2001). Repair of pectus excavatum deformities in children: A new perspective of treatment using minimal access surgical technique. *Archives of Surgery*, 136 (4), 419–424.

Zallen, G. S., & Glick, P. L. (2004). Miniature access pectus excavatum repair: Lessons we have learned. *Journal of Pediatric Surgery*, 39 (5), 685–689.

IV

Nursing Care of Children with Congenital Abdominal Conditions

18

Abdominal Wall Defects

By Beth T. Zimmermann

Congenital abdominal wall defects are found in many forms. All of the defects are related to the development of the umbilical cord. Abdominal wall defects include gastroschisis, omphalocele, bladder and cloacal exstrophy, prune-belly syndrome, urachal remnants, and omphalomesenteric duct malformations, such as patent arches and Meckel's diverticulum. Congenital malformations are an imbalance between cell proliferation and apoptotic cell death (Vermeij-Keers, Hartwig, & Van Der Werff, 1996). This chapter reviews the operative and nursing care of infants born with gastroschisis and omphalocele, both of which are defects that allow herniation of the intra-abdominal contents through the abdominal wall.

Gastroschisis is a Greek word that translates as "belly rent" and is classified as an abdominal wall defect (Moore, 1977). The defect is located lateral to the umbilical cord, commonly on the right. Typically, the defect is small, less than 4 cm. It presents as a herniation of intestine and other abdominal contents through the opening. The cause of this defect is unknown. Possible theories include ruptured omphalocele in utero, premature obliteration of the umbilical ring, deficiency of the embryonic mesenchyme, thrombosis of the omphalomesenteric artery, and accidental tear at the base of the cord from unknown causes (Tunell, 1993). Epidemiologic studies have noted an in-

creasing incidence of gastroschisis, especially in mothers who are under 20 years of age (Laughon et al., 2003; Houghland, Hanna, Meyers, & Null, 2005; Suita et al., 2000). Additionally, there is speculation that early prenatal exposure to drugs, particularly pseudoephedrine, during the first trimester increases risk ("Gastroschisis and Pseudoephedrine During Pregnancy," 2004).

During gestation, the unprotected bowel is exposed to amniotic fluid, including urine, leading to thickening and shortening of the bowel and development of a fibrous outer peel, resulting in damage to the intestine. The exposure of the bowel is the precursor to prolonged paralytic ileus and hypomotility, each affecting long-term feeding and prognosis. Constriction of the bowel at the defect can cause twisting or ischemia, leading to stenosis, atresia, or volvulus. Figure 18-1 depicts a gastroschisis in the newborn.

Omphalocele results from failure of the intestines to return to the abdomen during the second-stage rotation of the midgut loop, occurring during the eighth to 10th week of gestation (Moore, 1977). The covering of the hernial sac is the amnion of the umbilical cord with the arteries and veins inserted into the defect's apex. Varying sizes occur, with giant defects (> 10 cm) involving stomach, liver, spleen, and intestines (Fig. 18-2). In contrast

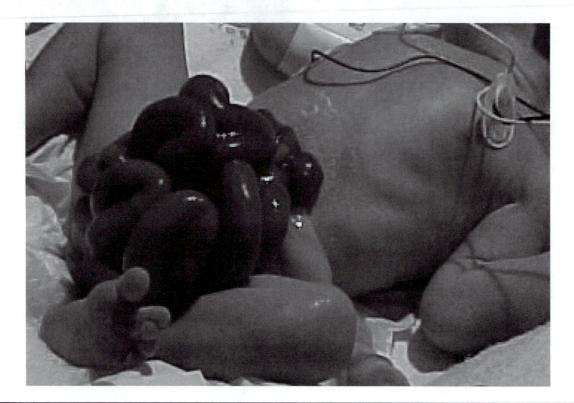

Figure 18-1 Gastroschisis.

to gastroschisis, the presence of the amnion covering the omphalocele provides protection for the intestine. The omphalocele sac may be ruptured, giving an impression of gastroschisis and increasing difficulty in managing the defect.

Incidence

Gastroschisis carries an incidence of 1:2 per 10,000 births, with an increasing incidence over the past few years. This defect is rarely seen in the infants of mothers older than 30 years (King & Askin, 2003; Houghland et al., 2005; Suita et al., 2000; Laughon et al., 2003). Babies with gastroschisis have a low incidence of extra-abdominal malformations. The recurrence risk of gastroschisis is low in families with this single congenital defect. In families of children with multiple defects, the risk of recurrence increases as a familial cluster effect (Yang et al., 1992). Current thinking about etiology postulates an early tear of the umbilical cord before complete closure of the umbilical ring, which occurs between the fourth and eighth weeks of gestation. A tear, not an embryologic problem, explains the lack of associated defects (Alexander, 1993). Intestinal atresia occurs in approximately 10% of infants

with gastroschisis, the result of ischemia secondary to pinching of the mesentery. Atresias associated with gastroschisis may be singular or multiple, involving the large or small intestine (Alexander).

Omphalocele carries an incidence of 1:3,200 to 10,000 births (Molenaar & Tibboel, 1993). Although the exact cause of omphalocele remains unknown, the most common theory is the failure to fuse of the cephalic, caudal, and lateral folds (Klein, 2005). Cardiac anomalies occur in 30% to 50% of infants and chromosomal anomalies in 10% to 40% of infants with omphalocele (Alexander, 1993). Structural, renal, limb, and facial anomalies may occur. Syndromes such as Beckwith-Wiedemann and pentalogy of Cantrell may also be present (Langer, 1996). The National Center on Birth Defects has reported that the use of multivitamins during pregnancy reduces the occurrence of nonsyndromic omphalocele (Botto, Mulinare, & Erickson, 2002).

Special Cases

Pentalogy of Cantrell may be present with an omphalocele. Pentalogy of Cantrell is a defect of the cephalic fold and a lateral defect in the central tendon of the diaphragm

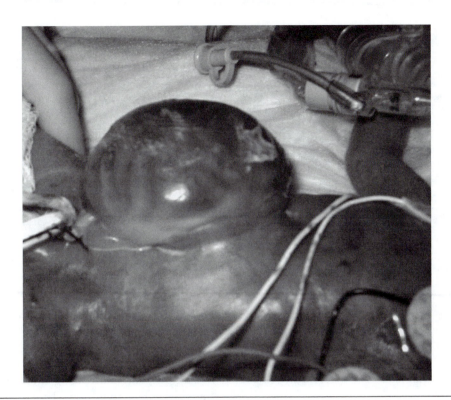

Figure 18-2 Giant omphalocele.

and the pericardium. The anomaly includes upper midline omphalocele, anterior diaphragmatic hernia, sternal cleft, ectopia cordis, and cardiac anomalies. The heart protrudes into the omphalocele sac, the sternum is split (cleft), and there is an intracardiac defect.

Omphalocele has also been reported to occur with cloacal exstrophy or imperforate anus (Fig. 18-3) (Gaines, Holcomb, & Neblett, 2000). Defects of the caudal fold include bladder or cloacal extrophy, imperforate anus, colonic atresia, vesicointestinal fistula, sacral vertebral anomalies, and meningomyelocele.

◼ Diagnosis

Abdominal wall defects are often diagnosed prenatally. Maternal alpha-fetoprotein levels are significantly greater than normal in gastroschisis or omphalocele and are a useful diagnostic indicator (Touloukian & Hobbins, 1980). Normal levels of alpha-fetoprotein are < 40 µg/L, stratified by weeks of gestation, and vary according to different laboratories. Elevated alpha-fetoprotein levels signal the need for thorough ultrasound examination of uterine contents. Prenatal diagnosis allows for tertiary center delivery with surgeons and neonatologists in attendance at the birth.

The identification of the defect (i.e., gastroschisis vs. omphalocele) is important because of the increased risk of associated anomalies with omphalocele. Echocardiography is recommended both pre- and postnatally in omphalocele infants (Gibbin, Touch, Broth, & Berghella, 2003). When an abdominal wall defect is identified, amniocentesis is indicated to identify chromosomal anomalies. The results of chromosomal studies are used for parental counseling, including the prognosis of the affected infant and the possibility of pregnancy termination in the presence of lethal malformations (Dykes, 1996). Highly unusual umbilical cords seen at delivery should remain unclamped until the presence of an abdominal wall defect is ruled out.

◼ Parental Counseling

Prenatal diagnosis allows for preparation and care of the family and infant. Continuing controversy exists regarding vaginal versus cesarean and/or early delivery of these infants. A recent study at the Montreal Children's Hospital found no improvement in the outcome of delivery by cesarean section except in those instances in which fetal distress is noted (Puligandla, Janvier, Flageole, Bouchard, & Laberge, 2004). To date, specific benefits of early or

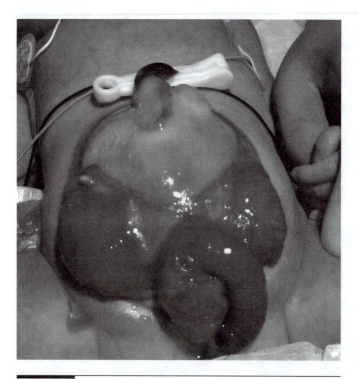

Figure 18-3 Cloacal extrophy.

cesarean delivery are unidentified (Dykes, 1996; Howell, 1998). Regardless of the defect, arrangements are made for delivery in the level III center, facilitating immediate surgical care. In those cases in which the defect is unidentified before delivery, the infant is stabilized and transferred via ground or air ambulance to provide surgical care as soon as possible.

Predelivery consultations with the neonatal care team, pediatric surgeon, neonatologist, and advanced practice nurses are facilitated. Tours of the neonatal intensive care unit decrease family stress and encourage decisions for the baby's care. The prenatal consultation outlines complications of the defect, surgery, and long-term outcomes. Additional discussions regarding hospitalization, blood donation, breast feeding, insurance, discharge planning/home care, and general pediatric care are advisable. Infants with abdominal wall defects spend from 1 week to many months in the hospital. A collaborative relationship among the family, advanced practice nurse, neonatologist, surgeon, and primary pediatrician is the hallmark of quality care.

■ Transport and Admission

Infant transport is preferentially in utero. If the child is delivered at an outlying center, the guidelines for trans-

port developed by the American Academy of Pediatrics (1993) should be followed. Key interventions for delivery room care of infants with gastroschisis and omphalocele are essentially the same other than specific care of the exposed bowel of the child with gastroschisis. The infant with omphalocele should not have the defect wrapped in moist gauze because this leads to unnecessary heat loss. However, the infant should be placed in the bowel bag for protection and visualization (Klein, 2005). The patient with gastroschisis needs the bowel kept moist and also benefits from the bowel bag. The purpose of the bowel bag (Steri-Drape 3M) is to decrease conductive and evaporative heat and fluid losses. Additionally, the bag allows observation of the defect within a sterile environment. The infant should be placed into the bag feet first up to the nipple line and the ties secured. The defects may be supported by rolled blankets on either side of the bag's exterior to prevent twisting and kinking. The goals of nursing care are to maintain the airway, obtain vital signs, prevent hypothermia, insert an orogastric or nasogastric decompression tube, place the infant in a bowel bag, and obtain intravenous access (Howell, 1998; Strodtbeck, 1998). Additionally, care is taken to avoid kinking of the exposed bowel of the infant, tearing the amnion of the omphalocele, or exerting pressure on either, thus preventing further ischemia and damage.

Neonatal intensive care unit admission care includes calling the surgical team for introductions and consent, weighing and stabilizing the patient, and orienting the family to the facility. The family is informed of the date, time, and location of the surgery. Optimally, the parents have experienced bonding time with the infant, including touching and caressing. Information regarding blood (directed donor), visiting hours, and family amenities is provided. If the mother is at another location, she is contacted and her phone number is documented.

Nursing care of the surgical neonate requires ongoing assessment and timely intervention (Harjo, 1998). Major factors include oxygenation, acid-base balance, thermoregulation, fluid and electrolyte balance, and pharmacologic support (Kenner, Amlung, & Flandermeyer, 1998). Specific care of the infant with an abdominal wall defect is outlined in Table 18-1.

■ Operative Procedure

The preferred repair for the infant with gastroschisis is within the first 24 hours; he or she is at risk for fluid loss,

Table 18-1	Preoperative Nursing Care of the Infant with an Abdominal Wall Defect

- **Prevent Infection**

  Use sterile barriers & sterile gloves; Administer antibiotics as ordered

- **Prevent Hypothermia**

  Cover/protect with bowel bag; Warm all solutions; Maintain temperature above 36.5°C; Use warmed humidified oxygen

- **Protect Bowel**

  Use bowel bag or protective covering; Prevent kinking of bowel; Large lumen soft silastic gastric decompression tube

- **Fluid Therapy**

  Weigh infant; Moniter I & O; Obtain laboratory tests (complete blood count, arterial blood gases, electrolytes, glucose, calcium, type and cross-match); Intravenous access; Provide fluids: maintenance plus 1.5–2X as needed; Monitor blood pressure and urine

- **Respiratory Support**

  Keep SaO_2 equal/greater than 95%; Avoid bag and mask as it will distend bowel; Auscultate breath sounds bilaterally

terventions before surgery occurs. The severity of accompanying defects determines the timing and the type of surgery. The size of the defect and the preoperative condition of the baby, including other possible congenital anomalies and respiratory distress, influence the surgical procedure used for each infant.

A primary closure is considered the optimum treatment of an abdominal wall defect. The bowel is emptied of meconium from top to bottom to ease closure. To cover the defect without closing the fascia, the abdominal wall may be stretched or skin flaps may be used (Vegunta, Cooney, & Cooney, 1993). If a ventral hernia is created by the skin flaps, it is repaired several years later and skin grafts may be used to cover the defect (Dillon & Cilley, 1993). Closure accomplished with tension requires close observation for vascular compromise of abdominal contents, decreased renal perfusion, and subsequent drop in urine output. Respiratory difficulties may be noted as a result of immobilization of the diaphragm and inability to properly ventilate the infant because of the increased intra-abdominal pressure (Howell, 1998).

A staged or gentle reduction occurs over a period of days with definitive closure, taking place within 7 to 10 days to decrease the incidence of infection. The first stage of repair places a Silastic silo around the exposed abdominal contents (Fig. 18-4), although some centers continue to use a Silastic wrap (Fig. 18-5). In cases in which the wrap is used, surgeons may wish to keep the wrap bathed in antibacterial agents or sterile wrappings at the base. Care is taken to avoid accidental expulsion of the silo or the wrap. However, if expulsion occurs, the silo is usually replaced at the bedside (Wu et al., 2003). The wrap may require a return to the operating room for a sterile replacement. Gravity and the mounting pressure from the pouch or wrap force the viscera to slowly move back into the expanding abdominal cavity. The covering may be lightly tied down carefully daily, avoiding pulmonary and bowel compression. The amount reduced each time can be gauged by monitoring intragastric or bladder pressure. Other methods of monitoring the pressure include visual inspection of the color and distention of the abdominal wall, urine output, distal pulses, and presence or absence of increased ventilator pressure with decreasing oxygenation. Once the viscera are reduced to skin level, the infant is taken to the operating room, the Silastic is removed, and the fascia is closed (Langer, 1996; Wu et al.). The use of the preformed silo has been shown to effectively decrease complications (Schlatter et al., 2003; Jona, 2003).

temperature instability, and infection. However, the use of a spring-loaded Silastic silo is an alternative to immediate repair, leading to a more gentle and gradual approach (Wu et al., 2003; Schlatter, Norris, Uitvlugt, DeCou, & Connors, 2003). The exposed bowel is placed into the silo and the encircling spring under the skin. Suturing is not required, and a simple Xeroform or gauze dressing can be placed around the base of the silo. Intermittent tie-down of the silo gently pushes the bowel into the abdominal cavity. When the bowel reaches skin level, the child is taken to the operating room, and the defect is closed primarily under sterile conditions.

The omphalocele infant is stabilized and additional tests are completed to rule out cardiac, renal, limb, and chromosomal anomalies (Langer, 1996). In either gastroschisis or omphalocele, a small defect is repaired in one stage or in one trip to the operating room, and larger defects require two stages of repair. Frequently, the first stage is nonoperative placement of a Silastic silo at the bedside. The alternative method to the spring-loaded silo is the suturing of a protective covering around the base of the defect with intermittent tie-downs and final closure.

Infants with additional defects (more common in omphalocele) require additional tests, consultations, and in-

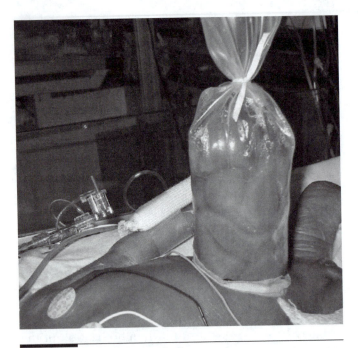

Figure 18-4 Gastroschisis with silo.

Additional surgical procedures may include the placement of mesh to close the wall of the abdomen, repair of an intestinal atresia, placement of central venous catheters, and placement of a gastrostomy tube. If possible, surgery is delayed to avoid the use of mesh, decreasing the possibility of infection. The presence of bowel atresias is addressed during the primary closure. If atresias are present, a diverting stoma is frequently necessary (Dillon & Cilley, 1993). The need for long-term nutrition sup-

port is a possibility in gastroschisis due to the presence of hypomotility and/or short-gut syndrome (Langer, 1996; Dillon & Cilley; Taylor, 1994). Central venous access and/or a gastrostomy tube for nutritional support are important adjuncts to the nutritional plan. Table 18-2 outlines the postoperative care of the patient with an abdominal wall defect.

Giant Omphalocele

The giant omphalocele poses problems that are different from the more common, smaller omphalocele. The giant omphalocele contains liver and other intestinal structures that protrude through a defect that may be 8 to 10 cm wide. Because of the lack of development of the lateral skin and the decreased size of the abdominal cavity, visceral contents of the giant omphalocele cannot be returned to the abdomen primarily, necessitating a process of gradual return of abdominal contents over months of time. Care must be taken to avoid the rupture of the amnion. Epithelialization is encouraged, leading slowly to the primary closure. Surgically removing the amnion and placing a silo can lead to overwhelming sepsis and death.

The use of a topical agent followed by covering with gauze and a compressive wrap gently leads to development of skin and growth of the abdominal cavity, allowing acceptance of the intestinal organs and closure of the defect (Nagaya, 1997; Belloli, Gattaglino, & Musi, 1996). Various topical agents have been used, with Silvadene being the most common. The purposes of the topical agent are to desiccate and shrink the amnion, to aid in the development of skin over the amnion, and to provide protection from infection until the defect can be closed. During this time, the child may go home with his or her parents, who are taught how to apply the agent and the wrapping. Additional instructions include use of the correct car seat, bathing techniques, antireflux precautions, and developmental stimulation not involving ventral positioning. Developmental issues regarding the abdominal muscles arise during this long period and once closure is accomplished. Physical therapy services are required (Gaines et al., 2000; Klein, 2005). Figs. 18-6A through E document the progression of a giant omphalocele wrap and closure. Table 18-3 outlines the principles of management of the giant omphalocele.

Nutrition

Hyperalimentation is started early as bowel function returns slowly, especially in the infant with gastroschisis. Feedings are begun when there is full bowel function,

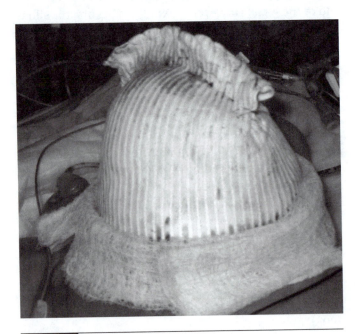

Figure 18-5 Gastroschisis with wrap.

Table 18-2	Postoperative Care of the Patient with an Abdominal Wall Defect
Respiratory Support	Respiratory distress may develop at any point but is likely to worsen as the staged reduction progresses and always occurs after a primary closure; Monitor pulse oximetry and arterial blood gases; Increase O_2 to maintain documented parameters; Administer paralytic (intubation required) and sedation agents as needed to maximize relaxation; Auscultate, suction, and administer chest therapy.
Infection Prevention	Silo integrity and care requires 2 people to avoid tension on bowel; Administer antibiotics as ordered; Bathe silo with warmed antibiotic solution/ointment and/or wrap with gauze/Xeroform (surgeon's preference); Sterile technique for dressing changes; Monitor/report separation, redness, or drainage at base of silo or suture site; Monitor labs and report abnormal results; Meticulous central venous access care.
Fluid Therapy	Fluid/protein is translocated from bowel into the silo; Administer albumin as needed; Maintain patency of Foley catheter, monitor hourly urine output (minimum: 0.5–1 mL/kg/hr); Dopamine (renal dose) as needed; Maintain decompression tube patency on low continuous suction, document aspirate and irrigant; Monitor, record, and replace glucose and electrolytes.
Pain Management	Assessment of signs and symptoms of pain completed hourly in postop period. Note increasing heart rate, decreasing SaO_2, changes in blood pressure or behavior; Administer narcotics to effect adequate dose response; Use behavioral interventions such as, pacifier, parent touch-vocalization, and decreased stimulation; Wean narcotics when appropriate
Skin Care	Increased abdominal pressure may impede circulation to the lower extremities; Observe pulses, temperature, and color; Use specialized mattress to decrease pressure; Keep infant and all linens warm and dry; Remove povidone-iodine and other solutions from skin with warmed normal saline to avoid chemical burns; Use pectin-based barriers under all tape to avoid epidermal stripping; Note the normal reddened appearance of the suture line, report drainage or dehiscence immediately; Keep sutured area clean with warmed normal saline and dry
Gastrointestinal Decompression	A non-functioning decompression tube will fail to decrease pressure causing pain, aspiration, and possible rupture; Irrigate decompression tube with air through the air port and normal saline through the succus port (4–5 mL every 4 hours and PRN); Dual lumen decompression tubes run on low constant suction; Clarify whether nurses or surgeons replace non-functioning decompression tubes; Document output minus irrigant and replace fluid losses as directed (usually mL per mL)
Plan of Care	Anticipate and plan for a daily silo reduction until the final closure; Document expected time of daily intervention; Gather requested supplies; Medicate infant prior to reduction to prevent increased discomfort; Observe carefully and document response to procedure

including stool passing. Continuous nasogastric, gastrostomy tube, or measured oral feedings begin with clear liquids and are advance as tolerated to breast milk or elemental formulas in the case of malabsorption. Formula additives may be needed, depending on the type and the brand of formula and the infant's nutritional needs. Growth curve maintenance and full enteral feedings are desirable but may be unobtainable before discharge. Some children are discharged on total parenteral nutrition (Taylor, 1994). The importance of breast milk is twofold: the decreased incidence and severity of necrotizing enterocolitis (Covert, 1995) and the mother's unique contribution to her infant's welfare (Zimmermann, 1995). Breast-feeding dyads should be assisted by the lactation specialist. Feedings advance slowly, either by concentration or by volume, with one change per time. Bilious vomiting, residuals greater than 10 mL/kg, guaiac-positive stools, and/or stool Clinitest greater than 2% may be signs of necrotizing enterocolitis or obstruction and are reported to the surgery service. Nonnutritive sucking is encouraged early and often during tube feedings. Sucking and swallowing difficulties are managed by the pediatric speech therapist.

Discharge Planning and Parent Care

The goal of discharge planning is a well-bonded family with the ability, desire, and knowledge to provide proper care for their infant. Home care needs depend on the presence of other anomalies and the condition of the infant.

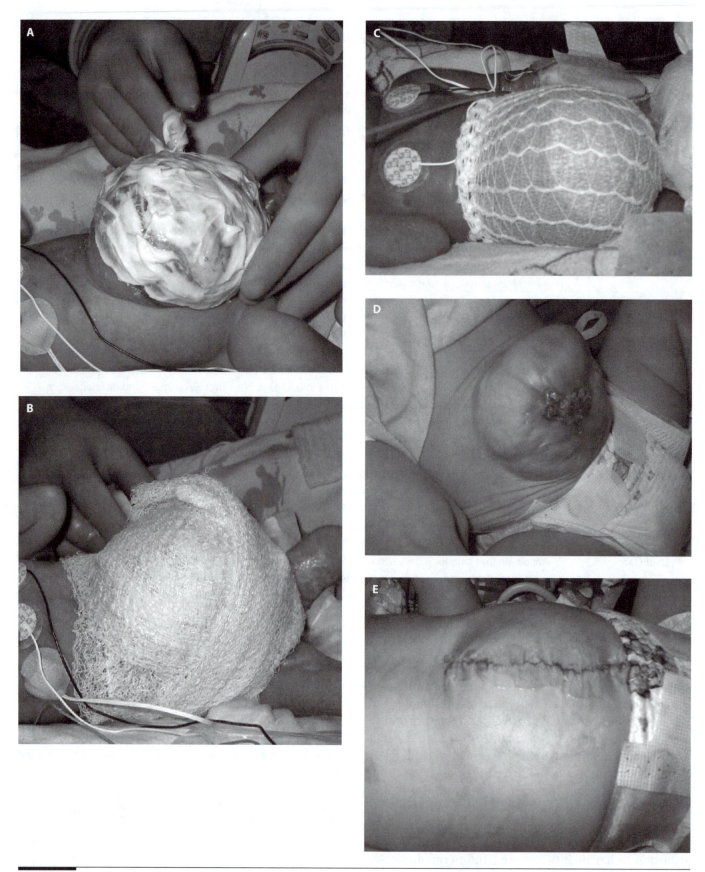

Figure 18-6 A, Application of topical agent. B, Application of gauze wrap. C, Application of pressure dressing. D, Presurgical closure. E, Postsurgical closure.

Table 18-3	Principles of Management of the Giant (>10 cm) Omphalocele
Infection	*Avoid* rupture of the amnion; Use sterile gloves and barriers; Maintain sterility of sclerosing agent; Administer antibiotics as ordered.
Prevent Hypothermia	Cover or protect with bowel bag; Moist gauze unnecessary as it leads to heat loss; Warm topical agent and wraps (see below); Maintain temperature above 36.5°C; Warmed humidified O_2
Protect Bowel	Apply topical agent (drying and bacteriostatic); Cover entire omphalocele, avoiding healthy skin; Wrap supportively but gently with Kerlex; Wrapping includes: under the back, around the caudal and cephalad portions of the defect and then under and over; Poor perfusion lower extremities, decreased urine output, pressure marks on skin, increased edema, and respiratory difficulties indicate increased intra-abdominal pressure; Pressure wrap with Flexinet, Ace-wrap, or Coban; Maintain gentle pressure and support upright to encourage gravity, may need rolls at the sides; Place decompression tube to low constant suction; AVOID: scratching, tearing, infecting or injuring amnion.
Fluid Therapy	Begin and maintain patent venous access; Draw labs; Deliver fluids at maintenance rate: will not lose as much fluid as gastroschisis; Monitor urine output, minimum of 1 mL/kg/hr (abdominal pressure indicator); I & O.
Respiratory Support	Keep SaO_2 equal or greater than 95%; Avoid bag and mask ventilation to prevent bowel distention. Intubation is preferred for ventilatory support; Auscultate lung fields bilaterally and suction as needed.
Associated Anomalies	Complete all additional tests; Echo, Chromosomal, Head ultrasound; Follow prescribed therapies as appropriate.
Daily Dressing Changes	Surgery service will do original dressings, staff and family will be taught and assisted; Opiates and sedatives are helpful; Gently remove previous dressing; Clean off all excess agent and any drainage with soft, moistened gauze; Do not remove eschar; Gently and thoroughly inspect all areas of amnion; Report tears and changes; Recover amnion with warmed agent and avoid healthy developed skin; Maintain sterility in the hospital, clean technique at home; Re-wrap and gently add additional pressure; As the baby matures and tolerates the pressure, Flexinet and Ace wrap may be used to assist in a tighter wrap; Use gravity as an assistant; Turn the infant to the side and support structure with rolls or foam; Use rings under head to avoid flattening of skull and occipital pressure; Sponge baths; Parents should hold and bond with infant; Physical therapy to guide movement and positioning
Discharge Planning	Teach parents independence in the wrap procedure; Sponge bathing; CPR training; Car seat test or horizontal car safety bed; Contact primary care physician with infant's information; Infant will be followed in Pediatric Surgery Clinic at regular intervals; Primary closure will take place when the fascia and skin can be drawn over the defect primarily. This process will take months.

Verification of financial and insurance status and investigation regarding the possibility of home nursing care should take place early in the hospitalization. The family should be referred to social services for financial guidance and emotional support. The family should choose a primary pediatrician who is apprised of the child's condition and who reviews the surgical reports. If the child requires a tube for enteral feeds or venous access for parenteral feedings at discharge, family education is intense. Equipment should be ordered as early as possible to facilitate delivery and family education. Complex social and educational needs may be ameliorated if identified and addressed early in the planning process.

Complications and Long-Term Outcomes

Educate families early as to the signs of complications: bilious emesis, abdominal distention, poor appetite, elevated temperature, constipation, diarrhea, and changes in behavior. These may be signs of obstruction or midgut volvulus.

Most infants with an abdominal wall defect lead healthy normal lives with few complications. The long-term survival, especially in gastroschisis, is greater than 95% (Davies & Stringer, 1997).

The most common complications are bowel obstruction and ventral hernias. A ventral hernia is defined as a loop of bowel protruding through the abdominal musculature that may occur in the area of the surgical scar. Surgical repair of ventral hernias or adhesive obstructions are required in approximately one third of cases (Langer, 1996). If complications occur, they are most common in children under 7 years of age (Tunell, Puffinbarger, Tuggle, Taylor, & Mantor, 1995).

It is imperative that parents know their baby's "normals" in order to recognize complications in a timely manner. Encourage parents to visit their hospitalized infant frequently for long periods of time at various times of the day. "Make parents experts on their babies wants and needs" (Harjo, 1995). Infants without coexisting anomalies who survive the surgical repairs (approximately 80%–90%) have a normal quality of life (Vergunta et al., 1993; Tunell et al., 1995).

The survival of infants with omphalocele is different. Their survival depends on the size of the defect, maintaining an intact amnion at birth, the severity of the associated anomalies, and respiratory function (Pacilli, 2005). When omphalocele children survive to discharge, a continuing concern is the presence of malrotation and possible volvulus. Parents should know the signs and symptoms of obstruction.

Conclusion

Omphalocele and gastroschisis are abdominal wall defects that require nursing care provided in the special care nursery at a tertiary center. The infant's long-term survival and quality of life depend on early interventions and care. Nurses have the opportunity to provide surgical patients and their families multidimensional care leading to optimal short- and long-term outcomes.

Dedication

This chapter is lovingly dedicated to the memory of Liv Sandvik. It is her family's and my hope that lessons learned from her courageous spirit will continue as nurses provide evidenced-based care to infants with giant omphalocele.

Acknowledgments

The author would like to thank Gina Lee and Andrew Sandvik for photos of their daughter used in preparation of this chapter. The author also thanks Hiwot Bekele Woldgeorgis for her assistance in conducting the literature search for this chapter.

Educational Materials

APSNA invites you to download the following diagnosis-related teaching tool for Chapter 18, Abdominal Wall Defects: Abdominal Wall Defects. This teaching tool is available at the APSNA Web site (www.apsna.org) and the Jones and Bartlett Web site (www.jbpub.com). All teaching materials are available in English and Spanish and are free of charge. APSNA encourages their use for your patients and families.

References

Alexander, F. (1993). Anterior abdominal wall defects. In R. Wyllie & J. W. Hyams (Eds.), *Pediatric gastrointestinal disease: Pathophysiology, diagnosis, and management* (pp. 506–514). Philadelphia: W.B. Saunders.

American Academy of Pediatrics. (1993). *Task force on interhospital transport: Guidelines for air and ground transport of neonatal and pediatric patients.* Elk Grove, IL: Author.

Belloli, B., Gattaglino, F., & Musi, L. (1996). Management of giant omphalocele by progressive external compression: Case report. *Journal of Pediatric Surgery, 31*(12), 1719–1720.

Botto, L. D., Mulinare, J., & Erickson, J. D. (2002). Occurrence of omphalocele in relation to maternal multivitamin use: A population based study. *Pediatrics, 109*(5), 904–908.

Covert, R. (1995, May). *The effects of breastmilk: Incidence of NEC.* Paper presented at the meeting of the Society of Pediatric Research, San Diego, CA.

Davies, B. W., & Stringer, M. D. (1997). The survivors of gastroschisis. *Archives of Disease in Childhood, 77*, 158–160.

Dillon, P. W., & Cilley, R. E. (1993). Newborn surgical emergencies: Gastrointestinal anomalies, abdominal wall defects. *Pediatric Clinics of North America Pediatric Surgery 40*(6), 1307–1314.

Dykes, E. H. (1996). Prenatal diagnosis and management of abdominal wall defects. *Seminars in Pediatric Surgery, 5*(2), 90–94.

Gaines, B. A., Holcomb, G. W., & Neblett, W .W. (2000). Gastroschisis and omphalocele. In K.W. Ashcraft (Ed.), *Pediatric surgery* (pp. 639–648). Philadelphia: W.B. Saunders.

Gastroschisis and pseudoephedrine during pregnancy. (2004). *Prescrire International, 13*, 141–143.

Gibbin, C., Touch, S., Broth, R. E., & Berghella, V. (2003). Abdominal wall defects and congenital heart disease. *Ultrasound in Obstetrics & Gynecology, 21*(4), 334–337.

Harjo, J. (1998). The surgical neonate. In C. Kenner, J. W. Lott, & A. A. Flandermeyer (Eds.), *Comprehensive neonatal nursing* (2nd ed., pp. 781–787). Philadelphia: W.B. Saunders.

Howell, K. K. (1998). Understanding gastroschisis: An abdominal wall defect. *Neonatal Network, 17*(8), 17–25.

Hougland, K. T., Hanna, A. M., Meyers, R., & Null, D. (2005). Increasing prevalence of gastroschisis in Utah. *Journal of Pediatric Surgery, 40*(3), 535–540.

Jona, J. Z. (2003). The "gentle touch" technique in the treatment of gastroschisis. *Journal of Pediatric Surgery, 38*(7), 1036–1038.

Kenner, C., Amlung, S. R., & Flandermeyer, A. A. (1998). Surgical neonate. *Protocols in neonatal nursing* (pp. 575–589). Philadelphia: W.B. Saunders.

King, J., & Askin, D. F. (2003). Gastroschisis: Etiology, diagnosis, delivery options, and care. *Neonatal Network, 22*(4), 7–12.

Klein, M. D. (2005). Congenital abdominal wall defects. In K. W. Ashcraft, G. W. Holcomb, & J. P. Murphy (Eds.), *Pediatric surgery* (4th ed., pp. 659–669). Philadelphia: W.B. Saunders.

Langer, J. C. (1996). Gastroschisis and omphalocele. *Journal of Pediatric Surgery, 5*(2), 124–128.

Laughon, M., Meyer, R., Bose, C., Wall, A., Otero, E., Heerens, A., & Clark, R. (2003). Rising birth prevalence of gastroschisis. *Journal of Perinatology 23*(4), 291–293.

Moore, K. L. (1977). *The developing human; Clinically oriented embryology* (2nd ed.). Philadelphia: W.B. Saunders.

Molenaar, J., & Tibboel, D. (1993). Gastroschisis and omphalocele. *World Journal of Surgery, 17*(3), 337–341.

Nagaya, M. (1997). Current status of management of omphalocele and gastroschisis. *Journal of Japanese Surgical Society, 98*(12), 1013–1017.

Pacilli, M. (2005). Staged repair of giant omphalocele in the neonatal period. *Journal of Pediatric Surgery, 40*(5), 785–788.

Puligandla, P. S., Janvier, A., Flageole, H., Bouchard, S., & Laberge, J. M. (2004). Routine cesarean delivery does not improve the outcome of infants with gastroschisis. *Journal of Pediatric Surgery, 39*(5), 742–745.

Schlatter, M., Norris, K., Uitvlugt, N., DeCou, J., & Connors, R. (2003). Improved outcomes in the treatment of gastroschisis using a preformed silo and delayed repair approach. *Journal of Pediatric Surgery, 38*(3), 459–464.

Strodtbeck, F. (1998). Understanding gastroschisis: An abdominal wall defect. *Neonatal Network, 17*(8), 17–25.

Suita, S., Okamatsu, T., Yamamoto, T., Handa, N., Nirasawa, Y., Watanbe, Y., et al. (2000). Changing profile of abdominal wall defects in Japan: Results of a national survey. *Journal of Pediatric Surgery, 35*(1), 66–72.

Taylor, D. V. (1994). The infant with gastroschisis. *Sutureline, 2*(3), 1–2.

Touloukian, R. J., & Hobbins, J. C. (1980). Maternal ultrasonography in the antenatal diagnosis of surgically correctable fetal abnormalities. *Journal of Pediatric Surgery, 14*, 373–377.

Tunnell, W. P. (1993). Omphalocele and gastroschisis. In K. W. Ashcraft & T. M. Holder (Eds.), *Pediatric surgery* (2nd ed., pp. 546–556). W.B. Philadelphia: Saunders.

Tunnell, W. P., Puffinbarger, N. K., Tuggle, D. W., Taylor, D. V., & Mantor, P. C. (1995). Abdominal wall defects in infants: Survival and implications for adult life. *Annals of Surgery, 221*(5), 525–530.

Vegunta, R. K., Cooney, D. E., & Cooney, D. R. (1993). Surgical management of abdominal wall defects in infants. *AORN Journal, 58*(1), 53–63.

Vermeij-Keers, C., Hartwig, N. G., & Van Der Werff, J. F. A. (1996). Embryonic development of the ventral body wall and its congenital malformations. *Seminars in Pediatric Surgery, 5*(2), 82–89.

Wu, Y., Vogel, A. M., Sailhamer, E. A., Somme, S., Santore, M. J., Chwals, W. J., et al. (2003). Primary insertion of a silastic spring-loaded silo for gastroschisis. *American Surgeon, 69*(12), 1083–1086.

Yang, P., Beaty, T., Khoury, M. J., Chee, E., Stewart, W., & Gordis, L. (1992). Genetic-epidemiologic study of omphalocele and gastroschisis: Evidence of heterogenicity. *American Journal of Medical Genetics, 44*, 668–675.

Zimmermann, B. T. (1995, April). *The maternal impact of breastfeeding a preterm infant in the post-discharge period.* Paper presented at the meeting of National Association of Neonatal Nurses: International Research Conference, Seattle, WA.

19

Intestinal Atresias, Duplications, and Meconium Ileus

Judith J. Stellar and Kelli B. Young

Intestinal obstruction in the neonate is most often due to a congenital anomaly rather than to an acquired condition. These patients present a clinical challenge. Symptoms may be acute, as with intestinal atresia, or gradual, as in anomalies that result in partial obstruction, such as duplications and meconium ileus. In addition to the wide scope of clinical presentation, many of these anomalies are associated with other life-threatening and/or genetic conditions that require thorough evaluation and meticulous nursing care. Because intestinal atresias, duplications, and meconium ileus all have the potential for associated anomalies, good understanding of anatomy, physiology, and embryonic development is required. Although most of these conditions unto themselves have a good prognosis overall, their high association with other anomalies and diseases contributes to potentially greater morbidity and mortality. The nurse provides expert clinical care, offers the family support and education, and provides continuous case management through discharge and along the life continuum.

■ Intestinal Atresias

Atresia of the intestinal tract is characterized by total obstruction of the intestinal lumen. A stenosis, on the other hand, is an incomplete obstruction or narrowing of the intestinal lumen. Excluding esophageal atresia and anorectal malformations, small bowel atresias account for 20% of all neonatal obstructions (Skandalakis & Gray, 1994). Overall, the incidence of intestinal atresia (all types) is reported as 1 in 3,000 (Touloukian, 1993). Of all intestinal atresias, duodenal atresia accounts for 40% of the cases, followed by ileal atresia, 35%; jejunal atresia, 20%; and colonic atresia, less than 5% (Skandalakis & Gray). Sex distribution is equal (Skandalakis & Gray; Touloukian). Duodenal atresia is far more likely to be associated with other anomalies (Harris, Kallen, & Robert, 1995; Stauffer & Schwoebel, 1998). No true familial tendency has been identified, but there have been reports of intestinal atresias occurring in twins and siblings (Gross, Armon, Abu-Dalu, Gale, & Schiller, 1996; Moore, de Jongh, Bouic, Brown, & Kirsten, 1996; Rothenberg, White, Chilmonczyk, & Chatila, 1995; Yokoyama et al., 1997). Table 19-1 outlines the distinctions between various intestinal atresias.

Embryology

It is theorized that duodenal atresia has a different embryologic mechanism than jejunal, ileal, and colonic atresia. Skandalakis and Gray (1994) group the embryogenesis of intestinal atresia as follows.

Table 19-1 Distinctions Between Various Intestinal Atresias

Type of Atresia	Etiology/Embryology	Incidence	Associated Anomalies
Duodenal (40%)	Primary atresia Failure of recanalization of lumen during late 8th to 10th wk	1:6,000–1:10,000	High rate of associated anomalies include: trisomy 21 (up to 40% of cases); malrotation; annular pancreas; congenital heart disease; VACTERL association; abdominal wall defects; preduodenal portal vein; biliary tree anomalies; immunodeficiency
Jejunal (20%) Ileal (35%)	Secondary atresia Result of fetal accident or ischemic event at 10 wk to 4 mo (intrauterine thrombosis, intussusception, volvulus)	1:750–1:5,000	Low rate of associated anomalies include: cystic fibrosis; meconium ileus; malrotation; renal dysplasia; ocular anomalies; Hirschsprung's disease; microcephaly; immunodeficiency
Colonic (< 5%)	Secondary atresia Ischemic event as above	Rare 1:20,000–1:40,000	Moderate rate of associated anomalies include: limb anomalies; Hirschsprung's disease; ocular anomalies; cardiac anomalies; abdominal wall defects

Abbreviation: VACTERL, vertebral, anorectal, cardiac, tracheal, esophageal, renal, limb.

Primary Atresia

Primary atresias are due to a defect in fetal development. During the second month of gestation, there is tremendous growth of epithelial lining cells of the intestine, so much so that the intestinal lumen is obliterated. By the end of the eighth to 10th week, the lumen undergoes recanalization. Failure of recanalization is theorized to be the cause of duodenal atresia and esophageal and rectal atresia. Another defect in the developmental process that results in atresias is the resorption of a segment of ileum during the assimilation of the vitelline duct at the fifth week of gestation.

Secondary Atresia

Secondary atresias are thought to be the result of an intrauterine ischemic event. In normal fetal development, bile secretion and swallowing of amniotic fluid begin at the 11th to 12th week of gestation. Autopsies of fetuses with jejunoileal atresia revealed bile and lanugo hairs in the intestinal segments distal to the atresia, thus indicating that the event causing these atresias occurred later than the recanalization period as described previously. In addition, defects in the arteriomesenteric arcade were also identified, supporting an ischemic event. In experimental models, in-utero ligation of a mesenteric vessel leads to an intestinal atresia. Causes of secondary atresias include scar formation after an intrauterine intestinal perforation in meconium ileus, intrauterine intussusception and volvulus, and intestinal snaring through the umbilical ring during bowel reentry into the abdominal cavity.

Secondary atresias can also be the result of bowel herniation through various mesenteric defects or localized infarction/thrombosis of the vascular supply to a segment of bowel, resulting in necrosis and subsequent atresia. Jejunoileal atresia and colonic atresia are considered the secondary result of an ischemic event, usually occurring much later in fetal development than duodenal atresia.

Classification

Intestinal atresias are classified as follows (Skandalakis & Gray, 1994; Stauffer & Schwoebel, 1998; Touloukian, 1993) (Fig. 19-1).

Type I

Intraluminal web, membrane, or diaphragm consisting of mucosa and submucosa, completely obstructing the lumen. The muscularis is intact. This is the most common type of duodenal atresia. The "windsock anomaly" is a type I atresia in which the mucosal membrane has elongated or stretched out into the distal segment because of peristalsis.

Type II

Proximal and distal blind ends connected by a fibrous cord with mesentery intact. Type II anomalies occur in both duodenal atresia and jejunoileal atresia.

Type IIIa

Proximal and distal blind ends separated by a defect, usually V shaped, in the mesentery.

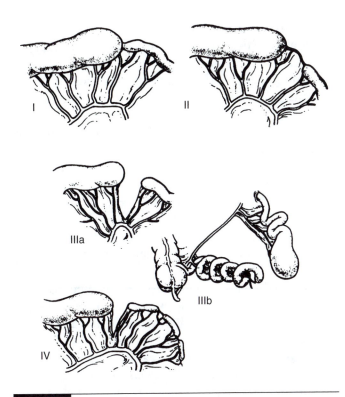

Figure 19-1 Classification of intestinal atresia.
(From *Pediatric Surgery*, 5th ed. O'Neill, J. A., Rowe, M. I., Grosfeld, J. L., Fonkalsrud, E. W., & Coran, A. G. Vols. I & II. 1998. Figure 74-5: Classification of Intestinal Atresia, pg. 1150.)

Type IIIb

Proximal blind end with distal segment coiling around single ileocolic vessel (apple peel or Christmas tree anomaly).

Type IV

Blind proximal end with multiple, isolated, distal segments (string of sausages).

Types III and IV are most often found in jejunal and ileal atresia. Multiple atresias of the duodenum are extremely rare. Types III and IV jejunal anomalies commonly result in short-bowel syndrome; types I and II usually result in normal intestinal length (Skandalakis & Gray, 1994). Type III and IV anomalies of the ileum may not result in short-bowel syndrome because of the ileum's ability to adapt to the shortened length.

Specific Types of Atresias

Duodenal Atresia

In a recent review, Stauffer and Schwoebel (1998) reported that duodenal atresia occurs in 1 in 6,000 to 1 in 10,000 live births. They reported the first documented case in the literature in the 18th century, but it was not until 1914 that the first successful repair was performed by Danish surgeon Ernst. One third of these cases have associated

Down syndrome, and, of these, there is a significant incidence of congenital heart disease. There is also an association with Hirschsprung's disease. Because this is a proximal intestinal obstruction, there is usually a history of polyhydramnios. As high as 50% to 65% of cases of duodenal atresia have associated prematurity because of the onset of premature labor as a result of severe polyhydramnios (Nakayama, 1997a; Ross, 1994; Skandalakis & Gray, 1994).

Pathophysiology Duodenal obstruction occurs as a result of stenosis, atresia, or extrinsic causes, such as annular pancreas, malrotation with volvulus, preduodenal portal vein, or duplications. A preduodenal portal vein is a condition in which the portal vein lies anterior to the duodenum. This anomaly is frequently associated with rotational abnormalities and situs inversus, which are, in turn, associated with duodenal obstruction (Ross, 1994). Annular pancreas is a condition that results from abnormal development of the pancreas during the second month of gestation, resulting in thin, flat segments of the pancreas surrounding the duodenum and causing a partial or complete obstruction. Stenosis and extrinsic causes result in partial obstruction and in some cases symptoms may not appear until later in life. Atresia, on the other hand, results in a complete obstruction and occurs with an acute onset of symptoms within hours after birth. The exception to this is the case of a type I atresia in which an intraluminal membrane or diaphragm perforates, resulting in a partial duodenal obstruction. Approximately 80% of duodenal atresias occur in the first and second portions of the duodenum, below the level of the bile ducts (Skandalakis & Gray, 1994). The proximal duodenum is greatly dilated with thickened, hypertrophied walls. The stomach and pylorus are also dilated. The distal duodenal segment is narrowed (because of disuse) and thin walled. Occasionally, the discrepancy in circumference of proximal and distal segments can be great, with the proximal segment measuring as much as 10 times that of the distal segment. Duodenal atresia rarely occurs above the level of the ampulla of Vater, with the most common site being at the ampulla. Occasionally, anomalies of the bile ducts and biliary tree are present.

Prenatal Diagnosis Duodenal and proximal jejunal obstruction often result in maternal polyhydramnios. Ultrasonography demonstrates a dilated, fluid-filled stomach and proximal duodenum. Absence of these findings does not necessarily rule out duodenal atresia, but patients with these findings should be closely monitored with subsequent ultrasonography. Amnioreduction is indicated in cases of severe polyhydramnios, threatening preterm labor. If this procedure is performed, an aliquot of amniotic fluid is usually sent for karyotyping to rule out trisomy 21. Duodenal stenosis is more difficult to diagnose prenatally because the amniotic fluid passes through the stenotic segment and is absorbed in the distal ileum. In cases in which duodenal atresia is suspected before birth, the family should be prepared for a transfer to a tertiary care center for the genetic work-up and postnatal surgical management and intervention (Nakayama, 1997a; Ross, 1994; Stauffer & Schwoebel, 1998).

Clinical Presentation Infants with duodenal atresia exhibit signs of an acute, proximal obstruction in the first few hours after birth. This is in contrast to more distal intestinal atresias in which the development of obstructive signs may occur gradually over the first 24 to 48 hours of life. Table 19-2 contrasts the history and presentation of infants with intestinal obstruction. Signs of obstruction may not develop in infants with duodenal stenosis until months or years later. Occasionally, signs of obstruction develop when there is a change in the consistency in feedings from liquids to pureed, soft, or semisolid foods. The introduction of liquid feedings is able to pass beyond the stenotic segment, but solid foods cause or reveal a partial obstruction. Infants with complete obstruction caused by duodenal atresia exhibit bilious emesis soon after birth or with the first feeding or have a bile-stained gastric aspirate. Exceptions to this are cases in which a high-level web occurs proximal to the ampulla, in which case emesis would be nonbilious. Gastric aspirate in excess of 30 mL indicates a high-level obstruction. An abdominal examination may reveal fullness in the area of the epigastrium and, otherwise, the belly is flat or scaphoid because of the lack of gas throughout the gastrointestinal (GI) tract. Occasionally, the stomach is so distended that the abdomen appears to have generalized distention. Decompression of the stomach with a vented orogastric/nasogastric (OG/NG) tube, such as a Replogle or Salem sump tube, relieves the distention and leaves the infant with a scaphoid abdomen. Patients with duodenal atresia pass meconium, in contrast to those with a more distal obstruction, in which meconium is scant. The infant may be jaundiced, with increased unconjugated or indirect hyperbilirubinemia. Other abnormal laboratory findings include electrolyte disturbances caused by dehydration and a hypochloremic alkalosis when persistent vomiting occurs.

Diagnostic Work-Up/Differential Diagnosis A plain, supine radiograph is indicated as part of the initial diagnostic work-up. An abdominal plain film may reveal a dilated, fluid-filled and air-filled stomach and proximal duodenum that appear as the classic "double-bubble" sign. The first part of the "double bubble" is the dilated stomach; the second part is the dilated duodenum. Beyond the dilated duodenum, the abdomen is gasless. This "double-bubble" sign combined with a gasless abdomen is diagnostic for duodenal atresia. Occasionally, a large amount of fluid in the stomach may obscure interpretation of the film. In this situation, an OG/NG tube is placed, and gastric fluid is aspirated. Then, 50 to 60 mL of air is instilled into the stomach through the tube. This amount of air usually provides sufficient contrast to demonstrate the double-bubble sign more clearly. In cases of complete duodenal obstruction caused by atresia, there is no role for a contrast study.

When duodenal stenosis or a partial high-level obstruction is suspected, a "double bubble" may be seen, but gas is also seen throughout the abdomen. In this case, two radiologic views of the abdomen should be obtained:

Table 19-2 Gastrointestinal Obstruction in the Neonate

	Proximal	Distal
1. Polyhydramnios	Yes	No
2. Prematurity	Frequent	Occasional
3. Onset of symptoms	Early (hours, after first feeding)	Late (24–48 hr)
4. Vomiting		
Character	± Bilious	+ Bilious
Volume	Large	Small
Timing	Early	Late
5. Distention	Mild, localized	Severe, generalized
6. Jaundice	Yes	Yes/no
7. Plain films	"Double bubble" or few dilated loops	Multiple dilated loops
8. Meconium	Adequate	Scant
9. Microcolon	No	Yes

a flat plate and a left lateral decubitus or cross-table lateral. Whenever even a scant amount of gas is seen distal to the obstruction, rotational abnormalities must be ruled out. Malrotation with midgut volvulus can cause compression of the superior mesenteric artery and resultant bowel ischemia within a few hours (see Chapter 24). Because of the possibility of bowel ischemia and necrosis, an upper GI series is performed promptly to rule out rotational abnormalities. Ultrasonography can be helpful in diagnosing an annular pancreas or may reveal a "whirlpool sign," which is characteristic of volvulus (Stauffer & Schwoebel, 1998).

Jejunoileal Atresia

Jejunoileal atresia is a congenital obstruction of either the jejunum or the ileum. These small intestinal atresias occur in 1 in 5,000 infants (Rowe, O'Neill, & Grosfeld, 1995). The incidence of associated congenital anomalies is lower with jejunoileal atresia, but the associated findings include being small for gestational age, meconium peritonitis/ileus, imperforate anus, renal dysplasia, cardiovascular defects, and a 7% association with chromosomal abnormalities (Herman & McAlister, 1995; Kimble, Harding, & Kolbe, 1997; Sanders, Blackmon, Hogge, & Wolfsberg, 1996; Slee & Goldblatt, 1996). Of note, 25% of neonates with jejunoileal atresia have cystic fibrosis.

Prenatal Diagnosis Diagnosis of midgut intestinal atresia may be suspected with maternal polyhydramnios and detected by fetal ultrasonography. Because amniotic fluid is absorbed in the distal ileum, a maternal history of polyhydramnios is less common in jejunoileal atresia than in duodenal atresia. Ultrasonography obtained at 24 weeks gestation demonstrates multiple dilated fluid-filled bowel loops proximal to the stenotic/atretic segment (Sanders et al., 1996), later in gestation than duodenal atresia.

Clinical Presentation The classic signs of jejunoileal atresia include bilious vomiting, abdominal distention, and failure to pass normal amounts of meconium. This obstructive picture, associated with jejunoileal atresia, usually does not present until after the first feeding or by 24 hours of life (Ross, 1994). An earlier presentation of obstruction would be suspect for a higher intestinal obstruction. Of note, the presence of bile in gastric aspirates suggests an obstruction distal to the ampulla of Vater, where the bile ducts empty into the duodenum, and is associated to a greater degree with jejunal atresia. The infant exhibits generalized abdominal distention. The greater the abdominal distention, the more distal the intestinal obstruction. In addition, in more distal obstruction, the passage of meconium becomes more scant. This is due to the lack of succus entericus passing through the distal segment.

Diagnostic Work-Up/Differential Diagnosis Abdominal radiographs, flat and erect or lateral decubitus, reveal air-fluid levels and multiple dilated proximal loops of bowel. A contrast enema may be helpful in diagnosing microcolon. Because the colon never fills with meconium, it remains underexpanded or unused, resulting in a colon smaller in diameter than the normal colon. In addition, a contrast enema helps to differentiate small- versus large-bowel distention or ileal stenosis and may evaluate intestinal rotation. Hirschsprung's disease should also be included in the differential diagnosis of distal ileal atresia, and a contrast enema should be obtained to identify a possible transition zone. Ultrasonography is helpful in distinguishing meconium ileus from ileal atresia. Ileal atresia presents as dilated loops filled with fluid and air (Neal, Seibert, Vanderzalam, & Wagner, 1997). On ultrasonographic examination, meconium ileus is demonstrated by a thick, echogenic fluid in the intestine. This meconium-filled bowel is described as a "soap bubble" or "ground glass" appearance, where air is mixed with thick, inspissated meconium. These are important radiologic findings because meconium ileus may be treated medically with hyperosmolar enemas, whereas intestinal atresias require surgery.

Colonic Atresia

Colonic atresia is the rarest form of intestinal atresia, occurring in about 1 in 20,000 live births and accounting for < 5% of all atresias (Oldham, 1998; Skandalakis & Gray, 1994). Successful repair with diverting colostomy reportedly was performed in 1922 by Gaub. Dr. Potts was the first to perform successful primary anastomosis in 1947. Colonic atresia is associated with skeletal, ocular, and cardiac anomalies; Hirschsprung's disease; and other intestinal atresias (Croaker, Harvey, & Cass, 1997; Oldham).

Embryology The embryogenesis of colonic atresia is thought to be the same as jejunoileal atresia: in utero vascular compromise. Possible causes of vascular compromise include incarcerated hernias, colonic volvulus, and intussusception. The classification of small bowel atresia is also applied to colonic atresia (Oldham, 1998; Skandalakis & Gray, 1994). See Figure 19-1.

Clinical Presentation A prenatal history of polyhydramnios is not usually present in colonic atresia because amniotic fluid is absorbed in the distal ileum. The infant with colonic atresia is seen with signs of a high-grade distal obstruction. These signs include generalized distention, feeding intolerance, and bilious vomiting. Because there is little intestine distal to the atresia, passage of meconium is scant or absent (Oldham, 1998; Ross, 1994; Touloukian, 1993).

Diagnostic Work-Up Abdominal plain films reveal multiple, large, dilated loops with a "cut-off sign" and air-fluid levels. A cut-off sign is the point at which the intestinal gas pattern abruptly ends. The proximal intestinal loops are distended, and no gas is in the rectum or distal colon. Colonic atresia presenting as a perforation is common. In this case, pneumoperitoneum is seen on plain films. A contrast enema, with either barium or a water-soluble agent, demonstrates a microcolon with a cut-off of contrast medium (contrast ends abruptly) at the atretic point and proximal, dilated bowel. The contrast enema establishes a definitive diagnosis of colonic atresia and can help identify an associated distal obstruction, such as short-segment Hirschsprung's disease.

Preoperative Management

The infant with a complete proximal intestinal obstruction requires aggressive gastric decompression, fluid resuscitation and replacement, and correction of electrolyte abnormalities. Moderate-to-severe hypochloremic alkalosis may be present, which, if untreated, can lead to cardiac dysrhythmia. Monitoring of bilirubin levels is indicated because of increased unconjugated or indirect hyperbilirubinemia. Once stabilized, the infant is a candidate for surgical repair. Associated problems, such as congenital heart disease or respiratory distress syndrome, should be identified before operative intervention. Malrotation should be ruled out, as described earlier. A thorough physical examination is performed before the operation to rule out associated anomalies, such as the VACTERL association (V = vertebral, A = anorectal, C = cardiac, T-E = tracheal-esophageal, R = renal, L = limb anomalies) (Skandalakis & Gray, 1994; Touloukian, 1993) and others as listed in Table 19-1. When an atresia is associated with an obvious VACTERL anomaly as evidenced on physical examination such as radial dysplasia or imperforate anus, further investigation for other associated anomalies within the VACTERL association should be performed.

Preoperative laboratory studies include electrolytes, complete blood count, type and cross-match, and bilirubin levels. Electrolyte imbalances are corrected or communicated to the anesthesia team. Packed red blood cells are available for use during surgery, although the actual need for transfusion is uncommon. Perioperative antibiotics are given intravenously. Before the child is taken to the operating room, a plan for long-term intravenous access should be considered, because in some cases, progression to full enteral feedings may not occur for some time.

The support and education of the family in this preoperative period are crucial. The family is not only adjusting to the arrival of a new infant, but they are also adjusting to the diagnosis, to the information regarding the upcoming surgery, and perhaps to the concomitant diagnosis of trisomy 21, congenital heart disease, and/or other associated anomalies. Collaboration among surgery, cardiology, genetics, and other subspecialties to provide consistent, timely information to the family at this time is imperative.

Operative Intervention

Once stabilized, the infant is a candidate for surgical repair. Options for surgical repair depend on the type of anomaly and the preference of the surgeon. The goal of surgical intervention is to establish intestinal continuity and eliminate or prevent functional obstruction.

Duodenal Atresia Repair

Excision of Duodenal Web (Fig. 19-2) Excision of the duodenal web is performed through a right upper-quadrant transverse incision. The dilated proximal duodenum is

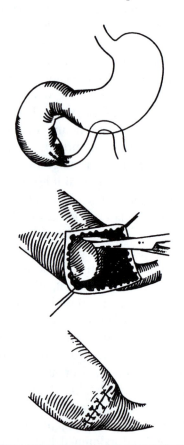

Figure 19-2 Excision of a duodenal web through a longitudinal incision across the area of obstruction.
(From *Pediatric Surgery*, 5th ed. O'Neill, J. A., Rowe, M. I., Grosfeld, J. L., Fonkalsrud, E. W., & Coran, A. G. Vols. I & II. 1998. Figure 73-10: Duodenal Web.)

identified. Because the muscularis is intact, the only finding is that of discrepant size of duodenal segments that are contiguous. A transpyloric tube is passed in the operating room in type I anomalies to rule out a wind-sock anomaly. When gentle pressure is placed on the tube, there is an indentation seen in the outer layer of the bowel at the point of the attachment of the membrane. A longitudinal incision is made at the site of obstruction. The web is identified, and the lateral portion is excised. The medial portion of the web is left intact because of the great risk of damaging the ampulla of Vater, which is often located at the site of the web attachment medially. The location of the ampulla can be detected by applying gentle pressure on the gallbladder. After excision of a portion of the web, a catheter is passed distally, and saline is instilled until it empties into the colon. This passage of fluid rules out multiple distal webs (Nakayama, 1997a; Ross, 1994; Stauffer & Schwoebel, 1998).

Duodenoduodenostomy (Fig. 19-3) In a duodenoduodenostomy, a transverse right upper-quadrant incision is made. The hepatic flexure of the colon is mobilized, and the proximal, dilated portion of the duodenum is identified and freed from its attachments. Careful note is made of the presence of a preduodenal portal vein, abnormal pancreas, or abnormalities in rotation. If malrotation exists, a

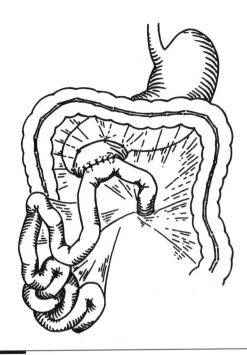

Figure 19-4 Duodenojejunostomy.
(From *Pediatric Surgery*, 5th ed. O'Neill, J. A., Rowe, M. I., Grosfeld, J. L., Fonkalsrud, E. W., & Coran, A. G. Vols. I & II. 1998. Figure 73-11: Duodenojejunostomy.)

Ladd's procedure is performed (see Chapter 24). The distal duodenal segment is identified and mobilized. A transverse incision is made in the proximal segment carefully placed above the level of the ampulla of Vater. A longitudinal incision is made in the distal duodenal segment. Before closure of the anastomosis, a catheter is passed into the distal segment, and saline is instilled until it empties into the colon. This is done to rule out multiple distal atresias (Cilley & Coran, 1995; Ross, 1994; Stauffer & Schwoebel, 1998). The proximal transverse incision and distal longitudinal incision allow creation of a diamond-shaped anastomosis (Kimura et al., 1990). If an annular pancreas exists, the segment of duodenum and aberrant pancreatic tissue is bypassed with the duodenoduodenostomy. The pancreatic tissue is not divided off the duodenum because of the risk of fistula formation, pancreatitis, and possible damage to underlying bile ducts (Cilley & Coran, 1995; Nakayama, 1997a; Stauffer & Schwoebel, 1998).

Duodenojejunostomy (Fig. 19-4) Occasionally, duodenojejunostomy may be required if the atresia involves the distal portion of the duodenum. A duodenojejunostomy consists of freeing up the proximal dilated duodenal segment and performing a retrocolic end-to-side anastomosis to the jejunum. In performing the duodenojejunostomy, consideration is given to placement of a gastrostomy tube, transanastomotic tube, and central line.

Tapering Duodenoplasty (Fig. 19-5) In cases in which the proximal duodenal bulb is extremely dilated and

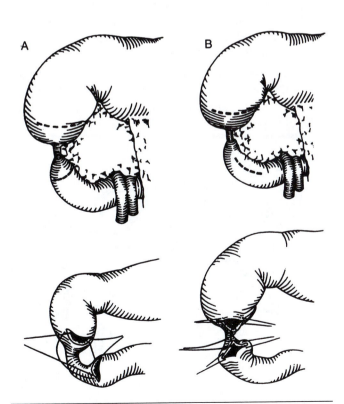

Figure 19-3 Duodenoduodenostomy.
(From *Pediatric Surgery*, 5th ed. O'Neill, J. A., Rowe, M. I., Grosfeld, J. L., Fonkalsrud, E. W., & Coran, A. G. Vols. I & II. 1998. Figure 73-12: Duodenoduodenostomy, pg. 1141.)

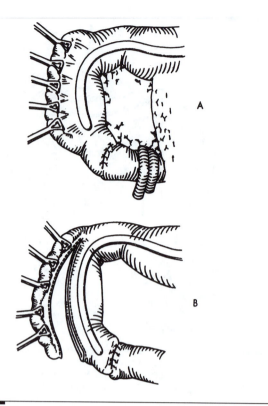

Figure 19-5 Tapering duodenoplasty in cases with excessive floppy and distended proximal duodenum.
(From *Pediatric Surgery*, 5th ed. O'Neill, J. A., Rowe, M. I., Grosfeld, J. L., Fonkalsrud, E. W., & Coran, A. G. Vols. I & II. 1998. Figure 73-14: Tapering Duodenoplasty, pg. 1142.)

floppy, a tapering procedure is considered to better approximate the proximal and distal portions of the repair. This procedure encourages earlier function of the dilated proximal segment and prevents stasis and dysmotility of the proximal end. This technique consists of autostapling and excising the antimesenteric portion of the dilated proximal segment longitudinally. Plication of the distended segment can also be performed over a dilator (Cilley & Coran 1995; Touloukian, 1993). An alternative plication procedure consists of performing an elliptical excision of the seromuscular section of the distended duodenum. The mucosa, which is left intact, is then inverted or imbricated (arranged in a regular pattern with overlapping edges). This technique avoids a long suture line but still tapers the dilated segment. It has been used to treat both duodenal and jejunal atresia (Kimura, Perdzynski, & Soper, 1996).

Jejunal-Ileal Atresia Repair

Jejuno-Jejunostomy An exploratory laparotomy is accomplished through a right upper-quadrant transverse supraumbilical incision. The atresia is identified, and the operative choice of procedure depends on the pathological type of obstruction. In cases of high jejunal atresia,

the atonic, atretic segment of proximal jejunum is resected back to the ligament of Treitz, and an end-to-oblique anastomosis is performed (Fig. 19-6). Leaving an extremely dilated proximal segment of intestine in any type of anastomosis usually results in a functional obstruction (Grosfeld, 1998). This is thought to be due to smooth muscle hyperplasia in the proximal segment, which in turn causes ineffective peristalsis. Inefficient contractions and propulsion lead to a chronic, obstructive state. In extreme cases, this results in decompensation of the segment of intestine and obstruction. Whenever possible, this dilated portion is resected.

Tapering Jejunoplasty (Fig 19-7) In cases in which intestinal length is limited, resection may not be possible. Instead, an antimesenteric-tapering jejunoplasty may be performed. Alternatively, an imbrication tapering technique can also be performed to reduce the caliber of distended intestine and facilitate restoration of function. The advantage of this technique is that the mucosa is left intact; the disadvantage is breakdown of the imbrication and recurrent dilation. The goal of either tapering procedure is to decrease the lumen size of dilated segment while preserving intestinal length. Similar to duodenal atresia, some surgeons consider placement of a transanastomotic feeding tube for proximal jejunal atresia, allowing for early enteral feedings.

Ileal Atresia Repair In cases of ileal atresia, primary anastomosis is preferred. However, in cases of ileal atresia associated with volvulus or where vascular integrity of the remaining bowel is in question, or in cases associated with meconium peritonitis, resection of the atretic ileal segment and exteriorization of bowel occurs. Examples of exteriorization procedures are demonstrated in Figure 19-8.

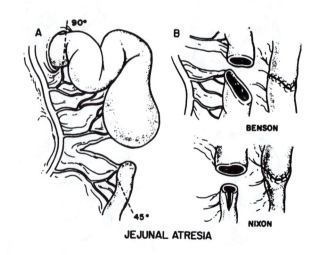

Figure 19-6 Jejuno-jejunostomy.
(From *Pediatric Surgery*, 5th ed. O'Neill, J. A., Rowe, M. I., Grosfeld, J. L., Fonkalsrud, E. W., & Coran, A. G. Vols. I & II. 1998. Figure 74-6: Jejunal Atresia.)

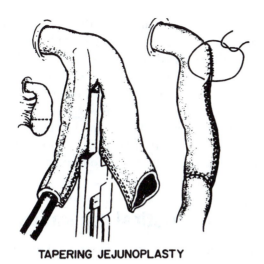

Figure 19-7 Tapering jejunoplasty.
(From *Pediatric Surgery*, 5th ed. O'Neill, J. A., Rowe, M. I., Grosfeld, J. L., Fonkalsrud, E. W., & Coran, A. G. Vols. I & II. 1998. Figure 74-6: Tapering Jejunoplasty.)

Colonic Atresia Repair A transverse supraumbilical incision is used to allow the greatest exposure. Resection of the vastly dilated proximal end, with end-to-oblique primary anastomosis, is performed in cases in which no perforation or spillage has occurred and the infant is generally stable. If the infant is unstable and/or there is significant fecal spillage or peritonitis, a diverting colostomy and a staged repair are performed. If the infant does not have severe cardiac or respiratory disease, prognosis and functional outcome are good. In either approach, the colonic specimen is evaluated for the presence of ganglion cells to rule out coexisting Hirschsprung's disease (Nakayama, 1997a; Oldham, 1998; Ross, 1994).

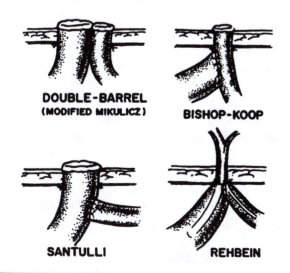

Figure 19-8 Exteriorization procedures.
(From *Pediatric Surgery*, 5th ed. O'Neill, J. A., Rowe, M. I., Grosfeld, J. L., Fonkalsrud, E. W., & Coran, A. G. Vols. I & II. 1998. Figure 74-7: Ileal Atresia, pg. 1153.)

Nutritional Support

The decision to place a gastrostomy tube is based on the overall condition of the infant and the individual surgeon's preference. Other indications for a gastrostomy tube may include complex congenital heart disease, Down syndrome, and severe prematurity. A transanastomotic nasojejunal or gastrojejunal tube is sometimes placed, with the goal of initiation of earlier enteral feedings. Some surgeons believe that this is not necessary and has not been effective in terms of initiating feedings earlier. For patients who do require a gastrostomy tube and if the surgeon prefers a transanastomotic tube, a side-by-side transgastric, transanastomotic tube is placed for early initiation of feedings. Occasionally, a surgical jejunostomy is performed for patients with complex anomalies or extreme prematurity. Finally, placement of a central line is considered at the time of operation for those patients who may require parenteral nutrition, who have critical associated anomalies, and/or who are small for age (Grosfeld, 1998; Touloukian, 1993).

Postoperative Management

Acute postoperative management includes the following: (1) oro/nasogastric decompression and drainage; (2) intravenous fluid administration, including replacement of gastric output and third-space losses; (3) administration of intravenous antibiotics for 48 hours; (4) serial abdominal examinations, including assessment of surgical incision; (5) serial laboratory evaluation; (6) assessment of return of bowel function, as evidenced by passage of stool (alert surgeon if stool is acholic or if stools are light tan or clay colored because of lack of bile, specifically choleic acid), decreasing NG aspirate, clearing of NG aspirate color from bilious to clear; and (7) pain management achieved by judicious administration of intravenous narcotics (morphine) and/or ketorolac, advancing to acetaminophen, as tolerated, or use of an epidural catheter managed in collaboration with the anesthesia pain team (see Chapter 5 for more information about postoperative pain management in the neonate).

Initiation of enteral feedings occurs when the ileus has resolved, the anastomosis begins to "open up" (GI secretions passing through the anastomosis), and the infant exhibits signs of return of bowel function as described previously. In particular, decreased gastric output that is lightening in color is a sign that the reanastomosed bowel has begun to function. Early signs of sepsis, including thrombocytopenia, temperature instability, increased white blood cells, and peritoneal signs herald an anastomotic leak (Nakayama, 1997a). In situations in which a transanastomotic feeding tube is placed or surgical jejunostomy is performed, slow continuous feedings can be started on the first postoperative day. Enteral feedings are initiated slowly and with caution, assessing for any signs of obstruction or anastomotic dysfunction. Initial enteral feedings consist of low-volume, clear, oral rehydration solution every 2 to 3 hours, with a gradual increase in volume. The feeding regimen goal is 150 mL/kg/day of 20 calorie per ounce formula or full-strength breast milk, which translates to 100 kcal/kg/day. Bolus feedings of full-strength 20 calorie per ounce formula or breast milk, given every 2 to 3 hours, are increased by 5 mL each day to goal. Alternatively, continuous feedings of full-strength formula are increased by 1 mL/day to goal. Once goal is reached at 150 mL/kg/day, formula or breast milk can then be concentrated if added calories are needed. Increased frequency of stools and reducing substances found in stool are signs of intolerance. The most common reason for failure to progress feedings is altered peristalsis. This results from the size discrepancy in blind ends, especially in cases in which a tapering procedure was not performed. Because of this anatomic problem, some patients may take up to 14 days for anastomotic function and bowel function to return. Another reason for delayed feeding is actual anastomotic dysfunction, in which reoperation and anastomotic revision is required. For patients with ileal atresia who have delayed passage of stool, Hirschsprung's disease should be considered. A suction rectal biopsy can assess for ganglion cells when there is a suspicion of Hirschsprung's disease.

Long-term survival of infants with intestinal atresia has improved over the past decades. As high as 95% of infants with isolated duodenal atresia survive (Stauffer & Schwoebel, 1998). Most causes of death are attributed to associated cardiac disease (Touloukian, 1993). Late complications of duodenal atresia include megaduodenum, which can be treated with a tapering procedure. Other complications include dysmotility, duodenogastric reflux, gastritis, peptic ulcer disease, and gastroesophageal reflux disease, all of which can be treated medically with motility-enhancing agents (bethanechol, metoclopramide) and acid suppression (ranitidine, omeprazole). Other rare complications include choledochal cyst, cholelithiasis, and cholecystitis. As with duodenal atresia, 95% of infants with isolated jejunoileal atresia can also be expected to survive. The exception is type IIIb (apple peel deformity) and type IV multiple atresias (string of sausages). In these cases, there is often significant loss of intestinal length resulting in short-bowel syndrome. Infants with less than 10 to 20 cm of small bowel have a poor prognosis and often succumb to complications of treatment

for short-bowel syndrome, including central line sepsis or total parenteral nutrition–associated liver failure. In addition, those infants who have lost distal ileum often experience B_{12} deficiency with resultant megaloblastic anemia and gallstones. However, most infants have an excellent outcome and at most need medical management and follow-up for dysmotility, bacterial overgrowth, and pseudo-obstruction (Bianchi, Crombleholme, & Dalton, 2000; Grosfeld, 1998; Touloukian, 1993).

■ Gastrointestinal Duplications

The term duplications encompasses GI anomalies that are either cystic or tubular and are associated in some way with the GI tract. Three traits are common to duplications: a coating of smooth muscle, an epithelial lining, and an attachment to the GI tract. Cystic duplications are usually closed and do not communicate with the GI tract, whereas tubular duplications usually do communicate with the GI tract, with the communication most often occurring at the caudal end. Duplications may arise anywhere along the GI tract from the base of the tongue to the anus. Seventy-five percent of GI duplications are abdominal, 20% are thoracic, and 5% are thoracoabdominal. Associated anomalies include vertebral anomalies, esophageal atresia, jejunal atresia, anal defects, and genitourinary fistulas. GI duplications can be extensive. Ten percent of GI duplications have more than one duplicated segment.

Embryology

There are varied theories concerning the embryology of GI duplications (Skandalakis & Gray, 1994). One theory is failure of regression of certain embryonic structures. A second theory is failure of recanalization, similar to the duodenal atresia embryogenesis, occurring at about the fifth to eighth week of gestation, where proliferation of epithelial cells obliterate the lumen of the intestine. A third embryologic process theorized to result in duplications occurs during the fourth week of gestation. During this time, the gut endoderm separates from the notochord. This notochord is the precursor of the vertebral column. Abnormal adherence of a cord of gut endoderm to a portion of the notochord results in the formation of GI duplications that are cystic, tubular, or diverticular.

Clinical Presentation

Gastrointestinal duplications typically are seen by 2 years of age. In utero diagnosis of duplication is considered in patients with suspicious fetal ultrasonograms, including signs of proximal bowel obstruction, as evidenced by polyhydramnios. Some duplications do not become symptomatic until adulthood, and still others are never symptomatic and are not found until autopsy. Clinical presentation depends on location and size. The symptoms may lead the clinician to suspect the more common diagnoses of intestinal atresia/stenosis, intussusception, volvulus, or Meckel's diverticulum. The typical presentation includes signs of partial intestinal obstruction, abdominal pain, and GI bleeding. Signs of obstruction, including abdominal distention, pain, and vomiting, occur as a result of the duplication compressing the lumen of the adjacent intestine (Ross, 1994; Stauffer & Schwoebel, 1998; Templeton, 1995). Pain is the result of intraluminal distention and bowel necrosis caused by compression of the mesenteric vasculature. GI bleeding is most often caused by ectopic gastric mucosa in the lining of the duplication, which in turn causes peptic ulceration. If ulceration progresses, erosion, perforation, and peritonitis may ensue. Thoracic or thoracoabdominal duplications present with respiratory distress from airway compression, heartburn, and melena. Pyloric or duodenal duplications may mimic hypertrophic pyloric stenosis, with emesis and failure to gain weight (Grosfeld, Boles, & Reiner, 1970; Ramsey, 1957). Duodenal duplications, which are rare, present with bleeding, obstruction, and jaundice as a result of obstruction at the ampulla of Vater. Symptoms may range from jaundice to high intestinal obstruction, pancreatitis, and hemorrhage. Colonic duplications may present with signs of constipation, rectal prolapse, and associated perirectal abscess (LaQuaglia et al., 1990).

Diagnostic Work-Up

Tubular GI duplications are most often identified on contrast studies. Cystic duplications can be identified with ultrasonography. In either situation, further radiographic studies, such as computed tomography with oral and intravenous contrast, may be necessary to rule out multiple duplications. Gastric duplications cause external compression on the greater curvature of the stomach, producing a filling defect on an upper GI examination. The contrast material does not fill that area of the stomach at the point where the duplication impinges on the greater curvature. An intestinal duplication cyst may be distinguished from an abdominal mass/tumor, such as neuroblastoma, because the cyst absorbs contrast only along the wall, whereas a tumor absorbs contrast material throughout the mass. A technetium scan is used to detect ectopic gastric lining (Grosfeld, 1998; Ross, 1994; Stauffer & Schwoebel, 1998; Templeton, 1995).

Operative Management

Treatment depends on symptoms and location. Primary resection and end-to-end anastomosis are attempted whenever possible. Because of the frequent presence of ectopic gastric mucosa in the duplication lining, mucosal stripping is performed in all cases to prevent peptic ulceration and carcinogenesis. The goals of surgery are to establish intestinal continuity, relieve obstruction, and preserve intestinal length.

Thoracic and thoracoabdominal duplications require excision. This is accomplished by resection and primary anastomosis or staged repair with communication with the GI tract for drainage. For gastric duplications, complete excision is recommended. If this is not possible, partial excision with stripping of the mucosa or excision of the common wall to facilitate drainage is performed. Duodenal duplication is the rarest and most difficult to treat, primarily because of the proximity to the biliary and pancreatic ductal systems. The compression of the first or second portions of the duodenum requires complete excision of the duplication or duodenotomy for internal drainage. A duodenotomy creates an opening that allows decompression and drainage from the duplication of the duodenum into the true, patent duodenum. Large cystic duplications that occur on the mesenteric side of the bowel or close to the ampulla of Vater may require a drainage procedure, such as a cystoduodenostomy or cystojejunostomy, in which the cyst is drained into the GI tract. This drainage strategy is used when excision is not possible because of the location of the duplication along or adjacent to integral structures (Skandalakis & Gray, 1994).

Small-intestine duplication is most common and is usually located in the ileum. There is usually a shared common muscular wall and a common blood supply with the native bowel. Treatment includes primary resection with end-to-end anastomosis, segmental resection (along with the adjacent intestine), or partial resection with internal drainage at the distal end. There are situations in which primary resection and end-to-end anastomosis are not possible. These situations include lengthy tubular duplications, in which resection would sacrifice a large portion of adjacent true GI tract. In these cases, in which the communication is often at the caudal end, the proximal end can be opened to create a "double barreled" segment of intestine.

Finally, colonic or rectal duplication has been classified as type I, those occurring above the peritoneal reflection, and type II, those associated with the urinary and genital tracts (Dodds & Kottra, 1971). Type I requires resection with primary anastomosis, whereas type II may not require surgery if internal communication is adequate. Some rectal duplications may benefit from a transanal exposure of the cyst and stripping of the cyst wall.

Postoperative Management

Postoperative care of an infant after repair of GI duplication is similar to the care after atresia repair as outlined earlier. This includes postoperative antibiotics, gastric decompression until the ileus is resolved, pain management, and slow advancement of enteral feedings. For older children, early ambulation is instituted, which helps hasten the return of bowel function. In addition, assessment for signs of infection and skin and ostomy care (if needed) are priorities after surgery.

■ Meconium Ileus

History, Incidence, and Associated Anomalies

Andrassy and Nirgiotis (1993) and Rescorla (1998) outlined the history and treatment of meconium ileus as follows. Meconium ileus was first described in 1905 by Landsteiner. It was considered a fatal condition until 1948, when Hiatt and Wilson performed the first successful enterotomy. Meconium ileus is the third most common reason for bowel obstruction in the neonate. Nearly all infants with meconium ileus have cystic fibrosis (CF). CF is an autosomal recessive disease affecting approximately 30,000 Americans of every ethnic population. In Caucasians, it is considered the most common lethal genetic disorder. About 10% to 15% of patients with CF present with meconium ileus as neonates (Andrassy & Nirgiotis; Rescorla). Thus, all patients with meconium ileus should be evaluated for CF. This evaluation should include a sweat test and genetic testing.

Pathophysiology/Diagnosis/Classification

CF is the result of mutations in the gene that codes for the cystic fibrosis transmembrane regulator (CFTR) protein. CFTR protein plays a major role in the transport of chloride, sodium, and water across the apical membrane of the epithelial cells (Andrassy & Nirgiotis, 1993). This aberration results in abnormal airway secretions, causing decreased mucociliary clearance, chronic bronchial infections, and abnormal gastrointestinal secretions, which cause problems with digestion and absorption of food, as well as blockage in the bowel.

Prenatal ultrasonography after 20 weeks' gestation that reveals an echogenic bowel may indicate a meco-nium ileus. This same finding before 20 weeks' gestation is considered normal (Rescorla, 1998). Making the diagnosis of CF includes a comprehensive clinical examination because the sweat test and genetic testing can be inconclusive. Initially, a patient with meconium ileus has abdominal distention, bilious emesis, and no passage of meconium. As part of the differential diagnosis, volvulus, intestinal atresias, Hirschsprung's disease, and perforation should be ruled out. In some cases, volvulus or perforation can occur as a result of meconium ileus. The latter is referred to as *complicated meconium ileus*. Perforation can occur before birth and results in ascites and peritonitis. Perforations that go undiagnosed and thus untreated can result in calcifications and adhesions. If volvulus is present, ischemia and necrosis may result (Andrassy & Nirgiotis, 1993; Nakayama, 1997b; Rescorla; Ross, 1994).

Radiographically, meconium ileus is characterized by dilated loops of proximal small bowel and a distal ileum packed with meconium. The distal portion of the ileum and ascending colon may be beaded with meconium. In about one third of the cases, air fluid levels are not present, because the meconium sticks to the lumen of the intestinal wall (Rescorla, 1998). The collection of meconium in the bowel has a granular appearance radiographically and thus is referred to as "ground glass" or "soap bubble" appearance (Rescorla). Distal to the obstruction, the colon is unused or described as a microcolon when visualized with contrast and radiography.

Preoperative Care/Medical Management

When meconium ileus is suspected, an OG/NG tube should be placed and connected to low, continuous suction to decompress the stomach. The patient should be adequately hydrated, and antibiotics should be started prophylactically. In an effort to clean out the thick, inspissated meconium, a hyperosmolar solution known as Gastrografin can be administered by means of an enema (Rescorla, 1998). This solution is radiopaque, and, therefore, the first dose is delivered during a radiographic study to assist in the diagnostic work-up. Gastrografin enemas have been successful in breaking up the meconium and resolving the obstruction. Hyperosmolar solutions cause a shift of fluids from the intravascular space into the bowel lumen, thus facilitating clearing of the thick meconium. Because of the hyperosmolar nature of Gastrografin, electrolytes and hydration status require close monitoring. Acetylcysteine (Mucomyst), a mucolytic, has also been used successfully to break up meconium and relieve the meconium ileus (Nakayama, 1997b; Rescorla; Ross, 1994).

Surgical Interventions

In situations in which meconium ileus cannot be relieved by medical management, surgical intervention is necessary. There are four methods of surgical intervention for meconium ileus: enterotomy and irrigation or resection and ileostomy by the Bishop-Koop, Santulli and Blanc, or the Mikulicz method (Fig. 19-9) (Rescorla, 1998). Survival of patients with meconium ileus who have undergone the Bishop-Koop procedure has dramatically increased over the past several decades (Del Pin, Czyrko, Ziegler, Scanlin, & Bishop, 1992). Enterotomy and irrigation (Fig. 19-10), currently the treatment of choice for uncomplicated meconium ileus, are accomplished by placing a purse-string suture on the antimesenteric wall of the dilated ileum near the *transition* zone. A small rubber catheter is placed through the enterotomy. The bowel is then irrigated with warm saline, acetylcysteine solution, or Gastrografin solution. Most of the meconium is removed through the enterotomy. The remaining meconium is flushed into the colon and is excreted (Rescorla).

In situations of complicated meconium ileus or meconium ileus not resolved by enterotomy and irrigation, an ileal resection is necessary. One of the following procedures is performed: the Bishop-Koop resection of the dilated ileal segment and the proximal end-to-distal ileal anastomosis with distal ostomy or Mikulicz resection with a double-barrel ileostomy. These procedures create temporary ileostomies that can be reversed when the meconium ileus is resolved (Rescorla, 1998). Timing for closure of an ostomy depends on the infant's general health, adequate growth, and assessment for a patent distal limb.

Postoperative Management

Postoperative management consists of GI decompression until the ileus resolves, respiratory support, and administration of antibiotics. Once GI function has resumed as described in earlier sections, enteral feedings are initiated. The diagnosis of CF should be made before the initiation of feedings because pancreatic enzyme supplements may be necessary to help with digestion and absorption of nutrients. From a surgical perspective, these patients do very well. The pulmonary team should be involved in the management strategies as soon as the diagnosis of CF is made. Occasionally, older children with CF develop a

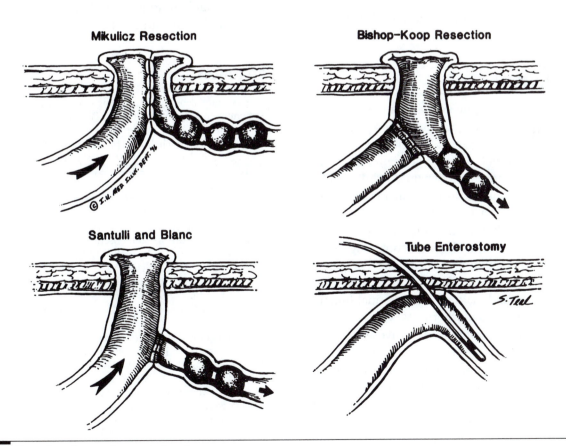

Figure 19-9 Procedures for treating meconium ileus.
(From Rescorla, F. J. & Grosfeld, J. L. Contemporary Management of Meconium Ileus, *World Journal of Surgery*, *17*, 318, 1993. With kind permission of Springer Science and Business Media.)

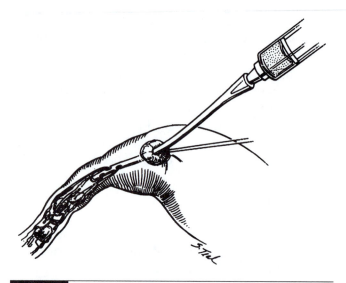

Figure 19-10 Tube enterostomy and irrigation.
(From Rescorla, F. J. & Grosfeld, J. L. Contemporary Management of Meconium Ileus, *World Journal of Surgery, 17,* 318, 1993. With kind permission of Springer Science and Business Media.)

condition termed *meconium ileus equivalent* that mimics meconium ileus of the newborn, in which GI obstruction occurs because of thick, viscous stool. Treatment consists of enemas and washouts with solutions that break up the stool.

Conclusion

Intestinal obstruction in the neonate caused by atresia, stenosis, duplications, or meconium ileus presents the nurse with multiple management challenges. Preoperative treatment priorities include establishment and maintenance of respiratory and hemodynamic stability and decompression of a dilated gastrointestinal tract. Because of the high rate of associated anomalies, the nurse must be a strong patient advocate in coordinating care with a variety of subspecialists, including neonatology, genetics, cardiology, and pulmonary medicine. The goals of surgery include relieving the obstruction, establishing intestinal continuity, and maximizing intestinal function. Surgical intervention in a newborn poses a crisis for families. This crisis may be minimized by involving the parents in discussion with the various disciplines, providing prenatal and preoperative teaching and counseling, and referring parents to appropriate support groups. After surgery, management strategies include assessment for return of bowel function, slow advancement of feedings, assessment for infection, and evaluation and continued education and support of the family. Discharge planning must be comprehensive, especially if coexisting anom-

alies or disease exists. Most patients with isolated atresias or duplications have a good prognosis. Those with associated anomalies or chronic conditions have higher morbidity and mortality. These diagnoses may continue to challenge the patient throughout the life span, so early referral to community resources and accessibility to specialized care is imperative.

Acknowledgment

The authors would like to acknowledge the contributions of Susan K. Von Nessen to this chapter in the first edition of this textbook.

Educational Materials

APSNA invites you to download the following diagnosis-related teaching tools for Chapter 19, Intestinal Atresias, Duplications, and Meconium Ileus: 1) Duodenal atresia; 2) Intestinal atresia. These teaching tools are available at the APSNA Web site (www.apsna.org) and the Jones and Bartlett Web site (www.jbpub.com). All teaching materials are available in English and Spanish and are free of charge. APSNA encourages their use for your patients and families.

References

Andrassy, R. I., & Nirgiotis, J. G. (1993). Meconium disease of infancy: meconium ileus, meconium plug syndrome, and meconium peritonitis. In K. W. Ashcraft (Ed.), *Pediatric surgery* (pp. 331–340). Philadelphia: W.B. Saunders.

Bianchi, D. W., Crombleholme, T. M., & Dalton, M. E. (2000). *Fetology-diagnosis and management of the fetal patient.* New York: McGraw-Hill.

Cilley, R. E., & Coran, A. G. (1995). Duodenoduodenostomy. In L. Spitz & A. G. Coran (Eds.), *Pediatric surgery* (5th ed., pp. 328–332). London: Chapman & Hall.

Croaker, G. D., Harvey, J. G., & Cass, D. T. (1997). Hirschsprung's disease, colonic atresia, and absent hand: A new triad. *Journal of Pediatric Surgery, 32*(9), 1368–1370.

Del Pin, C. A., Czyrko, C., Ziegler, M. M., Scanlin, T. F., & Bishop, H. C. (1992). Management and survival of meconium ileus. *Annals of Surgery, 215,* 179–185.

Dodds, W. J., & Kottra, J. J. (1971). Duplication of the large bowel. *American Journal of Roentgenology, 113,* 310.

Grosfeld, J. L. (1998). Jejunoileal atresia and stenosis. In J. A. O'Neill, M. I. Rowe, & J. L. Grosfeld (Eds.), *Pediatric surgery* (pp. 1145–1158). St. Louis, MO: Mosby.

Grosfeld, J. L., Boles, E. T., & Reiner, C. (1970). Duplication of pylorus in the newborn: A rare cause of gastric outlet obstruction. *Journal of Pediatric Surgery, 5,* 365–369.

Gross, E., Armon, Y., Abu-Dalu, K., Gale, R., & Schiller, M. (1996). Familial combined duodenal and jejunal atresia. *Journal of Pediatric Surgery, 31*(11), 1573.

Harris, J., Kallen, B., & Robert, E. (1995). Descriptive epidemiology of alimentary tract atresia. *Teratology, 52*(1), 15–29.

Herman, T. E., & McAlister, W. H. (1995). Familial type I jejunal atresias and renal dysplasia. *Pediatric Radiology*, 25(4), 272–274.

Kimble, R. M., Harding, J., & Kolbe, A. (1997). Additional congenital anomalies in babies with gut atresia or stenosis: When to investigate, and which investigation. *Pediatric Surgery International*, 12(8), 565–570.

Kimura, K., Mukohara, N., Nishijima, E., Muraji, T., Tsugawa, C., & Matsumoto, Y. (1990). Diamond-shaped anastomosis for duodenal atresia: An experience with 44 patients over 15 years. *Journal of Pediatric Surgery*, 25, 977.

Kimura, K., Perdzynski, W., & Soper, R. T. (1996). Elliptical seromuscular resection for tapering the proximal dilated bowel in duodenal or jejunal atresia. *Journal of Pediatric Surgery*, 31(10), 1405–1406.

LaQuaglia, M. P., Ghavimi, F., Penenberg, D., Mandell, L. R., Healey, J. H., Hadju, S., et al. (1990). Rectal duplications. *Journal of Pediatric Surgery*, 25, 980.

Moore, S. W., de Jongh, G., Bouic, P., Brown, R. A., & Kirsten, G. (1996). Immune deficiency in familial duodenal atresia. *Journal of Pediatric Surgery*, 31(12), 1733–1735.

Nakayama, D. K. (1997a). Duodenal atresia and stenosis. In D. K. Nakayama, C. L. Bose, & N. Chescheir (Eds.), *Critical care of the surgical newborn* (pp. 321–333). Armonk, NY: Futura.

Nakayama, D. K. (l997b). Meconium ileus, meconium peritonitis, and meconium plug. In D. K. Nakayama, C. L. Bose, & N. Chescheir (Eds.), *Critical care of the surgical newborn* (pp. 347–365). Armonk, NY: Futura.

Neal, M. R., Seibert, J. J., Vanderzalam, T., & Wagner, C. W. (1997). Neonatal ultrasonography to distinguish between meconium ileus and ileal atresia. *Journal of Ultrasound in Medicine*, 16(4), 263–268.

Oldham, K. T. (1998). Atresia, stenosis, and other obstructions of the colon. In J. A. O'Neill, M. I. Rowe, & J. L. Grosfeld (Eds.), *Pediatric surgery* (pp. 1361–1368). St. Louis, MO: Mosby.

Ramsey, G. S. (1957). Enterogenous cyst of the stomach simulating hypertrophic pyloric stenosis. *British Journal of Surgery*, 44, 643.

Rescorla, F. J. (1998). Meconium ileus. In J. A. O'Neill, M. I. Rowe, & J. L. Grosfeld (Eds.), *Pediatric surgery* (pp. 1159–1171). St. Louis, MO: Mosby.

Ross, A. J. (1994). Intestinal obstruction in the newborn. *Pediatrics in Review*, 15(9), 338–347.

Rothenberg, M. E., White, F. V., Chilmonzyk, B., & Chatila, J. E. (1995). A syndrome involving immunodeficiency and multiple intestinal atresias. *Immunodeficiency*, 5(3), 171–178.

Rowe, M. A., O'Neill, J. S., & Grosfeld, J. L. (1995). *Essentials of pediatric surgery*. St. Louis, MO: Mosby.

Sanders, R. C., Blackmon, L. R., Hogge, W. A., & Wolfsberg, E. A. (1996). *Structural fetal abnormalities: The total picture*. St. Louis, MO: Mosby.

Skandalakis, J. E., & Gray, S. W. (1994). *Embryology for surgeons*. Baltimore: Williams & Wilkins.

Slee, J., & Goldblatt, J. (1996). Further evidence for a syndrome of "apple peel" intestinal atresia, ocular anomalies and microcephaly. *Clinical Genetics*, 50(4), 260–262.

Stauffer, U. G., & Schwoebel, M. (1998). Duodenal atresia and stenosis: Annular pancreas. In J. A. O'Neill, M. I. Rowe, & J. L. Grosfeld (Eds.), *Pediatric surgery* (pp. 1133–1143). St. Louis, MO: Mosby.

Templeton, J. J. (1995). Gastrointestinal obstruction in the neonate. Resident Lecture Series. Philadelphia: The Children's Hospital of Philadelphia.

Touloukian, R. I. (1993). Intestinal atresia and stenosis. In K. W. Ashcraft (Ed.), *Pediatric surgery* (pp. 305–319). Philadelphia: W.B. Saunders.

Yokoyama, T., Ishizone, S., Momose, Y., Terada, M., Kitahara, S., & Kawasaki, S. (1997). Duodenal atresia in dizygotic twins. *Journal of Pediatric Surgery*, 32(12), 1806–1808.

20

Hirschsprung's Disease

By Melinda Klar

Hirschsprung's disease, also know as aganglionic or congenital megacolon, is a form of chronic intestinal obstruction caused by the absence of the intramural ganglia in the distal bowel. The intramural ganglia or ganglion cells are located throughout the gastrointestinal tract from the mouth through the esophagus and intestines down to the rectum. These cells cause the peristalsis of the muscles in the intestine to move food and by-products down to the rectum. Without ganglion cells, the intestine cannot push the waste out of the rectum. In 1886, Harold Hirschsprung, a pediatrician from Copenhagen, presented his classic description of this obstructive disease that now bears his name. More than five decades later, the actual cause of the obstruction was discovered and a definitive surgical treatment devised (Swenson & Bill, 1948).

■ Incidence

Hirschsprung's disease has a population incidence of 1 in 5,000 live births (Stewart & von Allmen, 2003). The male-to-female ratio is approximately 4:1 among patients with short-segment disease and approximately 1:1 among patients with long-segment disease. There is significant variation among race: Caucasians, with 1.5 cases; African Americans, with 2.1 cases; and Asians, with 2.8 cases per 10,000 live births (Amiel & Lyonnet, 2001).

Hirschsprung's disease most commonly presents as an isolated condition (70% of cases), which arises sporadically although it can be familial. Sporadic cases usually present with short-segment aganglionosis and carry a recurrence risk to siblings ranging from 1.5% and 3.3%. Siblings of patients presenting with long-segment aganglionosis have a risk ranging from 2.9% to 17.6% (Tam & Garcia-Barcelo, 2004). The highest risk is for a male sibling of a female with long-segment Hirschsprung's disease (Amiel & Lyonnet, 2001).

■ Embryology

In normal embryologic development, intestinal ganglion cells originate from neuroblasts that are formed during early fetal development. The cells migrate from the neural crest to the upper end of the alimentary tract and then proceed in the caudal direction. Hirschsprung's disease is a failure of these neural crest cells to colonize the hindgut enteric nervous system throughout its entire length. Therefore Hirschsprung's disease is classified as a "neurocristopathy" (Stewart & von Allmen, 2003).

Pathology

The physical appearance of the intestine in Hirschsprung's disease varies with the duration of the untreated disease. In the neonatal period, the intestine may appear fairly normal. As the child ages, the proximal normal ganglionic bowel hypertrophies and becomes thicker and longer than normal. The transition zone, where ganglionic and aganglionic intestine intersect, may be tunnel-like and variable in length (Fig. 20-1). Although the distal bowel appears grossly normal, the absence of ganglion cells in the distal intestine is the key feature of the disease. The ganglion cells are absent in both the submucosal (Meissner's) plexus and the intermuscular (Auerbach's) plexus. Associated with this finding is a marked increase in nerve fibers, which extend into the submucosa. Classically, the aganglionosis is found in the rectosigmoid region in approximately 80% of cases (Langer et al., 2003). In 10% of cases, the disease involves a greater length of the colon, and in 4%, it extends throughout the colon and may also involve a significant part of the small intestine. The process of aganglionosis is almost always continuous. A few rare cases have documented ganglion cells found intermittently in the colon, but this is extremely unusual.

Associated Anomalies

Seventy percent of Hirschsprung's disease cases are isolated disorders of full-term, otherwise healthy infants (nonsyndromic). Thirty percent of cases are associated with other congenital anomalies (syndromic) (Stewart & von Allmen, 2003). A chromosomal abnormality is associated with Hirschsprung's disease in 12% of cases, with more than 90% of those being trisomy 21. The remaining 18% of the syndromic cases are comprised of associated congenital anomalies, including gastrointestinal malformations, cleft palate, cardiac defects, polydactyly, and craniofacial anomalies (Amiel & Lyonnet, 2001). Although rates of associated urogenital anomalies have been reported to be as high as 23%, it is unknown whether these are primary defects or the result of an enlarged rectum that compresses the bladder neck, leading to obstruction and megacystis. Bladder function in these patients may mimic that of patients with spinal lesions (Holschneider & Ure, 2000).

Atresia of the large and small intestine has also been noted in Hirschsprung's disease. The cause of this association is unknown; it may be the result of a vascular accident with a blockage of ganglion cell migration to the distal intestine (Akgur, Tanyel, Buyukpamukcu, & Hicsonmez, 1993). In this instance, the diagnosis of Hirschsprung's disease is often delayed until after intestinal continuity is established and an obstructive pattern develops (Ikeda & Goto, 1984; Moore, Rode, Miller, & Cywes, 1990). Several clearly defined syndromes are known to be associated with Hirschsprung's disease, such as Waardenburg-Shah syndrome, congenital central hypoventilation syndrome (Ondine's curse), multiple endocrine neoplasia 2A, Goldberg-Shprintzen syndrome and Smith-Lemli-Opitz syndrome (Stewart & von Allmen, 2003; Amiel & Lyonnet, 2001; Dasgupta & Langer, 2004).

Pathophysiology

Normally, a motility reflex is present in the distal rectum. A mildly distending bolus in the distal rectum initiates a contraction above the bolus and a relaxation below the bolus allowing for the passage of the stool. Such a reflex is intrinsic to the intestine itself. The absence of ganglion cells leads to constant contraction of that segment of bowel and an inability to accept the bolus of stool. The segment of bowel that is normally innervated proximal to the aganglionic segment fills with stool and becomes distended. At the same time, it develops hypertrophy of its muscular layers as it tries to force the stool into the contracted distal segment, resulting in a very large dilated proximal segment, which is called megacolon (Filston, 1982).

Nitric oxide has recently been recognized as a neurotransmitter that mediates relaxation of the smooth muscle. The absence of nitric oxide–producing neurons is

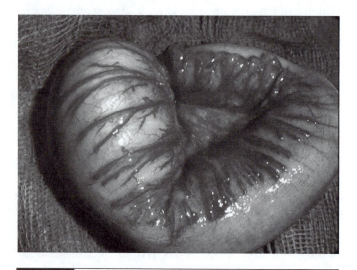

Figure 20-1 Proximal, hypertrophic ganglionic bowel in an infant with Hirschsprung's disease.
(Reprinted with permission by H.C. Filston, M.D.)

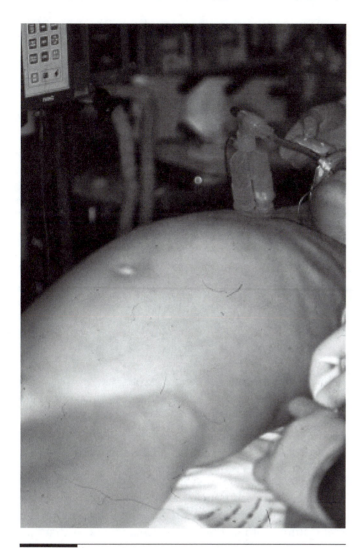

Figure 20-2 Abdominal distention in an older child with Hirschsprung's disease.

thought to be the reason that the aganglionic bowel does not relax (Holschneider & Ure, 2000). Another pathophysiologic feature of Hirschsprung's disease is the association between the congenital absence of ganglion cells and an increase of acetylcholinesterase in the affected tissue. Active research continues into the precise molecular mechanisms responsible for the dramatically increased levels of acetylcholinesterase in the aganglionic segments and its significance (Moore & Johnson, 2005).

■ Genetics

The most recent advances in the understanding of the pathogenesis of Hirschsprung's disease have been in the area of molecular genetics. Recent research has shown that DNA alterations may interfere with the colonization of the neural crest cells in the intestine, which may represent a

primary etiology for Hirschsprung's disease and other neurocristopathies. As work in this area continues, the prediction is that behavior of the gut neural crest stem cells will become better understood, making it possible to treat Hirschsprung's disease by transplanting neural crest stem cells directly into the aganglionic gut (Tam & Garcia-Barcelo, 2004). The advances in genetics have also refined the predictive accuracy of incidence and recurrence for clinicians. To date, nine genes and four loci for Hirschsprung's disease susceptibility have been identified (Brooks, Oostra, & Hofstra, 2005). Understanding and identifying not only the individual genes but how they interact will allow predictions about length of aganglionosis and prognosis after surgery (Stewart & von Allmen, 2003). Currently standard genetic testing in every Hirschsprung's disease patient is a time-consuming and costly activity with limited clinical consequences since surgical repair is reasonably available and very successful.

■ Diagnosis

Hirschsprung's disease should be considered in any child who has a history of constipation dating back to the newborn period. The age at which children are diagnosed with Hirschsprung's disease has decreased over the past several decades. The usual presentation of the disease in newborns consists of a history of delayed passage of stool within the first 48 hours of life, bilious vomiting, and abdominal distention (Khan, Vujanic, & Huddart, 2003). Rectal examination reveals a tight anus but an empty rectal ampulla (Holschneider & Ure, 2000). There may be an explosive discharge of gas and stool after the rectal examination, which may provide temporary relief of the obstruction (Albanese, Harrison, & Sydorak, 2003). Breastfed infants may go through the neonatal period with few or no symptoms. They present later with chronic constipation around the time of weaning or starting of solid foods.

Older children, along with the history of chronic constipation, may present with sluggishness, wasted extremities, flared costal margins, and a grossly distended abdomen (Fig. 20-2). These children have a history of dependence on enemas without significant encopresis. Affected children of any age may also present with enterocolitis or toxic megacolon. This is a potentially life-threatening illness, in which patients have a sepsis-like picture with fever, vomiting, foul-smelling diarrhea, and abdominal distention. Approximately 10% of children with Hirschsprung's disease present with diarrhea due to enterocolitis. Because Hirschsprung's disease is generally thought of as causing constipation, the diagnosis may be overlooked (Dasgupta & Langer, 2004).

Radiology Studies

Plain Radiographs

Flat and upright or decubitus abdominal films commonly show several distended loops of bowel. In the neonate, the initial presentation may be free air on a plain abdominal radiograph, which indicates a perforation of the intestine. It is the periappendiceal area that most commonly perforates proximal to the aganglionic colon (Arliss & Holgersen, 1990). Because this is an emergent event, it is important to consider Hirschsprung's disease with any form of spontaneous perforation in the neonatal period. The morbidity and mortality are high if the diagnosis is delayed or missed (Stewart & von Allmen, 2003).

Barium Enema

A barium enema may be helpful in making a diagnosis. This study involves the insertion of a small Foley catheter into the rectum. The colon is then filled with barium solution, and a series of radiographic films are taken. This allows the radiologist to evaluate the anatomy of the distal bowel and the capacity of the colon. The catheter should be inserted just inside the anus without inflating the catheter balloon because this would obliterate a low transition zone. In addition, it is important to avoid rectal examinations and enemas before the study, which could also distort a low transition zone (Stewart & von Allmen, 2003).

In newborns with suspected meconium ileus or meconium plug syndrome, a water-soluble contrast medium is preferred to barium and may actually serve as a treatment for these conditions (Dasgupta & Langer, 2004). A postevacuation film and 24-hour postevacuation film complete the study. These demonstrate whether the child adequately evacuates the remaining contrast or the colon remains dilated. A classic case of Hirschsprung's disease shows a spastic distal intestinal segment with a dilated proximal bowel (Figs. 20-3 and 20-4). The barium enema in the newborn period may fail to show a transition zone. A barium enema should not be obtained during a clinical episode of enterocolitis, because perforation may result. If the child does not pass any stools within 48 hours, a rectal washout may be necessary, because barium can become firm and difficult to pass.

Anorectal Manometry

Anorectal manometry is another method of diagnosing Hirschsprung's disease. A balloon catheter is placed in-

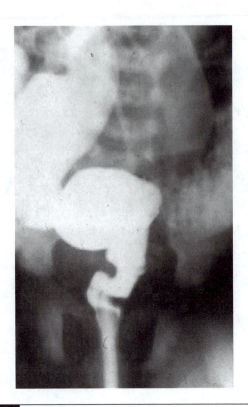

Figure 20-3 Anteroposterior view of barium enema of an infant. (Reprinted with permission by H.C. Filston, M.D.)

side the rectum, and pressures within the distal colon are measured. The technique relies on demonstrating the absence of a relaxation reflex after a distending bolus in the rectal lumen of patients with Hirschsprung's disease. Swenson initially advocated the technique as a first approach to children with this disorder (Swenson, 1964; Swenson, Fisher, & Gherardi, 1959; Swenson, Shennan, Fisher, & Cohen, 1975). Examination during an abnormal state, such as sepsis or hypothyroidism, may yield an inaccurate result (Yunis, Dibbins, & Shennan, 1976). Artifacts may be created by moving or crying and accuracy rates vary widely among reported series (Taxman, Yulish, & Rothstein, 1986; Yunis et al.). There are few complications or side effects with the procedure.

Rectal Biopsy

A rectal biopsy is the definitive method of diagnosing Hirschsprung's disease. Swenson first described the method of a full-thickness rectal biopsy in 1959. The tissue obtained with this technique involves both the submucosal and the intermuscular layers. This allows the pathologist to closely examine the muscle layers of the colon and identify whether ganglion cells are present. In 1960, Gherardi demonstrated that the level of aganglionosis was similar in the submucosa and the myenteric plexus.

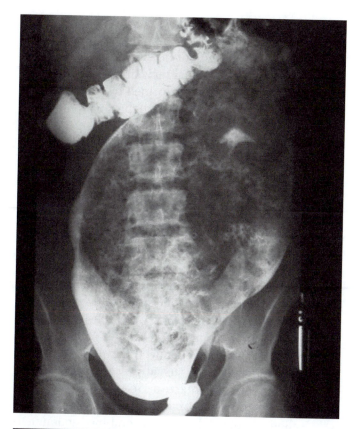

Figure 20-4 Barium enema of an older child with long-standing Hirschsprung's disease.
(Reprinted with permission by H.C. Filston, M.D.)

This allowed a submucosal piece of tissue to be used to make the diagnosis. Refinement of the technique led to the development of the suction biopsy by Dobbins and Bill (1965) and Noblett (1969). Use of the suction rectal biopsy has greatly facilitated the diagnosis of Hirschsprung's disease. Biopsies may be performed at the bedside or in a clinic. The diagnostic accuracy has been reported to be as high as 99.7%. The most common problem is an inadequate specimen with an insufficient amount of submucosa for the identification of ganglion cells. Another problem is a biopsy taken too close to the sphincter. The normal anus has an absence of ganglion cells at the level of the internal sphincter. The accepted practice is to obtain two or three specimens by suction rectal biopsy at least 2 cm above the anal valves. The tissue specimen may be obtained by rectal forceps, which clip a piece of mucosa from the lining of the colon or a suction biopsy instrument.

In Hirschsprung's disease, an intense staining of the biopsy specimens reveals hypertrophied nerve fibers throughout the muscle layers and the absence of ganglion cells. Specimens may also be stained for acetylcholines-

terase. If a suction rectal biopsy is inadequate or if the child is older, a full-thickness biopsy with the use of biopsy forceps may be performed. A full-thickness biopsy is obtained in the operating room with the child under general anesthesia. This specimen involves all the muscular layers of the colon. It provides a more substantial tissue sample for the pathologist to review. The risks of the procedure include bleeding, scarring, and infection.

■ Differential Diagnosis

Intestinal obstruction may be clinically difficult to determine from a variety of other causes of mechanical or functional obstruction at different ages in infants and children. The differential diagnosis approach will vary depending on the age and presenting picture (Table 20-1).

■ Preoperative Management

Once symptomatic, patients require gastrointestinal decompression as a first step (Holschneider & Ure, 2000). This is usually accomplished by placing a nasogastric tube for stomach decompression and repeated emptying of the rectum using rectal tubes and irrigations. Some surgeons prefer to add 1% neomycin to the final irrigation before the operative procedure. Patients with sepsis and/or dehydration must be stabilized with intravenous fluids and antibiotics. With a rate of associated anomalies at 18% in sporadic cases and as high as 39% in familial cases,

Table 20-1	**Differential Diagnosis of Hirschsprung's Disease**
Mechanical Obstruction	**Functional Obstruction**
• Meconium ileus	• Prematurity
• Ileal or colonic atresia	• Small left colon syndrome
• Meconium plug syndrome	• Sepsis
• Small intestine stenosis	• Pseudo-obstruction
• Congenital band	• Psychological /behavioral disorders
• Anorectal malformation	• Intestinal smooth muscle and other myopathic disorders
• Malrotation	• Medical causes (hypothyroidism, electrolyte imbalances, drugs, uremia, diabetes, etc.)

additional preoperative work-up should include careful evaluation for recognizable syndromes by a trained dysmorphologist (Amiel & Lyonnet, 2001). If the child is to undergo a multistage procedure requiring an ostomy, then discussion about ostomies and their care should begin with the parents before surgery.

■ Surgical Techniques

Clinical management of children diagnosed with Hirschsprung's disease is changing as new surgical techniques evolve. The treatment of Hirschsprung's disease involves the surgical resection of the aganglionic bowel, followed by mobilization of the proximal colon and anastomosis of the ganglionic bowel to the distal rectum, commonly called a *pull-through*. Traditionally, the approach for correction has been a two- or three-staged procedure in which a leveling colostomy is first performed for decompression. A staged procedure with a leveling colostomy may need to be used in cases of patients with enterocolitis or in those with large, dilated loops of bowel at the time of surgery. This occurs more commonly in children who had a delay in diagnosis. The colostomy remains for 3 to 12 months before the pull-through procedure is performed. This allows the dilated bowel to decompress and the child to grow.

Greater awareness of Hirschsprung's disease, suction rectal biopsies, specialized intensive care units, improved anesthesia care, and a larger number of pediatric pathologists have led to earlier diagnosis and treatment of these patients. Earlier diagnosis leads to less proximal bowel distention and less time for enterocolitis to occur. This has made it possible to complete the repair for Hirschsprung's disease in one stage, avoiding an ostomy.

Despite the advantages and good results with one-stage procedures, there are still indications for a diverting stoma in selected patients. These include associated life-threatening anomalies, deteriorating general health, severe enterocolitis, marked dilatation of the proximal bowel, long-segment aganglionosis, or a difficult or tenuous pull-through.

■ Operative Procedures

Three endorectal pull-through procedures with their modifications are presently being used. At the time of surgery, a biopsy specimen is obtained to confirm the presence of ganglion cells at the anastomotic site. Figure 20-5 illustrates the common surgical approaches in the definitive treatment of Hirschsprung's disease.

1. Swenson and Bill first described their curative operation for Hirschsprung's disease in 1948. The aganglionic section of the bowel is first removed through an abdominal incision. Then an end-to-end anastomosis is performed by prolapsing the rectum and the pulled-through, ganglionic bowel through the anus. Essential to this operation is careful dissection immediately adjacent to the rectal wall to avoid injury to the pelvic nerves responsible for rectal and bladder innervation and sexual function. This technique leaves the smallest amount of aganglionic bowel.

2. Duhamel introduced the retrorectal pull-through technique in 1956. In this procedure, the dissection is limited to the retrorectal space, where the dissection avoids potential injury to the pelvic nerves. Normally, the innervated (ganglionic) bowel is brought down posteriorly and anastomosed end to side to the aganglionic segment (Teitelbaum & Coran, 2003). The connecting wall between the two segments is cut, usually by a stapling device. This creates a neorectum, in which the anterior wall is aganglionic and the posterior wall is ganglionic (Duhamel, 1960). A combined abdominal-perineal approach is used.

3. Soave introduced the endorectal pull-through in 1964 in an attempt to avoid injury to the pelvic nerves. The mucosal layer is dissected away from the muscular layer of the aganglionic segment. This preserves the important sensory fibers and the integrity of the internal sphincter. The ganglionic segment is then pulled down through the aganglionic muscular cuff. Leaving aganglionic muscle to surround normal intestine theoretically leads to a higher incidence of constipation, but this has not been the case (Teitelbaum & Coran, 1995).

Advances in endoscopic surgery and instrumentation have lead to all three types of pull-through procedures being performed primarily (one stage) using laparoscopic techniques. The advantages are less pain, shorter time to feedings, shorter hospital stay, and lower costs (Somme & Langer, 2004). The procedure involves the use of three to four trocars (3.5-mm trocars for infants and 5-mm trocars for older children) for visualization and mobilization of the colon. The transition zone is identified and a liberalized resection is performed to include the entire transition. The remainder of the procedure is performed transanally.

Pediatric surgeons De la Torre-Mondragon and Ortega-Salgado first described a totally transanal endorectal pull-through in the newborn in 1998. Since then, many other

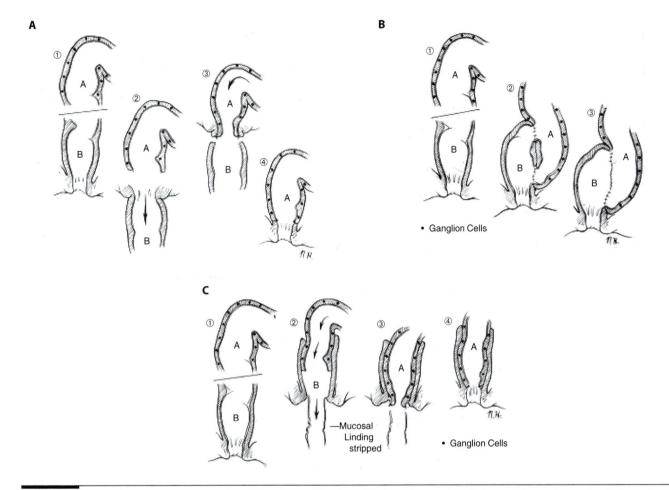

Figure 20-5A, B, and C   A, Swenson procedure. B, Martin modification of Duhamel procedure. C, Soave-Boley endorectal pull-through.
(Reprinted with permission by H.C. Filston, M.D.)

surgeons have begun to use this approach. Such a procedure has the potential advantages of lower cost, less risk of damage to pelvic structures, and the absence of any abdominal incisions. Short-term results show this approach to be safe and effective (Webster & Rintala, 2004). The long-term outcomes of this procedure have yet to be reported.

Postoperative Management

Nasogastric suction is used for 24 to 48 hours. Hydration is maintained with peripheral intravenous therapy. Clear liquids are started once bowel function has returned, and diet is advanced as tolerated. Pain is managed initially with intravenous narcotics and acetaminophen.

A Foley catheter is left in place for 24 to 48 hours after extensive pelvic dissection. If a colostomy has been performed, the stoma should be assessed for color, size and return of function. Stoma teaching with the family should be initiated the first postoperative day because of the short length of hospitalization.

It is important for the patient to have nothing placed in the rectum in the initial postoperative period. This includes thermometers, suppositories, and catheters. A sign to that effect should be placed on the patient's bed. Rectal dilations are withheld for 3 weeks and are restarted during outpatient visits (Marty et al., 1995). Some pediatric surgical practices are performing rectal wash-outs for the first 3 to 4 months in an effort to decrease the incidence of enterocolitis.

Frequent, loose stools (as many as 7–12 per day) may be expected after surgery, making anorectal skin care extremely important. The family should be instructed in good perineal care. Frequent tub soaks may be helpful in the weeks after surgery, as well as air drying of the perineum when possible. Skin barrier products including zinc oxide-based creams, such as Desitin (Pfizer, New York) or Critic-Aid (Coloplast Corp., Marietta, GA), should be applied with each diaper change. If the skin is denuded and moist, Ilex (Medcon, Princeton, NJ), a protective skin barrier, may be useful. Ilex is applied to clean, dry skin. It is topped with a layer of petroleum jelly or skin lotion to prevent the diaper from pulling the Ilex off. The cream should not be completely removed with each diaper change, because this will cause more irritation to the skin. Instead, the family should be instructed to wipe away the stool with a soft moist cloth and use more Ilex to patch exposed areas. There are other commercially available creams that may be helpful. If a yeast-type rash develops, a light dusting of antifungal powder should be applied directly to the skin with the protective ointment on top. Parents need support to get through this difficult period.

Continence and the issues regarding toilet training are always the ultimate concern of the child and the family. Initially, it is not possible to determine when or even whether the child will have a normal bowel movement pattern or when toilet training should begin. It is recommended that parents try to have a relaxed attitude regarding toilet training. It is unlikely that a child with Hirschsprung's disease will potty train as early as another child or sibling.

Many researchers have studied the long-term results of the various procedures for Hirschsprung's disease. Different definitions of normal bowel function and lack of precise measurements of complications, such as enterocolitis, make it difficult to state the superiority of any one procedure. Ongoing studies are looking at results of the newer, primary (one-stage), and completely transanal procedures. So far, these procedures appear to have results that are as good as or better than those performed in two or three stages (Engum & Grosfeld, 2004). It is important to note that regardless of the procedure, many children have needed a bowel training program using enemas and/or laxatives to completely evacuate the colon. Families should be aware that surgery is not the end of the disease process, and that irregular bowel patterns may persist throughout the child's life. Refer to Chapters 9 and 21 for further information on bowel management programs.

■ Complications

Four major complications are associated with Hirschsprung's disease: enterocolitis, anastomotic leak, stenosis, and bowel obstruction. Hirschsprung's enterocolitis remains the major cause of significant morbidity and mortality. The incidence varies from 5% to 35%, and it usually occurs in the year after surgery, but it may occur at any time. Patients with trisomy 21, long-segment disease, associated anomalies (cardiac, gastrointestinal, genitourinary, central nervous system), and anorectal steno-

sis or stenosis at the anastomotic site are at higher risk. The diagnosis of enterocolitis is made on the basis of a clinical history of diarrhea, vomiting, fever, and often lethargy (Elhalaby, Coran, Blane, Hirschi, & Teitelbaum, 1995). On physical examination, the children often have a distended abdomen, hyperactive bowel sounds, and explosive diarrhea after a rectal examination. The odor of the stool may be described as more foul smelling than usual. The color of the stool may also change to a darker green or gray. Along with the history and physical examination, the finding of an "intestinal cutoff sign" on abdominal radiographic films has a high degree of sensitivity for enterocolitis. A "cutoff sign" is a segment of large dilated intestine proximal to a markedly narrow segment of distal bowel.

Pathologically, enterocolitis is defined as an acute inflammatory infiltrate into the crypts and mucosa of the colonic or small intestinal epithelium. As the disease progresses, the mucosal epithelium becomes ulcerated, and the lumen of the intestine becomes filled with fibrinopurulent debris. If this process is left untreated, perforation of the intestine may occur (Teitelbaum, Qualman, & Caniano, 1988). The pathological process may be seen in ganglionic and aganglionic intestine (Elhalaby, Teitelbaum, Coran, & Heidelberger, 1995; Teitelbaum et al.).

Often, the family assumes that because the aganglionic portion of intestine has been removed, their child is "cured." If signs and symptoms of enterocolitis are reviewed at the time of discharge, parents seek treatment more quickly. It is important that the family seek medical advice from a physician familiar with Hirschsprung's disease, such as a pediatric surgeon or gastroenterologist, because mortality associated with Hirschsprung's enterocolitis may be as high as 39% (Vieten & Spicer, 2004).

The treatment of Hirschsprung's disease–associated enterocolitis begins with fluid resuscitation to correct fluid and electrolyte imbalances, decompression of the stomach with a nasogastric tube, and series of aggressive washouts using a rectal tube to decompress the colon above the anal sphincter (Table 20-2). Enemas alone are ineffective because they do not allow for adequate decompression of the colon. Either intravenous antibiotics or oral metronidazole (Flagyl) should accompany these serial washouts. Rectal washouts should be performed with care during fulminate disease because of the risk of perforation. Enterocolitis may recur, possibly due to mucosal changes that occurred early in life (Fujimoto & Puri, 1988; Lifschitz & Bloss, 1985). The practice of early prophylactic rectal washouts starting 3 weeks after the pull-through appears to decrease the incidence of enterocolitis (Vieten & Spicer, 2004).

Table 20-2 Protocol to Administer Rectal Washouts

The purpose of rectal irrigation is to remove stool and gas from the bowel using small amounts of normal saline every 4 hours until the bowel is clean. Rectal irrigation is different from an enema, in which a larger amount of water is given at a time.

Supplies Needed

1. Red Robinson all-purpose catheter with two additional holes cut in the sides of the catheter. Size of the catheter used depends on the weight of the child:

   newborn 16 Fr

   5–10 kg 20 Fr

   > 10 kg 22 Fr

2. A 60-mL Toumy syringe for administering the irrigation.

3. Normal saline at room temperature may be used for the irrigation. The volume used is 10 mL/kg. Example: 10 kg child $\times$ 10 mL/kg = 100 mL total volume.

Insertion of the Catheter

Position the patient on the left side when possible. An infant may be on the back with the legs in a frog position. A water-soluble lubricant may be used to help with the insertion of the catheter. Insert the catheter into the rectum until resistance is met. The normal saline may need to be instilled into the rectum as the catheter is advanced.

Irrigation

Fill the Toumy syringe with one-fourth total volume of normal saline. Push this amount into the rectum and aspirate back. Disconnect the syringe and discard this saline. Repeat three times until the total volume is used. If unable to aspirate, remove the syringe and drain. This procedure may be performed every 4 hours.

It is imperative that the family is taught to perform rectal washouts by an experienced member of the pediatric surgery service once the rectal anastomosis has healed. Passing dilators, rectal tubes, or thermometers through the rectum in the early postoperative period can damage the rectal anastomosis.

Oral antibiotic therapy may be used in conjunction with rectal washouts to treat mild cases of enterocolitis. Metronidazole has been found to be effective in the treatment of serious infections caused by susceptible anaerobic bacteria and is effective in the treatment of enterocolitis. The length of therapy is determined by the patient's symptoms. This drug requires compounding for administration to infants and young children. The addition of cherry base syrup makes the medication more palatable. When prescribing any medication that requires compounding, provide the family with the prescription a few days before it is needed, if possible, and direct the family to a pharmacy that can provide the necessary elixir form. As with any medication, the family should be educated about the potential side effects.

Another serious complication of Hirschsprung's disease is leak at the point of surgical anastomosis, probably due to vascular compromise. Presenting symptoms include fever, toxicity, increasing pain, and peritonitis. A water-soluble contrast enema or computed tomography scan can often diagnose this problem. For a mild leak,

keeping the child NPO and treating with intravenous antibiotics should suffice. For more severe leaks, a diverting colostomy is necessary (Holschneider & Ure, 2000).

A third potential complication is mild-to-moderate stenosis either at the anastomosis or through the length of the cuff. Generally, an anastomotic stenosis is treatable with dilations. To prevent stenosis, rectal dilations are begun 2 to 3 weeks after the pull-through. In general, these dilations are performed without anesthesia. Parents are instructed in performing daily dilations at home. A red rubber catheter or a calibrated dilator of either metal or plastic (Specialty Surgical Products, Hamilton, MT) may be used to prevent strictures. The dilations are continued until the anastomotic scar is supple, which may take up to 6 months.

Bowel obstruction resulting from adhesions may occur after any abdominal surgery. Obstructive symptoms may occur at any time throughout the child's life. The patient and family should be instructed to seek medical attention if symptoms of abdominal pain or vomiting persist for longer than 24 hours.

It is important for families, school nurses, and primary care physicians to recognize that although a child has had surgery for Hirschsprung's disease, the disease has not been eliminated. There may continue to be issues regarding stool patterns and constipation or recurrent enterocolitis. It is common for toilet training to be delayed in children with Hirschsprung's disease compared with siblings or friends. Toilet training is often a trigger for stool retention, which can then lead to constipation, staining of underwear, or gas bloat syndrome. Early symptoms of enterocolitis as previously described should be reported to a specialist immediately.

A common gastrointestinal virus that may cause mild symptoms of diarrhea or vomiting in a healthy child may have exaggerated effects on a child with Hirschsprung's disease. Symptoms of diarrhea that persist beyond a few days should be evaluated.

Other Forms of Hirschsprung's Disease

Total colonic aganglionosis accounts for about 5% to 10% of all patients with Hirschsprung's disease. These children are a unique subset of patients because of increased morbidity and mortality. Without the colon, the child's ability to reabsorb fluid and store stool is markedly impaired. Many infants with total colonic Hirschsprung's disease require parenteral nutrition for an extended period of time, making sepsis, failure to thrive, stomal dysfunction, electrolyte imbalance, and dehydration common problems.

Near-total intestinal aganglionosis is extremely rare, making up less than 1% of all children with Hirschsprung's disease. Some of these children experience enough adaptation to eventually wean from total parenteral nutrition, but those children who must remain on parenteral nutrition for extended periods of time are at risk for total parenteral nutrition–induced cholestasis leading to liver failure. Small-bowel transplantation may be the only chance of survival (Dasgupta & Langer, 2004) (see Chapter 30).

Variant Hirschsprung's disease is a term used to describe conditions that resemble Hirschsprung's disease in their presentation and course, but that are not characterized by the absence of ganglion cells on rectal biopsy (Puri, 1997). One of the more commonly described examples of variant Hirschsprung's disease is intestinal neuronal dysplasia. Intestinal neuronal dysplasia has been associated with Hirschsprung's disease in 25% to 35% of cases by some investigators; however, others believe that intestinal neuronal dysplasia is a secondary phenomenon induced by congenital obstruction and inflammatory disease (Puri & Rolle, 2004).

Hypoganglionosis is another form of variant Hirschsprung's disease, in which the ganglia that are present in the biopsy specimen are sparse and small. The corrective treatment is the pull-through procedure. Hypoganglionosis is not to be confused with immature ganglia that are seen in preterm infants and does not need surgical intervention (Dasgupta & Langer, 2004).

Ultra-short-segment Hirschsprung's disease is limited to the anal ring and usually presents at 6 to 9 months of life with chronic constipation resistant to therapy. The treatment of choice has been either internal sphincter dilatation or a partial myectomy of the distal internal sphincter (Angerpointner, 2005).

Long-Term Results

Although many children with Hirschsprung's disease have a good outcome after surgical treatment, long-term studies have identified several concerns. The most common long-term problems identified are constipation, incontinence, enterocolitis, and psychological issues (Engum & Grosfeld, 2004). In some cases, the problems of constipation and incontinence may improve as the child enters adolescence; however, the use of a good bowel management program, including the antegrade continence enema procedure, may be necessary for many years after surgery (see Chapters 9 and 21). If patients continue to have severe constipation with conservative bowel management, a repeat rectal biopsy may be needed. If the biopsy shows aganglionosis, a redo pull-through procedure may be needed. Incontinence rates have been reported from zero to 74% (Bai, Chen, Hao, Huang, & Wang, 2002). The cause of incontinence in Hirschsprung's disease patients is still perplexing; however, increasing appreciation of the importance of preserving the bulk of the internal anal sphincter has decreased its incidence (Engum & Grosfeld).

Any operation in the pelvis can cause injury to the nerves affecting bladder and sexual function. Bladder or sexual function complications are reported but are thought to be rare (Moore, Albertyn, & Cywes, 1996). It is suspected that the numbers of cases with bladder or sexual dysfunction may be much higher, but these data have been difficult to obtain because most children with Hirschsprung's disease are not followed up to the age at which they become sexually active. Problems with bladder or sexual function may be seen by other subspecialists who do not report the dysfunction as being related to the surgical repair for Hirschsprung's disease.

Recently, more attention has been given to the quality-of-life outcomes for patients with Hirschsprung's disease. The most common cause of a negative quality of life is due to fecal soiling, which is physically, socially, and psychologically disabling. One study reports that bowel function and quality of life were poorer for children with Hirschsprung's disease than those of healthy children (Bai et al., 2002). Another study demonstrated that a large proportion of children with congenital anorectal malformations (including Hirschsprung's disease) tended to be depressed and the severity of depression increased with age (Funakosi et al., 2005). These studies stress the importance of maintaining a long-term connection with the patient and the family. Access to a good bowel management program, psychological counseling, and a family support network are essential.

■ Conclusion

Increased awareness and improvement of diagnostic techniques have made an important impact on the treatment of Hirschsprung's disease. The average age of diagnosis has shifted from childhood to early infancy. This increased awareness has led to a prompt initiation of treatment, resulting in a decrease in mortality. The refinements in surgical treatments and postoperative care have significantly improved the long-term outcome for these patients.

■ Acknowledgments

I would like to acknowledge the important contributions made by Jennifer Chamberlain and Daniel Teitelbaum, who co-authored this chapter for the 1st edition of this textbook.

■ Educational Materials

APSNA invites you to download the following diagnosis-related teaching tool for Chapter 20, Hirschsprung's disease: Hirschsprung's disease. This teaching tool is available at the APSNA Web site (www.apsna.org) and the Jones and Bartlett Web site (www.jbpub.com). All teaching materials are available in English and Spanish and are free of charge. APSNA encourages their use for your patients and families.

References

Akgur, F. M., Tanyel, F. C., Buyukpamukcu, N., & Hicsonmez, A. (1993). Colonic atresia & Hirschsprung's disease association shows further evidence for migration of enteric neurons. *Journal of Pediatric Surgery, 28*(4), 635–636.

Albanese, C. T., Harrison, M. R., & Sydorak, R. M. (2003). Congenital gastrointestinal lesions. In L. W. Way & G. M. Doherty (Eds.), *Current surgical diagnosis & treatment* (11th ed.). USA: McGraw-Hill.

Amiel, J., & Lyonnet, S. (2001). Hirschsprung's disease, associated syndromes, and genetics: A review. *Journal of Medical Genetics, 38*, 729–739.

Angerpointner, T. A. (2005). Diagnosis and therapy of ultrashort Hirschsprung's disease. *Journal of Pediatric Surgery, 40*(7), 1217.

Arliss, J., & Holgersen, L. O. (1990). Neonatal appendiceal perforation and Hirschsprung's disease. *Journal of Pediatric Surgery, 25*(6), 694–695.

Bai, Y., Chen, H., Hao, J., Huang. Y., & Wang, W. (2002). Long-term outcome and quality of life after the Swenson procedure for Hirschsprung's disease. *Journal of Pediatric Surgery, 37*(4), 639–642.

Brooks, A. S., Oostra, B. A., & Hofstra, R. M. (2005). Studying the genetics of Hirschsprung's disease: Unraveling an oligogenic disorder. *Clinical Genetics, 67*(1), 6–14.

Dasgupta, R., & Langer, J. C. (2004). Hirschsprung's disease. *Current Problems in Surgery, 41*(12), 942–988.

De la Torre-Mondragon, L., & Ortega-Salgado, J. A. (1998). Transanal endorectal pull-through for Hirschsprung's disease. *Journal of Pediatric Surgery, 33*(8), 1283–1286.

Dobbins, W. O., & Bill, A. H. (1965). Diagnosis of Hirschsprung's disease excluded by rectal suction biopsy. *New England Journal of Medicine, 272*, 990.

Duhamel, B. (1960). A new operation for the treatment of Hirschsprung's disease. *Archives of Diseases of Childhood, 35*, 38–40.

Elhalaby, E. A., Coran, A. G., Blane, C. E., Hirschi, R. B., & Teitelbaum, D. H. (1995). Enterocolitis associated with Hirschsprung's disease: Clinical-radiological characterization based on 168 patients. *Journal of Pediatric Surgery, 30*(1), 76–83.

Elhalaby, E. A., Teitelbaum, D. H., Coran, A. G., & Heidelberger, K. P. (1995). Enterocolitis associated with Hirschsprung's disease: A clinical histopathological correlative study. *Journal of Pediatric Surgery, 30*(7), 1023–1027.

Engum, S. A., & Grosfeld, J. L. (2004). Long-term results of treatment of Hirschsprung's disease. *Seminars in Pediatric Surgery, 13*(4), 273–285.

Filston, H. C. (1982). Specific problems: Hirschsprung's disease. *Surgical problems in children: Recognition & referral* (1st ed., p. 81). St. Louis, MO: Mosby.

Fujimoto, T., & Puri, P. (1988). Persistence of enterocolitis following diversion of fecal stream in Hirschsprung's disease. A study of mucosal defense mechanisms. *Pediatric Surgery International, 3*, 141–146.

Funakosi, S., Hayashi, J., Kamiyama, T., Vena, T., Ishii, T., Wada, M., et al. (2005). Psychosocial liaison-consultation for the children who have undergone repair of imperforate anus and Hirschsprung's disease. *Journal of Pediatric Surgery, 40*(7), 1156–1162.

Gherardi, G. J. (1960). Pathology of the ganglionic-aganglionic junction in congenital megacolon. *Archives of Pathology, 69*, 520.

Holschneider, A., & Ure, B. M. (2000). Hirschsprung's disease. In K. Ashcroft, J. P. Murphy, R. J. Sharp, D. L. Sigalet, & C. L. Snyder (Eds.), *Pediatric surgery* (3rd ed.). Philadelphia: W.B. Saunders.

Ikeda, K., & Goto, S. (1984). Diagnosis and treatment of Hirschsprung's disease in Japan. An analysis of 1628 patients. *Annals of Surgery, 199*(4), 400–405.

Khan, A. R., Vujanic, G. M., & Huddart, S. (2003). The constipated child: How likely is Hirschsprung's disease? *Pediatric Surgery International, 19*(6), 439–442.

Langer, J. C., Durrant, A. C., De la Torre, L., Teitelbaum, D. H., Minkes, R. K., Caty, M. Q., et al. (2003). One-stage Transanal Soave pullthrough for Hirschsprung's disease: A multicenter experience with 141 children. *Annals of Surgery, 238*(4), 569–585.

Lifschitz, C. H., & Bloss, R. (1985). Persistence of colitis in Hirschsprung's disease. *Journal of Pediatric Gastroenterology and Nutrition, 4*(2), 291–293.

Marty, T. L., Sea, T., Matlak, M. E., Sullivan, J. J., Black, R. E., & Johnson, D. G. (1995). Gastrointestinal function after surgical correction of Hirschsprung's disease: Long-term follow-up in 135 patients. *Journal of Pediatric Surgery, 30*(5), 655–658.

Moore, S. W., & Johnson, G. (2005). Acetylcholinesterase in Hirschsprung's disease. *Pediatric Surgery International*, 21(4), 255–263.

Moore, S. W., Albertyn, R., & Cywes, S. (1996). Clinical outcome and long-term quality of life after surgical correction of Hirschsprung's disease. *Journal of Pediatric Surgery*, 31(11), 1496–1502.

Moore, S. W., Rode, H., Miller, A. J., & Cywes, S. (1990). Intestinal atresia and Hirschsprung's disease. *Pediatric Surgery International*, 5, 182–184.

Noblett, H. R. (1969). A rectal suction biopsy tube for use in the diagnosis of Hirschsprung's disease. *Journal of Pediatric Surgery*, 4(4), 406–410.

Puri, P. (1997). Variant Hirschsprung's disease. *Journal of Pediatric Surgery*, 32(2), 149–157.

Puri, P., & Rolle, U. (2004). Variant Hirschsprung's disease. *Seminars in Pediatric Surgery*, 13(4), 293–299.

Soave, F. (1964). Hirschsprung's disease: A new surgical technique. *Archives of Diseases of Childhood*, 39, 116–122.

Somme, S., & Langer, J. C. (2004). Primary versus staged pull-through for the treatment of Hirschsprung's disease. *Seminars in Pediatric Surgery*, 13(4), 249–255.

Stewart, D. R., & von Allmen, D. (2003). The genetics of Hirschsprung's disease. *Gastroenterology Clinics of North America*, 32(3), 819–837.

Swenson, O., & Bill, A. H. (1948). Resection of rectum and rectosigmoid with preservation of the sphincter for benign spastic lesions producing megacolon. *Surgery*, 24, 212–220.

Swenson, O., Fisher, I. H., & Gherardi, G. J. (1959). Rectal biopsy in the diagnosis of Hirschsprung's disease. *Surgery*, 45, 690–695.

Swenson, O., Shennan, I., Fisher, I., & Cohen, E. (1975). The treatment and postoperative complications of congenital megacolon: A 25 year follow-up. *Annals of Surgery*, 182, 266–273.

Swenson, O. (1964). Partial internal sphincterotomy in the treatment of Hirschsprung's disease. *Annals of Surgery*, 160, 540–550.

Tam, P. K., & Garcia-Barcelo, M. (2004). Molecular genetics of Hirschsprung's disease. *Seminars in Pediatric Surgery*, 13(4), 236–248.

Taxman, T. L., Yulish, B. S., & Rothstein, F. C. (1986). How useful is the barium enema in the diagnosis of infantile Hirschsprung's disease? *American Journal of Diseases of Children*, 140, 881–884.

Teitelbaum D. R., & Coran, A. G. (2003). Primary pull-through for Hirschsprung's disease. *Seminars in Neonatology*, 8(3), 233–241.

Teitelbaum, D., & Coran, A. (1995). Hirschsprung's disease. In I. Spitz & A. Coran (Eds.), *Rob & Smith's operative surgery, pediatric surgery* (pp. 471–494). London: Chapman & Hall.

Teitelbaum, D. H., Qualman, S. I., & Caniano, D. A. (1988). Hirschsprung's disease: Identification of risk factors for enterocolitis. *Annals of Surgery*, 207(3), 240–244.

Vieten, D., & Spicer, R. (2004). Enterocolitis complicating Hirschsprung's disease. *Seminars in Pediatric Surgery*, 13(4), 263–272.

Wester, T., & Rintala, R. J. (2004). Early outcome of transanal endorectal pull-through with a short muscle cuff during the neonatal period. *Journal of Pediatric Surgery*, 39(2), 157–160.

Yunis, E. I., Dibbins, A. W., & Shennan, F. E. (1976). Rectal suction biopsy in the diagnosis of Hirschsprung's disease in infants. *Archives of Pathology & Laboratory Medicine*, 100(6), 329–333.

Anorectal Malformations in Children

By Kathleen O'Connor Guardino

Expert nursing care of the child born with an anorectal malformation is essential to achieving optimal results in all stages of the disease process. The natural history of these defects, diagnostic methods, and medical and surgical therapy are reviewed in this chapter. The nurse is familiarized with the assessment and management of children with anorectal malformations. The role of nursing from diagnosis through surgical correction to bowel training and management is emphasized.

Anorectal malformations occur in 1 of every 4,000 newborns (Peña, 1990b). The term *anorectal malformation* encompasses multiple congenital anomalies of the rectum, urinary, and reproductive structures with varying degrees of complexity. They require different types of treatments with variable prognoses for bowel, urinary, and sexual function. Most children with anorectal malformations have an abnormal communication between the rectum, the genitourinary tract, and the perineum. These communications are called *fistulas*.

Generally, children with complex malformations have poor sphincter tone, a flat perineum, and no clear midline intergluteal groove in addition to an absent anal opening. These children need a three-stage repair: (1) creation of a diverting colostomy, (2) the main repair or pull-through procedure, and (3) colostomy closure. The most

frequent surgical repair used is the posterior sagittal anorectoplasty (PSARP). Those children with relatively benign malformations, or "low" defects, simply need an anoplasty without a colostomy.

■ Physical Examination/Work-Up

The diagnosis of an anorectal malformation is most commonly made in the delivery room on examination of the infant after birth or in the newborn nursery when the nurse attempts to take a rectal temperature and no anus is visible.

Coordinated with the routine nursing examination, the infant with imperforate anus (absent anal opening) should be assessed for the following: abdominal distention, vomiting, presence of meconium in the perineum of a male infant or in the genitalia of a female infant, voiding pattern, and presence of meconium in the urine of a male baby, as detected by filtering urine through a gauze pad placed at the tip of the penis or by urinalysis.

Once the diagnosis of imperforate anus has been established, the goals of care are as follows: provision of general medical support, evaluation of potential associated defects that require immediate attention, determination of whether the infant needs a temporary colostomy (high defects) or whether the defect can be treated by a minor procedure called *anoplasty*, and provision of education and emotional support for the parents, including relevant information concerning the diagnosis, tests, treatment, and prognosis.

General Support

General support of the infant includes administration of antibiotics, insertion of a nasogastric (NG) tube for gastric decompression, administration of vitamin K, administration of intravenous fluids, avoidance of feedings by mouth or feeding tube (NPO), and strict monitoring of intake and output.

Associated Defects

The most frequently associated defects that require immediate attention are those of the urinary tract (Peña, 1997). Therefore, every infant with an anorectal malformation requires an ultrasound examination of the abdomen to detect urinary obstruction. If the ultrasound examination is abnormal, a more detailed urologic evaluation is indicated. Other associated defects include those of the gastrointestinal tract, including esophageal atresia and tracheoesophageal fistula, vertebral, cardiac, and skeletal anomalies (Shaul & Harrison, 1997). All infants should have a cardiac evaluation with echocardiogram before surgery (Kiely & Peña, 1998). A spinal ultrasound also demonstrates the presence of a tethered cord.

Colostomy Creation Versus Anoplasty

Some minor (low) anorectal malformations can be treated with a one-stage surgical repair called an *anoplasty*. However, in infants with high defects, the creation of an intestinal diversion called a *colostomy* is necessary to decompress the bowel. This diversion also helps prevent infection during the postoperative period after the pull-through procedure. A colostomy is indicated in most malformations as delineated in Tables 21-1 and 21-2. The decision to perform a colostomy is generally made after 24 hours of observation (Wilkins & Peña, 1988).

Traditionally, a study called an *invertogram* or upside-down film (Wangensteen & Rice, 1930) was obtained after 24 hours of life. The radiographic examination was performed at this time so that the infant would have enough intraluminal pressure in the bowel to distend the most distal blind portion of the rectum with gas. Today, a cross-table lateral film is obtained with the infant in the prone position and the pelvis elevated (Narasimharao, Prassad, & Katariya, 1983). The gas inside the distended blind rectum gives a radiolucent image. The distance between the radiopaque marker (placed on the skin) and the blind rectum is measured. This film provides objective information concerning the height of the defect and the position of the colon in relationship to the infant's anal sphincter. While this study is being performed, the infant should be kept wrapped to prevent hypothermia and assessed for vomiting or cyanosis.

Education and Emotional Support

Most parents of a child with an anorectal malformation suffer from emotional stress due to the birth of a child with a congenital defect. The family should be provided with emotional support and information so that they can begin the process of adjustment. Specific resources and support groups are listed in the Resource chapter of the textbook.

Table 21-1 **Types of Male Defects**

Diagnosis	Initial Treatment	Final Treatment	Incidence of Associated Defects	Bowel Control (%)	Urinary Control (%)
Perineal fistula	No colostomy	Minimal PSARP	<10%	100	100
Rectobulbar urethral fistula	Colostomy	PSARP	30%	85	100
Rectoprostatic urethral fistula	Colostomy	PSARP	60%	60	100
Rectobladder neck fistula	Colostomy	PSARP with laparotomy	90%	15	100
Imperforate anus without fistula	Colostomy	PSARP	50% Down syndrome	85	100
Rectal atresia and stenosis	Colostomy	PSARP	Undetermined	100	100

Table 21-2 **Types of Female Defects**

Diagnosis	Initial Treatment	Final Treatment	Incidence of Associated Defects
Perineal fistula	No colostomy	Minimal PSARP	<10%
Vestibular fistula	Colostomy	PSARP	30%
Imperforate anus without fistula	Colostomy	PSARP	50% Down syndrome
Rectal atresia	Colostomy	PSARP	Undetermined
Persistent cloaca	Colostomy	PSARVUP	90%

Abbreviations: PSAP, posterior sagittal anoplasty, PSARP, posterior sagittal anorectoplasty; PSARVUP, posterior sagittal anorecto-vagino-urethroplasty.

■ Description of Specific Defects

Perineal Fistula

When the rectum opens into the perineum (Fig. 21-1), it is a low malformation called a *perineal fistula*. This is a benign condition that does not require a protective colostomy, and the child has an excellent prognosis for normal bowel function. Surgical repair involves a limited posterior sagittal anoplasty, usually performed during the newborn period. During the first 24 hours of life, these infants usually pass meconium through a small fistula opening on the perineum. This orifice is located in the midline anterior to the anal dimple; in the perineum, at the base of the scrotum; or sometimes at the base of the penis. Sometimes, the defect is a midline "black ribbon-like" subepithelial meconium fistula. At other times, the defect has a prominent midline skin tag located in the anal dimple, below which one can pass an instrument.

This last defect is called a "bucket handle" malformation (Fig. 21-2) (Paidis & Peña, 1997).

Rectourinary Fistulas

Approximately 80% (Rich, Brock, & Peña, 1988) of the male patients with anorectal malformations have an abnormal communication between the rectum and the urinary tract called a *rectourinary fistula*. The specific location of the fistula has important therapeutic and prognostic implications.

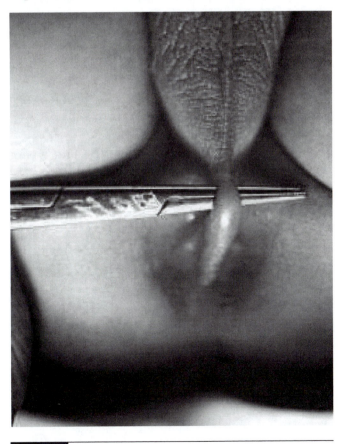

Figure 21-2 Low malformation in male: "bucket handle malformation."

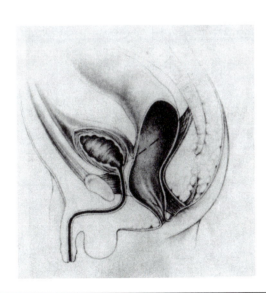

Figure 21-1 Low malformation in male: perineal fistula.

Rectourethral Bulbar Fistula

In a rectourethral bulbar fistula (Fig. 21-3), the rectum communicates with the lower posterior portion of the urethra called the *bulbar urethra*. Usually, meconium can be detected in the urine by placing a gauze pad at the tip of the penis to filter the output. The results can be confirmed by urinalysis. Passing meconium through urine usually occurs after 16 to 24 hours of life. This time frame allows intraluminal bowel pressure to develop and force the meconium through the fistula. In these cases, a colostomy is indicated, followed by a definitive repair. The most common repair performed is the PSARP, which is performed on an elective basis, usually within the first year of life.

Rectourethral Prostatic Fistula

In a rectourethral prostatic fistula, the rectum communicates with the upper part of the posterior portion of the urethra, passing through prostatic tissue (Fig. 21-4). The passage of meconium through the urethra follows the same pattern described for rectourethral bulbar fistula cases. The perineum tends to be flat, with little prominence of the midline groove. Surgical management is the same as described for the bulbar-urethral fistula, but the prognosis for future bowel control is not as good.

Rectobladder Neck Fistula

A rectobladder neck fistula is the highest defect in male patients. In these cases, the rectum communicates with the bladder neck, and the sacrum is usually abnormal (Fig. 21-5). Children with this defect sometimes experience urinary incontinence. This indicates the existence of a serious nerve deficiency that translates into a poor

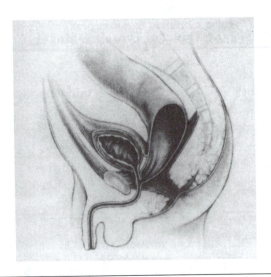

Figure 21-4 High malformation in male: prostatic fistula.

prognosis for future bowel control. The definitive repair in these cases is generally performed in the first year of life on an elective basis. The surgical procedure includes a PSARP plus laparotomy to mobilize a rectum that cannot be reached from below. This defect represents only approximately 10% of all the male cases (Peña, 1988).

Imperforate Anus Without a Fistula

Imperforate anus without a fistula is an unusual malformation that occurs in less than 10% of all patients (Narasimharao et al., 1983). The rectum is completely blind and ends approximately 2 cm from the perineum. No meconium is present in the urine. Diagnosis is confirmed by radiologic study to determine the height of the malformation. This defect is frequently associated with Down syndrome

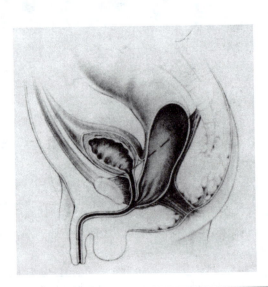

Figure 21-3 Low malformation in male: bulbar urethral fistula.

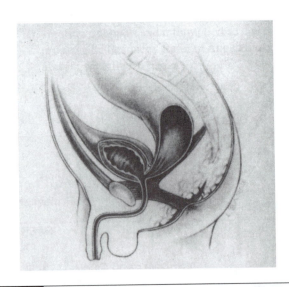

Figure 21-5 High malformation in male: bladder neck fistula.

(Torres, Levitt, Tovilla, Rodriguez, & Peña, 1998). The treatment, prognosis, perineal appearance, characteristics of the sacrum, and frequency of associated urologic defects are the same as in cases of rectourethral bulbar fistulas.

Rectal Atresia and Stenosis

Rectal atresia and stenosis are unusual defects that occur in approximately 1% of all cases of anorectal malformations. There is no communication with the urinary tract (Peña, 1990b). The perineum looks normal, including a normal-looking anus. Complete obstruction atresia or a decrease in the caliber (stenosis) of the rectum is present approximately 2 cm above the anal opening. These are usually the cases in which the diagnosis is delayed and established by a nurse while trying to take a rectal temperature. The sacrum and sphincters are normal, and, therefore, the prognosis for bowel function is excellent. A temporary colostomy is indicated, followed by a main repair (PSARP), usually performed within the first year of life on an elective basis.

Anorectal Malformations in Female Infants

Approximately 95% of female infants with imperforate anus have a fistula to the genitalia or to the perineum. Thus, the clinical diagnosis of the specific type of defect and the decision concerning the creation of a colostomy in cases of female patients are usually easier than in male patients (Peña, 1990b).

Perineal Fistula

Perineal fistula is the most benign of all the defects seen in female patients (Fig. 21-6). The rectum opens through an abnormal orifice (fistula) located in the perineum between the genitalia and the anal dimple (Truffler &

Wilkinson, 1962). These patients have an excellent functional prognosis.

Vestibular Fistula

Vestibular fistula is the most frequent defect seen in females (Peña, 1992). The rectum opens through an abnormally narrow orifice located in the vestibule of the genitalia, that is, immediately outside the hymen (Fig. 21-7). Meconium does not pass through the genitalia before 20 hours of life (Peña). More than 90% of these patients achieve bowel control when adequately managed. Most surgeons believe that a colostomy is indicated during the first few days of life.

Vaginal Fistula

Vaginal fistula is an exceptionally rare malformation. Most of the cases reported in the literature as "vaginal fistulas" are cases of vestibular fistulas that have been erroneously diagnosed. To correctly establish this diagnosis, one must see the meconium coming through the vagina from inside the hymen orifice. These patients must also receive a colostomy and subsequently a PSARP as in cases of vestibular fistula (Peña, 1992).

Imperforate Anus Without Fistula and Rectal Atresia and Stenosis

The characteristics of imperforate anus without fistula and rectal atresia and stenosis, as well as treatment and prognosis, are identical to those previously discussed in male patients.

Persistent Cloaca

Persistent cloaca, a complex malformation, is defined as a defect in which the rectum, vagina, and urinary tract

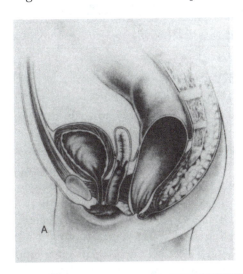

Figure 21-6 Low malformation in female: perineal fistula.

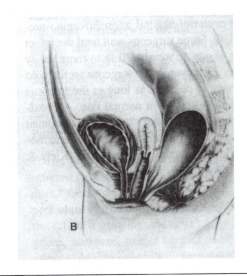

Figure 21-7 Low malformation in female: vestibular fistula.

are fused together into a single common channel that communicates exteriorly through a single perineal orifice located at the normal urethral site (Fig. 21-8). The diagnosis of persistent cloaca is easily established purely on clinical assessment. The patient's genitalia appear to be smaller than normal (Fig. 21-9). Meticulous inspection of the small labia discloses a single perineal orifice, which is the characteristic of this defect. Urologic defects occur at a rate of 90% in children with a cloaca anomaly and may require immediate attention (Rich et al., 1988). These patients represent a potential urologic emergency. An abdominal and pelvic ultrasound examination must always be performed. Based on the results of the study, a urologic work-up may be needed before the surgical creation of a colostomy. These infants require a diverting colostomy and concomitant urinary diversion (vesicostomy, ureterostomy) or vaginal diversion (vaginostomy) in cases of an obstructed, distended vagina (Rich et al.). When the infant is older than 3 months, the entire malformation is repaired with a surgical procedure called posterior sagittal anorectovagino-urethroplasty (PSARVUP). Some surgeons wait until the infant is older than 1 year of age or weighs 20 lb to facilitate the visualization of the anatomy. If the child is thriving and maintaining a normal growth curve, some surgeons may prefer to perform the PSARVUP as early as possible. In approximately 40% of cases, it is necessary to open the abdomen simultaneously with the posterior approach to reach and mobilize a very high rectum and/or vagina (Kiely & Peña, 1998).

Rare Anorectal Malformations in Male and Female Infants

Cloacal Exstrophy

Cloacal exstrophy is a rare malformation, occurring about once in every 250,000 births. Cloacal exstrophy is a com-

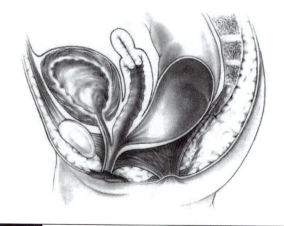

Figure 21-8 High malformation in female: cloaca.

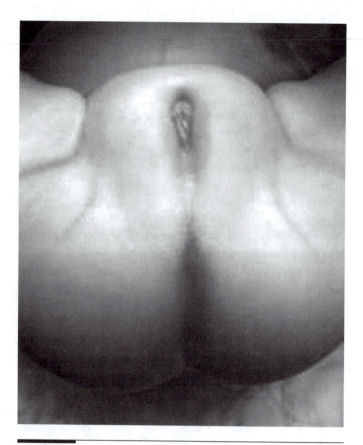

Figure 21-9 Perineum of a patient with a persistent cloaca.

plex anomaly that includes omphalocele, two exstrophied hemibladders with cecum between them, imperforate anus, and abnormalities of the sexual structures. Children with this malformation generally undergo multiple surgical procedures throughout their life in an attempt to provide for the most normal gastrointestinal, urinary, and sexual functioning possible (Hendren, 1997).

■ Treatment

Anoplasty

Anoplasty is performed in infants born with low defects or perineal fistulas that do not require a protective colostomy (Peña, 1988). Before surgery, the child must refrain from feedings for at least 4 hours or in accordance with individual anesthesia guidelines. The surgical procedure involves moving the fistula opening into the anatomically correct position at the center of the anal sphincter. A larger anal opening is then created. After surgery, the child should not have anything inserted in the rectum. A sign at the beside provides clear guidelines for care providers. Antibiotic ointment should be applied to the perineum three times per day for 2 weeks. Intravenous antibiotics are administered for 2 to 3 days. Feedings are resumed immediately after surgery. Breast feeding is encouraged because it is unlikely to cause constipation. Infants receiving a synthetic formula may require a stool softener and occasionally a laxative.

At the 2-week check-up, a program of anal dilations is initiated. The dilation schedule is described in detail later in the text.

Colostomy Creation

When a colostomy is needed, a descending colostomy is usually created, with a functioning stoma and a mucous fistula (nonfunctioning stoma). It is optimal if there is enough skin between the two stomas to allow an ostomy bag to cover the functional site only (Wilkins & Peña, 1988) (Fig. 21-10). This helps to avoid complications from stool leakage from the stoma. Creating a colostomy high on the sigmoid loop allows for easy mobilization during the pull-through procedure (Wilkins & Peña).

After the operation, the child has a nasogastric tube for approximately 48 hours and receives intravenous antibiotics to treat enteric pathogens. Colostomy and skin care, as well as assessment of vital signs, are important during the postoperative period. Postoperative pain is generally managed with a nonsteroidal anti-inflammatory medication administered intravenously (ketorolac [Toradol]) every 6 hours for 48 hours. Intravenous nar-

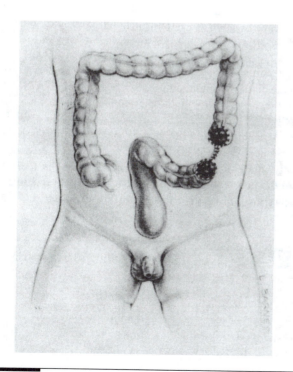

Figure 21-10 Descending colostomy with separated stomas in the left lower quadrant of the abdomen.

cotics, such as morphine, can be used for breakthrough pain. The expected length of stay is 4 to 5 days.

The advanced practice nurse, primary nurse, and an enterostomal therapist may assess and address the educational and discharge needs of the family. The parents must learn stoma care before the infant's discharge. Some institutions do not use stoma bags in infants with a lower colon colostomy because the stool is more formed and less irritating. Instead, they allow the stool to empty directly into the diaper. Some parents prefer this method. In these cases, preventative skin care is imperative. Use of a barrier ointment on the abdominal skin surfaces should be started immediately. However, most parents find that the use of a stoma bag prevents skin breakdown.

The initial reaction from parents who see their infants' colostomy for the first time and realize that they will be responsible for the care of it is usually one of anxiety. The nurse plays an important role in reassuring and teaching the parent. With patience, support, understanding, and clinical expertise from the nurse, the parents learn stoma management and become experts in their child's care in a short period of time.

Pre-PSARP Care

Nursing care and assessment are essential during the preoperative stage. Before the PSARP, a distal colostogram is performed to determine the location of the most distal part of the bowel and document the presence and location of a fistula between the bowel and the urogenital tract. This study is obtained in an outpatient setting (Gross, Wolfson, & Peña, 1991).

Preoperative preparation may occur in the hospital or home setting. Visiting nurses may assist the family in the home setting. Bowel preparation includes irrigation of the distal stoma (nonfunctional, mucous fistula) with warm normal saline solution with the aid of a Foley catheter. The purpose of this irrigation is to remove colonic fecal matter distal to the colostomy and to avoid contamination at the time of the pull-through. Irrigations are continued until the fluid return is clear.

Posterior Sagittal Anorectoplasty

The posterior sagittal anorectoplasty is more commonly referred to as the PSARP (Peña, 1992), or the "Peña procedure." Generally, this second stage of the surgical repair is performed in patients older than 1 month of age, provided that the infant is growing and developing normally. Some surgeons prefer to wait until the baby is 6 to 12 months old. The operation is performed in the prone position (face down) with a Foley catheter inserted in the bladder. A midline posterior sagittal incision is made, running from the middle portion of the sacrum to the anterior edge of the external sphincter. The sphincter mechanism is divided in a midline incision, thereby preserving the nerve fibers and decreasing the amount of postoperative pain. The back of the child's buttocks is opened like a book, and all internal structures are exposed. The rectum is then meticulously separated from the genitourinary tract and is mobilized to reach its normal site without tension. The fistula site is then closed. With the use of an electrical muscle stimulator, the limits of the sphincter mechanism are determined, and the rectum is placed in its optimal location to achieve the best functional results. If the child is known to have a very high defect or the child's rectum is unreachable with this approach, the abdomen must also be opened (laparotomy).

The postoperative course for this surgical procedure is relatively benign. If a laparotomy was not needed, the child may drink fluids after the surgery and have a regular diet the next day. The intravenous line must be preserved for the administration of antibiotics for 2 to 3 days. Some surgeons continue antibiotics for several more days. In males and in females with cloaca, the Foley catheter remains in place 5 to 10 days. This protects the suture line in the urethra, where the communication between the bowel and urethra is located. If the catheter is removed inadvertently, the nurse should never replace it. The surgeon should be notified. If the infant is unable to void, a suprapubic tube is inserted. The children do not need to be in any particular position; they may simply find the best position for themselves. Instruct the parents to apply triple antibiotic ointment to the perineum with every diaper change to prevent local infection. Continue the antibiotic ointment for 2 weeks until the child's first postoperative visit. The expected length of stay is 2 to 3 days.

Postoperative Care in Cases of PSARP plus Laparotomy

Children experience more postoperative pain and a longer hospital stay if a laparotomy is needed with the PSARP (Peña, 1992). A laparotomy is generally performed if the rectum is too high to be visualized and mobilized from a posterior approach. These children return from the operating room with an intravenous line and an NG tube. The NG remains in place for approximately 3 days or until active bowel sounds are heard. Pain is managed with intravenous nonsteroidal anti-inflammatory medications (ketorolac) every 6 hours around the clock for 48 hours. Narcotic analgesia may be used for breakthrough pain. In selected cases, a lumbar epidural may enhance pain

control. The skin care of the perineum remains the same, with antibiotic ointment as described earlier.

Two-Week Postoperative Visit

Two weeks after surgery, the stitches are removed, and the antibiotic ointment is discontinued. At this time, the process of anal dilations is initiated (Paidis & Peña, 1997). The dilations prevent anal strictures from forming. It is imperative for the parents to adhere to the guidelines given to them. The surgeon generally passes the first dilator, and then the surgeon or advanced practice nurse teaches the parents the dilation process. Position the child with the knees flexed close to the chest. Lubricate the tip of the anal dilator and insert it 3 to 4 cm into the rectum. Repeat this procedure twice a day for approximately 30 seconds each time. Every week, the size of the dilator is advanced. After 6 to 8 weeks, the "desired size" is reached (Table 21-3). Then colostomy closure is planned.

Dilation Schedule (after the Desired Size Has Been Reached)

Dilations continue, with decreasing frequency, after the PSARP for a total period of approximately 6 months. The parent must continue passing the last desired size of dilator twice per day until the dilator passes easily and without pain. Then, the parent can begin decreasing the frequency of dilations on the following schedule (Peña, 1992):

- One time a day for 1 month
- Every other day for 1 month
- Two times a week for 1 month
- Once a week for 1 month
- Once a month for 3 months

Colostomy Closure

When the child is ready to undergo colostomy closure, preoperative preparation may occur in the hospital or home setting. Irrigations are necessary for the proximal (functional) stoma and are performed in the same manner as those for the distal (nonfunctioning) stoma before

Table 21-3	Anal Dilator Selection Criteria
Child's Age	**Hegar Dilator Size**
1–4 months of age	Number 12
4–8 months of age	Number 13
8–12 months of age	Number 14
1–4 years of age	Number 15
> 4 years of age	Number 16

the PSARP. The child receives a clear liquid diet on the day before surgery. Broad-spectrum antibiotics are administered before surgery, preferably 1 hour before the first incision time. The surgery entails taking down both stomas and performing a bowel anastomosis to reestablish the colon continuity. After surgery, the child may experience more pain than after the pull-through procedure if a laparotomy was not required. The child returns to the pediatric unit with intravenous fluids and a Salem sump NG tube placed for low continuous suction. Intravenous antibiotics are routinely given for 3 to 7 days. Scheduled pain medications are given, and breakthrough doses are administered as needed. The use of pediatric pain scales assists the care team in evaluating the level of comfort by providing objective assessments. The child remains NPO, on intravenous hydration and with an NG tube for 1 to 3 days or until bowel sounds are heard. Once flatus is passed, clear liquids or breast milk can be started. The diet is then advanced as tolerated. After surgery, the expected length of stay is 4 to 5 days.

Children are not discharged until they pass stool from the anus. Stools are often small, liquid, and very frequent during the immediate postoperative period. Perianal excoriation is a serious complication that often occurs. Preventative skin care must be a nursing goal. Discussing skin care with the family several weeks before the colostomy closure is very helpful.

One relatively natural preparation to prepare the skin before the colostomy closure can be accomplished by coating the perineum with a paste and then adding a small amount of stool from the colostomy for 15 minutes, three times a day for approximately 2 weeks. After surgery, a variety of "butt pastes" can be ordered to protect and heal the perineum. For example, one useful paste consists of vitamin A & D ointment, aloe, zinc, and Mylanta (to help the ointment stick to the skin and help form a paste). A petroleum-based barrier cream (i.e., Ilex®) has also proved helpful in anecdotal studies. This is applied 3 to 4 times a day and covered with petroleum jelly at each diaper change. No other diaper creams should be used with this product because the effectiveness could be altered. Although this product can become tacky, holding stool, it should not be removed by scrubbing. Removal with mineral oil makes this process easier. An antifungal cream or powder (only with a prescription) can be added if a yeast infection occurs (Paidis & Peña, 1997). This would be evidenced by a migrating, raised, erythematous rash that often causes itching. Mixing the petroleum based–skin barrier (Ilex®) 1:1 with the antifungal cream or ointment is very effective in treating fungal skin problems. Eventually, the number of bowel movements decreases, and

the diaper rash is no longer a concern (Peña, 1992). As the number of bowel movements per day decreases over the next several weeks, the skin begins to heal nicely.

At that point, constipation becomes a concern. Constipation is the most frequent sequela in children born with anorectal malformations (Peña & El Behery, 1993). A laxative-type diet is recommended to prevent constipation and fecal impaction. The family is given a detailed list of fiber-rich foods. If the diet does not result in regular soft stools, a laxative medication or stool softener, such as senna, docusate sodium, or mineral oil, is prescribed to ensure that the patient empties his or her rectum every day (Poenaru et al., 1997) (see Bowel Management, Chapter 9).

■ Postoperative Bowel Function

Children who undergo surgical repair of anorectal malformations experience variable degrees of bowel control. Children with anorectal malformations also become toilet trained for stool later than children with normal anatomy. There are some signs, however, that the surgeon can use before that age to predict the possibility of the child's success with toilet training.

Patients born with good prognostic types of malformations and showing good prognostic signs as described earlier in this chapter are expected to achieve success with toilet training. Alternatively, patients born with poor prognostic malformations or showing bad prognostic signs are offered a bowel management program (Peña, 1990a, 1992; Peña et al., 1998). The goal of a bowel management program is social continence for children who are unlikely to become toilet trained.

Toilet Training

Toilet training for stool is the long-term goal for children with anorectal malformations, although this is not always possible. Parents should be encouraged to use the same strategies for toilet training as in children with normal anatomy. Between 2 and 3 years of age, the parents are instructed to sit the child on the toilet after every meal. The parents are encouraged to do it as a game and not as a punishment. The child should sit in front of a little table and play with favorite toys. The parents should be encouraged to sit with the child and not to argue or force the child to remain seated. However, if the child gets up, the parents should put the toys away. The child should be rewarded for a bowel movement or voiding while on the toilet. If the child is not successfully toilet trained by school age, there are two alternatives: (1) do not send the child to school for one more year and continue attempts at toilet training or (2) try the bowel management program (Peña et al., 1998) for 1 year, assuming that it will be implemented on a temporary basis. Then, during the next summer vacation, the parents can again attempt to toilet train the child.

It is unacceptable to send a child with fecal incontinence to school in diapers when his classmates are already toilet trained (Peña, 1997). Children who require diapers or who have accidents while in school because of fecal incontinence are exposed to ridicule from their peers that can lead to adverse psychological sequelae (Poenaru et al., 1997).

■ Bowel Management Program

To achieve fecal continence, three components are necessary: sensation within the rectum, good motility of the colon, and good voluntary muscle or sphincter control (Peña, 1992). Children with anorectal malformations lack all or some of these essential components.

First, children born with anorectal malformations lack the intrinsic sensation to feel stool or gas passing through their rectum. Therefore, many times the child may unknowingly soil.

Second, the child needs to have good motility of the colon. Normally, the rectosigmoid remains quiet for periods of 24 to 48 hours, followed by a massive peristaltic wave that promotes the complete emptying of the colon. Patients with anorectal malformations have abnormal peristaltic waves in the rectosigmoid colon that result in stagnant stool or an overactive colon. The child then develops constipation or encopresis (overflow incontinence). Alternatively, a very active colon may provoke a constant passing of stool, which may significantly interfere with bowel continence.

Third, the child needs good voluntary muscles or sphincteric mechanism. These muscles allow for good control and retention of stool.

Children who have fecal incontinence after repair of imperforate anus can be divided into two well-defined groups that require individualized treatment plans: (1) children with constipation are mainly those who underwent operations in which the rectum was preserved (anoplasty, PSARP, and sacroperineal pull-through), and (2) children with diarrhea are mainly those who underwent operations in which the rectum and, at times, the sigmoid colon were resected (abdominoperineal procedure, endorectal resection). Sometimes, the child has lost a portion of the colon for some other reason or has a condition that produces diarrhea.

The basis of the bowel management program consists of teaching the parents or patient to clean the colon every day by the use of enemas or colonic irrigations followed by finding a method to keep the colon quiet for the following 24 hours. This prevents soiling episodes and involuntary bowel movements. Success of the bowel management program is enhanced with specific diets or medications, such as Lomotil® or Imodium®. Success is usually achieved within a week of a trial-and-error process (Peña et al., 1998).

Children with Constipation

A guide to help parents manage children with constipation is imperative. Identify a quiet, relaxed time of day for the enema program. After dinner often works well for families. Administer the enemas 1 hour after eating to take advantage of the gastric-colic reflex. Ask the child to sit on the toilet for 30 to 45 minutes. The use of phosphate enemas (Fleet®) is most convenient. However, pure saline enemas are often just as effective. Children older than 8 years of age or heavier than 65 lb may receive one adult phosphate enema daily. Children between 3 and 8 years of age or 35 and 65 lb may receive one pediatric phosphate enema a day. Patients should never receive more than one phosphate enema a day because of the risk of phosphate intoxication and hypocalcemia and hyponatremia (Peña et al., 1998). Symptoms of hyperphosphatemia are associated with the symptoms of the related hypocalcemia and include tetany, paresthesias, and Q-T wave prolongation. Treatment of hyperphosphatemia includes elimination of any excess intake, use of aluminum hydroxide antacids, and administration of intravenous saline (Weigle & Tobin, 1992). The phosphate enema administered on a regular basis should result in a bowel movement followed by a period of 24 hours of complete cleanliness (Fig. 21-11).

If one enema is not enough to clean the colon, then the patient requires a more aggressive treatment, and a saline (only) enema is administered. If the addition of the saline enema still results in inadequate results, then high colonic washings are indicated with a Foley catheter attached to the bottle of the Fleet® enema. A 20 to 24 Fr Foley catheter is lubricated and gently introduced through the anus as far as possible (Fig. 21-12). The catheter is flexible so the parents can maneuver it into the colon of children with severe impaction. If the catheter does not pass up into the bowel, insert the tube a few centimeters and inflate the balloon with 20 to 30 mL of water. Pull on the catheter, occluding the colonic lumen with the balloon acting as a plug. This enables the enema solution to go up into the bowel with minimal leakage (Fig. 21-13A

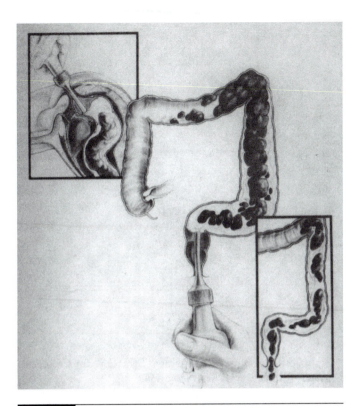

Figure 21-11 Colonic irrigation technique: without a tube.

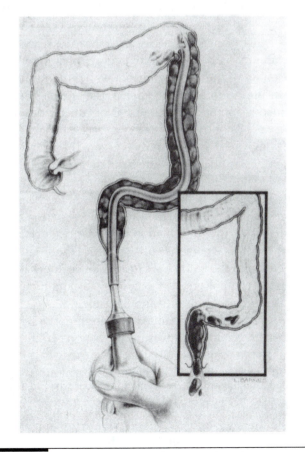

Figure 21-12 Colonic irrigation technique: with a tube.

through C). If the child soils at any point during the following 24 hours, the bowel washout was incomplete, and a more aggressive technique is required. Parents can increase the volume of the enema or administer a second saline enema 30 minutes later. The program must be individualized while the parents and children learn to look at the consistency and amount of stool obtained after the enema to determine effectiveness.

Position the child to take advantage of gravity. High colonic washing can increase the efficacy of the enema. Young children can be positioned over the parent's lap for administration. In older children, instill the enema with the children on their knees, with the buttocks up and their head close to the floor (Fig. 21-14A through C). Encourage the child to sit on the toilet for 30 to 45 minutes after the administration of the enema until he or she feels that the colon is empty. A portable television, books, homework, or games can make this time pass faster. Constipated children have a colon and a rectosigmoid with decreased motility. Frequently, all they may need is a good enema or colonic irrigation to remain clean for 24 hours (Peña et al., 1998).

A second group of children who experience severe constipation are those who have undergone a surgical repair for an anorectal malformation with an adequate sacrum and sphincters. The history reveals an operation that was performed successfully, without complication and a preserved rectosigmoid segment. Yet these children can have severe constipation associated with a megasigmoid (Peña & El Behery, 1993). Parents describe that the interval between bowel movements is greater than a week and then the child is incontinent of stool. A contrast enema demonstrates the presence of a giant sigmoid colon. These children require an aggressive program of enemas to be clean. Another alternative is surgery that involves resecting the most dilated portion of the megasigmoid. The procedure makes the patient fecally continent and demonstrates that the problem was severe constipation with secondary encopresis or overflow pseudo-incontinence (Peña & El Behery). If the constipation is not extreme, administration of laxatives may have the same effect as the operation.

Children with Diarrhea

Management of children with diarrhea is a separate challenge. Patients with a history of diarrhea often have an overactive colon. Children with anorectal malformations who had the rectosigmoid colon resected have no reservoir for stool. Rapid transit of stool results in frequent episodes of diarrhea. Stool passes so rapidly from the cecum to the descending colon that they are unable to main-

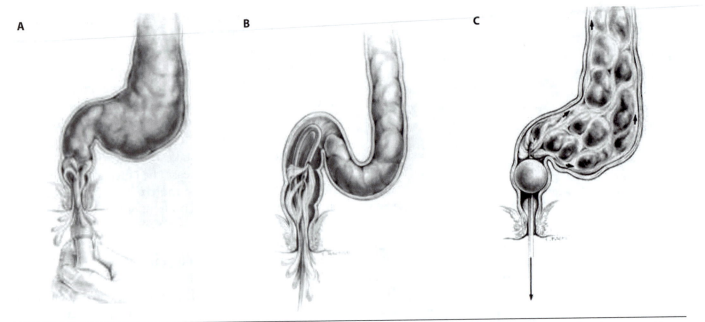

Figure 21-13 A–Irrigation tube is obstructed by fecal material. B–Irrigation tube has been turned back by fecal impaction. C–Enema with colonic irrigation technique using a Foley ballon inflated.

tain continence, even after administration of an enema. A constipating diet and/or medications to slow down the colon, such as loperamide (Imodium®), are recommended. Provide parents with a list of constipating foods to promote a regular diet and a list of laxative foods to be avoided. Most parents know which meals provoke diarrhea and which constipate their child. Despite the best efforts of all, some children never develop social continence. This rare group of children may benefit from a permanent colostomy (Peña et al., 1998).

Children who do not achieve successful bowel management with enemas and diet require medication. To determine the combination that will be successful for the child, the following plan is recommended. (1) Start the treatment with enemas, a very strict constipating diet, and a high dose of loperamide. Most patients respond to this aggressive management within 24 hours. The child should remain on a strict diet until clean for 24 hours 2 to 3 days in a row. (2) Allow the child to choose one new food every 2 to 3 days and observe the effect on his or her colonic activity. If the child soils after eating a newly introduced food, eliminate that food from the diet. However, find the most liberal diet possible for the child. (3) If the child continues to be clean with a more liberal diet, gradually reduce the medication to the lowest dose effective to keep the child clean for 24 hours.

If incontinence appears again, it means that something has changed in the child's habits and a meticulous evaluation is needed. The first thing to question is whether the enemas are still effective. The questions are: "Is the child emptying himself/herself properly?" "Is he/she emptying the colon less successfully than before?" To fully evaluate this change, it is necessary to have an x-ray study of the abdomen to analyze the quantity of stool present in the colon. If the x-ray study shows a large amount of stool in the colon after the enema, the enema needs to be adjusted (increased volume and/or concentration) to the new needs of the child. After a week of trial and error in which a daily x-ray study is taken, the practitioner and family should have a better understanding of the individual issues. On the other hand, if the plain radiograph shows a clean colon, the "accidents" may have been due to increased motility. Medications that slow the colon and a constipating diet plan may be reintroduced. It is imperative to evaluate the consistency of the stool: feces that remain in the colon for a long time becomes harder and stickier; therefore, it is necessary to carefully evaluate both the stool quantity and consistency.

Change in a child's habits plays an important role in bowel management: changes in the diet on certain occasions, like birthdays, holidays, and so on, may have repercussions, especially in children with hypermotility. In the same way, stressful factors can play a role in bowel function (e.g., moving from one's house, divorces, changes of school). In some adolescents, there are predictable circumstances that influence bowel function, such as examinations and school stress. Administering a medication,

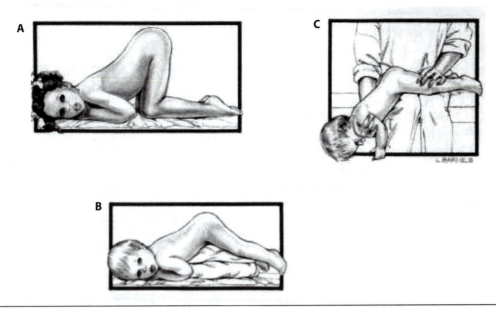

Figure 21-14 A through C, Ideal positioning for patients for the administration of enemas.

such as loperamide, the day before an examination may help decrease bowel motility.

Additional Bowel Management Strategies for Children with Anorectal Malformations

Another strategy for managing fecal incontinence in children is the creation of a continent appendicostomy for the administration of an antegrade enema. This procedure is effective in children who experience fecal incontinence despite success with a bowel management program (Curry, Osborne, & Malone, 1998; Fukunaga, Kimura, Lawrence, Soper, & Phearman, 1996; Graf et al., 1998; Meier, Foster, Guzzetta, & Colin, 1998; Webb, Barraza, & Crump, 1997; Wilcox & Kiely, 1998) (see Bowel Management, Chapter 9).

Another adjunct to a bowel management program is biofeedback. Biofeedback therapy may help children who are able to recognize sensation in the rectum to distinguish between solids, liquids, and gas. The goal is control of bowel movements. Biofeedback involves inserting a probe into the child's anus and asking him or her to perform Kegel exercises. A computer screen provides a visual image that displays periods of contraction and relaxation, the pelvic muscle activity. Continence is improved in children who are able to follow directions, are self-motivated, and are willing to practice the new skills at home in addition to the training sessions. A carefully planned diet supplements a biofeedback program. Although the use of biofeedback is not widespread in children with anorectal malformations (Paidis & Peña, 1997;

Poenaru et al., 1997), it has been shown to be effective in some children (Iwai, Iwata, Kimura, & Yanagihara, 1997). It may also be worthwhile to use behavior modification techniques in children who are toilet training, having two to three bowel movements per day, and soiling in between these bowel movements (Paidis & Peña).

Children with complex or high anorectal malformations require a bowel management program for the remainder of their lives (Hendren, 1997; Peña, 1992; Truffler & Wilkinson, 1962). Children with less severe defects may remain socially continent with a disciplined diet of regular meals to provoke bowel movements at a predictable time. It is never too late to consider a bowel management program. Children who initially fail to achieve continence at ages 3 to 5 years may successfully achieve continence in the early school-aged years. Encourage children with some potential for bowel control to gain control of their bowel movements without enemas over the summer vacation. Parents and children who commit to this process must stay at home, socialize little, and maintain a regular diet and schedule to achieve success. Encourage the child to sit on the toilet after every meal and try to pass stool. In addition, the child must remain alert all day while trying to learn to discriminate the feeling of an imminent bowel movement. Children with constipation may benefit from a daily laxative to provoke a single bowel movement per day. Adjust the dosage of the laxative as needed to avoid uncontrolled diarrhea. Start with a laxative-type diet. Then, add a bulk-forming product, such as a stool softener. If these medications do not work, a laxative with an active ingredient is indicated. After a few days or weeks, the family and the child are in a position to decide whether they want to continue with that regimen or whether they would prefer to go back to the bowel management program.

The bowel management program is an ongoing process that is responsive to individual patient and family needs. The success of the bowel management program depends on the dedication, determination, and consistency of everyone involved. Children who have completed the bowel management program and remain clean for 24 hours experience a new sense of confidence based on an improved quality of life.

■ Conclusion

The variety of anorectal malformations can have significant differences in continence outcomes. An understanding of the diagnosis and management of the various types of malformations guides the care of these children and their families. Unfortunately, these children may continue to have some degree of bowel dysfunction after surgery. A variety of treatment modalities exist to assist the child in achieving continence. The success of any of these strategies, the bowel management program, biofeedback, and surgical intervention, requires collaboration between the family, the child, and the health care team.

■ Educational Materials

APSNA invites you to download the following diagnosis-related teaching tool for Chapter 21, Anorectal Malformations in Children: Posterior sagittal anorectoplasty (PSARP). This teaching tool is available at the APSNA Web site (www.apsna.org) and the Jones and Bartlett Web site (www.jbpub.com). All teaching materials are available in English and Spanish and are free of charge. APSNA encourages their use for your patients and families.

References

Curry, J. L., Osborne, A., & Malone, P. S. (1998). How to achieve a successful Malone antegrade continence enema. *Journal of Pediatric Surgery*, 33(1), 138–141.

Fukunaga, K., Kimura, K., Lawrence, J., Soper, R. T., & Phearman, L. A. (1996). Button device for antegrade enema in the treatment of incontinence and constipation. *Journal of Pediatric Surgery*, 31(8), 1038–1039.

Graf, J. L., Strear, C., Bratton, B., Housley, H. T., Jennings, R. W., Harrison, M. R., et al. (1998). The antegrade continence enema procedure: A review of the literature. *Journal of Pediatric Surgery*, 33(8), 1294–1296.

Gross, G. W., Wolfson, P. J., & Peña, A. (1991). Augmented-pressure colostogram in imperforate anus with fistula. *Pediatric Radiology*, 21, 560–562.

Hendren, W. H. (1997). Management of cloaca malformations. *Seminars in Pediatric Surgery*, 6(4), 217–227.

Iwai, N., Iwata, G., Kimura, O., & Yanagihara, J. (1997). Is a new biofeedback therapy effective for fecal incontinence in patients who have anorectal malformations? *Journal of Pediatric Surgery*, 32(11), 1626–1629.

Kiely, E. D., & Peña, A. (1998). Anorectal malformations. In J. S. O'Neill, M. I. Rowe, J. L. Grosfeld, E. W. Fonkalsrud, & A. G. Coran (Eds.), *Pediatric surgery* (Vol. 2, 5th ed., p. 1425). St. Louis, MO: Mosby.

Meier, D. E., Foster, M. E., Guzzetta, P. C., & Colin, D. (1998). Antegrade continent enema management of chronic fecal incontinence in children. *Journal of Pediatric Surgery, 33*(7), 1149–1152.

Narasimharao, K. A., Prassad, G. R., & Katariya, S. (1983). Prone cross-table lateral view: An alternative to the invertogram in imperforate anus. *American Journal of Roentgenology, 140*, 227–229.

Paidis, C. N., & Peña, A. (1997). Rectum and anus. In K. T. Oldham, P. M. Colombani, & R. P. Foglia (Eds.), *Surgery of infants and children: Scientific principles and practice* (p. 1323). Philadelphia: Lippincott-Raven.

Peña, A. (1988). Posterior sagittal anorectoplasty: Results in the management of 332 cases of anorectal malformations. *Pediatric Surgery International, 3*, 94–104.

Peña, A. (1990a). Advances in the management of fecal incontinence secondary to anorectal malformations. In L. M. Nyhus (Ed.), *Surgery annual* (pp. 143–167). Norwalk, CT: Appleton & Lange.

Peña, A. (1990b). *Atlas of surgical management of anorectal malformations* (p. 1). New York: Springer-Verlag.

Peña, A. (1992). Current management of anorectal anomalies. *Surgical Clinics of North America, 72*(6), 1393–1416.

Peña, A. (1997). Preface: Advances in anorectal malformations. *Seminars in Pediatric Surgery, 6*(4), 165–169.

Peña, A., & El Behery, M. (1993). Megasigmoid: A source of pseudo incontinence in children with repaired anorectal malformations. *Journal of Pediatric Surgery, 28*, 1–5.

Peña, A., Guardino, J. M., Tovilla, M. A., Levitt, G., Rodriguez, G., & Tones, R. (1998). Bowel management for fecal incontinence in patients with anorectal malformations. *Journal of Pediatric Surgery*, 33(1), 133–137.

Poenaru, D., Roblin, N., Bird, M., Duce, S., Groll, A., Pietak, D., et al. (1997). The pediatric bowel management clinic: Initial results of a multidisciplinary approach to functional constipation in children. *Journal of Pediatric Surgery*, 32(6), 843–848.

Rich, M. A., Brock, W. A., & Peña, A. (1988). Spectrum of genitourinary malformations in patients with imperforate anus. *Pediatric Surgery International, 3*, 110–113.

Shaul, D. B., & Harrison, A. (1997). Classification of anorectal malformations: Initial approach, diagnostic tests, and colostomy. *Seminars in Pediatric Surgery, 6*(4), 187–195.

Torres, P., Levitt, M. A., Tovilla, J. M., Rodriguez, G., & Peña, A. (1998). Anorectal malformations and Down's syndrome. *Journal of Pediatric Surgery*, 22(2), 1–5.

Truffler, G. A., & Wilkinson, R. H. (1962). Imperforate anus: 147 cases. *Canadian Journal of Surgery*, 5, 169–177.

Wangensteen, O. H., & Rice, C. O. (1930). Imperforate anus: Determining the surgical approach. *Annals of Surgery*, 92, 77.

Webb, H. W., Barraza, M. A., & Crump, J. M. (1997). Laparoscopic appendicostomy for management of fecal incontinence. *Journal of Pediatric Surgery*, 32(3), 457–458.

Weigle, C. G. M., & Tobin, J. R. (1992). Metabolic and endocrine disease in pediatric intensive care. In M. C. Rogers (Ed.), *Textbook of pediatric intensive care* (Vol. 2, 2nd ed., p. 1235). Baltimore: Williams & Wilkins.

Wilcox, D. T., & Kiely, E. M. (1998). The Malone (Antegrade Colonic Enema) Procedure: Early experience. *Journal of Pediatric Surgery*, 33(2), 204–206.

Wilkins, S., & Peña, A. (1988). The role of colostomy in the management of anorectal malformations. *Pediatric Surgery International, 3*, 105–109.

V

Nursing Care of Children with Abdominal Problems

Hypertrophic Pyloric Stenosis

By Kimberly O'Dowd

Hypertrophic pyloric stenosis (HPS) is a common surgical disorder in infancy that produces nonbilious emesis as its hallmark symptom (Rowe, O'Neill, Grosfeld, Fonkalsrud, & Coran, 1995). Classically, the disease presents at approximately 2 to 3 weeks of age with nonbilious vomiting that may be described as forceful or projectile, occurring 30 to 60 minutes after feeding. This emesis usually appears as stale, curdled milk or may be clear. It may also have a coffee-ground appearance that is associated with bleeding from proximal gastritis (Puri & Lakshmanadass, 2003). The projectile nature of the vomiting is described as being forcefully ejected 1 to 4 feet from the child. The emesis is even more projectile when the infant is in a side-lying position. Most infants with HPS experience vomiting in small amounts at about 2 weeks of life because of partial obstruction, and as the disease progresses, nearly complete obstruction of the pylorus develops by the second to fourth week of life (Rowe et al.).

Pathophysiology

HPS is defined as an acquired condition in which the circumferential muscle of the pyloric sphincter becomes thickened, resulting in elongation and obliteration of the pyloric channel. This process produces a high-grade gastric outlet obstruction, with compensatory dilation, hypertrophy, and hyperperistalsis of the stomach (Magnuson & Schwartz, 2005).

HPS has been reviewed and the clinical features and pathology discussed by many. In the 19th century, Dr. Hirschsprung described two cases of HPS that established it as a discrete clinical entity. The first successful surgical treatment of HPS was performed by Dr. Lobker in 1898, using a gastrojejunostomy. In 1911, Dr. Ramstedt developed and described the pyloromyotomy that remains the standard surgical procedure today for treatment of HPS (Dudgeon, 1993).

Etiology

The cause of HPS has long been debated. In Ireland in 1987, sonographic studies were obtained on 1,400 newborns to determine whether HPS is acquired rather than congenital. These studies confirmed that pyloric muscle hypertrophy visualized on ultrasonography is not present in the early newborn period of infants who later developed infantile HPS. This suggests that HPS is an acquired disease (Rollins, Shields, Quinn, & Wooldridge, 1989; Puri & Lakshmanadass, 2003).

Multiple theories of etiology include immature or degenerated pyloric neural elements, variations of infant feeding regimens, and excess production of gastrin in either mother or infant (Dudgeon, 1993; Rowe et al., 1995). Other hypotheses include a theory of dyscoordination between gastric peristaltic activity and pyloric relaxation, causing inappropriate pyloric contraction in the face of elevated intragastric pressures. This results in work-related hypertrophy of the pyloric muscle, initiating a cycle of increasing pyloric obstruction and gastric contractions (Magnuson & Schwartz, 2005). Recent theories of abnormalities in the enteric nervous system and abnormalities in the distribution of neuropeptides and neurotransmitters have also been reviewed (Magnuson & Schwartz). Hypotheses exploring involvement of a reduction in the neuronal nitric oxide synthase in the hypertrophic circular layer of the pylorus suggest that nitric oxide is a potent inhibitory neurotransmitter that induces relaxation of smooth muscle. Therefore, absence of the enzyme producing nitric oxide implies that the gastric outlet obstruction of HPS might be related to a defect of pyloric relaxation (Vanderwinden et al., 1996).

In recent studies, an association has been suggested linking maternal and infant exposure to erythromycin and the development of HPS (Cooper, Ray, & Griffin, 2002; Magnuson & Schwartz, 2005; Mahon, Rosenman, & Kleiman, 2001; Sorensen et al., 2003).

■ Incidence

The incidence of HPS ranges from 0.1% to 1% in the general population. HPS has a significant male predominance of 4:1. The incidence varies with ethnic origin, being more predominant in Caucasians and encountered less often in infants of Asian or Indian descent (Magnuson & Schwartz, 2005; Puri & Lakshmanadass, 2003; Rowe et al., 1995).

The development of HPS also appears to involve the variable transmission of an inheritable trait between generations, with the transmission of the trait being more common from mothers than from fathers (Magnuson & Schwartz, 2005).

■ Presentation

HPS is most commonly seen in full-term male infants, at approximately 3 to 6 weeks of age. Initial symptoms may begin as early as 2 to 3 weeks of life. Parents describe a previously well infant who begins to vomit. Initially, the infant may intermittently regurgitate after a feeding.

However, as the pyloric obstruction increases, the vomiting occurs with every feeding. This emesis is described as progressive, projectile, and nonbilious. Commonly, the infant appears ravenous and eager to eat immediately after the previous episode of emesis (Dudgeon, 1993). Some infants may appear well on early presentation. However, infants who are symptomatic for several days before diagnosis may have weight loss, slight jaundice, and significant dehydration, and they appear quite ill. On clinical examination, palpation of the hypertrophied pylorus is diagnostic.

■ Differential Diagnosis

Many differential diagnoses are considered in the initial examination of an infant who is vomiting, including feeding intolerance, milk allergy, overfeeding, and gastroesophageal reflux. Other disease entities, such as pylorospasm, primary gastric atony, salt-wasting adrenogenital syndrome, central nervous system lesions with increased intracranial pressures, gastric antral web, pyloric atresia, pyloric duplication cyst, ectopic pyloric pancreas, and pancreatic adenomas, may also be considered in the differential diagnosis (Dudgeon, 1993). It is the persistent, forceful, and progressive nature of the nonbilious emesis, the abrupt onset of the disease in a previously healthy infant, and the degree of illness in the presenting infant that usually lead to the consideration of HPS as the primary diagnosis.

■ Physical Examination

On physical examination, the infant may or may not appear acutely ill and dehydrated. Other clinical manifestations include projectile vomiting, weight loss, and persistent hunger despite the recent emesis. Palpation of a small oval mass, olive-like in nature, in the midepigastrium is usually diagnostic of pyloric stenosis. Most clinicians believe that if this "olive" is unequivocally palpated in the midepigastrium, no further diagnostic studies are indicated. However, palpation of this mass is not always possible. Palpating the olive should be attempted when the infant is not crying and the abdominal muscles are relaxed. An empty stomach during palpation, such as after an episode of emesis or nasogastric decompression, is helpful. The practitioner should elevate or gently bend the infant's knees or move the infant's lower extremities while the infant is sucking on a pacifier or bottle. This technique promotes increased abdominal muscle relaxation (Rowe et al., 1995). Palpation begins just over the spine and above the umbilicus. Two or three fingers are pressed lightly into the deeper tissues in a sweeping motion superiorly to inferiorly. The pyloric olive is smooth, hard, oblong, and usually about 1 to 2 cm long.

Another technique that aids in the diagnosis of HPS is observation of the infant during feeding. Peristaltic waves moving across the infant's abdomen from left to right just before emesis occurs may be observed, thus providing an opportunity to assess the forcefulness and character of the emesis.

■ Serum Laboratory Work

Serum laboratory work in an infant with HPS may demonstrate hypochloremia and hypocalcemia with metabolic alkalosis, hypoglycemia, and elevated unconjugated bilirubin (Magnuson & Schwartz, 2005). Persistent vomiting results in loss of fluid and hydrochloric acid from the stomach. The gastric mucosa produces hydrochloric acid that is lost with the vomitus, but the bicarbonate continues to enter the blood and is not buffered by the hydrogen equivalent. This causes metabolic alkalosis. Hypokalemia results from the distal renal tubules responding to the renin-aldosterone system. This process promotes the excretion of potassium and hydrogen in exchange for sodium and continues to exacerbate the metabolic alkalosis by producing hypokalemia and increasing distal bicarbonate reabsorption associated with hydrogen ion secretion. The hyperbilirubinemia is associated with a decrease in hepatic glucuronyl transferase activity (Magnuson & Schwartz).

■ Diagnostic Studies

HPS can be clinically diagnosed easily by a skilled clinician. In most cases, radiologic confirmation of HPS is not required. However, both contrast studies and ultrasonography can aid in the diagnosis of HPS. Contrast studies, such as an upper gastrointestinal series, are favored by some surgeons who believe they are more cost-effective than ultrasonography because they may demonstrate many other disease entities (Hulka, Campbell, Harrison, & Campbell, 1997). Upper gastrointestinal contrast studies can diagnose gastroesophageal reflux, pylorospasm, and delayed gastric emptying. An upper gastrointestinal tract study is diagnostic of HPS by demonstrating an elongated and narrowed pyloric channel, an enlarged stomach, and minimal transit of contrast through the pylorus. This is commonly referred to as the "string sign," defining one narrow channel, or a "railroad track

sign," defining two narrow channels (Fig. 22-1). Other characteristic findings on upper gastrointestinal studies include visualization of the "shoulders" of the hypertrophied pylorus bulging into the gastric lumen (Magnuson & Schwartz, 2005).

Some criticize the use of upper gastrointestinal studies compared with ultrasonographic studies in diagnosing HPS because upper gastrointestinal contrast studies expose an infant to ionizing radiation. There is also the risk of aspiration of gastrointestinal contents and barium if the infant undergoes surgery with general anesthesia (Dudgeon, 1993).

In 1977, ultrasonography was used in making the diagnosis of HPS, and today it is favored by many as a reliable, inexpensive, noninvasive diagnostic study in the evaluation of HPS (Fig. 22-2) (Magnuson & Schwartz, 2005; Hernanz-Schulman et al., 1994; Hernanz-Schulman, 2003). The abdominal ultrasonogram measures the length and the diameter of the pyloric muscle. An overall diameter of 17 mm or more, a muscular wall thickness of 4 mm or more, and a channel length of 17 mm or more confirm the diagnosis of HPS. In infants who are less than 30 days of age, smaller measurements are used as the criteria for the diagnosis of HPS (Magnuson & Schwartz).

Godbole, Sprigg, Dickson, and Lin (1996) compared ultrasonography with clinical examination in diagnosing HPS. Their findings indicated that ultrasonographic study was useful in cases in which the clinical examination was

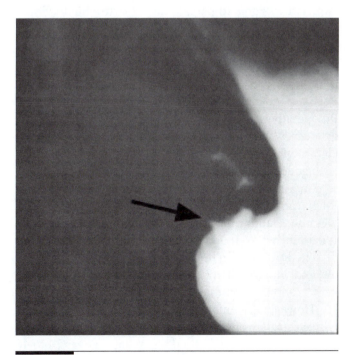

Figure 22-1 "String sign" indicating pyloric stenosis from upper gastrointestinal series.

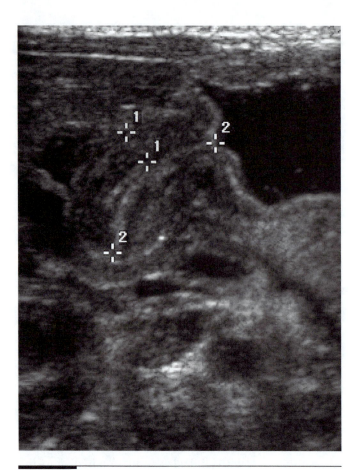

Figure 22-2 Pyloric stenosis shown on ultrasound.

negative. However, it was not necessary if an experienced clinician was able to palpate the hypertrophied pylorus (Godbole et al.).

■ Recommended Therapy

Recommended therapy for HPS is surgical intervention. Preoperative preparation of the infant with HPS is critical because most of these infants experience significant electrolyte abnormalities, making a surgical procedure with general anesthesia risky.

Surgical correction of HPS is not an emergency. An infant can be stabilized by rehydrating and correcting any electrolyte abnormalities with intravenous fluids while remaining without oral feedings. An infant without signs of dehydration, with normal glucose and electrolyte levels, and with excellent urine output may proceed to surgery as soon as possible.

However, the infant who is significantly dehydrated with electrolyte imbalances and metabolic alkalosis needs aggressive preoperative fluid resuscitation over 24 to 48 hours. The infant should have normal serum chloride, potassium, and bicarbonate levels, as well as normal vi-tal signs and good urine output, suggesting adequate fluid repletion, before proceeding to surgery (Magnuson & Schwartz, 2005).

■ Operative Considerations/Surgical Procedure

The surgical treatment most commonly used in infants with HPS is the Rammstedt pyloromyotomy (Greason, Thompson, Downey, & Sasso, 1995). The most common surgical approach used when performing a pyloromyotomy is to enter the peritoneal cavity through a transverse incision in the right upper quadrant over the rectus muscle at or above the liver edge (Garcia & Randolph, 1990; Rowe et al., 1995). The pyloromyotomy is a longitudinal incision made down to the mucosa, splitting the hypertrophied muscle where the pylorus is thickest and fibers most easily separate (Fig. 22-3) (Magnuson & Schwartz, 2005).

During the pyloromyotomy, extreme care is taken to avoid gastric mucosal tears because duodenal perforations are a potential complication in infants with HPS (Hulka, Harrison, Campbell, & Campbell, 1997; Poon, Zhang, Cartmill, & Cass, 1996). If a gastric mucosal tear is recognized, it can be repaired without associated morbidity or compromise to the pyloromyotomy. However, if a mucosal tear is not recognized during the surgery, associated postoperative complications, such as peritonitis, may occur. This increases the infant's overall risk of morbidity (Magnuson & Schwartz, 2005). After surgery, the nasogastric tube is removed as soon as the infant awakens from anesthesia unless the duodenal mucosa was perforated. In this case, the nasogastric tube should remain in place for an additional 24 to 48 hours to ensure gastric decompression (Rowe et al., 1995).

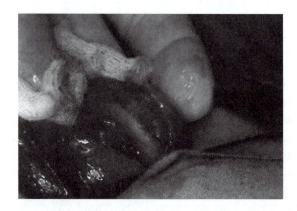

Figure 22-3 Intraoperative picture of the pyloromyotomy incision.

Another surgical option used in infants with HPS is laparoscopic pyloromyotomy. Greason et al. (1995) reported a case series of 11 infants with HPS comparing open pyloromyotomy with the laparoscopic approach. The findings indicated laparoscopic surgery to be equally safe and effective with superior cosmetic results. Surgical times or postoperative time until feedings were initiated was not significantly different. Although open pyloromyotomy is the most consistently successful operation ever described, the authors of this study are supportive of laparoscopic pyloromyotomy as an excellent alternative procedure in the management of HPS (Greason et al.).

Complications associated with pyloromyotomy are rare. Children treated for HPS using a standard surgical procedure by an experienced pediatric surgeon, with expert anesthesia, and appropriate preoperative resuscitation have minimal risk of mortality (Magnuson & Schwartz, 2005). However, rare postoperative complications may occur, including duodenal perforation, wound infections, and postoperative vomiting. Most infants experience some postoperative vomiting. This is not considered a true complication unless the vomiting continues for more than 48 hours (Hulka, Harrison, et al., 1997). If persistent vomiting continues for greater than 2 weeks, then a contrast study should be performed to rule out a gastric leak or fluid collection obstructing the gastric outlet, or an incomplete myotomy (Magnuson & Schwartz).

Developmental Considerations

Developmental concerns foremost in the nurse's mind in caring for the infant and parents of the infant with HPS include caring for a newborn infant and family, with the added psychological stresses of a hospitalization and impending surgery. Infants are first seen with HPS anywhere from 2 to 4 weeks of age; that is just enough time for parents to begin to establish some routine with their newborn child at home. Parents are recovering from the birth process and now are confronted with multiple new issues and adjustments. These might include sleep deprivation, fatigue, learning to breastfeed, sibling rivalry, and possibly entertaining family and friends who are admiring the new infant. This family is already stressed to some degree. A social service consultation may be indicated and is supportive for many of these families.

Many parents may feel that they have caused their infant to be sick in some way, possibly by overfeeding, by giving the wrong formula or by not choosing to breastfeed. Other parents may feel guilty knowing that there is a hereditary link to HPS. Nevertheless, this family and infant need intense support and encouragement. These parents may have an extremely high anxiety level. Therefore, information may need to be reinforced repeatedly. Specific data should be shared with the parents to help decrease anxiety, such as length of procedure, postoperative care, and what to expect perioperatively.

Separation, interrupted bonding, and not feeding a hungry infant are concerns that many parents experience before surgery. In some cases, the infant may still be allowed to feed small amounts of dextrose water or breast milk until a few hours before surgery.

Breast-feeding mothers should be encouraged to pump, save the breast milk, and have skin-to-skin contact to console the infant. Parents should be advised of the anticipated time of surgery. Parental education should also include the need for correction of any dehydration and electrolyte abnormalities before surgery. After surgery, parents need to be taught that many infants continue to intermittently vomit for a few feedings and may continue to do so for a few days. This is normal and expected. If this information is not reinforced, parents may believe that the pyloromyotomy was not successful, resulting in heightened parental anxiety.

Preoperative and Postoperative Nursing Considerations

Preoperative nursing considerations in caring for the child with HPS include obtaining an accurate nursing assessment of the infant and family on admission. Family support systems, family dynamics, and recent stresses should be discussed. Admission time is crucial for the nurse to establish a therapeutic relationship with the family and to assess and educate the parents. Vital signs and accurate intake and output should be recorded, including the last wet diaper and stool pattern, weight before illness, and current weight. Other key assessments should include the onset of the symptoms in the infant and a description of the vomiting. Invasive procedures during admission include starting intravenous fluids and drawing blood and may include placing a nasogastric tube.

The patient should have blood chemistry studies done, including sodium, potassium, chloride, carbon dioxide, glucose, blood urea and nitrogen, and creatinine levels. Bilirubin levels may also need to be evaluated. Other preoperative laboratory tests, such as prothrombin time, partial thromboplastin time, and complete blood count with platelets, are sometimes assessed as well. If the patient is extremely ill and dehydrated, specific tests may be ordered to assess the infant's acid base balance, such as arterial blood gases, because these babies can develop metabolic alkalosis.

Routine postoperative care includes frequent assessments of the infant's vital signs and pain, assessments of the infant's dressing for bleeding or drainage, and accurate assessment of intake and output. If the infant is having difficulty tolerating feedings and the abdomen is full and distended, abdominal girth measurements may be obtained.

Traditionally, postoperative feeding regimens have varied from overnight NPO status with limited amounts of formula, to a shortened 6 to 8 hour NPO time with set feeding times and amounts. Georgeson, Corbin, Griffen, and Breaux (1993) retrospectively reviewed the feeding regimens of 223 infants who underwent pyloromyotomy for HPS. The authors concluded that delaying feedings overnight or advancing feedings slowly every 4 hours did decrease the incidence and amount of postoperative vomiting. However, the authors were supportive of initiation of feedings 6 hours after surgery and advancing feedings every 2 hours. The authors suspected that the latter feeding regimen increased the incidence of postoperative vomiting but did not delay the eventual tolerance for ad libitum feedings. This feeding regimen was not associated with any increased incidence in postoperative complications, and both overall hospital stay and hospital charges decreased.

Recent studies have shown that although a shorter NPO time after surgery does result in an increase in postoperative emesis, this figure is not statistically significant. In addition, with feedings given ad libitum, hospital stay, associated costs, and morbidity were not significantly affected. Babies who underwent uncomplicated pyloromyotomy were able to leave the hospital sooner, tolerating full feeds without problems (Kretz, Watfa, & Sapin, 2005; Morash, 2002; Puapong, Kahng, Ko, & Applebaum, 2002).

An example of a postoperative feeding regimen for an infant with HPS is as follows: "nothing by mouth" status for 6 hours after surgery, followed by an initial feeding of 30 mL of Pedialyte or glucose water. The feedings are then progressed slowly or ad libitum until 60 to 90 mL of formula is tolerated, with care being taken not to overfeed. If the infant is breastfed, breast milk is substituted for formula. To help the breastfed infant successfully resume breast feeding, consider allowing the infant to go directly to the breast. Two effective means of quantifying the volume of breast milk consumed by the breast-feeding infant are the use of a supplemental nursing system and the use of a breast-feeding scale. A supplemental nursing system allows the clinician to offer an approximate volume of breast milk to be administered at the mother's breast while the infant nurses. A breast-feeding scale is also helpful by accurately assessing the infant's pre– and post–breast-feeding weight, thus allowing a fairly accurate calculation of volume intake. If vomiting occurs with feedings, the feeding may be held for 2 hours, and then the regimen is reinitiated. Intravenous fluids may be infused and tapered accordingly as the infant tolerates the feeding regimen (Adzick et al., 1998).

◼ Discharge Needs

Once the infant tolerates the feeding regimen and appears well, discharge teaching may be initiated. The nurse should review anticipated pain management, signs and symptoms of infection, the current feeding regimen, plans for progression, and adequate urine and stool outputs. Parents should be instructed to call for fever, persistent emesis, abdominal pain demonstrated by persistent crying, tenderness to touch, the infant pulling the legs up, lethargy, decreased urine or stool output, wound drainage or redness, and any other concern or question that arises. The nurse should remind the parents that intermittent emesis is normal after surgery. If persistent emesis occurs with every feeding, the parents should be instructed to call their primary care provider and the pediatric surgeon.

Follow-up appointments should be arranged with the infant's primary care provider and pediatric surgeon. The infant and family should follow up with their primary care provider within a few days of discharge and the pediatric surgical team within 1 to 2 weeks after discharge (Puri & Lakshmanadass, 2003).

◼ Conclusion

Infants diagnosed with HPS have an excellent prognosis. Nursing care focuses on the management of fluid and electrolytes and on education and support to the parents. Although some vomiting does occur after surgery, most infants achieve normal feeding patterns and good weight gain by their first postoperative visit. Parents can then begin to focus on the normal growth and development of their infant.

◼ Acknowledgment

The author would like to recognize the work of Joanna Joyce Morganelli, author of "Hypertrophic Pyloric Stenosis" in the first edition of this textbook.

■ Educational Materials

APSNA invites you to download the following diagnosis-related teaching tool for Chapter 22, Pyloric Stenosis: 1) Pyloric Stenosis. This teaching tool is available at the APSNA Web site (www.apsna.org) and the Jones and Bartlett Web site (www.jbpub.com). All teaching materials are available in English and Spanish and are free of charge. APSNA encourages their use for your patients and families.

■ References

Adzick, N. S., Wilson, J. M., Caty, M. G., Fishman, S. J., Saenz, N. C., Jennings, R. W., et al. (1998). *Department of surgery's house officer's manual* (10th ed.). Boston: Children's Hospital.

Cooper, W. O., Ray, W. A., & Griffin, M. R. (2002). Prenatal prescription of macrolide antibiotics and infantile hypertrophic pyloric stenosis. *Obstetrics & Gynecology, 100*(1), 101–106.

Dudgeon, D. L. (1993). Lesions of the stomach. In K. Ashcraft & T. Holder (Eds.), *Pediatric surgery* (pp. 289–304). Philadelphia: W.B. Saunders.

Garcia, G. F., & Randolph, J. G. (1990). Pyloric stenosis: Diagnosis and management. *Pediatrics in Review, 11*(10), 292–295.

Georgeson, K. E., Corbin, T. J., Griffen, J. W., & Breaux, C. W. (1993). An analysis of feeding regimens after pyloromyotomy for hypertrophic pyloric stenosis. *Journal of Pediatric Surgery, 28*(11), 1478–1480.

Godbole, P., Sprigg, A., Dickson, J. A. S., & Lin, P. C. (1996). Ultrasound compared with clinical examination in infantile hypertrophic pyloric stenosis. *Archives of Disease in Childhood, 75*, 335–337.

Greason, K. L., Thompson, W. R., Downey, E. C., & Sasso, B. L. (1995). Laparoscopic pyloromyotomy for infantile hypertrophic pyloric stenosis: Report of 11 cases. *Journal of Pediatric Surgery, 30*(11), 1171–1574.

Hernanz-Schulman, M. (2003). Infantile hypertrophic pyloric stenosis. *Radiology, 227*, 319–331.

Hernanz-Schulman, M., Sells, L. L., Ambrosino, M. M., Heller, R. M., Stein, S. M., & Neblett, W. W. (1994). Hypertrophic pyloric stenosis in the infant without a palpable olive: Accuracy of sonographic diagnosis. *Pediatric Radiology, 193*, 771–776.

Hulka, F., Campbell, J. R., Harrison, M. W., & Campbell, T. J. (1997). Cost-effectiveness in diagnosing infantile hypertrophic pyloric stenosis. *Journal of Pediatric Surgery, 32*(11), 1604–1608.

Hulka, F., Harrison, M. W., Campbell, T. J., & Campbell, J. R. (1997). Complications of pyloromyotomy for infantile hypertrophic pyloric stenosis. *The American Journal of Surgery, 173*, 450–452.

Kretz, B., Watfa, J., & Sapin, S. (2005). Our experience in "Ad Libitum" feeding after pyloromyotomy (review of 97 cases). *Archives of Pediatrics, 12*(2), 128–133.

Magnuson, D. K., & Schwartz, M. Z. (2005). Acquired abnormalities of the stomach and duodenum. In K. T. Oldham, P. M. Colombani, R. P. Foglia, & M. A. Skinner (Eds.), *Surgery of infants and children* (pp. 1152–1156). Philadelphia: Lippincott-Raven.

Mahon, B. E., Rosenman, M. B., & Kleiman, M. B. (2001). Maternal and infant use of erythromycin and other macrolide antibiotics as risk factors for infantile hypertrophic pyloric stenosis. *Journal of Pediatrics, 139*(3), 380–384.

Morash, D. (2002). An interdisciplinary project that changed practice in feeding methods after pyloromyotomy. *Pediatric Nursing, 28*(2), 113–118, 137.

Poon, T., Zhang, A., Cartmill, T., & Cass, D. (1996). Changing patterns of diagnosis and treatment of infantile hypertrophic pyloric stenosis: A clinical audit of 303 patients. *Journal of Pediatric Surgery, 31*(12), 1611–1615.

Puapong, D., Kahng, D., Ko, A., & Applebaum, H. (2002). Ad libitum feeding: Safely improving the cost-effectiveness of pyloromyotomy *Journal of Pediatric Surgery, 37*(12), 1667–1668.

Puri, P., & Lakshmanadass, G. (2003). Hypertrophic pyloric stenosis. In Puri, P. (Ed.), *Newborn surgery* (2nd ed., pp. 389–395). New York: Oxford University Press.

Rollins, M. C., Shields, M. D., Quinn, R., & Wooldridge, M. (1989). Pyloric stenosis: Congenital or acquired? *Archives of Disease in Childhood, 64*, 138–139.

Rowe, M., O'Neill, J., Grosfeld, J., Fonkalsrud, E., & Coran, A. (1995). *Essentials of pediatric surgery* (pp. 481–485). St. Louis, MO: Mosby.

Sorensen, H. T., Skriver, M. V., Pedersen, L., Larsen, H., Ebbesen, F., & Schonheyder, H. C. (2003). Risk of infantile hypertrophic pyloric stenosis after maternal postnatal use of macrolides. *Scandinavian Journal of Infectious Disease, 35*, 104–106.

Vanderwinden, J., Liu, H., Menu, R., Conreur, J. L., De Laet, M. H., & Vanderhaeghen, J. J. (1996). The pathology of infantile hypertrophic pyloric stenosis after healing. *Journal of Pediatric Surgery, 32*(11), 1530–1537.

Gastroesophageal Reflux Disease: Recognition and Management

By Frances N. Price

Gastroesophageal reflux (GER) is a physiologic occurrence in all individuals. GER is a normal event in which gastric contents regurgitate into the esophagus. GER is considered pathological when it interferes with normal growth, causes damage to the esophageal lining, or interferes with breathing. Gastroesophageal reflux disease (GERD) is the focus of this chapter. In order to correctly assess and treat the child with GERD, it is important that the practitioner understand the physiologic basis for the disease and the treatment modalities available.

■ Pathophysiology

The lower esophageal sphincter (LES) is an anatomic area formed by the confluence of muscle fibers from the esophagus and the stomach (Fig. 23-1). Release of acetylcholine from the vagus nerve provides a normal resting pressure sufficient to act as a sphincter, preventing reflux of stomach contents into the esophagus. Although LES pressure in infants may be low (< 5 mm Hg), they usually develop a normal pressure (15–20 mm Hg) by the age of 15 months. Infants typically outgrow GER between the ages of 9 and 24 months, due in part to the maturation of the LES (Ostlie & Holcomb, 2002). In children with GERD, LES pres-

sure is inadequate, allowing gastric contents to continue to reflux into the esophagus.

Esophageal peristalsis provides timely clearance of substances through the esophagus. In the case of GERD, esophageal motility can be compromised, allowing irritating gastric acids to be in contact with the esophageal mucosa for longer periods of time. Prolonged contact can lead to inflammation of the mucosa and cause ulceration and scarring of the esophagus with potential stricture development.

Delayed gastric emptying may also play a role in GERD (Henry, 2004; Spitz & McLeod, 2003). If the stomach empties poorly, feedings accumulate and do not empty normally. An increase in stomach volume then places more pressure on an already incompetent LES, resulting in GER.

Although the specific cause of GERD is unknown, it is theorized that some or all of the barriers to GER are compromised (Henry, 2004; Spitz & McLeod, 2003). Several groups of children are especially prone to pathogenic GERD. These include children with neurologic impairment, cystic fibrosis, bronchopulmonary dysplasia, repaired esophageal atresia, and those who require gastrostomy feedings (Henry; Hillemeier, 1996; Rudolph et al., 2001).

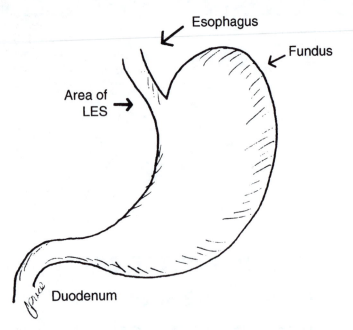

Figure 23-1 Anatomy of the stomach including area of the lower esophageal sphincter.

Table 23-1	Clinical Manifestations of Gastroesophageal Reflux Disease
Constitutional	Failure to thrive
	Weight loss
Gastrointestinal	Irritability associated with feedings
	Vomiting
	Dysphagia
	Esophageal stricture
Respiratory	Recurrent pneumonia
	Apnea spells
	Reactive airway symptoms
Hematologic	Anemia
	Hematemesis

■ Clinical Presentation

The clinical presentation of GERD varies according to the severity of the child's disease and symptoms and may range from mild to severe. Often, GER may be "silent" for a time, with no obvious symptoms until esophageal inflammation becomes severe enough to cause strictures or dysphagia. Most symptoms are caused by excessive or prolonged contact of acid on esophageal mucosa. GERD may be the most common cause of failure to thrive in infants, with vomiting being the most common clinical sign (Armentrout, 1995; Beattie, 2003; Spitz & McLeod, 2003). Vomiting can lead to aspiration pneumonia, as well as failure to thrive when the infant cannot retain a sufficient amount of calories for growth. Irritability caused by esophagitis from acid irritation is another common symptom. Severe esophagitis is associated with hematemesis, anemia, and esophageal strictures. Sandifer's syndrome, an association of GERD with spastic torticollis and dystonic body movements, may occur (Armentrout).

Respiratory symptoms associated with GERD may be as mild as coughing or as severe as wheezing, recurrent pneumonia, apnea, or acute life-threatening events. GERD may also be associated with sudden infant death syndrome (Foglia, 1997; Rudolph et al., 2001). Gastric acid in the tracheobronchial tree can lead to apnea, pneumonia, bronchitis, and reactive airway disease (Foglia). Table 23-1 summarizes the clinical manifestations of GERD (Armentrout, 1995; Berube, 1997; Rudolph et al.).

■ Differential Diagnosis

The symptoms associated with GERD can be caused by other processes. The patient should be evaluated for metabolic, infectious, anatomic, or neurologic causes of the vomiting. For instance, bilious vomiting signifies obstruction, whereas projectile nonbilious emesis could indicate pyloric stenosis or a central nervous system etiology. Some metabolic disorders present with vomiting in infancy. The respiratory symptoms associated with GERD may also be caused by asthma, cystic fibrosis, central apnea, seizures, central nervous system trauma or malformations, congenital heart disease, allergies, or primary lung disease. Symptoms may be due to peptic ulcers or nonspecific irritability (Henry, 2004; Orenstein, 1999; Spitz & McLeod, 2003).

■ Diagnostic Studies

Once the need for further evaluation has been established, certain diagnostic studies are indicated (Henry, 2004; Orenstein, 1999). Although no single study can consistently identify children with GERD, careful choice of the diagnostic tools available can provide sufficient information to allow the practitioner to determine the appropriate treatment.

The primary diagnostic tools in the work-up of GERD in the pediatric population are upper gastrointestinal (UGI) series, 12 to 24 hour pH probe monitoring and radionucleotide gastric emptying study, esophagoscopy, and bronchoscopy (Orenstein, 1999; Spitz & McLeod, 2003).

The "gold standard" for diagnosing GERD is the 12 to 24 hour pH monitor (Armentrout, 1995; Hillemeier, 1996; Henry, 2004). This study involves positioning a thin antimony probe in the child's esophagus and leaving it in place for 12 to 24 hours. During this time, the child is fed normally and feedings are recorded. At the end of the study period, three main parameters are measured: number of reflux episodes per day, number of episodes lasting longer than 5 minutes, and total percent of time that esophageal pH is less than 4. These parameters, along with normal values, are shown in Table 23-2 (Sondheimer, 1994). A new technique called multi-intraluminal impedance is gaining popularity. This study is similar to a pH study; however, the technique uses electrical conductivity to determine the difference between air and liquid in the esophagus, thereby leading to a more definitive diagnosis of acid reflux (Condino et al., 2006; Wenzl et al., 2002).

An UGI is a radiographic examination that may demonstrate GER fluoroscopically, as well as the presence of a stricture, hiatal hernia, or variations in esophageal motility as well as other causes for delayed gastric emptying: pyloric stenosis, duodenal obstruction, and malrotation. It is not diagnostic for GERD (Georgeson & Tekant, 2006). Figure 23-2 depicts an UGI that demonstrates GER. Note the barium refluxing into the esophagus. UGI studies should be obtained in all children with a history of recurrent pneumonia because of the association with GERD. Dysfunctional swallowing with primary aspiration of ingested food can also lead to recurrent pneumonia. GERD treatment does not rectify a swallowing disorder, and these children are referred to occupational or speech therapists to address problems of swallowing dysfunction.

Some centers use scintigrams, or radionucleotide gastric emptying studies, to determine whether the stomach empties at a normal rate. The child either drinks or is gavaged a radiopaque liquid meal, and gastric emptying is monitored. A normal range for gastric emptying is 40 to 60 minutes (Foglia, 1997). Many children with GERD, primarily those with neurologic deficits, diagnostically exhibit prolonged gastric emptying times (Fonkalsrud et al., 1995).

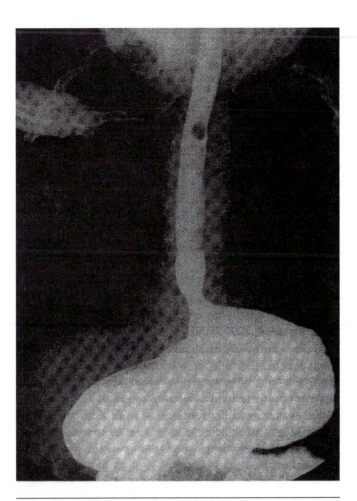

Figure 23-2 Upper gastrointestinal study showing gastroesophageal reflux.

Esophagoscopy can be useful in determining the degree of esophageal irritation as well as the presence of Barrett's esophagus, a precancerous esophageal dysplasia associated with severe acid reflux. Clinicians use bronchoscopy to assess for lipid-laden macrophages, an indication of aspiration of stomach contents into the trachea.

■ Medical Management

Once the diagnosis of GERD has been established, treatment can begin. The goal in the treatment of GERD is to control reflux, decrease symptoms, and prevent complications. Medical antireflux therapy is effective in approximately 80% of children with reflux disease (Foglia, 1997). However, medical management is not indicated for children who have severe symptoms, such as esophageal strictures or near-death episodes from aspiration. These children should be referred directly for surgical treatment (Rudolph et al., 2001).

Table 23-2	**Extended pH Study: Normal Values**
Parameter	**Normal Value (per day)**
No. reflux episodes/day	< 35
No. reflux episodes > 5 minutes	< 7
Percent time with esophageal pH < 4	< 6

The cornerstones of medical management are upright or prone-elevated positioning, thickening feeds, delivering smaller volumes of feeds at more frequent intervals, and prescribing pharmacologic agents, such as histamine receptor blockers and prokinetic agents (Armentrout, 1995; Henry, 2004; Spitz & McLeod, 2003; Rudolph et al., 2001).

Reflux can be exacerbated by supine, seated, or head-down position. For this reason, parents should hold infants in the upright position or place in a prone position with head elevated at a 30-degree angle for at least 30 minutes to an hour after feeding. The head of the infant's crib can be raised on blocks and elevated to about 30 to 45 degrees. The bed elevation, along with gravity, helps decrease the risk of stomach contents refluxing into the lungs (Foglia, 1997; Rudolph et al., 2001). The American Academy of Pediatrics guidelines recommend that infants be laid supine or in a side-lying position to avoid the risk of sudden infant death syndrome, except in cases of severe GERD (Rudolph et al.).

Thickening the infant's formula can help reduce reflux. A common technique for thickening feeds includes adding rice cereal, approximately 1 tablespoon of cereal per 4 to 6 ounces of formula. The nipple of the bottle may be widened so that the infant can suck easily, being careful not to make the opening so wide that the child receives too much. In some cases, using postpyloric feedings (jejunal or duodenal tube feedings) may be an effective way to increase nutrient absorption and decrease symptoms, allowing time for the infant to outgrow the reflux (Armentrout, 1995; Berube, 1997; Rudolph et al., 2001).

Another intervention is to decrease feeding volume to allow the infant's stomach to empty thoroughly between feeds. If the stomach contains large volumes of formula, reflux is more likely to occur. Allowing the stomach to empty alleviates pressure and therefore decreases these episodes. Teaching parents to give smaller, more frequent feedings using proper positioning techniques may help control GER.

Pharmacologic interventions include histamine$_2$ (H$_2$) antagonists, such as ranitidine, famotidine, and cimetidine; prokinetic agents, including metoclopramide; and proton pump inhibitors, such as omeprazole and lansoprazole. H$_2$ antagonists decrease the gastric secretion from the parietal cells. Prokinetic agents promote gastric emptying by improving motility, and proton pump inhibitors increase gastric pH by blocking hydrogen ion production (Henry, 2004; Orenstein, 1999).

Nonoperative treatments are successful in managing GERD in most children. Infants and children with complications related to GERD as well as neurologically devastated children and those with anatomic abnormalities of the gastrointestinal tract are more likely to fail to respond to medical management. These children are candidates for surgical intervention. (Orenstein, 1999; Rudolph et al., 2001; Henry, 2004).

■ Surgical Intervention

Operative indications include unremitting emesis with failure to thrive after 2 to 3 months of intensive medical therapy, recurrent pneumonia, apnea, an acute life-threatening event secondary to GERD, refractory airway disease, severe esophagitis or stricture, or Barrett's metaplasia (Foglia, 1997; Powers et al., 2003).

The most widely used antireflux procedure in the pediatric population is the Nissen fundoplication (Rothenberg, 2002). The Nissen fundoplication (Fig. 23-3) is a circumferential wrap of the fundus of the stomach around the intraabdominal esophagus. The goal of the operation is to create an area of high pressure at the LES. After antireflux surgery, the portion of the stomach that is wrapped around the esophagus temporarily acts as a one-way valve when gastric pressure increases, thereby preventing reflux into the esophagus. When gastric pressure returns to normal, the wrap relaxes and does not impinge on resting esophageal function (Foglia, 1997; Rowe, O'Neill, Grosfeld, Fonkalsrud, & Coran, 1995; Pacilli, Chowdbury, & Pierro, 2004).

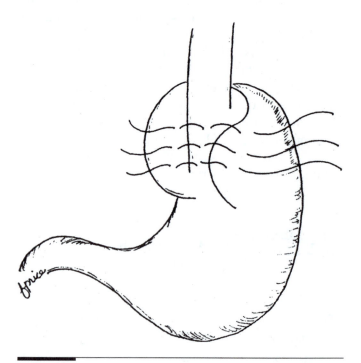

Figure 23-3 Nissen fundoplication showing circumferential wrap of lower esophagus.

The success rate of antireflux surgery approaches 80% to 90% (Kimber, Kiely, & Spitz, 1998). Pulmonary symptoms frequently improve or are alleviated. The children gain weight, and esophagitis substantially resolves (Foglia, 1997). Laparoscopic technique for fundoplication has become popular because there is decreased need for postoperative analgesia, decreased length of hospitalization, and better cosmetic results (Lima et al., 2004; Ostlie & Holcomb, 2002; Rothenberg, 2002; Sydorak & Albanese, 2002).

Some children with delayed gastric emptying require a pyloroplasty. This is a procedure in which the pylorus muscle is partially divided, thereby enlarging the outlet of the stomach and facilitating gastric emptying. This procedure is performed in conjunction with fundoplication (Fonkalsrud et al., 1995; Rothenberg, 2002).

Many children who require antireflux procedures also require a gastrostomy for feeding access or for temporary protection of the wrap. A gastrostomy is a surgically created tract that allows direct access to the stomach for feeding and decompression. A gastrostomy tube or skin-level device is placed, either open percutaneously or laparoscopically. Refer to Chapter 7 for care and maintenance of gastrostomies.

Complications of the antireflux procedures include small-bowel obstruction, wrap failure, gastric perforation, dumping syndrome, gastric outlet obstruction, damage to vagus nerve, bloating, diarrhea, dysphagia, choking, retching, and paraesophageal hernia. The child with developmental delay is particularly at risk for these complications, in part because of the combination of poor esophageal motility and delayed gastric emptying (Broscious, 1995; Pacilli et al., 2004; Lima et al., 2004; Raffensperger, 1990; Rothenberg, 2002).

■ Preoperative Care

If surgery is needed, the nurse prepares the child and family for the upcoming operation. Preoperative preparation of the child for surgery is discussed in detail in Chapter 1. Routine preoperative laboratory studies are no longer indicated. However, children with respiratory or other medical conditions may require chest radiographic examination, complete blood count, or electrolyte level determinations. Children who have had hematemesis or anemia may warrant additional blood tests for type and screen or type and cross for a potential blood transfusion.

Preoperative education about gastrostomy care, feeding, and gastric decompression helps caregivers anticipate and participate in the postoperative decision making.

Whenever possible, encourage the child to play with a nasogastric (NG) tube, gastrostomy devices, masks, or other surgical paraphernalia. If appropriate, it is helpful to allow the older child to choose the gastrostomy device if one is indicated.

■ Postoperative Care

Routine interventions after fundoplication include monitoring for return of gastric function, gastric decompression via NG or gastrostomy device, pain management, and care of the incision and tubes (Bordewick, Bildner, & Burd, 2002; Broscious, 1995; O'Brien, Davis, & Erwin-Toth, 1999). For children who undergo an antireflux procedure without gastrostomy, an NG tube is placed in the operating room for gastric decompression until gastric function returns. The patency of the tube is maintained by regulating the suction and irrigation/aspiration of the tube. Manipulation of a surgically placed tube is not recommended. If the NG tube malfunctions, the nurse should notify the surgeon rather than reposition the tube and risk damage to the wrap. If a gastrostomy is performed in conjunction with the antireflux procedure, the gastrostomy device may be used for stomach decompression (Armentrout, 1995).

Gastrostomy complications include dislodgement, stomach perforation, exacerbation of gastroesophageal reflux, skin or stoma infection, gastric outlet obstruction, and intestinal obstruction (Bordewick et al., 2001; Coldicutt, 1994). Refer to Chapter 7 for complete care of gastrostomy devices.

Postoperative Feeding

Whether or not the child has a gastrostomy as part of the surgical procedure, feeding concerns remain the primary focus in the postoperative period. Feedings are initiated slowly as bowel function returns. At first, avoid feeding the child large amounts despite the need to regain caloric losses. The child's stomach will adjust slowly to the larger, desired volume, but initially, feeding can be quite uncomfortable. Balancing the caloric needs and fluid requirements is challenging. Input from the nurse and family is vital. Once the child adjusts to the feedings, average-sized meals should be well tolerated.

For those children who are fed exclusively by gastrostomy, developmental, social, and speech issues are addressed (Chaplen, 1997; Sharpe, 2000). These include warming the formula to a comfortable temperature and simulating normal feeding patterns. Cold formula can cause cramping. Feed the child over 30 to 45 minutes, just like a child being fed orally. Feeding times should be appropriate to the age of the child. For example, feed a toddler three meals and two snacks (Arrowsmith, 1996; Chaplen; Sharpe). Sometimes, the child requires continuous feedings delivered by a feeding pump. The child can later transition to larger volume bolus feedings once the stomach becomes acclimated to larger volumes. Bolus feedings are more similar to a normal feeding pattern, but not all children tolerate them.

After a fundoplication, it may be difficult for some children to burp or vomit. For these children, it may be necessary to decompress the stomach by opening the gastrostomy. Decompressing the stomach after a few ounces of formula minimizes the child's discomfort during feedings. The gastrostomy device should remain vented for approximately 15 to 30 minutes after feedings to allow gas to escape from the stomach (Arrowsmith, 1996; Sharpe, 2000). One method of venting the stomach is to attach a large syringe with the plunger removed to the gastrostomy device. The syringe is held upright, which allows air to escape. Formula may also fill the tube during the venting process and returns to the stomach as the air is evacuated. If gagging and retching occur during continuous feeds, the use of a Farrell Bag® provides continuous decompression during feeding administration.

Offering an infant a pacifier helps to stimulate sucking and to develop oral motor skills (Arrowsmith, 1996; Radford, Thorne, & Bassingthwaighte, 1997). When medically safe, oral feeding provides oral stimulation and reinforces the connection between eating and a full stomach. Obtain a modified barium swallow examination before oral feedings are started. Children who aspirate need further intervention before they begin oral feedings. In some cases, oral feedings are contraindicated (Sharpe, 2000).

Normal interactions between the child and siblings should be encouraged. Siblings may be included in the care of the child with GERD to foster sibling bonding. Mealtime provides a rich environment for learning. Tube feeding the child at the table with the rest of the family promotes mealtime rituals and rules (Spalding & McKeever, 1998; Radford et al., 1997).

Nursing Interventions

The success of the surgical procedure is greatly influenced by the instructions provided to the parents. It is important for staff and families to understand the surgical procedure and its effect on the child. After the antireflux procedure, the child may not be able to vomit, and the act of retching increases the pressure on the fundoplication sutures. An NG tube or gastrostomy can be used to decompress the stomach in situations of prolonged retching (Arrowsmith, 1996).

Tube feedings should be administered slowly. Rapid infusion of formula into the stomach may cause cramping and discomfort to the child. If feeding by gravity, the higher the tube, the faster that the feeding infuses (Arrowsmith, 1996; Sharpe, 2000). Positioning the child right side down helps with the emptying of the stomach and can decrease cramping. A bloated or distended abdomen may indicate obstruction or feeding intolerance and should be reported to the physician. Monitoring stool patterns in the postoperative period helps identify complications such as constipation, dumping syndrome, or intestinal obstruction. Refer to Chapter 7 for additional help to solve gastrostomy problems.

Transitioning to Home

Despite mastering the postoperative Nissen fundoplication and gastrostomy care in the hospital, families become very anxious and overwhelmed at the prospect of managing complicated feeding regimens at home. Support from a visiting nurse provides encouragement, additional educational opportunity, and growth assessments.

Finally, it is important to acknowledge that in addition to the physical considerations of caring for a child with feeding problems, there are far more complex, long-term emotional family coping issues. Families of children who have had fundoplication face technical, emotional, physical, and social long-term problems related to eating. It is important to provide resources for caregivers before making the transition to home. These complicated children require coordinated, comprehensive, long-term follow-up care with the multidisciplinary team. This team includes colleagues from gastroenterology, nutrition, pulmonology, physical therapy, occupational therapy, and surgery, in addition to the primary care team. Ongoing evaluation avoids readmission for feeding problems and helps the child and family to cope at home (Sharpe, 2000; Thorne, Radford, & Armstrong, 1997).

■ Research

Dealing with a chronic disease such as GERD is taxing for families and staff. If the child is hospitalized frequently for GERD complications, he or she may fall far behind in reaching development milestones. Further research that studies the effect of GERD on children's development directs medical management therapies. Early identification of children with severe GERD may decrease physical and developmental deficits that result from repeated hospitalizations

(Berube, 1997; Thorne et al., 1997). Quality-of-life issues related to the morbidity of antireflux procedures warrant further investigation. Finally, research that evaluates bonding issues in families of children with special feeding problems might improve long-term outcomes.

Conclusion

Nurses assist with the diagnosis and treatment of children with GERD. Families require information and emotional support to follow the medical and/or surgical treatment plan. Both the medical and the surgical approaches require a time commitment. The success of each child's plan is based on parental involvement and commitment to the plan. Consistent, clear, written and verbal instructions provide an easier transition to home and better long-term outcome. With timely diagnosis and proper intervention, children with GERD can achieve excellent outcomes with optimal quality of life.

Acknowledgment

The author gratefully acknowledges the collaboration of Maureen Smith on the previous edition of this chapter.

Educational Materials

APSNA invites you to download the following diagnosis-related teaching tool for Chapter 23, Gastroesophageal Reflux Disease: Recognition and Management: Gastroesophageal Reflux. This teaching tool is available at the APSNA Web site (www.apsna.org) and the Jones and Bartlett Web site (www.jbpub.com). All teaching materials are available in English and Spanish and are free of charge. APSNA encourages their use for your patients and families.

References

Armentrout, D. (1995). Gastroesophageal reflux in infants. *Nurse Practitioner, 20*(5), 54–63.

Arrowsmith, H. (1996). Nursing management of patients receiving gastrostomy feeding. *British Journal of Nursing, 5*(5), 268–273.

Beattie, R. M. (2003). Managing gastro-esophageal reflux in infants and children. *Journal of Family Health Care, 13*(4), 98–101.

Berube, M. (1997). Gastroesophageal reflux. *Journal of the Society of Pediatric Nursing, 2*(1), 43–46.

Bordewick, A. J., Bildner, J. I., & Burd, R. S. (2002). An effective approach for preventing and treating gastrostomy tube complications in newborns. *Neonatal Network, 20*(2), 37–40.

Broscious, S. K. (1995). Preventing complications of PEG tubes. *Dimensions of Critical Care Nursing, 14*(1), 37–41.

Chaplen, C. (1997). Parents' views of caring for children with gastrostomies. *British Journal of Nursing, 6*(1), 34–38.

Coldicutt, P. (1994). Children's options. *Nursing Times, 90*(13), 54–56.

Condino, A. A., Sondheimer, J., Pan, Z., Gralla, J., Perry, D., & O'Connor, J. A. (2006). Evaluation of infantile acid and nonacid gastroesophageal reflux using combined pH monitoring and impedance measurement. *Journal of Pediatric Gastroenterology & Nutrition, 42*(1), 16–21.

Foglia, R. P. (1997). Gastroesophageal reflux. In K. T. Oldham, P. M. Colombani, & R. P. Foglia (Eds.), *Surgery of infants and children: Scientific principles and practice* (pp. 1035–1047). Philadelphia: Lippincott-Raven.

Fonkalsrud, E. W., Ellis, D. G., Shaw, A., Mann, C. M. Jr., Black, T. L., Miller, J. P., et al. (1995). A combined hospital experience with fundoplication and gastric emptying procedure for gastroesophageal reflux in children. *Journal of the American College of Surgeons, 180*, 449–455.

Georgeson, K. E., & Tekant, G. T. (2006). Gastroesophageal reflux disease. In J. L Grosfeld, J. A. O'Neill, E. W. Fonkalrud, & A. G. Coran (Eds.), *Pediatric surgery* (pp. 1121–1140). Philadelphia: Mosby-Elsevier.

Henry, S. M. (2004). Discerning differences: Gastroesophageal reflux and gastroesophageal reflux disease in infants. *Advances in Neonatal Care, 4*(4), 235–247.

Hillemeier, A. C. (1996). Gastroesophageal reflux: Diagnostic and therapeutic approaches. *Pediatric Gastroenterology, 43*(1), 197–212.

Kimber, C., Kiely, E. M., & Spitz, L. (1998). The failure rate of surgery for gastro-oesophageal reflux. *Journal of Pediatric Surgery, 33*(1), 64–66.

Lima, M., Bertozzi, M., Ruggeri, G., Domini, M., Libri, M., Parigi, C. B., et al. (2004). Laparoscopic antireflux surgery in neurologically impaired children. *Pediatric Surgery International, 20*(2), 114–117.

O'Brien, B., Davis, S., & Erwin-Toth, P. (1999). G-tube site care: A practical guide. *RN, 62*(2), 52–56.

Orenstein, S. R. (1999). Gastroesophageal reflux. *Pediatrics in Review, 20*(5), 174–183.

Ostlie, J., & Holcomb, G. W., 3rd. (2002). Laparoscopic fundoplication and gastrostomy. *Seminars in Pediatric Surgery, 11*(4), 196–204.

Pacilli, M., Chowdbury, M. M., & Pierro, A. (2004). The surgical treatment of gastroesophageal reflux in neonates and infants. *Seminars in Pediatric Surgery, 38*(6), 886–891.

Powers, C. J., Levitt, M. A., Tantoco, J., Rossman, J., Sarpel, U., Brisseau, G., et al. (2003). The respiratory advantage of laparoscopic Nissen fundoplication. *The Journal of Pediatric Surgery, 38*(6), 886–891.

Radford, M. J., Thorne, S., & Bassingthwaighte, C. (1997). Long-term gastrostomy in children: Insights from expert nurses. *Issues in Comprehensive Pediatric Nursing, 20*(1), 35–50.

Raffensberger, J. G. (1990). *Swensen's pediatric surgery* (5th ed., pp. 811–822). Norwalk, CT: Appleton & Lange.

Rowe, M. I., O'Neill, J. A., Grosfeld, J. L., Fonkalsrud, E. W., & Coran, A. G. (1995). *Essentials of pediatric surgery* (pp. 422–427). St. Louis, MO: Mosby.

Rothenberg, S. S. (2002). Laparoscopic Nissen procedure in children. *Seminars in Laparoscopic Surgery, 9*(3), 146–152.

Rudolph, C. D., Mazur, L. J., Liptak, G. S., Baker, J. T., Colletti, R. B., Gerson, W. T., et al. (2001). Guidelines for evaluation and treatment of gastroesophageal reflux in infants and children. *Journal of Pediatric Gastroenterology and Nutrition, 32*[Suppl. 2], S1–S31.

Sharpe, G. (2000). Assessment of eating and drinking in a child with a gastrostomy. *British Journal of Nursing, 9*(12), 770–772, 774, 776–778.

Sondheimer, J. M. (1994). Gastroesophageal reflux in children. Clinical presentation and diagnostic evaluation. *Gastrointestinal Endoscopy Clinics of North America, 4*, 55–74.

Spalding, K., & McKeever, P. (1998). Mothers' experiences caring for children with disabilities who require a gastrostomy tube. *Journal of Pediatric Nursing, 13*(4), 234–243.

Spitz, L., & McLeod, E. (2003). Gastroesophageal reflux. *Seminars in Pediatric Surgery, 12*(4), 237–240.

Sydorak, R. M., & Albanese, C. Y. (2002). Laparoscopic antireflux procedures in children: Evaluating the evidence. *Seminars in Laparoscopic Surgery, 9*(3), 133–138.

Thorne, S. E., Radford, M. J., & Armstrong, E. A. (1997). Long-term gastrostomy in children: Caregiver coping. *Gastroenterology Nursing, 20*(2), 46–53.

Wenzl, T. G., Moroder, C., Trachterna, M., Thomson, M., Silny, J., Heimann, G., et al. (2002). Esophageal pH monitoring and impedance measurement: A comparison of two diagnostic tests for gastroesophageal reflux. *Journal of Pediatric Gastroenterology and Nutrition, 34*(5), 511–512.

Malrotation and Volvulus

By Jeannette A. Diana-Zerpa and Tina J. Shapiro-Stolar

■ Description

Malrotation is an asymptomatic anatomical variant that occurs as a result of failure to complete normal rotation and fixation of the bowel (Aiken & Oldham, 2005; Stockmann, 2005). Malrotation becomes a surgical emergency and a potentially life-threatening situation when the midgut twists or kinks in a clockwise direction around the superior mesenteric artery, causing an intestinal obstruction known as volvulus. This condition is one of the most serious surgical emergencies seen in the neonate or infant, and delayed surgical intervention may have catastrophic results (Aiken & Oldham; Hajivassiliou, 2003; Shelton, 1999; Stockmann). Midgut volvulus may lead to widespread intestinal ischemia and progress rapidly to necrosis of the bowel, perforation, shock, respiratory failure, and death (Aiken & Oldham; D'Agostino, 2002).

■ Incidence

The true incidence of malrotation is difficult to estimate because only children with complications of the anomaly present with symptoms, most during the neonatal period. Estimates of the occurrence are reported at 1 in 6,000 live births (Aiken & Oldham, 2005; Malek & Burd, 2005;

Stockmann, 2005). Many of these patients remain undiagnosed until well into childhood or adult life when, after years of chronic abdominal complaints, malrotation is discovered (D'Agostino, 2002; Imamoglu, Cay, Sarihan, & Sen, 2004; Kume, Fumino, Shimotake, & Iwai, 2004; Malek & Burd; Prasil et al., 2000). Malrotation is more common in boys than girls in children diagnosed at less than 1 year of age (Aiken & Oldham; Stockmann).

Most patients with midgut volvulus are infants. Ninety percent of clinical symptoms occur in children less than 1 year of age. Of those children, 50% to 75% present during the first month of life, specifically the first week of life (Aiken & Oldham, 2005; Hajivassiliou, 2003; Kimura & Loening-Baucke, 2000; Kume et al., 2004; Stockmann, 2005).

■ Embryology

During embryologic life, two important events occur related to normal intestinal development. These two events, rotation of the duodenojejunal loop and rotation of the cecocolic loop, take place simultaneously but are described here as two separate events (Aiken & Oldham, 2005; Stockmann, 2005). At about the fourth week of embryonic life, the gut begins to change from a straight-line structure to an elongated tube herniating into the umbilical cord (Gray & Skandalakis, 1972). The upper portion of this elongated structure, the duodenojejunal loop, eventually develops into duodenum and jejunum. The lower portion, known as the cecocolic loop, later becomes the terminal ileum, cecum, and colon. The superior mesenteric artery, which provides the blood supply to this portion of the bowel, is the main pivotal point.

During this time, the duodenojejunal loop lies above the superior mesenteric artery (SMA). The loop begins to rotate 90 degrees counterclockwise to the right of the SMA, then another 90 degrees to beneath the SMA. Finally, the loop rotates 90 degrees across the spine and upward so that the duodenojejunal junction lies in the left upper quadrant in an area to be marked by the ligament of Treitz (Aiken & Oldham, 2005; Stockmann, 2005) (Fig. 24-1).

The cecocolic loop originates beneath the SMA and begins rotation counterclockwise also in 90-degree intervals. The first rotation places this loop to the left of the SMA. Next, the loop rotates 90 degrees above the artery. The last 90-degree rotation of the cecocolic loop is a downward movement to the right of the SMA, where the cecum becomes fixed in the right lower quadrant. At this point, the left colon lies to the left of the SMA, the transverse colon crosses the artery, and the right colon lies to the right of the SMA with the cecum in the right iliac fossa (Aiken & Oldham, 2005; Stockmann, 2005) (Fig. 24-2).

With normal rotation completed, the intestines return from the umbilical cord to the abdominal cavity, where fixation commences from the 10th to 12th week of gestational life and continues postnatally (Aiken & Oldham, 2005; Kimura & Loening-Baucke, 2000; Stockmann, 2005). The normal fixation of the mesentery of the midgut is best illustrated in Figure 24-3. As shown in Figure 24-3, the broad-based mesentery is maintained in position after normal rotation and fixation occur by the ligament of Treitz (*A*) and the ileocecal junction (*B*). The duodenum becomes securely fixed to the retroperitoneum as the C-loop. In addition, the ascending and descending colon are attached retroperitoneally. The bowel is now stabilized by the broad-based mesentery preventing any twisting or kinking of the intestines from occurring.

The process of rotation and fixation is complex in nature and has been broken down in this text as a series of events. In reality, intestinal rotation is a spectrum with a multitude of stages occurring almost simultaneously.

■ Pathophysiology of Malrotation

Malrotation of the intestines was described as early as 1761 by Morgagni. In 1923, Dott first correlated the clinical picture of this malformation with embryologic theory (Dott, 1923). In 1932, Dr. William E. Ladd wrote the classic article explaining the pathophysiology of malrotation with volvulus, including surgical correction (Ladd, 1932). Dr. Ladd's subsequent article, written in 1936, described releasing the constricting peritoneal bands in what is now known as a *Ladd's procedure* (Ladd, 1936).

Malrotation is a term that describes a number of different rotational errors. The most common of these anomalies occurs with an incomplete rotation of 180 degrees instead of the normal 270-degree rotation. When the previously described normal 270-degree rotation of the bowel is interrupted or deviated, the duodenum lies behind the superior mesenteric artery or fails to cross the midline. The cecum does not reach the right iliac fossa but lies anterior to the duodenum, and adhesions form running from the cecum across the duodenum to the right lateral wall of the abdomen (Fig. 24-4). These adhesions are called *Ladd's bands*, and they obstruct the duodenum (D'Agostino, 2002).

■ Pathophysiology of Midgut Volvulus

Midgut volvulus occurs as a complication of malrotation. Because the intestines are not fixed normally and do not have a broad-based mesentery, there is a high incidence of twisting of the midgut on its narrow pedicle. Volvulus usually involves a 360-degree or more turn of the intestines on the narrow stalk containing the superior mesenteric vessels. The entire arterial and venous blood supply

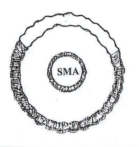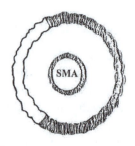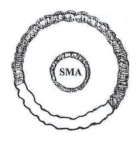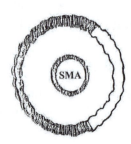

Figure 24-1 Rotation of the duodenojejunal loop.

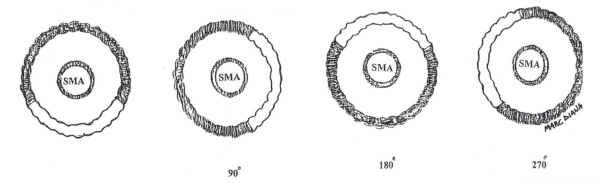

Figure 24-2 Rotation of the cecocolic loop.

is contained in this pedicle or stalk. The twisting causes vascular obstruction, and complete necrosis of the midgut develops rapidly over 1 to 2 hours (D'Agostino, 2002). Unless immediate diagnosis and surgical treatment are initiated, the necrosis may quickly lead to shock and death (Fig. 24-5).

Clinical Presentation

Malrotation may present as a chronic problem with asymptomatic periods combined with episodes of abdominal pain and vomiting. The bands across the duodenum may lead to varying degrees of obstruction manifested as recurrent episodes of vomiting. Often, children are not diagnosed with malrotation until well into adolescence, when chronic symptoms warrant a gastrointestinal work-up, and the anomaly is discovered (Hajivassiliou, 2003; Kume et al., 2004; Stockmann, 2005).

Malrotation with midgut volvulus, however, presents with acutely intense symptoms. The typical clinical picture is that of a healthy infant who begins to suddenly vomit. At first, the vomiting may consist of gastric contents but quickly becomes bilious. Bilious vomiting in a neonate who is otherwise well should alert the clinician

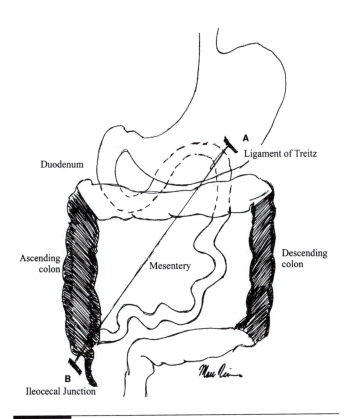

Figure 24-3 Normal fixation of the mesentery.

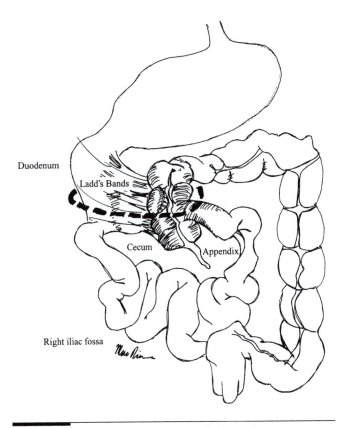

Figure 24-4 Ladd's bands with duodenal obstruction.

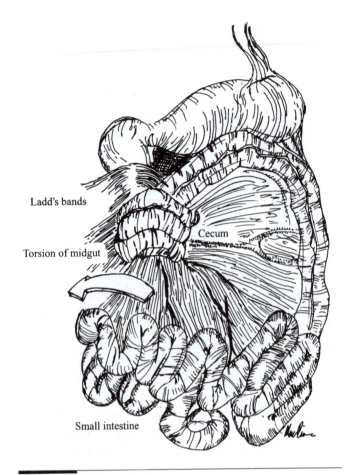

Ladd's bands

Torsion of midgut

Cecum

Small intestine

Figure 24-5 Midgut volvulus.

to the possibility of midgut volvulus or other high-grade small-bowel obstruction (Aiken & Oldham, 2005; D'Agostino, 2002; Hajivassiliou, 2003; Kimura & Loening-Baucke, 2000; Kume et al., 2004; McCollough & Sharieff, 2003; Millar, Rode, & Cywes, 2003; Stockmann, 2005). As a result of vomiting, pancreatic secretions, gastric secretions, and bile are lost, resulting in rapid electrolyte imbalance and dehydration (Shelton, 1999).

Initial examination of the abdomen may be normal in 50% of babies, but the clinical picture deteriorates rapidly. The infant appears pale and in acute distress with abdominal pain, distention, and grunting respirations. Passage of bloody stools is a late symptom and is indicative of a gravely ill baby (Aiken & Oldham, 2005; McCollough & Sharieff, 2003; Stockmann, 2005).

Differential Diagnosis

The differential diagnosis for midgut volvulus generally includes sepsis, duodenal atresia, duodenal stenosis, duodenal webs, and jejunoileal atresia (Aiken & Oldham, 2005; Kimura & Loening-Baucke, 2000; McCollough &

Sharieff, 2003; Stockmann, 2005). The possibility of pyloric stenosis may be considered with a healthy baby who suddenly begins to vomit; however, this diagnosis is quickly ruled out when the emesis becomes bilious.

Work-Up

The work-up for an infant with malrotation differs according to the severity of symptoms. If the infant is not acutely ill, malrotation may be discovered during an elective upper gastrointestinal series (UGI) to rule out pyloric stenosis or gastroesophageal reflux. However, if midgut volvulus is suspected, the work-up must be initiated expeditiously. The work-up should include the following and be completed simultaneously: history and physical examination; emergent laboratory values with placement of intravenous access; intravenous hydration; stat flat and upright plain radiographs of the abdomen; and stat UGI series.

History and Physical Examination

The infant or child with malrotation may present as generally well appearing. History obtained from the parents usually describes an infant or child with chronic gastrointestinal upset, including intermittent vomiting, crampy abdominal pain, failure to thrive, constipation, bloody diarrhea, and even hematemesis or pancreatitis (Aiken & Oldham, 2005; D'Agostino, 2002; Malek & Burd, 2005; Stockmann, 2005).

On physical examination, the infant or child is alert and hydrated. The abdomen is rarely distended because the stomach is decompressed by occasional episodes of vomiting. The emesis may be secondary to duodenal obstruction by Ladd's bands, to the kinking of the abnormally positioned duodenum, or to intermittent torsion from the volvulus (Aiken & Oldham, 2005; Imamoglu et al., 2004).

The history of an infant with midgut volvulus is quite different. Usually, these parents present with the infant to the emergency room or to the pediatrician, describing a well baby who suddenly began to vomit. The vomiting is gastric contents at first, but soon becomes bilious. The parents may also report constipation or loose stools.

The physical examination reveals an infant in distress. The baby may be crying intensely; pulling up the legs; have grunting respirations, tachycardia, or tachypnea; may appear lethargic; and may be pale. Once the midgut becomes ischemic, the abdominal examination reveals evidence of distention and marked tenderness. Rectal bleeding or sloughed mucosal tissue per rectum may occur from vascular compromise of the intestines (Aiken & Oldham, 2005; D'Agostino, 2002; McCollough

& Sharieff, 2003; Millar et al., 2003). The abdomen becomes increasingly tender as the ischemia involves the serosal surface of the bowel and as sequestration of fluid in the abdomen results in peritoneal irritation. On rectal examination, stool is usually absent, but if present, is guaiac positive or shows gross blood (Aiken & Oldham).

Laboratory Work

A complete blood count, type and screen, and electrolyte levels are obtained when evaluating an infant for midgut volvulus. Electrolyte imbalance is expected in a child diagnosed with volvulus due to vomiting and to third spacing of fluid into the bowel and abdominal cavity (Aiken & Oldham, 2005; Shelton, 1999). Low hemoglobin and hematocrit values may be noted as well, from pooling of blood in the intestine. The correction of metabolic abnormalities and any necessary transfusions should begin as soon as possible.

Radiologic Diagnosis

An immediate radiologic evaluation is imperative if the infant or child presents with clinical signs of acute or chronic intestinal obstruction. However, intravenous fluid resuscitation is essential before any radiologic study in order to rehydrate the infant and correct electrolyte imbalance. The infant may subsequently deteriorate rapidly in the radiology department if proper fluids are not infused before and during the studies. Initially, flat and upright or lateral decubitus views plain-film abdominal x-ray studies are sufficient to evaluate intestinal obstruction, but the diagnosis of malrotation cannot be made on plain films alone (Stockmann, 2005). The plain films may show air in the stomach and proximal duodenum, a "double bubble" appearance, in an otherwise gasless abdomen, suggesting intestinal obstruction. The classic "double bubble" sign that is pathognomonic for duodenal atresia may be present in 20% of patients with malrotation and volvulus (Stockmann). Gastric and proximal duodenal dilation with air noted in the distal intestine suggests an incomplete obstruction consistent with malrotation (Aiken & Oldham, 2005; D'Agostino, 2002; Stockmann). The plain films may also show multiple dilated loops of small bowel with air/fluid levels, suggestive of intestinal strangulation (Aiken & Oldham).

Infants with clinical findings suggestive of impending bowel necrosis, such as bloody emesis and stools, abdominal tenderness, dehydration, and lethargy, in addition to plain films revealing duodenal obstruction, require ag-

gressive fluid resuscitation and immediate operation. No further radiologic studies are necessary (Aiken & Oldham, 2005; Stockman, 2005).

If the diagnosis is in doubt, and compromised bowel is not evident, a contrast study is the standard examination for malrotation. A UGI series is the preferred study rather than a barium enema (Aiken & Oldham, 2005; D'Agostino, 2000; Hajivassiliou, 2003; Kimura & Loening-Baucke, 2000; Millar et al., 2003; Stockmann, 2005; Strouse, 2004). A UGI series evaluates the position of the ligament of Treitz while a barium enema evaluates the position of the cecum and colon. In malrotation, the cecum and colon may sometimes be positioned normally, making the barium enema a less reliable study (Aiken & Oldham; Stockmann).

Malrotation of intestines presents with the following on UGI: (1) abnormal position of the ligament of Treitz, which is normally located on the left side of the spine; (2) partial obstruction of the duodenum, with a spiral or corkscrew appearance; and (3) proximal jejunum in the right abdomen.

When volvulus is present, the barium column is noted to end with a peculiar beaking effect. The beaking appearance is pathognomonic of a volvulus and is caused by twisting of the bowel into a sharp point resembling the beak of a bird (Fig. 24-6) (Aiken & Oldham, 2005; Stockmann, 2005; Strouse, 2004).

Other imaging studies, such as ultrasound (US) and computed tomography (CT), may be helpful in supporting the diagnosis of malrotation. An abnormal relation-

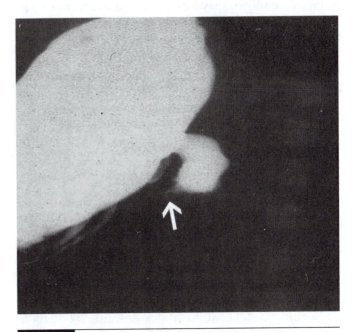

Figure 24-6 Upper gastrointestinal series with bird's beak.
(Reprinted with permission by Allen F. Browne.)

ship of the superior mesenteric vein (SMV) to the SMA is usually consistent with malrotation, and both US and CT may demonstrate this finding. In addition, as the SMV wraps around the SMA, a whirlpool sign is formed, rotating in clockwise direction, and is evident on color Doppler ultrasound (Aidlen, Anupindi, Jaramillo, & Doody, 2005; Millar et al., 2003; Patino & Munden, 2004; Strouse, 2004). However if US or CT demonstrates this reversed vasculature, a UGI study is still needed to confirm the diagnosis of malrotation due to inconsistencies with the studies, particularly with US. Malrotation may not always present with this aberrant anatomy. Conversely, normal SMA and SMV anatomy does not always exclude malrotation (Aiken & Oldham, 2005; Stockmann, 2005).

Treatment and Operative Considerations

Infants and children who present with acute symptoms of midgut volvulus require emergent surgical correction. Fluid resuscitation, placement of nasogastric decompression tube and Foley catheter, drawing blood for laboratory values, and administration of broad-spectrum antibiotics should all be initiated concurrently with diagnostic studies. Time is crucial, and delaying the surgery may affect viability of the bowel (Aiken & Oldham, 2005; Hajivassiliou, 2003; Kimura & Loening-Baucke, 2000; Stockmann, 2005). Patients with midgut necrosis at the time of surgery have a 50% mortality rate and those surviving children may be destined to a lifetime of permanent disability with short-bowel syndrome (Aiken & Oldham; Stockmann).

In children with asymptomatic malrotation, or in those with symptomatic malrotation without volvulus, surgical correction is indicated but may be performed on an elective or nonemergent basis. The symptomatic patient should undergo operative correction as soon as possible, especially if the child is less than 1 year of age because the risk for volvulus is greatest in this age group (Aiken & Oldham, 2005; Kume et al., 2004; Malek & Burd, 2005; Prasil et al., 2000).

The asymptomatic child has less urgency for immediate operation, and, in fact, the treatment remains somewhat controversial. Many surgeons believe that the surgery should be carried out in a timely manner because the predisposition for midgut volvulus still exists, regardless of age (Aiken & Oldham, 2005; Hahivassiliou, 2003; Kimura & Loening-Baucke, 2000; Malek & Burd, 2005, 2006; Stockmann, 2005). Others suggest that the surgery be performed if certain criteria exist, such as abnormal po-

sition of the ligament of Treitz and cecum, regardless of age (Prasil et al., 2000).

Surgical Procedure

The patient is expeditiously taken to the operating room for a Ladd's procedure. The laparotomy is performed through a transverse right upper quadrant incision, allowing for evisceration and assessment of the bowel. Volvulus occurs in a clockwise manner; therefore, the bowel is detorsed in a counterclockwise direction. After detorsion, the bowel is evaluated for viability. If the entire bowel turns pink and seems viable, the surgeon then releases the constricting duodenal and duodenojejunal bands (Fig. 24-7). The cecum and ascending colon must be totally mobilized and moved to the left side of the abdomen, thus returning the midgut to its fetal position (Fig. 24-8). Not only does this procedure relieve the existing obstruction, but it also minimizes the chance of a recurrent volvulus (Fig. 24-9). In addition, because of the abnormal position of the appendix in the left lower

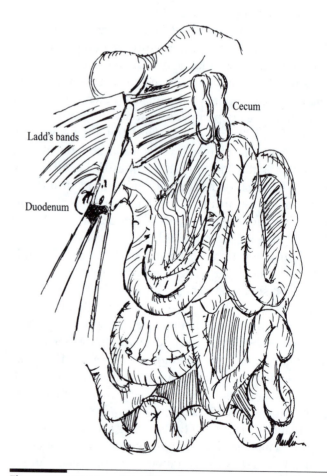

Figure 24-7 Division of Ladd's bands.

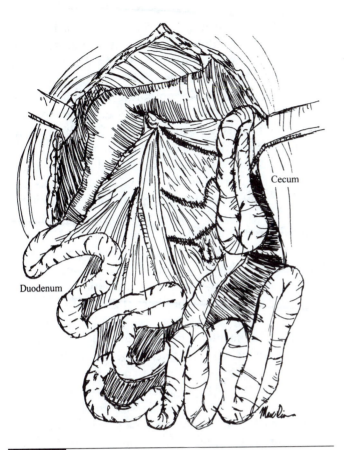

Figure 24-8 Placement of the small and large intestine in non-rotation.

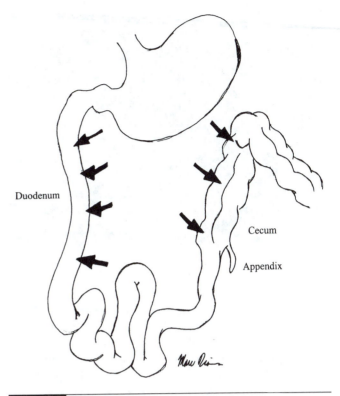

Figure 24-9 Spreading the mesentery with disassociation of the cecum and duodenum.

or left upper abdomen after the Ladd's procedure, most surgeons remove the appendix. Therefore, the possibility of acute appendicitis with symptoms in the left abdomen is eliminated (Aiken & Oldham, 2005; Stockmann, 2005).

If there is no question of viability of the intestine, the Ladd's procedure is carried out as described above. However, if the viability of the bowel is questioned, three events are possibly encountered. **First possible presentation:** a short segment of bowel is necrotic and the remaining intestine seems healthy. The necrotic bowel is resected, and an anastomosis is performed that preserves maximal length of intestines as the goal. **Second possible presentation:** a short portion of intestine is obviously necrotic, but after resection, varying lengths of proximal and distal bowel appear compromised. In this case, both ends of bowel may be brought to the skin as stomas. After 24 to 48 hours, second-look exploration and resection of further necrotic intestine is performed if the stoma ends still appear necrotic. **Third possible presentation:** a large segment of the small bowel seems necrotic, or regions of both necrotic and viable intestines are noted. The bowel is then put back into the peritoneal cavity without re-

section. A second operation is performed 24 hours later, the bowel is reassessed, and if necrotic bowel is present, resection is performed (Aiken & Oldham, 2005; Stockmann, 2005).

The guiding principal in any of the above situations is preservation of bowel length (Kimura & Leoning-Baucke, 2000; Stockmann, 2005). In some cases, the entire midgut is necrotic and unsalvageable (Fig. 24-10). The abdomen is closed, and the parents are told of the dismal prognosis due to this catastrophic event (Stockmann).

■ Preoperative Nursing Management

Patients with acute presentation of midgut volvulus require immediate and aggressive fluid resuscitation to correct hypovolemia and metabolic imbalance. In addition, blood samples for laboratory values should be drawn. Intravenous broad-spectrum antibiotics are given to avoid bacterial translocation through the necrotic bowel wall. A nasogastric tube is inserted to decompress the gastrointestinal tract and a Foley catheter placed to measure accurate urine output. These measures can be accomplished while the infant or child is in the process of obtaining radiologic studies. The patient should be kept

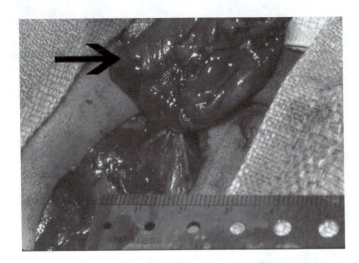

Figure 24-10 Ischemic bowel from volvulus.
(Reprinted with permission by Allen F. Browne.)

warm during all procedures, especially while in radiology. Operative preparations must be accomplished without delaying transport to the operating room because time is a critical factor in preventing ischemic bowel injury (Aiken & Oldham, 2005; Stockmann, 2005).

Particular care must be given to the parents of the infant or child at this time, especially before emergent surgery. Loss of the familiar parental role and the uncertainty of the surgical outcome are the most stressful aspects of hospitalization for the parents (Manworren & Fledderman, 2000). To decrease stress, all procedures should be explained to the parents by the surgeon with reinforcement of explanations by the pediatric surgical nurse. Timely updates from the operating room also help alleviate parental concerns. Social services may be contacted to provide additional family support during this crisis.

Postoperative Nursing Management

Postoperative care of the infant with midgut volvulus is similar to that of any infant undergoing intestinal surgery. Principles of fluid and electrolyte management, bowel decompression, and pain relief are instituted. Fluid and electrolyte balance must be carefully monitored. Adequate urine output of 1.0 cc per kilogram of body weight per hour is measured by Foley catheter or by weighing the infant's diapers on a gram scale.

A nasogastric tube (NGT) is inserted, placed to low intermittent suction, and left intact until bowel function returns. This tube should be monitored carefully and accurate outputs recorded every 4 hours. The NGT should be kept patent by flushing with 5 to 10 cc of normal saline every 2 hours. In addition, skin care at the nares and face is important because breakdown from NGT pressure may occur within 24 hours. A clear, adhesive dressing on the patient's cheek is useful in promoting good skin integrity, allowing visibility of the skin while securing the NGT in place. Abdominal girth and auscultation of bowel sounds should also be performed and results recorded.

Postoperative analgesia is achieved by administering morphine intravenously every 2 to 3 hours as necessary. The patient's vital signs are monitored continuously by cardiorespiratory and oxygen saturation monitors while receiving morphine. Acetaminophen (Tylenol) suppositories may also be administered for pain or fever. Developmental level is an important consideration in pediatric pain management, and distraction techniques may be used to augment the effect of analgesics (Mackey, 2000).

Parents of the infant should be informed about all aspects of their baby's care. Encouraging handling of the infant after surgery is beneficial to both parent and baby. Rocking and holding are nonpharmacologic comfort measures to be used along with analgesics. In older babies or children, early ambulation is mandatory in order to prevent respiratory sequelae and to promote the return of bowel function.

As soon as bowel function returns, feedings are started. Depending on the extent of the surgery, appropriate formula and amounts are ordered. Feedings are usually advanced as tolerated. If a large portion of necrotic bowel was removed, leaving a short-bowel situation, a gastrostomy feeding tube is placed at time of operation, along with a central venous catheter for parenteral feedings. Initial feedings via gastrostomy are usually started with very dilute elemental formula in small amounts. First, volume, then concentration, of formula is gradually increased until full-strength formula is tolerated. The feeding progression of an infant or child with short-bowel syndrome is a very tedious process with many setbacks of days or even weeks (Kasson, 2000). The setbacks are usually very frustrating to the parents as well as the nurse. In addition to enteral feedings, long-term parenteral nutrition may be necessary in the case of short-bowel syndrome.

Complications

Most serious and long-term complications of malrotation and midgut volvulus are related to delays in diagnosis and treatment. Intestinal ischemia and infarction, short-bowel syndrome, and recurrent intestinal obstruction are the direct result of delayed surgical treatment. Obstruction may occur from adhesive bands (Ladd's bands), recurrent volvulus, and intestinal dysmotility (Aiken & Oldham, 2005; Stockmann, 2005). Other devastating complications of necrotic bowel include sepsis, shock, multi-system organ failure, and death (Stockmann). Minor complications include those associated with any surgery, including postoperative bleeding and wound infection.

Prognosis

The prognosis for children who have undergone surgical correction of malrotation without bowel injury are excellent, with very low morbidity. Prompt diagnosis and treatment of malrotation with midgut volvulus can ensure normal life expectancy as well.

The mortality rate is increased for patients with necrotic bowel, associated congenital anomalies, or age less than 1 month. However, advances in pediatric surgical intensive care, enteral and parenteral nutrition, and skilled nursing care have decreased mortality and morbidity, even in the most complicated cases (Aiken & Oldham, 2005; Stockmann, 2005).

Conclusion

Malrotation is the result of an aberration in the complex embryologic development of the gastrointestinal tract. Volvulus is a life-threatening complication of malrotation. Bilious vomiting in a neonate may be the first sign of this very serious problem and requires immediate work-up to prevent catastrophic outcomes. In general, children with malrotation have a good prognosis. The prognosis for patients with midgut volvulus is variable, depending on the amount of damage sustained by the intestines. Nursing care includes family support and ongoing education.

Acknowledgments

We would like to thank the following people for their generous contributions in helping us complete this chapter: Marc Diana, Kara McGee, Elizabeth Ruiz, Dr. Malvin Weinberger, and Carlos Zerpa.

Educational Materials

APSNA invites you to download the following diagnosis-related teaching tool for Chapter 24, Malrotation & Volvulus: 1) Malrotation & Volvulus. This teaching tool is available at the APSNA Web site (www.apsna.org) and the Jones and Bartlett Web site (www.jbpub.com). All teaching materials are available in English and Spanish and are free of charge. APSNA encourages their use for your patients and families.

References

Aidlen, J., Anupindi, S. A., Jaramillo, D., & Doody, D. P. (2005). Malrotation with midgut volvulus: CT findings of bowel infarction. *Pediatric Radiology, 35*(5), 529–531.

Aiken, J. J., & Oldham, K. T. (2005). Malrotation. In K. W. Ashcraft, G. W. Holcomb, & P. Murphy (Eds.), *Pediatric surgery* (4th ed., pp. 435–447). Philadelphia: Elsevier Saunders.

D'Agostino, J. (2002). Common abdominal emergencies in children. *Emergency Medicine Clinics of North America, 20*(1), 139–152.

Dott, N. M. (1923). Anomalies of intestinal rotation: Their embryology and surgical aspects, with the report of five cases. *British Journal of Surgery, 11*, 251–286.

Gray, S. W., & Skandalakis, J. E. (1972). *Embryology for surgeons* (pp. 129–141). Philadelphia: Saunders.

Hajivassiliou, C. A. (2003). Intestinal obstruction in neonatal/pediatric surgery. *Seminars in Pediatric Surgery, 12*(4), 241–253.

Imamoglu, M., Cay, A., Sarihan, H., & Sen, Y. (2004). Rare clinical presentation mode of intestinal malrotation after neonatal period: Malabsorption-like symptoms due to chronic midgut volvulus. *Pediatric International, 46*(2), 167–170.

Kasson, B. R. (2000). Necrotizing enterocolitis. In B. V. Wise, G. Garvin, C. McKenna, & B. J. Harmon (Eds.), *Nursing care of the general pediatric surgical patient* (pp. 291–304). Gaithersburg, MD: Aspen.

Kimura, K., & Loening-Baucke, V. (2000). Bilious vomiting in the newborn: Rapid diagnosis of intestinal obstruction. *American Family Physician, 61*(9), 2791–2798.

Kume, Y., Fumino, S., Shimotake, T., & Iwai, N. (2004). Intestinal malrotation with midgut volvulus in a 10-year-old girl. *Journal of Pediatric Surgery, 39*(5), 783–784.

Ladd, W. E. (1932). Congenital obstruction of the duodenum in children. *New England Journal of Medicine, 206*, 277–283.

Ladd, W. E. (1936). Surgical diseases of the alimentary tract in infants. *New England Journal of Medicine, 215*, 705–708.

Mackey, W. L. (2000). Pain management and sedation in children. In B. V. Wise, G. Garvin, C. McKenna, & B. J. Harmon (Eds.), *Nursing care of the general pediatric surgical patient* (pp. 56–77). Gaithersburg, MD: Aspen.

Malek, M. M., & Burd, R. S. (2005). Surgical treatment of malrotation after infancy: A population-based study. *Journal of Pediatric Surgery, 40*, 285–289.

Malek, M. M., & Burd, R. S. (2006). The optimal management of malrotation diagnosed after infancy: A decision analysis. *American Journal of Surgery, 19*(1), 45–51.

Manworren, R. C. B., & Fledderman, M. (2000). Preparation of the child and family for surgery. In B. V. Wise, G. Garvin, C. McKenna, & B. J. Harmon (Eds.), *Nursing care of the general pediatric surgical patient* (pp. 3–15). Gaithersburg, MD: Aspen.

McCollough, M., & Sharieff, G. Q. (2003). Abdominal surgical emergencies in infants and young children. *Emergency Medicine Clinics of North America, 21*(4), 909–935.

Millar, A. J., Rode, H., & Cywes, S. (2003). Malrotation and volvulus in infancy and childhood. *Seminars in Pediatric Surgery, 12*(4), 229–236.

Patino, M. O., & Munden, M. M. (2004). Utility of the sonographic whirlpool sign in diagnosing midgut volvulus in patients with atypical clinical presentation. *Journal of Ultrasound Medicine, 23*(3), 397–401.

Prasil, P., Flageole, H., Shaw, K. S., Nguyen, L. T., Youssef, S., & Laberge, J. M. (2000). Should malrotation in children be treated differently according to age? *Journal of Pediatric Surgery, 35*(5), 756–758.

Shelton, B. K. (1999). Intestinal obstruction. *American Association of Critical-Care Nurses Clinical Issues, 10*(4), 478–491.

Strouse, P. J. (2004). Disorders of intestinal rotation and fixation ("Malrotation"). *Pediatric Radiology, 34*(11), 837–851.

Stockmann, P. T. (2005). Malrotation. In K. T. Oldham, P. M. Colombani, R. P. Foglia, & M. A. Skinner (Eds.), *Principles and practice of pediatric surgery* (Vol. 2, pp. 1283–1296). Philadelphia: Lippincott Williams & Wilkins.

CHAPTER

25

Intussusception

By Lynn E. Fagerman and Lynne D. Farber

Intussusception is the invagination or telescoping of one intestinal segment into another adjacent segment of bowel, which creates a mechanical obstruction. Although intussusception can occur at any age, it is the most common abdominal emergency in early childhood, particularly in children younger than 2 years of age. Roughly 60% of children are younger than 1 year old, and 80% are younger than 2. It is the second most common cause of intestinal obstruction after pyloric stenosis (Lloyd & Kenny, 2004).

The incidence of intussusception in the United States is 1.5 to 4 cases per 1,000 live births, with males more frequently affected (Sherman & Consentino, 1993). Without prompt medical attention and accurate diagnosis, intestinal perforation and bowel death can occur, creating significant morbidity. Because of the age of the child, an explanation of symptoms and discomfort may be mistaken for those of a benign illness. Intussusception should be high on the list of differential diagnoses when children, especially younger than 1 year of age, are seen with sudden onset of abdominal pain.

The cause of intussusception falls into one of three categories: idiopathic, lead point, or postoperative. The idiopathic type has no readily identifiable cause, although it is the most common type. Lead point is so named because an identifiable change in the intestinal mucosa can

be discovered, usually during surgical treatment for intussusception. Postoperative intussusception is not common but can occur after operative procedures involving the abdomen or even the chest.

■ Pathophysiology

The most common segment of bowel involved in intussusception is the ileocecal region. When small bowel (ileum) and the attached mesentery, lymphatic tissue, and blood vessels invaginate into the large bowel (cecum), the folding over of intestines and vessels impedes normal blood flow to the tissues (Raffensperger, 1990). This leads to further swelling, which in turn decreases blood flow further. If not recognized and treated, bowel death occurs and may involve significant portions of intestine.

Although there is no readily identifiable cause of idiopathic intussusception, it is not uncommon to obtain a history of recent upper respiratory or gastrointestinal illness. It is hypothesized that viral infection leads to hypertrophy of Peyer's patches, a type of lymphoid tissue in the intestinal wall, creating a slightly thickened segment, thereby encouraging invagination to occur (Rowe, 1995). Idiopathic intussusception is the most common form seen in infants. More than 50% of all cases occur before the age of 1 year, and 10% to 25% after the age of 2 years (Fallat, 2005). Intussusception has been theorized as a cause of small bowel atresia in premature infants (Mooney, Steinthorsson, & Shorter, 1996) and has been misdiagnosed as necrotizing enterocolitis, delaying operative intervention in some cases (Avansino, Bjerke, Hendrickson, Stelzner, & Sawin, 2003; Martinez Biarge et al., 2004). Lead point intussusception is the form more commonly found in children who are older than 2 to 3 years of age (Stevenson & Ziegler, 1993). It is estimated that between 2% and 12% of all intussusceptions in infants are due to a recognizable anatomic lead point or malformation in the intestinal mucosa (Meier, Coln, Rescorla, OlaOlorun, & Tarpley, 1996). Almost every patient has marked hypertrophy of the lymphoid tissue of the ileal wall of the *intussusceptum*, which is the proximal portion of the intestine. For all age groups, the list of anatomic lead points includes intestinal polyps, the appendix, ectopic pancreas or gastric mucosa, intestinal duplication, cysts, carcinoid tumors, foreign bodies, hemangioma, Meckel's diverticulum, non-Hodgkin's lymphoma, blunt abdominal trauma with intestinal hematomas, and submucosal hemorrhage resulting from Henoch-Schönlein purpura. Meckel's diverticulum is the most common lead point (Fallat, 2005). These malformations create points where invagination and subsequent telescoping of bowel can occur, with resulting obstruction, edema, and hemorrhage.

Children with cystic fibrosis and the characteristic changes in the bowel secondary to thick inspissated stool and mucus are also at risk for lead point–type intussusception (Rowe, 1995). The average age of this type of secondary intussusception is 9 to 12 years and might recur on several occasions.

Intussusception after surgical procedures in the abdomen or chest is thought to be due to the disordered motility that can occur after receiving general anesthesia or as a result of direct handling of intestinal tissue. Intussusception may also occur after placement of long tubes for decompression or direct feedings into the bowel (Rowe, 1995). Bowel obstruction, of which intussusception is one type, should be considered if there is an increase in nasogastric drainage 2 to 5 days after surgery, rather than the usual decrease in such output seen in the postoperative period.

■ Clinical Presentation

The typical clinical scenario is that of a usually healthy, well-nourished, and active child in later infancy who experiences a sudden onset of abdominal pain, which may also create a change in behavior. The child is seen drawing up his or her legs to the abdomen as if experiencing colicky pain and may not like being held or moved. This episode may occur in waves, with periods of rest in between. Initially, the child has no change in appetite but eventually becomes anorectic and may have vomiting that progresses to a bilious color. The child becomes increasingly more irritable and lethargic as the bowel becomes more compromised. Some children pass stools consisting of sloughed mucosa that have a dark red color with a mucoid consistency. These have been termed "currant jelly" stools (Fig. 25-1), which, although a classic sign of intussusception, are also a later appearing sign and indicates damage to the intestines (Stevenson & Ziegler, 1993).

The picture of an infant who is irritable yet lethargic, with decreased appetite and vomiting, and who seems to be in pain when the body is moved creates a confusing picture for many examiners. It is not unusual for such children to be evaluated for possible pneumonia, sepsis, or meningitis first.

■ Physical Examination

The physical examination of the child varies, depending on when in the course of the intussusception the child presents. Young children whose critical condition is less obvious to parents may be brought to medical attention late, at which time they have dehydration, lethargy, shock, or even coma. Symptoms of intussusception (vomiting, pain, abdominal mass, and bloody stools) are found to exist together in less than one half of children in whom the diagnosis is made (Kuppermann, O'Dea, Pinckney, &

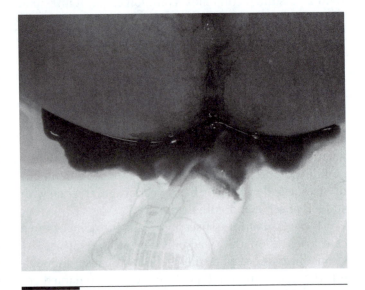

Figure 25-1 Current jelly stool.

Hoecker, 2000). The child initially vomits undigested food, eventually becoming bilious (Fallat, 2005). As the course progresses, the abdomen changes from soft to tender and distended. Between episodes of pain, with the child relaxed, it may be possible to palpate a sausage-shaped mass in the mid- to upper right abdomen. The lower right quadrant is empty. Palpation may be difficult because of the child's irritability. If the abdomen is auscultated during a crisis, hyperperistaltic rushes (borborygmi) may be heard. There are decreased or absent bowel sounds with significant ileus or peritonitis. Hematochezia (maroon-colored stool) is not always present. The rectal examination is significant if there is bloody mucus on the examiner's fingertip. Sixty percent to 90% of children have gross or occult blood on rectal examination, 20% to 50% have passed mucoid bloody stools, and the remaining have occult blood on testing (Losek & Fiete, 1991).

Vital signs are normal early in the course, but as abdominal distention and vomiting continue, with loss of fluid and bacteremia, the child becomes tachycardic and hypotensive and may have a temperature elevation. If fever is significant, the examiner must check for an extra-abdominal source. Specifically, pneumonia should be considered. The groin should be palpated for incarcerated hernia or torsion of the testicle or ovary as other possible sources of sudden onset of abdominal pain (Stevenson & Ziegler, 1993).

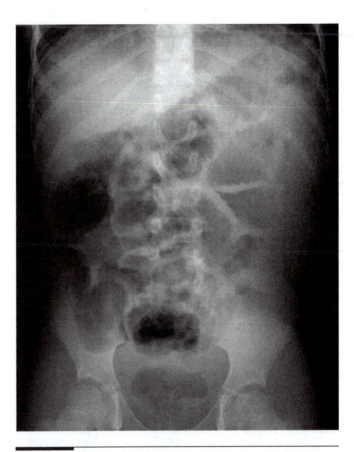

Figure 25-2 Small bowel obstruction with absence of colonic gas. (Reprinted with permission by Stephen P. Dunn, MD, Chief, Pediatric Surgery & Transplant, Alfred I. Dupont Hospital for Children.)

■ Laboratory Studies

Initial studies of the child should include complete blood count, electrolytes, and urinalysis. The white blood cell count is often elevated because of necrotic tissue and inflammation. Electrolyte imbalances should be expected if the child is acidotic or dehydrated from vomiting (Losek & Fiete, 1991). Urine output may be low (< 0.5 to 1.0 mL/kg/hr), with an elevated specific gravity in the dehydrated child as well.

■ Radiographs

Radiologic techniques may be not only diagnostic but therapeutic as well. After a thorough physical examination, supine and upright abdominal series may be ordered. If the intussusception is very early in the course, these may be relatively normal. With progression, a more obvious pattern of small-bowel obstruction with absence of gas in the colon is found (Fig. 25-2). The finding of a right upper quadrant soft tissue density is helpful in predicting intussusception. If these radiographic findings of

bowel obstruction are seen and are consistent with the history and physical examination, an air or barium enema is attempted if no intraperitoneal air has been detected. If intraperitoneal air is found, this indicates that intestinal perforation has occurred, and emergency surgery is indicated. The use of ultrasound has become increasingly more routine in the evaluation of suspected intussusception and is highly sensitive in verifying the diagnosis (Heller & Hernanz-Schulman, 1999).

Before the enema, intravenous access should be obtained to administer fluids, sedation, pain relief, and, in some cases, antibiotics. A nasogastric tube may also be placed for gastric decompression. The child should be well hydrated and stable before any radiologic reduction attempts are made.

The barium enema has long been considered the most reliable diagnostic technique for an ileocolic intussusception and is the accepted treatment for most children. Water-soluble contrast materials are of high osmolality and should not be used because of the risk of intravascular compartment shifts and hypovolemic shock (Heller & Hernanz-Schulman, 1999). The air enema is widely used and is considered safer and as effective in diagnosing and reducing an intussusception as barium (Menor, Cortina, Marco, & Olague, 1992).

Because of the risk of perforation a surgeon should be present during the barium enema. A noninflatable rectal tube is inserted into the rectum, and the buttocks are taped together. Contrast enters the rectosigmoid by gravity under fluoroscopic guidance. If air is used, it is delivered under constant pressure. The pressure instilled during the reduction must be carefully controlled, regardless of the material used, to avoid inadvertent perforation. Commonly, a concave filling defect is seen in the transverse colon that can be reduced to the cecum. As the intussusceptum is reduced through the ileocecal valve, contrast or air should reflux freely into the small intestine; this radiographic finding is essential to document a successful reduction. If the first enema is not successful, a second or third attempt may be made with periods of waiting while the child evacuates the barium or air. Usually, the intussusception is reduced after one or two attempts (Doody, 1997). Success rates with hydrostatic reduction have been reported to range between 70% and 90% of cases (Menor, Cortina, Marco, & Olague, 1992). The most common complication after radiologic reduction is recurrence of intussusception, which occurs soon after the reduction. For this reason, the child is sometimes admitted to the hospital for 24 hours of observation. Most children are able to tolerate a liquid diet and are discharged from the hospital within that period.

■ Surgical Treatment

Immediate surgery is indicated if barium or air reduction fails or if there is clinical evidence of peritonitis or bowel perforation on radiographic examination. A transverse right lower quadrant incision is made, and the intussusception is brought out into the wound (Fig. 25-3). Surgical reduction is accomplished by gently manually milking the intussusception proximally until the bowel is completely reduced (West & Grosfeld, 1999). Resection and end-to-end anastomosis are performed if manual reduction cannot be accomplished or if the reduced bowel is gangrenous or perforated. Resection is also performed if a specific lead point is found. Often during these surgical procedures, an incidental appendectomy is performed. Postoperative complications are rare except in those cases in which the child is in shock or when a significant amount of dead bowel is present. The complications are similar to those of other major abdominal surgeries, including wound infection, abscess formation, and pneumonia.

The incidence of recurrent intussusception is approximately 2% to 20%, with about one third occurring within 24 hours and the majority within 6 months of the initial episode (Fallat, 2005). Multiple recurrences can occur in the same patient. Early signs of recurrence are irritability and discomfort (Fallat). Recurrence rates of intussusception are lower if surgical reduction is performed, ranging between 1% and 4%. With all recurrences,

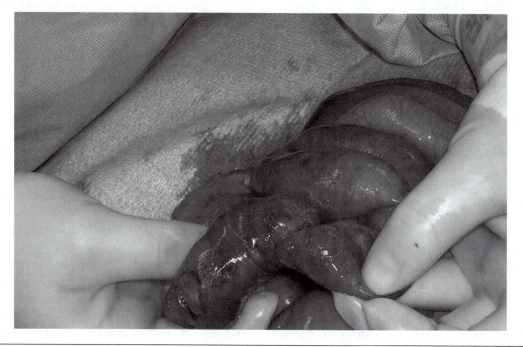

Figure 25-3 Intussusception.
(Reprinted with permission by Stephen P. Dunn, MD, Chief, Pediatric Surgery & Transplant, Alfred I. Dupont Hospital for Children.)

an underlying abnormality should be considered, such as is found in lead point type intussusception.

Indications for Referral

Anticipatory guidance with parents of hospitalized children can prevent long-term adverse reactions to invasive procedures and separation. Most children with intussusception requiring surgical treatment resume their healthy preoperative status fairly quickly. On postoperative follow-up, the child should have resumed the former eating pattern and should be gaining weight. If the child lost a significant amount of bowel when a resection was performed, special nutritional supplementation may be required for a time. These cases, although rare, often benefit from monitoring by a visiting nurse agency until the family is comfortable with any special care needs.

Research

In 1998, the first licensed rotavirus vaccine, RotaShield, was withdrawn from the U.S. market less than a year after its introduction because it was associated with intussusception, at an estimated rate of 1 incident per 10,000 vaccine recipients (Murphy et al., 2001; Peter & Myers, 2002). Fortunately, new clinical trials have reported promising results of two new rotavirus vaccines that significantly reduce the rate of severe gastroenteritis from any cause and are not associated with an increased risk of intussusception (Glass & Parashar, 2006; Ruiz-Palacios et al., 2006). Because rotavirus disease kills approximately half a million children annually and accounts for one third of hospitalizations for diarrhea worldwide, these trials generate hope for a vaccine that may prevent much of the severe diarrhea in children around the world (Velazquez et al., 2004).

The cause of intussusception remains vague, even for those children with lead point type intussusception. For example, most children who have upper respiratory viruses, gastrointestinal illnesses, or even a Meckel's diverticulum do not have intussusception develop. Research and epidemiologic studies should continue to search for those commonalities in children with intussusception, which may help primary care providers provide anticipatory guidance to families with young children.

Nursing Considerations

Nursing care of the child with intussusception includes strict attention to maintaining intravenous fluids, naso-gastric decompression of the stomach, and frequent assessment of hydration status by observation of strict intake and output records. Vital signs are also monitored closely, both before and after treatment of the intussusception, being mindful of the changes seen in young children with fluid volume deficit or shock. Age-appropriate pain assessment tools should be used to aid in the decision-making regarding the administration of ordered pain medications. Nonpharmacologic pain relief techniques are useful as adjunctive therapy, as well as possibly decreasing the need for frequent use of pain medications. Attention to the psychosocial care of the child and family is an equally important role for the nurse. Separation between the child and the primary support person(s) should be minimized and may be accomplished by facilitating rooming in. The child should be allowed to keep a transitional object, such as a favorite blanket or toy, at all times. Family caregivers should be encouraged to bring in the child's own pajamas, slippers, and clothes if the child is hospitalized. Explanations should be offered to the family at their level of understanding, and new situations should be explained to decrease anxiety and promote comfort for the child. The child should be provided with play opportunities as appropriate because play is necessary to his or her well-being. Assigning the same nursing personnel as much as possible provides continuity of care and decreases the number of strangers who come into contact with the child. Painful procedures should be performed in a treatment room whenever possible, thereby maintaining the concept of the child's bed or room as a safe haven.

Discharge Instructions

After a radiologic reduction, parents should be instructed to return with the child to a medical facility again if signs such as vomiting, abdominal pain, or bloody stools return. If surgical treatment has been necessary, the family should be instructed in the signs and symptoms of wound infection: fever, redness, swelling, or drainage from the incision, as well as symptoms of recurrence of the intussusception.

Conclusion

Intussusception is a serious mechanical bowel obstruction that is most commonly seen in children younger than 3 years of age. The symptoms may mimic other, more frequently occurring, illnesses in young children, which may hamper and delay the diagnostic process.

Barium or air-contrast enemas may be both diagnostic and therapeutic interventions. Intussusception must be diagnosed and treated quickly to prevent bowel ischemia and necrosis, which may lead to significant morbidity for the child.

■ Acknowledgment

The authors would like to acknowledge the work of Margaret Meyer who contributed to the "Intussusception" chapter in the first edition of this textbook.

■ Educational Materials

APSNA invites you to download the following diagnosis-related teaching tool for Chapter 25, Intussusception: 1) Intussusception. This teaching tool is available at the APSNA Web site (www.apsna.org) and the Jones and Bartlett Web site (www.jbpub.com). All teaching materials are available in English and Spanish and are free of charge. APSNA encourages their use for your patients and families.

■ References

Avansino, J. R., Bjerke, S., Hendrickson, M., Stelzner, M., & Sawin, R. (2003). Clinical features and treatment outcome of intussusception in premature neonates. *Journal of Pediatric Surgery, 38,* 1818–1821.

Doody, D. (1997). Intussusception. In K. T. Oldham, P. M. Colombani, & R. P. Foglia (Eds.), *Surgery of infants and children* (pp. 1241–1248). Philadelphia: Lippincott-Raven.

Fallat, M. (2005). Intussusception. In K. W. Ashcraft, G. W. Holcomb, & J. P. Murphy (Eds.), *Pediatric surgery* (4th ed., pp. 533–542). Philadelphia: Elsevier Saunders.

Glass, R. I., & Parashar, U. D. (2006). The promise of new rotavirus vaccines. *New England Journal of Medicine, 354*(1), 75–77.

Heller, R., & Hernanz-Schulman, M. (1999). Applications of new imaging modalities to the evaluation of common pediatric conditions. *The Journal of Pediatrics, 135,* 632–639.

Kuppermann, N., O'Dea, T., Pinckney, L., & Hoecker, C. (2000). Predictors of intussusception in young children. *Archives of Pediatric and Adolescent Medicine, 154*(3), 250–255.

Losek, J. D., & Fiete, R. I. (1991). Intussusception and the diagnostic value of testing stool for occult blood. *American Journal of Emergency Medicine, 9*(1), 1–3.

Lloyd, D. A., & Kenny, S. E. (2004). The surgical abdomen. In W. A. Walker, O. Goulet, R. E. Kleinman, et al. (Eds.), *Pediatric gastrointestinal disease: Pathopsychology, diagnosis, management* (4th ed., p. 604). Ontario: BC Decker.

Martinez Biarge, M., Garcia-Alix, A., Luisa del Hoyo, M., Alarcon, A., Saenz de Pipaon, M., Hernandez, F., et al. (2004). Intussusception in a preterm neonate; a very rare, major intestinal problem–systematic review of cases. *Journal of Perinatal Medicine, 32*(2), 190–194.

Meier, D. E., Coln, C. D., Rescorla, F. J., OlaOlorun, A., & Tarpley, J. L. (1996). Intussusception in children: International perspective. *World Journal of Surgery, 20*(8), 1035–1039; discussion 1040.

Menor, F., Cortina, H., Marco, A., & Olague, R. (1992). Effectiveness of pneumatic reduction of ileocolic intussusception in children. *Gastrointestinal Radiology, 17,* 339–343.

Mooney, D. P., Steinthorsson, G., & Shorter, N. A. (1996). Perinatal intussusception in premature infants. *Journal of Pediatric Surgery, 31*(5), 695–697.

Murphy, T. V., Gargiullo, P. M., Massoudi, M. S., Nelson, D. B., Jumaan, A. O., Okoro, C. A., et al. (2001). Intussusception among infants given an oral rotavirus vaccine. *New England Journal of Medicine, 344*(8), 564–572.

Peter, G., & Myers, M. G. (2002). Intussusception, rotavirus, and oral vaccines: Summary of a workshop. *Pediatrics, 110*(6), e67.

Raffensperger, J. G. (1990). Intussusception. In *Swenson's pediatric surgery* (5th ed., pp. 224–226). Stamford, CT: Appleton & Lange.

Rowe, M. I. (1995). *Essentials in pediatric surgery* (pp. 542–544). St. Louis, MO: Mosby.

Ruiz-Palacios, G. M., Perez-Schael, I., Velazquez, F. R., Abate, H., Breuer, T., Clemens, S. C., et al. (2006). Safety and efficacy of an attenuated vaccine against severe rotavirus gastroenteritis. *New England Journal of Medicine, 354*(1), 11–22.

Sherman, J. O., & Consentino, C. M. (1993). Intussusception. In K. M. Ashcraft & T. M. Holder (Eds.), *Pediatric surgery* (2nd ed., pp. 416–420). Philadelphia: W.B. Saunders.

Stevenson, R., & Ziegler, M. Z. (1993). Abdominal pain unrelated to trauma. *Pediatrics in Review, 14*(8), 302–311.

Velazquez, F. R., Garcia-Lozano, H., Rodriguez, E., Cervantes, Y., Gomez, A., Melo, M., et al. (2004). Diarrhea morbidity and mortality in Mexican children: Impact of rotavirus disease. *Pediatric Infectious Disease Journal, 23*[10 Suppl.], 149–155.

West, K. W., & Grosfeld, J. L. (1999). Intussusception. In R. Wyllie & J. S. Hyams (Eds.), *Pediatric gastrointestinal disease: Pathophysiology, diagnosis, management* (p. 427). Philadelphia: W.B. Saunders.

Appendicitis

By Cynthia A. Bishop and Mary Ellen Carter

Abdominal pain is a frequent complaint in the pediatric population and usually presents a diagnostic dilemma. The most common cause of abdominal pain is acute gastroenteritis, although more serious cases must be excluded. Acute appendicitis is the most common condition requiring emergency surgery in childhood and adolescence, with approximately 59,000 children undergoing appendectomies each year (Popovic, 2001). The diagnosis of appendicitis should be included in the differential diagnosis in all age groups complaining of abdominal pain, but it is most common during childhood and early adulthood, usually occurring between 4 and 15 years of age (O'Neill, Grosfeld, Fonkalsrud, Coran, & Caldmone, 2004). The incidence of appendicitis is greater in males than in females (Ashcraft & Holder, 1993).

■ Pathophysiology

Appendicitis is the result of obstruction of the lumen of the vermiform appendix. The lumen is usually obstructed by a fecalith, also called an *appendicolith*, a small hardened ball of feces, or less commonly by hyperplasia of submucosal follicles occurring after a viral infection. Pinworm infestation and carcinoid tumor are rare causes of obstruction. This obstruction of the lumen results in edema, mucosal secretion, venous engorgement, and increased intraluminal pressure. Ultimately, bacteria invade through the wall of the appendix and, along with arterial infarction, leads to gangrene and perforation (Lawrence, 1993).

■ Bacteriology

The organism most commonly found when an appendix becomes gangrenous or perforated is the aerobic organism *Escherichia coli*, a gram-negative rod. As symptoms progress, multiple organisms, including *Klebsiella*, *Streptococcus*, and *Pseudomonas* are found. The most common anaerobic pathogen is *Bacteroides fragilis*, a gram-negative organism (Mosdell, 1994).

■ Classification

The stages of appendicitis have five classifications. The stage is determined during appendectomy and microscopic evaluation of the pathological specimen. See Table 26-1 for a description of the various stages of appendicitis.

Table 26-1	Stages of Appendicitis

Acute/simple: The appendix shows mild hyperemia and edema; serosal exudate is not evident.

Suppurative: The appendix is edematous, vessels are congested, and fibrin exudates form. The peritoneal fluid may be clear or turbid.

Gangrenous: In addition to the findings of suppurative appendicitis, purple or black areas of gangrene appear in the appendix wall. There may be microperforations present on microscopic examination, and the peritoneal fluid is increased and cloudy.

Perforated: There is visible perforation of the appendix wall, and the peritoneal fluid may be purulent and odorous.

Abscess: Abscess formation occurs adjacent to the perforated appendix and contains fetid pus. The abscess location can be pelvic, retrocecal, or subcecal.

■ History

A careful history and thorough physical examination are paramount in the diagnosis of appendicitis. History should be taken from both the primary caregiver and the child. The classic presentation of appendicitis begins with a gradual onset of diffuse periumbilical or epigastric pain. This is usually followed by loss of appetite, then nausea and vomiting. In time, the pain localizes to the right lower quadrant and increases in intensity. Many patients describe a change in bowel habits, usually bouts of diarrhea, which is related to pelvic inflammation. However, the amount of diarrhea is less in volume than expected with gastroenteritis. Fevers of 38° to 39° Celsius are common; however, some children do not have fever. Temperatures greater than 39° Celsius with associated peritoneal signs usually suggest perforation (Rowe, 1995). An unusual location of the appendix results in varied symptoms and creates tremendous diagnostic confusion. A retrocecal appendix can cause flank pain. Urinary symptoms may occur when the appendix tip meets the bladder. Regardless of the location of the appendix, the first site of pain with appendicitis is usually periumbilical referred pain. When the pain shifts, it localizes on the site of the appendix.

■ Physical Examination

A child with appendicitis quite often appears ill, frightened, and apprehensive. Many children are found lying on their side with their knees drawn up and flexed. It is important to perform a complete physical examination, including neck, throat, and chest examination, because other conditions, such as streptococcus pharyngitis and right middle lobe pneumonia, can mimic the symptoms of appendicitis.

A cardinal sign of appendicitis is point tenderness. This is a defined area of maximum tenderness in the right lower quadrant. This often occurs at McBurney's point, which is one third of the distance along the line from the right anterior iliac spine to the umbilicus (Lawrence, 1992).

On examination, the child exhibits right lower quadrant tenderness with palpation, coughing, and shaking. As peritoneal irritation progresses, voluntary guarding (stiffening of the rectus muscle) and rebound tenderness (pain with release of pressure) occur. The inflamed appendix causes irritation of the psoas muscle. Pain with passive extension or flexion of the right leg is a positive psoas sign. If the inflamed appendix should lie on the obturator internus muscle, pain may be elicited on passive internal rotation of the flexed thigh. This is the obturator sign. A positive Rovsing's sign (pain in the right lower quadrant during palpation of the left lower quadrant) also suggests appendicitis (Bates, 1991). Auscultation generally demonstrates diminished bowel sounds, but an obviously silent abdomen suggests peritonitis (Bates). A rectal examination may also elicit tenderness of the right vault or a pelvic abscess. It can also rule out constipation and fecal impaction as a cause of abdominal pain. A rectal examination aids in diagnosing a pelvic mass. Teenage girls who are sexually active need a thorough pelvic examination to rule out bacterial infections.

■ Laboratory Findings

Laboratory tests may be helpful in the diagnosis of appendicitis when combined with physical findings. A white blood cell count greater than 10,000/cubic millimeter may be indicative of appendicitis but is not specific. The combination of an elevated white blood cell count along with an increased neutrophil ratio and elevated C-reactive protein has shown a higher positive predictive value (Anderson, 2004; Khan, Davie, & Irshad, 2004; Mohammed, Daghman, Aboud, & Oshibi, 2004; van den Broek, van der Ende, Bijnen, Breslau, & Gouma, 2004; Wu, Chang, & Lin, 2003). A urinalysis is also important because elevated white blood cells (10,000 to 20,000/cubic millimeter), hematuria, and nitrates may be consistent with a urinary tract infection, which may mimic appendicitis symptoms (Lawrence, 1993). Urinary tract symptoms may not totally exclude appendicitis, however, but may indicate positioning of the inflamed appendix in close proximity to the right distal ureter or bladder.

All adolescent and adult females should have a beta human chorionic gonadotropin level determination to rule out pregnancy.

■ Radiographic Findings

Several radiologic tests may aid in the diagnosis of appendicitis, including abdominal and chest radiography, abdominal ultrasonography, computed tomography, and barium enema. Abdominal radiographs are often nonspecific unless a calcified fecalith is visualized (Fig. 26-1). This occurs in a small percentage of patients. Other abdominal radiographic findings include mild distention of loops of small bowel and obliteration of the right psoas muscle shadow. Ultrasonography identifies an acutely inflamed appendix by visualizing a noncompressible, tubular structure at the point of maximal tenderness. If the appendix diameter is greater than 6 mm and evidence of free fluid is noted, appendicitis is confirmed (Fig. 26-2). Ultrasound can also be used to rule out pelvic inflammatory disease or ovarian torsion or cysts in females. Ultrasound may be limited by the position of the appendix (retrocecal), abdominal guarding, excessive bowel gas, obesity, inadequate bladder filling, or an uncooperative patient (Sivit, 1993). Results may also be dependent on the experience and the expertise of the sonographer.

When the diagnosis is still unclear, an abdominal computed tomographic scan (Figs. 26-3 and 26-4) should be obtained (Friedland, 1997). The use of oral, rectal, or intravenous contrast may increase the accuracy of results, but the accuracy of unenhanced, focused, helical

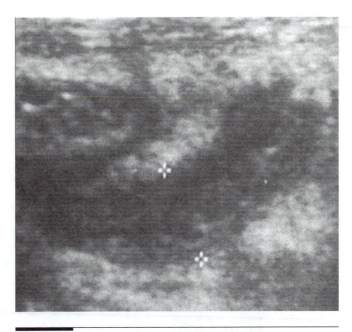

Figure 26-2 Ultrasound showing "thickened appendix" positive for appendicitis.

computed tomography without contrast has been reported to be similar to that of enhanced computed tomography in children (Hoecker & Billman, 2005; Rosendahl, Aukland, & Fosse, 2004). Barium enemas are rarely used in this era. Historically, if the lumen of the appendix does not fill with barium, or partially fills, indicating perforation, appendicitis is confirmed. A chest radiograph is needed to rule out right middle lobe pneumonia when abdominal pain and respiratory signs and symptoms are involved.

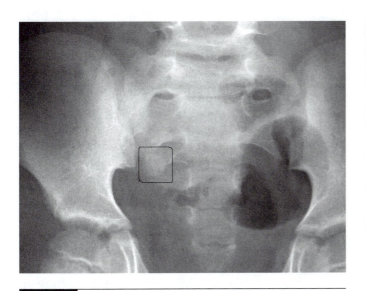

Figure 26-1 Radiograph showing appendicolith.

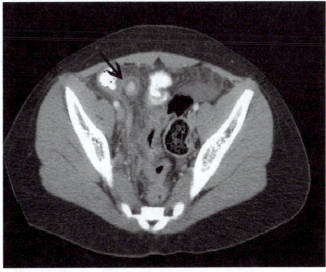

Figure 26-3 "Target sign," fecalith next to cecum filled with contrast.

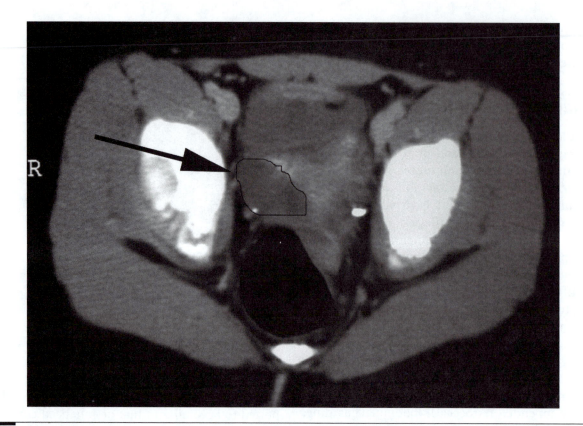

Figure 26-4 Free fluid between rectum and bladder with mesentery stranding, indicating perforation.

■ Differential Diagnosis

Gastroenteritis is the most common cause of abdominal pain in children and can often be mistaken for appendicitis (Mones, 1991). Children with gastroenteritis have abdominal pain that coincides with or occurs after vomiting. Diarrhea in gastroenteritis is usually high volume and frequent; diarrhea is low volume and irritative in appendicitis.

Fever, leukocytosis, and dysuria are common in patients with urinary tract infections and appendicitis. Careful examination, including evaluation of flank pain and urinalysis, may indicate urinary tract infection.

Constipation is a common cause of abdominal pain in the school-aged child and adolescent and can be accompanied by fever, vomiting, and leukocytosis. Usually, right lower quadrant pain experienced as a result of constipation persists but fails to progress. Fecal masses can sometimes be palpated in smaller children. Stool in the rectal vault can be noted on rectal examination. Abdominal radiographs can confirm constipation.

Pelvic inflammatory disease mimics appendicitis. Adolescents with pelvic inflammatory disease have pain in both lower quadrants and fever. Cervical and adnexal tenderness is noted on rectal examination. Pelvic examination may reveal cervical discharge and positive cultures.

Pneumonia of the right middle or lower lobe causes referred pain to the abdomen. Respiratory symptoms and associated radiographic findings can confirm appendicitis or pneumonia.

Intussusception is a common cause of abdominal pain in children younger than 3 years of age. The symptoms are usually intermittent severe colicky pain, abdominal mass in the right lower quadrant, and bloody stools. Radiologic intervention is diagnostic and often therapeutic.

Although uncommon in the child younger than 3 years, appendicitis must still be included in the differential diagnosis of infants and toddlers who present with abdominal pain, tenderness, and vomiting (Alloo, Gerstle, Shilyansky, & Ein, 2004). Mesenteric adenitis is a condition that is most likely due to viral infection and causes mild abdominal symptoms. Inflammation of the lymph nodes clustered in the mesentery of the terminal ileum is noted. This can be diagnosed by ultrasonography or is frequently confirmed during surgery. Other conditions that mimic appendicitis in childhood include ovarian cyst, midmonth cycle ovulation (mittelschmerz), inflammatory bowel disease, Meckel's diverticulum, cholecystitis, pancreatitis, and sickle cell disease with pain during crisis (Zitelli, 1992).

■ Treatment

The child with suspected appendicitis should be observed closely, including vital signs and temperature. Intravenous hydration should be administered while maintaining NPO status. Serial abdominal examinations should be performed and monitored along with follow-up diagnostic studies. Children with viral gastroenteritis usually improve with intravenous fluid hydration. The child with appendicitis usually does not improve, aiding in the confirmation of appendicitis.

Preoperative antibiotics should be administered to all patients with presumed appendicitis. Clinical experience demonstrates that prophylactic and perioperative antibiotics reduce the infectious complications of appendicitis (Soderquist-Elinder, 1995). Commonly, cephalosporins or triple antibiotics (ampicillin, gentamicin, and clindamycin) are administered (O'Neill et al., 2004).

■ Operative Procedure

Laparoscopic appendectomy has gained wide acceptance in recent years for the treatment of early and advanced appendicitis. Operative time and complication rates are essentially the same for laparoscopic and open procedures. Operative costs are generally slightly higher for laparoscopy but length of stay may be shorter (O'Neill et al., 2004; Sauerland, Lefering, & Neugebauer, 2004). Laparoscopy allows for better visualization and exploration of other intra-abdominal structures and is often advantageous in the obese patient (Emil et al., 2003; O'Neill et al.). Laparoscopic appendectomy can be performed through either a three-port, a two-port, or a one-port approach. With the three-port approach, a 12-French port is placed through the umbilicus or the left lower quadrant, with the umbilicus preferred from a cosmetic viewpoint. Two other 5-mm ports are placed, one in the right mid-abdomen and the other in the left lower quadrant or umbilicus, depending on where the first port was placed. A stapler is used to divide the mesoappendix and then across the base of the appendix (O'Neill et al.).

The two-port technique uses a 5-mm port in the umbilicus and a 10-mm port in the right lower quadrant. The appendix is brought up through the 10-mm site as the port is removed (Fig. 26-5), and an extracorporeal appendectomy is performed (O'Neill et al., 2004). Using

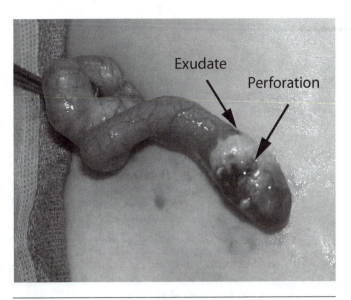

Figure 26-5 Inflamed appendix with inflammatory exudates and perforation.
(Reprinted with permission by Allen F. Browne.)

the one-port approach, the base of the appendix is tied and divided under the umbilical incision and held under direct vision. The appendix is then freed and delivered through the umbilical incision (Stomi et al., 2001).

Open appendectomy is performed using a transverse right lower quadrant incision. The abdominal muscle and peritoneum are opened. The cecum is identified. The inflamed appendix is identified, isolated, clamped, divided, and tied. A purse-string suture is placed in the cecal wall, and the base of the appendiceal stump is inverted into the cecal wall. The muscle layers are closed, and the skin layer is closed in a running subcuticular fashion (Rowe, 1995).

In the patient with perforated appendix, peritoneal cultures before irrigation have been shown to be of little benefit (Fig. 26-6) (O'Neill et al., 2004). Intraperitoneal drains may be placed in the pelvis and pericolic gutter to provide intra-abdominal abscess drainage (Chen, Botelho, Cooper, Hibberd, & Parsons, 2003). Few institutions continue the use of delayed primary closure of wounds in which the wound is left open and packed with wet-to-dry dressings. As healing and granulation occur, the skin is later closed. This usually necessitates delayed hospital discharge, frequent dressing changes, discomfort for the child, and less than satisfying cosmetic results (Chen et al.).

■ Appendiceal Abscess

Patients who have a perforated appendix and a walled-off abscess are managed conservatively with computed

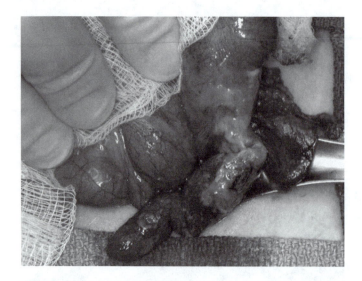

Figure 26-6 Grossly perforated appendix at operation.
(Reprinted with permission by Allen F. Browne.)

tomography-guided or ultrasound-guided percutaneous drainage of the abscess and/or drain placement. Parenteral antibiotics are administered until the fever defervesces and the white blood cell count diminishes. Normal diet is resumed when abdominal pain resolves and appetite returns. Drains are removed after output decreases. When pain is adequately controlled and diet is tolerated, the patient may be discharged to complete the course of parenteral antibiotics at home after placement of a peripherally inserted central catheter. Some practitioners prescribe an additional 1 to 2 weeks of oral antibiotics. An interval appendectomy is planned in 6 to 8 weeks when the inflammatory process has subsided (O'Neill et al., 2004).

■ Postoperative Management

In the immediate postoperative period, the child undergoing an appendectomy for acute appendicitis receives intravenous hydration and may, depending on surgeon preference, receive antibiotic therapy until the fever defervesces, usually 24 hours. Clear fluids are begun, and the child is advanced to a regular diet as tolerated. Pain medication is administered as needed. Ambulation is encouraged the first few hours after surgery. A dry, sterile dressing covers the incision or incisions as in the case of a laparoscopic procedure. These should be observed for any excess drainage. Minimal serosanguinous drainage is normal. Discharge usually occurs within 24 to 48 hours of surgery when the child is tolerating a regular diet, afebrile, and receiving effective pain control using oral medications (Borkowski, 1994). The patient with a gangrenous or perforated appendix requires more aggressive

postoperative management. Vital signs should be monitored every 4 hours, including temperature. Aggressive postoperative fluid rehydration should be provided at maintenance or maintenance and one half to maintain adequate urine output.

Antibiotic coverage for the child with gangrenous or perforated appendicitis remains controversial among pediatric surgeons. Choices of antibiotic, duration, and route of administration are variable. Broad-spectrum antibiotics are recommended with anaerobic and aerobic organisms. The standard of choice is the combination of ampicillin, gentamicin, and either clindamycin or metronidazole (Emil et al., 2003; Muehlstedt, Pham, & Schmeling, 2004). Penicillin-allergic children are treated with gentamicin and clindamycin. The use of single, broad-spectrum antibiotic therapy, piperacillin-tazobactam, is rising in use as its efficacy and ability to be used in the home care setting are documented (Fishman, Pelosi, Klavon, & O'Rourke, 2000).

Length of treatment also varies by physician preference, but the majority base termination of antibiotic coverage on clinical parameters. These indicators are resolution of ileus, normal white blood cell count and differential, and afebrile status for 24 hours (Chen et al., 2003; Muehlstedt et al., 2004). Others use an established protocol requiring administration of antibiotics for a set duration, with or without conversion to oral antibiotics in the home (Rice et al., 2001).

Fevers are expected in the first few days after surgery as a result of fluid shifts and because of the extent of the peritonitis from the perforation. A prolonged ileus may be expected after the surgery because of the irritation of bowel by the peritonitis. Many children require nasogastric tube decompression for the first few days. When bowel function resumes, the nasogastric tube is discontinued and a clear liquid diet is initiated. Diet is advanced slowly to regular as the child tolerates.

Pulmonary toilet, including incentive spirometry, coughing, deep breathing, and early ambulation, is encouraged. Children who have significant peritonitis may have a sympathetic pleural effusion develop in the base of either lung. This is another potential source of fever and requires aggressive pulmonary toilet and continued antibiotics. Meticulous wound inspection, whether it be a closed or open wound, with or without drains, is important. The site should be observed for erythema, warmth, purulent drainage, and increased tenderness.

Intravenous pain medication, morphine or ketorolac tromethamine (Toradol), is used during the first few days after surgery. The transition to oral pain medication occurs with tolerance of fluids.

Discharge Instructions

Families are instructed to notify the surgeon or primary care physician if the child has a fever greater than 38.5° Celsius, emesis, diarrhea, new onset of abdominal pain, or anorexia. They are also to notify the surgeon if erythema, warmth, increased tenderness, or purulent drainage is noted around the incision. Children are allowed to bathe 3 to 5 days after surgery with long soaks of the incision(s) occurring after 7 days. Children are usually able to return to school within 1 week after discharge. Physical education, recess, sports, and lifting of weights totaling greater than 5 to 10 pounds should be limited for 2 of 4 weeks after surgery because of healing of the abdominal muscles.

Complications

Over the past three decades, the mortality rate of appendicitis has diminished such that it is now almost never the primary cause of death in children. Complications relate to the duration of symptoms and the expediency of treatment and diagnosis. These factors are primary determinants of the likelihood of rupture (Kokoska et al., 1998).

Intra-abdominal abscess is considered in the patient after treatment for a perforated appendicitis with fever, abdominal pain, irritability, leukocytosis, anorexia, and emesis. A rectal examination may elicit tenderness, or a mass and focal tenderness on palpation may be helpful in the diagnosis of an abscess. An abdominal computed tomography or ultrasonography can confirm the presence, size, and location of the fluid collection. If the abscess is accessible, a percutaneous or transrectal drain is inserted into the collection under fluoroscopy, and antibiotic coverage is started (Jamieson, Chait, & Filler, 1997). Antibiotic coverage continues for 7 to 10 days and can be transitioned to the home environment once the patient reaches discharge criteria.

A wound infection can occur a few days after surgery and manifest with erythema, warmth, purulent drainage, and increased tenderness. If the wound is open and the pus is noted, cultures should be obtained and the wound should be irrigated and then packed to allow slow granulation and closure by secondary intention. Antibiotics may be reinstituted or changed on the basis of cultures and sensitivities.

A side effect of administering broad-spectrum antibiotics is *Clostridium difficile* colitis. Patients have profuse, liquid, foul-smelling diarrhea, abdominal pain, and fever. This occurs because broad-spectrum antibiotics disrupt the normal colonic flora, allowing *C. difficile*, a spore-forming anaerobe, to colonize the colon causing mucosal inflammation and subsequent diarrhea (Infection Control Newsletter, 1996). If *C. difficile* toxin assessment is positive, the treatment is oral metronidazole for 7 to 10 days and rehydration. Symptoms resolve within 24 to 48 hours of treatment.

Other noted complications that can arise in the child with appendicitis are pneumonia, adynamic ileus, and intestinal obstructions. Management of these entities is condition specific, and awareness of these complications is key to good patient care.

Research

Prospective studies, which encourage decreased length of stay and better use of health care dollars, need to continue in this time of managed care. This methodology may provide the means to reduce overall costs as well as to improve quality of care outcomes by minimizing variability in diagnosis and practice (Warner et al., 1998; Warner, Rich, Atherton, Anderson, & Kotagal, 2002). Quality clinical outcomes need collaborative initiatives to develop widely accepted standards of practice (Newman et al., 2003). Nurses must continue to actively participate and lead in the development and ongoing evaluation of these outcomes for children with acute appendicitis.

Conclusion

Children undergoing appendectomies account for a large percentage of pediatric surgical patients. The management of these children may seem routine to some but continues to change as evidence-based research refocuses our care. It is the experienced nurse who will continue to provide excellent care backed by strong clinical knowledge. Quality care must include family-centered educational and emotional support to the family and child undergoing this surgery.

Acknowledgment

The authors would like to recognize the contribution of Luanne Pelosi, who authored this chapter in this textbook's first edition.

Educational Material

APSNA invites you to download the following diagnosis-related teaching tool for Chapter 26, Appendicitis: 1) Appendectomy. This teaching tool is available at the

APSNA Web site (www.apsna.org) and the Jones and Bartlett Web site (www.jbpub.com). All teaching materials are available in English and Spanish and are free of charge. APSNA encourages their use for your patients and families.

■ References

Alloo, J., Gerstle, T., Shilyansky, J., & Ein, S. H. (2004). Appendicitis in children less than 3 years of age: A 28-year review. *Pediatric Surgery International, 19*, 777–779.

Anderson, R. E. (2004). Meta analysis of the clinical and laboratory diagnosis of appendicitis. *British Journal of Surgery, 91*, 28–37.

Ashcraft, K. W., & Holder, T. M. (1993). *Pediatric surgery* (2nd ed.). New York: W.B. Saunders.

Bates, B. (1991). *A guide to physical examination and history taking* (5th ed.). Philadelphia: Lippincott-Raven.

Borkowski, S. (1994). Common pediatric surgical problems. *Nursing Clinics of North America, 29*, 560–562.

Chen, C., Botelho, C., Cooper, A., Hibberd, P., & Parsons, S. K. (2003). Current practice patterns in the treatment of perforated appendicitis in children. *Journal of the American College of Surgeons, 196*, 212–221.

Emil, S., Laberge, J. M., Mikhail, P., Baican, I., Flageole, H., & Nguyen, I. (2003). Appendicitis in children: A ten-year update of therapeutic recommendations. *Journal of Pediatric Surgery, 38*, 236–242.

Fishman, S. J., Pelosi, L., Klavon, S. L., & O'Rourke, E. J. (2000). Perforated appendicitis: Prospective outcome analysis for 150 children. *Journal of Pediatric Surgery, 35*, 923–926.

Friedland, J. A. (1997). CT appearance of acute appendicitis in childen. *American Journal of Radiology, 168*, 439–441.

Hoecker, C. C., & Billman, G. F. (2005). The utility of unenhanced computed tomography in appendicitis in children. *The Journal of Emergency Medicine, 28*, 415–421.

Infection Control Newsletter. (1996). *Children's hospital, 4*(5).

Jamieson, D. H., Chait, P. G., & Filler, R. (1997). Interventional drainage of appendiceal abscesses in children. *American Journal of Radiology, 169*, 1619–1622.

Khan, M. N., Davie, E., & Irshad, K. (2004). The role of white cell count and c-reactive protein in the diagnosis of acute appendicitis. *Journal of Ayub Medical College, Abbottabad, 16*, 17–19.

Kokoska, E. R., Silen, M. L., Tracy, T. F., Dillon, P. A., Cradock, T. V., & Weber, T. R. (1998). Perforated appendicitis in children: Risk factors for the development of complications. *Surgery, 124*, 619–626.

Lawrence, P. F. (1992). *Essentials of surgery* (2nd ed.). Baltimore: Williams & Wilkins.

Lawrence, P. F. (1993). *Essential surgical specialties*. Baltimore: Williams & Wilkins.

Mohammed, A. A., Daghman, N. A., Aboud, S. M., & Oshibi, H. O. (2004). The diagnostic value of c-reactive protein, white blood cell count and neutrophil percentage in childhood appendicitis. *Saudi Medical Journal, 25*, 1212–1215.

Mones, R. L. (1991, August). Acute abdomen in children. Appendicitis and beyond. *Emergency Medicine*, 179–186.

Mosdell, D. M. (1994). Peritoneal cultures and antibiotic therapy in pediatric perforated appendicitis. *The American Journal of Surgery, 167*, 313–316.

Muehlstedt, S. G., Pham, T. Q., & Schmeling, D. J. (2004). The management of pediatric appendicitis: A survey of North American pediatric surgeons. *Journal of Pediatric Surgery, 39*, 875–879.

Newman, K., Ponsky, T., Kittle, K., Dyk, L., Throop, C., Gieseker, K., et al. (2003). Appendicitis 2000: Variability in practice, outcomes, and resource utilization at thirty pediatric hospitals. *Journal of Pediatric Surgery, 38*(3), 372–379.

O'Neill, J. A., Grosfeld, J. L., Fonkalsrud, E. W., Coran, A. G., & Caldmone, A. A. (Eds.). (2004). *Principles of pediatric surgery* (2nd ed.). St. Louis, MO: Mosby.

Popovic, J. R. (2001). 1999 national hospital discharge survey: Annual summary with detailed diagnosis and procedure data. *Vital Health Statistics Series 13, 151*, 1–206.

Rice, H. R., Brown, R. L., Gollin, G., Caty, M. G., Gilbert, J., Skinner, M. A., et al. (2001). Results of a pilot trial comparing prolonged intravenous antibiotics with sequential intravenous/oral antibiotics for children with perforated appendicitis. *Archives of Surgery, 136*, 1391–1395.

Rosendahl, K., Aukland, S. M., & Fosse, K. (2004). Imaging strategies in children with suspected appendicitis. *European Radiology, 14*, L138–L145.

Rowe, M. I. (1995). *Essentials of pediatric surgery*. St. Louis, MO: Mosby.

Sauerland, S., Lefering, R., & Neugebauer, E. A. (2004). Laparoscopic versus open surgery for suspected appendicitis. *The Cochrane Database of Systematic Reviews, 4*.

Sivit, C. J. (1993). Diagnosis of acute appendicitis in children: Spectrum of sonographic findings. *American Journal of Roentgenology, 161*, 147–152.

Soderquist-Elinder, C. (1995). Prophylactic antibiotics in uncomplicated appendicitis in childhood. *The European Journal of Pediatric Surgery, 5*, 282–285.

Stomi, A., Tanimizu, T., Takahashi, S., Kawase, H., Murai, H., Yonekawa, H., et al. (2001). One-port laparoscopy-assisted appendectomy in children with appendicitis: Experience with 100 cases. *Pediatric Endosurgery & Innovative Techniques, 5*(4), 371–377.

van den Broek, W. T., van der Ende, E. D., Bijnen, A. B., Breslau, P. J., & Gouma, D. J. (2004). Which children could benefit from additional diagnostic tools in cases of suspected appendicitis? *Journal of Pediatric Surgery, 39*, 570–574.

Warner, B. W., Kulick, R. M., Stoops, M. M., Mehta, S., Stephan, M., & Kotagal, U. R. (1998). An evidenced-based clinical pathway for acute appendicitis decreases hospital duration and cost. *Journal of Pediatric Surgery, 33*, 1371–1375.

Warner, B. W., Rich, K. A., Atherton, H., Anderson, C. L., & Kotagal, U. R. (2002). The sustained impact of an evidenced-based clinical pathway for acute appendicitis. *Seminars in Pediatric Surgery, 11*, 29–35.

Wu, H. P., Chang, C. F., & Lin, C. Y. (2003). Predictive inflammatory parameters in the diagnosis of acute appendicitis in children. *Acta Paediatrica Taiwanica, 44*, 227–231.

Zitelli, B. J. (1992). *Atlas of pediatric physical diagnosis* (5th ed.). Philadelphia: Lippincott-Raven.

Splenectomy, Cholecystectomy, and Meckel's Diverticulum

By Mary E. Otten and Marilyn Miller Stoops

Advances in pediatric surgery offer new approaches in the management of children requiring splenectomy, cholecystectomy, or a diverticulectomy and excision of Meckel's diverticulum. This chapter provides an overview of the indications for each of these surgical procedures, including the laparoscopic approach, and nursing care of children who undergo splenectomy, cholecystectomy, and excision of Meckel's diverticulum.

◼ Splenectomy

Embryology and Pathophysiology of the Spleen

Embryologic development of the spleen begins during the fifth week of gestation. It is lobulated at first and assumes its characteristic shape early in the fetal period (Moore & Persaud, 1993). As the spleen grows, it is carried into the left upper quadrant of the abdomen with visceral relationships to the greater curvature of the stomach, the tail of the pancreas, the left kidney, and the splenic flexure of the colon. The spleen consists of a capsule, connective tissue framework, and parenchyma. The normal size and weight of the spleen vary between children and closely correlate with the size of the child. The mean weight is 11 g at birth, 55 g by the age of 6 years, and 125 g by adult age. The tip of the spleen is palpable on deep inspiration in 3% to 5% of normal children and adolescents (Pearson, 2002). One way to assess normal splenic size is to measure the length of the spleen as compared with the left kidney by ultrasound, with the upper limit of normal for the spleen/kidney ratio being 1.25 (Loftus & Metreweli, 1998).

The spleen provides several important functions. It functions as the hematopoietic center until late fetal life and retains this potential for blood cell formation into adult life (Moore & Persaud, 1993). By birth, most blood cells are produced by the bone marrow. The spleen is the largest of the secondary lymphoid organs, with mononuclear phagocytes to filter and cleanse the blood and lymphocytes for immune response to blood-borne microorganisms. During the first few years of life, when specific circulating antibodies against polysaccharide-encapsulated organisms, such as *Streptococcus pneumoniae* and *Haemophilus influenzae*, have not developed, phagocytosis of these organisms during bacteremia occurs almost exclusively in the spleen. It is a major source of production of IgM and properdin as well as formation of antibodies against particulate intravenous antigens. The spleen may also play an important role in the production of autoantibodies, found in idiopathic thrombocytopenic purpura (ITP) and autoimmune hemolytic anemia (Pearson, 2002). To cleanse the blood, it performs a unique pitting role by removing a variety of intraerythrocytic red blood cell (RBC) inclusions (e.g., Howell-Jolly bodies and Heinz bodies).

The spleen is the principal site of the destruction of senescent RBCs, which cannot traverse the splenic cords. This RBC destruction can be greatly exaggerated in states associated with abnormally rigid RBC, such as spherocytosis, or in hemolytic anemias with antibody-coated RBCs (Pearson, 2002). It also serves as a blood reservoir (McCancre & Huether, 1990). The spleen contains about 50 mL of blood and about 30% of the circulating platelet pool. In people with splenomegaly, the splenic reservoir may be significantly increased, resulting in an apparent anemia, neutropenia, and thrombocytopenia (Pearson).

The spleen can be affected during fetal development (congenitally) or can develop functional problems after birth. During fetal development, rare congenital conditions of asplenia, polysplenia, and heterotaxia can occur, which are usually associated with congenital heart disease. Asplenic infants are at high risk for fulminant bacterial septicemia and should receive prophylactic antibiotics. Polysplenic infants are not at an increased infection risk but often develop biliary atresia (Pearson, 2002). A wandering spleen, *splenic ectopia*, refers to the spleen being mobile and present anywhere in the abdomen other than the left upper quadrant, probably related to failure of the suspensory ligaments to form properly. This condition is generally associated with either a sudden onset or chronic intermittent abdominal pain caused by torsion affecting perfusion. If the spleen is found to have viable and functional tissue, it can be salvaged with a splenopexy, which places it in the normal anatomic position (Rice, 2005).

Accessory spleens are found in as many as 10% to 15% of individuals. They resemble small nodules of splenic tissue that are most commonly found around the splenic hilum or the tail of the pancreas (Ein, 1993). They resemble lymph nodes but may be as large as 10 cm (Ein). Accessory spleens function in the same manner as the spleen, requiring them to be removed at the time of splenectomy for any reason other than trauma to avoid any future splenic-related complications (Ein). The spleen can be adversely affected by a number of disorders, such as sickle cell anemia, causing its function to diminish to the point of functional asplenia or hyposplenia which increases the risks of infection.

Hypersplenia occurs most commonly with congestive splenomegaly with peripheral cytopenias, despite effective bone marrow production, but it is observed in other disorders as well (Pearson, 2002). Because asplenic children are at great risk of developing overwhelming sepsis, splenectomies are performed only when absolutely necessary. There has been a recent trend toward partial splenectomy to retain the phagocytic properties of the remaining spleen.

Indications for Splenectomy

Indications for splenectomy can be divided into medical/hematologic and surgical categories. The common medical hematologic disorders that may necessitate splenectomy include congenital hemolytic anemias, hereditary spherocytosis and other severe hemolytic diseases, sequestration crisis of sickle cell anemia, acquired immunologic disease, chronic idiopathic thrombocytopenic purpura, autoimmune hemolytic anemia, hypersplenic syndromes, Gaucher's disease, thalassemia major and intermedia, and congestive splenomegaly. The common surgical reasons for splenectomy include splenic cysts, tumors, exposure shunting for portal hypertension, relief of mechanical symptoms because of size, as in chronic juvenile myelogenous leukemia and Hodgkin's disease, and splenic trauma (Pearson, 2002).

Splenectomies are largely performed on an elective basis and, rarely, emergently. One reason for emergency pediatric splenectomy is ITP with major bleeding in the central nervous system, especially intracranial bleeding. Acute ITP is a disease of children that often follows a viral infection. Acute ITP lasts a few weeks to 1 or 2 months and has no residual effects. Chronic ITP affects adolescents and adults, begins insidiously, and lasts longer. Corticosteroid treatment is usually effective, but, occasionally, splenectomy is the treatment of choice (Zamir et al., 1996). More than 80% of children affected with ITP respond to corticosteroid treatment within a few days to several weeks of treatment (Ben-Yehuda, Gillis, & Eldor, 1990). The spleen is a major organ for platelet destruction and a site for antiplatelet antibody production (Bussel, 1990). Splenectomy has long been used as an effective therapeutic modality, with complete remission being achieved in 75% to 90% of patients undergoing splenectomy (Ben-Yehuda et al.; Chirletti et al., 1992). The indications for splenectomy in ITP include lack of response to medical treatment, decrease in platelet count while attempting to taper the corticosteroids, or severe side effects of steroid therapy (Ben-Yehuda et al.). To aid in decisions about splenectomy, the response of a patient with chronic ITP to intravenous immunoglobulin (IVIG) treatment has been found to help predict the response to splenectomy (Holt et al., 2003).

Children who sustain a splenic injury undergo splenectomy if the injury is too severe for splenic salvage. Splenic trauma from blunt force can cause a wide range of injuries, from subcapsular hemorrhage to total fracture and maceration of the spleen, which can be diagnosed by splenic scintigraphy (TcScan), computed tomography, or ultrasound. Children with enlarged spleens, which are not protected by their rib cage, are at increased risk of splenic trauma after relatively minor incidences. Almost all other children with blunt splenic trauma can be managed conservatively with inpatient observation, bed rest, and transfusions as necessary to maintain circulatory stability. Long-term follow-up of children treated nonoperatively has not revealed significant numbers of late complications (Pearson, 2002).

A small number of children who cannot be clinically stabilized and those with multiple organ injury require surgery. Emergency situations can progress to massive internal hemorrhage, resulting in hypovolemic shock. In some instances, splenic repair or partial splenectomy may be possible (Pearson, 2002). If a trauma-related emergency splenectomy is indicated, it would typically be a traditional open splenectomy as opposed to a laparoscopic procedure. Splenosis, the growth of splenic tissue within the abdominal cavity, has been noted with the fragmentation of the spleen from trauma. Although the spleen tissue implants, grows, and appears histologically normal, the spleen immune function to clear encapsulated bacteria does not occur (Arzoumanian & Rosenthall, 1995; Soutter, Ellenbogen, & Folkman, 1994). These patients are treated as in asplenia with prophylactic antibiotics and vaccines. The incidence of mortality from septicemia is increased 50-fold in children who have undergone splenectomy after trauma (Peter, 1997).

There are many indications for elective splenectomy, but the most common are hereditary spherocytosis and sickle cell anemia. Spherocytosis is the presence of spherocytes in the blood. Spherocytes are completely hemoglobinated erythrocytes in the blood that are abnormally fragile and break down, leading to jaundice and splenomegaly. Some have mild cases of anemia, whereas others may experience acute aplastic and hemolytic crisis precipitated by infections and then require blood transfusions. Because of the risk of postsplenectomy sepsis in young children, the current recommendation is to wait until after the age of 5 to 6 years, unless severe anemia warrants early intervention, and to evaluate the gallbladder owing to the frequency of gallstone development (Mehta & Gittes, 2005).

Rice et al. (2003) reported successful partial splenectomy treatment in all 25 children in their study. Partial splenectomy appeared to control hemolysis while retaining splenic function in children with hereditary spherocytosis, as well as appearing to control symptoms and splenic sequestration in children with other hemolytic anemias. Partial splenectomy may decrease the initial need for blood transfusions while preserving immune function, but follow-up has shown only a short-term benefit due to regrowth of the splenic remnant, and the procedure is used only where the benefit of postponing the splenectomy is desired (de Buys Roessingh, de Lagausie, Rohrlich, Berrebi, & Aigrain, 2002).

Sickle cell disease is a hereditary, genetically determined hemolytic anemia, largely occurring in the African-American population, in which the erythrocytes are sickle shaped and become clumped in the vascular system, causing arthralgia, attacks of abdominal pain, and splenomegaly (Ein, 1993; Peter, 1997). When the erythrocytes sickle and become sequestered in the spleen, the spleen enlarges with progressive infarction and gradual loss of total function with atrophy, usually after approximately 10 years.

The most common indication for splenectomy is acute splenic sequestration crisis, in which severe anemia and splenomegaly develop with associated hypersplenism and thrombocytopenia so severe that it could lead to circulatory collapse and death. Though rare, acute splenic sequestration crisis is the leading cause of death in patients with sickle cell disease who are younger than 10 years. Severe acute splenic sequestration crisis attacks have a 40% to 50% risk of recurrence and a 20% mortality rate. After recovery from a severe attack or after two mild attacks, these patients should undergo splenectomy (Mehta & Gittes, 2005).

Sickle cell patients with significant transfusion requirements due to hypersplenism from splenomegaly may also require splenectomy to decrease their increased risks of transfusion complications. Partial splenectomy has been advocated in these patients because of their high risk of postsplenectomy sepsis (Idowu & Hayes-Jordan, 1998; Svarch et al., 1996). In up to 20% of sickle cell patients, abdominal surgery poses a significant risk of acute chest syndrome as a postoperative complication, whether the procedure has been performed laparoscopically or open (Wales, Carver, Crawford, & Kim, 2001). A study by Crawford, Speakman, Carver, and Kim (2004) reported an overall incidence of acute chest syndrome in 16% of their patients after splenectomy and cholecystectomy (7 of 48 splenectomy patients and 9 of 51 cholecystectomy patients). The mean onset was 49 hours after surgery with symptoms of cough and fever and an abnormal chest examination noted in all cases involving the basal lobes with a predilection for lung regions on the side of surgery.

Elective splenectomy may offer relief for patients with Gaucher's disease. Gaucher's disease is a genetically acquired storage disease that results in massive accumulation of glucocerebroside in the reticuloendothelial system, the bone marrow, and the central nervous system. Massive splenomegaly and hepatomegaly develop because of deposition of lipids in these organs. Holcomb and Greene (1993) noted that until recently, total splenectomy has been recommended to manage hypersplenism-associated anemia and thrombocytopenia. Currently, because the risk of postsplenectomy sepsis is so great, partial splenectomy has been used in the treatment of children with hypersplenism. Partial splenectomy for type I Gaucher's disease, which is the most common, has been found to be successful, whereas its use for type III Gaucher's disease, the rarest form of disease, remains in question (Holcomb & Greene). Studies have reported that total splenectomy offers considerable relief and improvement, but partial splenectomy may only temporize symptoms with a common finding of recurrence (Rice et al., 1996; Lorberboym et al., 1997). Type I Gaucher's disease is characterized by hepatosplenomegaly in almost all patients. Children with this form usually are seen in middle to late childhood and may have a normal life expectancy. Type III Gaucher's disease results in progressive neurologic decline early in life (Holcomb & Greene).

Thalassemia patients benefit from spleen procedures to improve symptoms of hypersplenism. The genetic hemoglobinopathies of thalassemia, classified as major, minor, or intermedia forms, can cause diffuse deposits of iron in the spleen and engorgement with destroyed red blood cells. In severe cases, transfusion requirements increase as more erythrocyte sequestration develops with hypersplenism. Partial splenectomy, partial splenic embolization, and partial dearterialization of the spleen have been offered in select patients to improve symptoms yet maintain the splenic immune function to protect against postsplenectomy sepsis. However, recurrence or splenic infection may still necessitate a total splenectomy (Mehta & Gittes, 2005).

Elective splenectomy may be indicated for the child with a chronic form of leukemia, such as juvenile myelogenous leukemia. These children become so physically compromised with extremely large spleens and livers that splenectomy is performed as a palliative procedure to help keep the child mobile and as comfortable as possible for as long as possible.

Splenic involvement can occur with patients with lymphoma. In Hodgkin's disease, the spleen may become involved with malignant cells but is rarely the primary site. When the spleen is infiltrated by tumor, splenomegaly may develop. In order to maintain the benefits of intact splenic function, splenectomy is no longer part of the therapy for Hodgkin's disease as it was in the past. Recently, chemotherapy has come to be used in all stages of Hodgkin's to reduce radiation therapy doses (Mehta & Gittes, 2005).

There is a staging system for Hodgkin's disease that ranges from stages I to IV. This system is fairly reliable because the disease almost always has one focus and then spreads by a pattern through the lymphatics. The disease progression to stage III includes involvement of lymph nodes on both sides of the diaphragm, localized involvement of an extralymphatic organ or site, and/or involvement of the spleen.

In the past, staging for Hodgkin's disease was necessary by laparotomy with splenectomy because the diagnostic testing was less sophisticated for identifying the extent of the disease. Recent advances in imaging have made the use of this procedure unnecessary unless the findings would greatly alter the treatment plan. Pediatric hematologists are more likely to rely on imaging studies than surgical intervention at present.

Splenic tumors, cysts, and abscesses are all relatively rare in children. Symptomatic tumors and cysts are surgically treated with partial or total splenectomy as indicated. Splenic abscesses may be responsive to antibiotic therapy with or without percutaneous drainage as amenable. If therapy is unsuccessful, splenectomy may be indicated (Mehta & Gittes, 2005).

Preoperative Preparation

Decisions for splenic surgical intervention always take into consideration the clinical safety of preservation of sufficient splenic immune function for young children who are at increased risk of postsplenectomy sepsis. In the case of elective surgery, a polyvalent vaccine against streptococcal pneumococcus and *Haemophilus influenzae* infection should be administered 10 days to 2 weeks before surgery (Peter, 1997). In addition, a vaccine for *Neisseria meningitidis* is also recommended for those patients older than 2 years. These vaccines are safely given together and are also effective when given after splenectomy if necessary, preferably before discharge. Revaccination after 2 years is also recommended and is well tolerated (Rutherford et al., 1995). The detailed recommendations for pneumococcal, *H. influenzae* type B, and meningococcal immunizations for children undergoing splenectomy are provided by the American Academy of Pediatrics (American Academy of Pediatrics [AAP], 2000). Patients with sickle cell anemia may be required to undergo preoperative blood transfusions to improve anemia and reduce their hemoglobin S level to avoid intraoperative bleeding complications.

Preoperative preparation for laparoscopic surgery and open surgery is the same because there is always the possibility that a laparoscopic approach may need to be abandoned in favor of an open approach. Some institutions recommend giving a bowel prep regimen the evening before surgery to decrease the chance of injuring the colon with the laparoscopic equipment. Prophylactic antibiotics are administered intravenously immediately before the procedure.

Operative Procedure

The operative approach to splenectomy has recently become more varied than an open or laparoscopic total splenectomy after the advancements of spleen-saving techniques such as partial splenectomy, splenic embolization, and splenorrhaphy (Mehta & Gittes, 2005).

Laparoscopic Surgery

Surgeons have been performing laparoscopic splenectomies in children since 1992 (Tulman, Holcomb, Karamanoukian, & Reynhout, 1993). The increased frequency of these procedures has resulted in the development of new instruments and techniques that make the technical aspects more reliable and easier to perform (Schleef, Morcate, Steinau, Ott, & Willital, 1997). Various techniques have also developed with the increased frequency of the procedure. Many surgeons consider laparoscopy to be the gold standard in children, offering safety with decreased postoperative length of hospital stay and lower analgesia requirements, particularly when the spleen size is normal or only slightly enlarged (Rescorla et al., 2002). The general technique starts with appropriate patient positioning for the operation to facilitate access and retraction for the procedure, with some surgeons preferring the supine position and others the right lateral decubitus position. A Foley catheter and nasogastric tube are placed for bladder and gastric decompression. Then, an incision is made through the umbilicus, a cannula is passed, and pneumoperitoneum or air is introduced into the peritoneal cavity to 10 to 15 mm Hg. Next, a laparoscope is inserted, and then three or four small ports are inserted at various points in the abdomen. The patient is put in a steep Trendelenburg position with the left side elevated. Before starting any dissection, many surgeons complete a thorough exploration for any accessory spleens, which may require removal as indicated for the patient's illness, particularly in cases of hemolytic anemia or ITP and in certain cases of hypersplenism. The vessels and ligaments are carefully dissected, cut, and stapled or

clipped to mobilize the spleen. Care is taken to avoid any damage to the tail of the pancreas, the left kidney, and the colon as the spleen is removed. An endoscopic, puncture-resistant bag (Cook Surgical, Inc., Indianapolis, IN) is then introduced, and the spleen is placed in the bag. During all manipulations, care is taken not to spill splenic fragments into the abdominal cavity to avoid any development of splenosis.

The splenic tissue is morselized or cut into strips and suctioned out of the sac to a point where the sac can be removed. The splenic bed and pancreas are examined to be sure there is no bleeding. The trocars are then removed and the sites sutured in the standard way. Finally, the Foley catheter and nasogastric tube are removed (Smith et al., 1994).

Schleef, Morcate, Steinau, Ott, & Willital (1997) have found that using a loop of umbilical band as an atraumatic way of grasping and manipulating the spleen is an improvement over grasping the spleen with forceps, which can cause damage to the capsule and intracapsular bleeding. An instrument called a harmonic scalpel facilitates the division of blood vessels and coagulation, thus reducing blood loss (Janu, Rogers, & Lobe, 1996). Additional instruments continue to be developed to improve laparoscopic procedures.

Open Surgery

Open splenectomy requires either a midline or a left subcostal incision. Moving or mobilizing the intestines exposes the spleen, and the vessels are tied off and cut (Fig. 27-1A and B) (Ashcraft, 1994). The spleen is removed (Fig. 27-1C). The abdomen is explored for any accessory spleens with removal as indicated if they may cause any future complications for the patient. If the accessory spleens are not excised during the initial procedure, further surgery is required. After removal of the spleen and any accessory spleens, the abdomen is closed.

Partial Splenectomy

Partial splenectomy and splenorrhaphy represent surgical alternatives to total splenectomy. It is the vascular anatomy of the spleen that allows segmental vessel ligation of the artery after it splits into its upper and lower pole arteries, providing a line of demarcation to follow for a partial splenectomy. Sutures and absorbable mesh help provide hemostasis. These splenic salvage procedures are supported by the need to maintain some level of splenic immune functions to prevent postsplenectomy sepsis in trauma and other indications as previously discussed. Splenic embolization can be used in patients with portal hypertension to ablate up to 80% to 90% of the

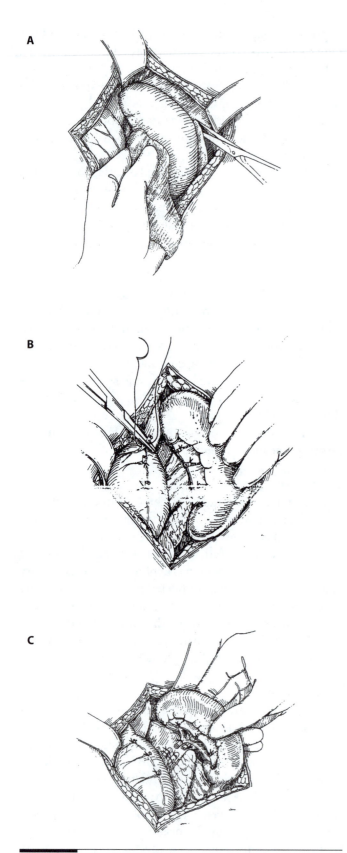

Figure 27-1 A, Open splenectomy. Exposure of spleen. B, Vessels tied off and cut. C, Removal of spleen.

(Reprinted from *Atlas of Pediatric Surgery* [2nd ed.], Ashcraft, Figures 22-3, A, B, and C, © 1994, with permission from Elsevier.)

spleen and avoid a total splenectomy in a patient with dangerously enlarged portal vein collaterals (Mehta & Gittes, 2005).

Postoperative Care

Laparoscopic patients may initially receive clear fluids a few hours after surgery and then are advanced as tolerated to a regular diet, usually by the following day. Discharge from the hospital is on day 2 or 3 with an antibiotic, usually penicillin, and analgesics.

After open surgery, the Foley catheter is removed by postoperative day 1. The nasogastric tube remains in place as needed until the return of bowel sounds. Clear liquids are given after removal of the nasogastric tube, and the diet is advanced to a regular diet as tolerated. The average hospital stay is 4 days.

Table 27-1 shows the advantages and disadvantages of laparoscopic splenectomy compared with traditional open splenectomy. Laparoscopic splenectomies appear to result in longer operative times but shorter lengths of stay, earlier first oral intake, and significantly fewer requirements for intravenous narcotics, providing a reduction in hospital charges compared with those of open splenectomy (Reddy et al., 2001). Minkes, Lagzdins, and Langer (2000) reported the hospital costs as comparable but also reported that the laparoscopic patients had a shorter length of stay.

Preventing Postsplenectomy Sepsis

Postsplenectomy sepsis, sometimes called overwhelming postsplenectomy infection (OPSI), is the most feared complication from a splenectomy because of its high mortality rates and its onset at anytime from a few days to approximately 2 years after the procedure. The risk of OPSI is greatest in infancy and slowly declines as the child reaches adulthood. Approximately 80% of OPSI occurs within 2 years after splenectomy (Ein, 1993). The more serious the underlying splenic disease, the greater the risk for the development of serious infection. Asplenic children have a morbidity rate of 1.5% to 80%, depending on the reason for which the spleen was removed (Ein). OPSI after splenectomy for trauma has the lowest rate and thalassemia has the highest rate, with all other diseases between these two extremes (Ein). The mortality rate in asplenic patients averages about 3% but can be as high as 11% (Ein). The infections are typically fulminant and are most often caused by the encapsulated organisms a healthy spleen could have produced antibodies against (Mehta & Gittes, 2005). The incidence of infection was decreased by 47% and the mortality rates were reduced by 88% with the use of routine preoperative vaccinations and pro-

Table 27-1	Advantages and Disadvantages of Laparoscopic Splenectomy in Children

Advantages of Laparoscopic Approach

- Smaller incisions, less painful than upper abdominal incisions
- Need for less pain medication after surgery
- Fewer respiratory complications
- Improved return of respiratory function
- Reduced or absent postoperative ileus
- Shorter hospital stay
- Faster return to unrestricted activities
- Small scars cosmetically more preferable
- Reduced operative exposure to bodily fluid

Disadvantages of Laparoscopic Approach

- Increased operative time
- More expensive cost of equipment
- May not be possible if splenomegaly is in advanced stage
- May require conversion to open procedure
- Possible complaints of shoulder pain

phylactic antibiotics, in a study that compared these patients with historical controls with no prophylaxis. Vaccine boosters were also a recommendation every 5 to 10 years for optimal protection (Jugenburg, Haddock, Freedman, Ford-Jones, & Ein, 1999).

Streptococcus pneumoniae is the most frequent bacteremia in infants and children older than 1 year of age (Ein, 1993). Prevention of overwhelming postsplenectomy infection caused by *Staphylococcus pneumoniae* (lancet-shaped, gram-positive diplococci) is achieved by administering pneumococcal vaccine about 2 weeks or more before the surgery (Ein). The vaccine is composed of 23 pneumococcal serotypes (Peter, 1997). There have been 84 pneumococcal serotypes identified thus far. The vaccine dose (0.5 mL) contains 25 mg of each polysaccharide antigen and is given either subcutaneously or intramuscularly. The effectiveness of this vaccine in preventing pneumonia has been demonstrated in healthy young adults and in children who are predisposed. Vaccinated children who have undergone splenectomy experience significantly less pneumococcal disease than unvaccinated children. Children 2 years of age and older should be vaccinated. The vaccine has limited immunogenicity in children younger than 2 years of age. Common side effects of the vaccine include erythema and pain at the infection site. Uncommon side effects include fever, myalgia, and severe local reactions. Anaphylaxis has rarely been reported (Peter).

Pneumococcus is the responsible organism in more than 50% of cases of OPSI. Other microorganisms causing OPSI include meningococcus, *Escherichia coli*, *H. influenzae*, *Staphylococcus*, and *Streptococcus* (Ein, 1993; Peter, 1997). Immunization with polyvalent capsular polysaccharide antigens of pneumococci (and possibly *H. influenzae* and meningococci) may be given at least several weeks before anticipated splenectomy because asplenic individuals have a diminished response to such immunization (Ein). If the child has received the entire three doses of *H. influenzae* type B vaccine, it is not necessary to revaccinate. If the child has not received the entire three doses, the immunizations should be completed before or after splenectomy. The vaccine for *N. meningitidis* is also recommended for those patients older than 2 years. All three of these vaccines are safely given together and are also effective when given after splenectomy if necessary, preferably before discharge (Rutherford et al., 1995). As noted in the preoperative discussion, the detailed recommendations for pneumococcal, *H. influenzae* type B, and meningococcal immunizations for children undergoing splenectomy are provided by the American Academy of Pediatrics (2000).

The Committee on Infectious Diseases of the American Academy of Pediatrics (Peter, 1994, 1997) emphasizes that vaccination does not guarantee protection from fulminant pneumococcal disease and death (case fatality rates are 50%–80%). Even though vaccines increase protection, continued high vigilance is needed because one study reported that 19% of asplenic patients developed disease by serotypes not included in current vaccines (Schutze et al., 2002). The onset of OPSI may be sudden, with fever, nausea, vomiting, and confusion being the initial symptoms. Left untreated, the illness may progress to seizures, shock, disseminated intravascular coagulation, coma, and death within hours in 50% to 75% of affected children (Ein, 1993). Therefore, asplenic patients with unexplained fever greater than 38.5°C or other manifestations of sepsis should receive prompt medical attention, including treatment for suspected bacteremia, the initial signs and symptoms of which may be subtle. Antimicrobials selected for therapy should be effective against *S. pneumoniae*, *N. meningitidis*, and beta-lactamase-producing *H. influenzae* type b (Peter, 1997).

In addition to vaccination, many experts recommend daily antimicrobial prophylaxis with oral penicillin G or V. Children younger than 5 years of age receive 125 mg twice daily and those older than 5 years of age, 250 mg twice daily. This prophylaxis may be continued through childhood and into adulthood, depending on the practitioner. Antimicrobial prophylaxis may be particularly useful in children younger than 2 years because they are not likely to respond to the vaccine.

Surgeons vary significantly in their practice about sending children back to school and resuming full activities. Some believe that resuming normal activities is best accomplished as soon as the child feels up to them. Others are more conservative in their beliefs and insist on a 4-week postoperative hiatus. School can be resumed anywhere from a week to 10 days after the surgery in most instances.

■ Cholecystectomy

Cholecystitis and gallstones are infrequent in children and have been historically associated with adolescent pregnancy or hemolytic disorders. However, the presence of gallstones is being reported with increased frequency in childhood. This changing incidence and spectrum of cholelithiasis over the last 30 years has resulted in an increased frequency of the cholecystectomy procedure (Balaguer, Price, & Burd, 2006). Obesity causes 8% to 33% of pediatric gallstones in all children, especially in

children with no underlying medical conditions. Obesity increases the risk of gallstones by over four-fold in children (Baker et al., 2005).

Embryology

The liver, gallbladder, and biliary duct system are formed from an outgrowth of the caudal portion of the foregut during the fourth week of gestation. This liver bud or hepatic diverticulum divides into a larger cranial portion, which becomes the liver. The smaller caudal portion becomes the gallbladder, with its stalk forming the cystic duct (Moore & Persaud, 1993). Congenital anomalies of the gallbladder itself are of significance to the surgeon who may be attempting to identify anatomy during a cholecystectomy or other surgical procedure (Shaffer, 1996).

Nonhemolytic Cholelithiasis

The conditions that predispose a child to cholelithiasis depend on the age of the child at presentation (Fig. 27-2). Nonhemolytic cholelithiasis refers to the formation of gallstones in the absence of a hemolytic disorder. The

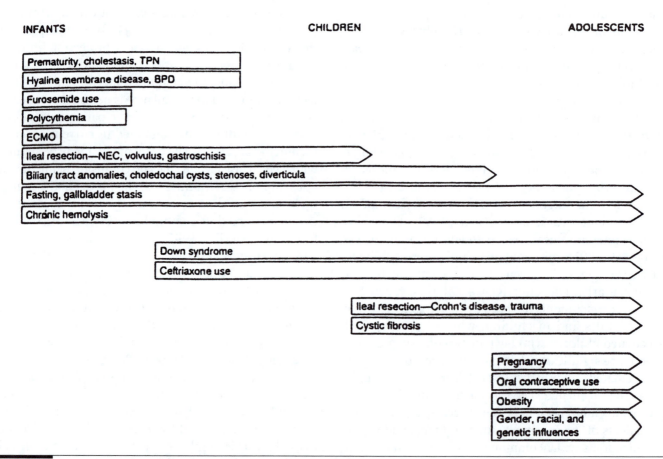

Figure 27-2 Predisposition to cholelithiasis at different stages of development. BPD, bronchopulmonary dysplasia; ECMO, extracorporeal membrane oxygenation; NEC, necrotizing enterocolitis; TPN, total parenteral nutrition.

use of long-term total parenteral nutrition (TPN) has been implicated as a significant contributing factor to the increasing incidence of cholelithiasis in the pediatric population. The lack of enteral feedings reduces the effectiveness of gallbladder contractions, thus reducing the flow of bile from the gallbladder and resulting in biliary stasis. In addition, some of the actual components of the TPN may contribute to cholelithiasis. One study found that 13% of pediatric patients requiring TPN for longer than 30 days had cholelithiasis develop (King, Ginn-Pease, Lloyd, Hoffman, & Hohenbrink, 1987). Other non-hemolytic factors contributing to the development of cholelithiasis include obesity, history of ileal resection, cystic fibrosis, oral contraceptive use, and pregnancy (Flake, 1997) (Fig. 27-2).

Hemolytic Cholelithiasis

Hemolytic cholelithiasis is the most common cause of gallstones at urban academic medical centers where there is a large population of children with sickle cell disease (Holcomb & Pietsch, 1998). More than 50% of children with sickle cell disease have evidence of cholelithiasis by the age of 18 years (Lachman, Lazerson, Starshak, Vaughters, & Werlin, 1979). Thalassemia and spherocytosis are also associated with an increased incidence of gallstones. The bile of patients with these disorders contains a large amount of unconjugated bilirubin. This can lead to the formation of gallbladder sludge, thus increasing the risk for cholelithiasis (Rescorla, 1997).

Biliary Dyskinesia and Acute Acalculous Cholecystitis

Other indications for cholecystectomy include biliary dyskinesia and acute acalculous cholecystitis. Biliary dyskinesia occurs when the gallbladder has poor contractility and emptying, perhaps with cholesterol crystals present within the bile in the gallbladder. This may be an early stage of the formation of cholesterol gallstones (Rescorla, 1997). In addition, Campbell, Narasimhan, Golladay, and Hirschl (2004) reported histologic findings of chronic cholecystitis in 86% of patients who underwent cholecystectomy for biliary dyskinesia, suggesting that the dysfunction of the gallbladder in biliary dyskinesia could be the result of some chronic process. These children present with a history of chronic abdominal pain but are otherwise healthy and have normal laboratory and radiologic studies. A nuclear medicine study using an injection of cholecystokinin is performed if biliary dyskinesia is suspected. Cholecystokinin induces contraction and emptying of the gallbladder and relaxation of the sphincter of Oddi. During this examination, an ejection fraction is mathematically calculated by measuring the initial and residual amounts of a radioactive bile marker in the gallbladder (Krishnamurthy, Bobba, & Kingston, 1981). An ejection fraction of less than 35% is considered abnormal (Rescorla). The exact time of the onset and relief of pain and its relation to the emptying of the gallbladder are important in establishing the diagnosis. Pain occurring outside the gallbladder-emptying phase could be nonbiliary in origin (Krishnamurthy & Krishnamurthy, 1997).

Cholecystectomy is the treatment of choice for cases of documented biliary dyskinesia. However, it is important to note that some patients may not have complete resolution of symptoms after the procedure. One study found that patients who exhibited the combined symptoms of abdominal pain, nausea, and a markedly decreased gallbladder ejection fraction of less than 15% benefited most from a cholecystectomy for biliary dyskinesia (Carney et al., 2004). This information can be used during preoperative discussions with patients and families who are considering a surgical procedure for the treatment of biliary dyskinesia.

In the pediatric population, acute acalculous cholecystitis generally occurs after episodes of sepsis or other severe infections. In acute acalculous cholecystitis, the gallbladder becomes acutely inflamed. In contrast to the children with biliary dyskinesia, patients with acute acalculous cholecystitis have fever, vomiting, and right upper quadrant pain. They may also have abnormal liver function test results and white blood cell counts (Tsakayannis, Kozakewich, & Lillehei, 1996). On ultrasonographic examination, the wall of the gallbladder is markedly thickened and contains debris. Cholecystectomy is the treatment of choice if the gallbladder becomes progressively distended or if the patient's clinical status deteriorates (Flake, 1997).

Clinical Presentation

Symptoms of gallstones vary, depending on the age of the patient. Occasionally, gallstones are found incidentally during an evaluation for another clinical problem. In infants, the presence of gallstones may result in fever and direct hyperbilirubinemia along with other abnormal liver function test results. Children tend to be initially seen with fever, abdominal pain, and an elevated white blood cell count. Older children complain of right upper quadrant or epigastric pain. This pain may radiate to the right scapula or shoulder, and the patient may experience nausea and vomiting. The pain and nausea may or may not occur in relation to meals or the ingestion of fatty foods.

On physical examination, pain may be elicited as the patient deep breathes while the examiner palpates the abdomen in the region of the gallbladder. This is referred to as Murphy's sign and is an indication of possible gallbladder disease. Differential diagnoses include other causes of upper abdominal or epigastric pain and other conditions that may result in jaundice or abnormal liver function tests.

The diagnostic studies that are performed depend on the age of the child, the presence of risk factors for the development of gallstones, and the presenting symptoms. Studies may include liver function tests, a complete blood count, abdominal radiography or ultrasonography, and perhaps a nuclear medicine study. If the radiologic studies do not indicate a gallbladder disorder but one is still suspected, an endoscopic retrograde cholangiopancreatography can be performed to evaluate the pancreas and common bile duct. During this procedure, an endoscope is passed through the esophagus into the duodenum. A catheter is then passed through the endoscope into the pancreatic duct and bile ducts. Contrast medium is injected through this catheter into the ducts, and the biliary tract is evaluated for an obstruction or other abnormality. If stones are found, the physician may decide to remove them during this procedure.

Management

Nonsurgical

The management of gallstones depends on the age of the child and the symptoms that are present. In infants, gallstones sometimes spontaneously resolve without any intervention (Jacir, Anderson, Eichelberger, & Guzzetta, 1986). If the infant is asymptomatic, the physician may closely observe the patient for a period of time. If the child is older than 2 years of age and presents with pain or abnormal diagnostic studies, cholecystectomy is the treatment of choice. Even if the older child is asymptomatic, some would advocate elective cholecystectomy to prevent any future problems, such as cholecystitis (Shaffer, 1996). Nonsurgical treatments, such as lithotripsy and oral dissolution therapy, are rarely used in children because of limited pediatric research trials using these techniques and the advancement of pediatric laparoscopic surgery (Holcomb & Pietsch, 1998).

Surgical

Laparoscopic cholecystectomy for children with cholelithiasis is being performed with increasing frequency, and studies have demonstrated its safety and effectiveness in the pediatric population (Holcomb et al., 1999; Esposito

et al., 2001). When the laparoscopic approach is used, all visualization of the operative field and tissues occurs through a small camera inserted through an incision in the umbilicus. A Foley catheter and nasogastric tube are placed before the first incision in the umbilicus. The abdomen is insufflated through the umbilical incision with an infusion of carbon dioxide. This helps to distend the abdomen and improve visualization. Three additional incisions are made at various locations in the abdomen (Fig. 27-3). These three incisions serve as port sites through which the surgeon inserts other instruments, such as grasping forceps and dissecting forceps, to perform the procedure. During the procedure, a cholangiogram may be performed by injecting radiopaque dye directly into the bile ducts. This helps the surgeon better identify the common bile duct and any structural abnormalities that may exist. Once the cystic duct, common bile duct, and other structures are identified, the gallbladder is removed through the umbilical incision. The instruments are removed from the other port sites in the abdomen with the laparoscope still in place to observe for any bleeding from the areas of the incisions. The laparoscope is then removed, the abdomen desufflated, and the incisions closed with absorbable, subcuticular sutures. Wound closure

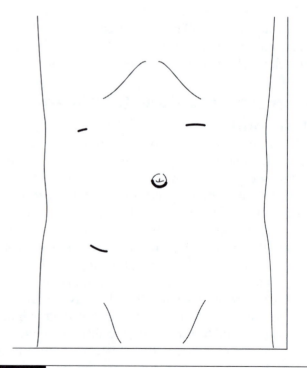

Figure 27-3 Example of potential locations of incisions for trocar placement for laparoscopic cholecystectomy.
(Reprinted from the *Journal of Pediatric Surgery*, 34(8): Holcomb et al., "Laparoscopic cholecystectomy in children: Lessons learned from the first 100 patients." © 1999, reprinted with permission from Elsevier. Drawing courtesy of Jan Warren, Cincinnati Children's Hospital Medical Center, Cincinnati, Ohio.)

strips or transparent tape and gauze are placed over each incision. The laparoscopic procedure may be contraindicated in a patient who has undergone previous abdominal surgery. In such a case, an open cholecystectomy can be performed through a traditional right upper quadrant incision (Monson, 1993).

Recent studies have compared laparoscopic and traditional operative or open cholecystectomy procedures in pediatrics. Kim, Wesson, Superina, and Filler (1995) compared both of these procedures, evaluating cost, length of stay, and use of parenteral analgesics after surgery. The average cost per patient, duration of hospitalization, and use of parenteral analgesics were all significantly less in the patients who underwent laparoscopic cholecystectomy. Another study has documented similar findings (Holcomb, Sharp, Neblett, Morgan, & Pietsch, 1994). In addition, laparoscopic surgery has a much better cosmetic result, and the children are able to return to normal activities much sooner, often within 1 week after surgery (Holcomb, Olsen, & Sharp, 1991).

Complications after laparoscopic or open cholecystectomy include wound infections, bleeding, and postoperative pneumonia as a result of immobility or poor pulmonary toilet. One of the most serious complications is a bile leak, which occurs as a result of disruption of a biliary duct. If the leak is very small, it may not be noticed in the operating room, and the patient may have symptoms in the postoperative period, including fever and abdominal pain. The leak may result in peritonitis. If the leak does not seal itself within a short time, diagnostic studies are performed to identify the exact location of the leak, and surgical repair may be necessary.

Nursing Considerations

The exact content of preoperative teaching for the patient and family depends on whether the procedure is performed on an urgent or elective basis. All teaching should include the routine information about surgery, as well as reinforcing specific details regarding the recovery time and the expected length of stay after surgery. If the procedure is scheduled to be performed laparoscopically, the family and patient should be aware that the procedure might be converted to an open cholecystectomy if indicated.

There are several conditions in which special preoperative circumstances exist. If the child has an acutely inflamed gallbladder, surgery may be delayed until the patient has received several days of antibiotics and the inflammation is decreased. If pain medication is required, morphine sulfate is avoided because it increases spasm of the sphincter of Oddi. When the sphincter of Oddi spasms, it obstructs the normal flow of bile into the intestine, resulting

in an increase in pain. If the child has sickle cell anemia, the patient should be admitted the day before surgery for hydration and a possible blood transfusion to ensure a hemoglobin level of 10 to 12 g/dL before surgery (Al-Salem & Nourallah, 1997). Other hemolytic disorders also may require some preoperative blood work.

For most elective procedures, the patient arrives at the hospital the day of surgery and is admitted after surgery. After recovering in the postanesthesia care unit, the child is transferred to the surgical floor. Nursing interventions for these patients are similar to those of any postoperative patient, consisting of vital sign assessment, pain management, intake and output recording, and wound assessment. If the procedure was performed laparoscopically, the child should be offered clear liquids the night of surgery. If the liquids are tolerated, the child is quickly advanced to a regular diet. The child is usually discharged the day after surgery if afebrile and tolerating a regular diet, and if pain can be managed with oral narcotics and the child is otherwise doing well.

In addition to incisional pain, the child may complain of shoulder pain after laparoscopic surgery. This is referred pain from the diaphragm caused by reabsorption of residual carbon dioxide used for insufflating the abdomen during the operative procedure (George, Hammes, & Schwarz, 1995). This excess carbon dioxide can irritate the diaphragm. The patient should be encouraged to cough and deep breathe, and the patient should be positioned with the head of the bed only slightly elevated.

If the procedure was performed open, the patient may require more pain medication and have a longer recovery time. Because of this, these patients are usually discharged 3 to 5 days after the procedure. Patients with sickle cell anemia may also have a longer hospitalization and recovery time because of potential pulmonary complications, as well as the risk for developing a sickle cell crisis.

On discharge, the nurse should provide the family and patient with information regarding pain medication, wound care, and activity. Narcotics are rarely needed past the first 4 to 5 postoperative days. The child can then transition to over-the-counter medications. Wound care, whether the surgery was performed laparoscopically or open, consists of keeping the sites dry, usually for less than 1 week, depending on the kind of dressing that was applied by the surgeon during surgery. The child can return to regular activity within a couple of weeks if the surgery was performed laparoscopically and within 4 to 6 weeks if an open procedure was performed. Patients should be advised that if they experience any pain as they begin to increase their activity, that specific activity should be stopped, and they should wait several days before attempting that activity again. Parents should be educated on the signs and symptoms of infection and encouraged to call the surgeon's office with any additional questions after discharge. Follow-up with the surgeon should be arranged approximately 2 weeks after surgery. If the child is doing well at that time, he or she needs to see the surgeon again only if additional concerns arise.

Meckel's Diverticulum

Embryology and Pathophysiology of Meckel's Diverticulum

Meckel's diverticulum is defined as a persistence in the omphalomesenteric duct or stalk of the yolk sac. The yolk sac develops on approximately day 10 in the inner mass of the embryo and expands to become both the primitive gut and the cavity of the chorion (which gives rise to the placenta). It does this by creating a passageway known as the omphalomesenteric duct. After supplying nourishment to the embryo, the yolk sac usually disappears between the fifth and ninth week of pregnancy, just before the midgut returns to the abdomen. If the stalk of the yolk sac or omphalomesenteric duct persists, it becomes a protuberant sac usually located within 100 cm from the ileocecal valve and the distal ileum, becoming known as *Meckel's diverticulum*. It is also referred to as *diverticulum ilei verum* or *omphaloileal* (Sawin, 2005; Brown & Stevenson, 2002). Meckel, a German anatomist and embryologist, is credited with this discovery in 1812.

Meckel's diverticulum occurs in 2% of the population and is usually asymptomatic. It is one of the most common anomalies of the digestive tract (Moore & Persaud, 1993). Other congenital anomalies of the omphalomesenteric duct remnant are related to their attachment to the small intestine and to the umbilicus. In 75% of cases, the duct remnant completely detaches from the umbilicus to become a Meckel's diverticulum (Brown & Stevenson, 2002). The blood supply to the remnant is a primitive vitelline artery that usually arises from the mesentery and may be quite prominent in patients with bleeding (Sawin, 2005; Schropp, 2005). Ectopic tissue has been identified in about half of all Meckel's diverticula, with 80% reported as gastric mucosa and 5% as pancreatic in origin (Brown & Stevenson). Grosthwaite & Leather (1997) stated that 95% of those who present with bleeding contain some gastric mucosa, whereas those who had a diverticulum removed who were asymptomatic had

findings of only 15% with gastric mucosa. Other studies have reported the asymptomatic ectopic tissue findings to be in a wide range from 5% to 65% (Sawin).

Rarely, carcinoid tumors arise from a Meckel's diverticulum in children, but most other tumor findings have been confined to adult patients (Brown & Stevenson, 2002). An increased incidence of Meckel's has been reported in patients with other anomalies, such as esophageal atresia, imperforate anus, omphalocele, and neurologic or cardiovascular malformations (Brown & Stevenson).

Meckel's diverticulum is clinically significant in two instances: when it produces symptoms and when it is found incidentally at the time of a laparotomy. More than half of the patients who present with symptoms do so by 2 years of age (Foglia, 1993). Only 15% of children with symptomatic Meckel's diverticulum are older than 4 years of age (Schropp, 2005; Brown & Stevenson, 2002). From the 2% of the population in which Meckel's diverticulum occurs, approximately 4% experience symptoms (Soltero & Bill, 1976). Meckel's diverticulum is the most common cause of serious lower gastrointestinal bleeding, necessitating aggressive approaches to treatment and diagnosis (Brown & Stevenson).

Clinical Presentation

The "rule of twos" has been helpful and has been often applied to describe Meckel's diverticulum because it occurs in 2% of the population, is located within 2 feet of the ileocecal junction, measures 2 inches in length and about 2 cm in diameter, has two types of ectopic mucosa (gastric and pancreatic), has a 2:1 male to female ratio, and is usually symptomatic before 2 years of age (Brown & Stevenson, 2002). The three most common presentations of a symptomatic Meckel's diverticulum are lower gastrointestinal bleeding, intestinal obstruction, and abdominal pain (Foglia, 1993). Meckel's diverticula are most commonly manifested in children by painless lower gastrointestinal bleeding and in adults as an inflammatory process or obstruction (Digiacomo & Cottone, 1993). Some clinical presentation statistics for Meckel's diverticulum have been reported as 40% to 60% for hemorrhage, 25% for obstruction, and 10% to 20% for diverticulitis (Schropp, 2005).

Bleeding is present in 25% to 56% of children with symptomatic lesions (Vane, West, & Grosfeld, 1987). Bleeding results from ulceration of the adjacent ileal mucosa by the acid secretions of the gastric or pancreatic tissue contained in the diverticulum (Caty & Gibson, 2005). Bleeding can be slight, with dark, tarry stools, or it may be massive, with a more reddish stool. There may be copious bright red blood per rectum with no stool. It may also have a mucoidlike currant jelly appearance because Meckel's diverticulum can be the lead point of an intussusception. Except in the case of intussusception, the bleeding is almost always painless and stops spontaneously. Excessive bleeding can lead to anemia, necessitating a blood transfusion (Foglia, 1993).

The child should be assessed for signs of hemodynamic instability because rectal bleeding is the most common presenting symptom. Frequently, however, the bleeding is slight and may not cause changes in the child's hemodynamic picture. Any young child with hemoglobin-positive stools and chronic iron deficiency anemia should be investigated for a bleeding Meckel's diverticulum (Schropp, 2005).

The second symptom, intestinal obstruction, occurs in about one third of all patients and is a frequent finding in younger patients. Besides acting as the lead point in an intussusception, Meckel's diverticulum can become the cause of a volvulus, a twisting of the bowel, or the cause of an internal hernia (Digiacomo & Cottone, 1993; Foglia, 1993). The Meckel's diverticulum may also become incarcerated within a hernia sac (Brown & Stevenson, 2002). In the older child (mean age of 8.2 years), the obstructive complications present as abdominal pain, distention, and obstipation, and the diagnosis of the cause as Meckel's diverticulum is usually made at laparotomy or laparoscopy (Brown & Stevenson).

In addition, the Meckel's diverticulum can become inflamed when the lumen is obstructed and can lead to diverticulitis symptoms, similar to the symptoms of appendicitis. The developing increased pressure within the diverticulum leads to decreased mucosal perfusion, tissue acidosis, and bacterial invasion, with potential progression to tissue gangrene and perforation. The ectopic gastric or pancreatic mucosa could contribute to the obstruction or could develop an area of ulceration, which leads to the bacterial invasion. The abdominal pain symptoms are similar to those of appendicitis, usually presenting as diffuse periumbilical and progressing to lower abdominal pain. Due to its variable location along the distal ileum, the peritoneal irritation pain can be anywhere in the lower abdomen, but it is commonly in the right lower or mid abdomen. Progression to perforation can cause a more serious peritonitis than appendicitis because of its mobile location and poor ability to wall off the infection. Frequently, the patient is thought to have appendicitis and is taken to the operating room, where the Meckel's diverticulitis is found. It is always recommended to look for this when the appendix is found to be noninflamed in cases of peritonitis (Sawin, 2005).

Work-Up

The "gold standard" for diagnosing Meckel's diverticulum is the "Meckel's scan," or scintigraphy (Foglia, 1993) (Fig. 27-4). A scintigraph is a picture produced by an imaging device that shows the distribution and intensity of radioactivity in various tissues and organs after the administration of a radiopharmaceutical. Technetium (Tc) pertechnetate, an isotope, is readily absorbed by gastric mucosa and appears anywhere gastric mucosa exists in the body. Because a symptomatic Meckel's diverticulum contains gastric mucosa in most instances, this scan accurately confirms diagnosis in 80% to 90% of cases. The scan has been reported to be 85% sensitive and 95% specific for Meckel's diverticulum (Brown & Stevenson, 2002; Caty & Gibson, 2005). Therefore, a negative scan result does not always exclude Meckel's diverticulum. The scan should be repeated if results are negative but suspicion remains high. Defects that include less than 1 cm of gastric mucosa in the diverticulum are beyond the resolution of the camera.

Some institutions premedicate with a histamine$_2$ blocker to lengthen the amount of time the radioisotope remains in the area of interest by slowing the isotope's removal, thereby aiding in the diagnosis (Foglia, 1993). In addition, some institutions may use pentagastrin to stimulate the isotope uptake by the ectopic mucosa and add glucagons to decrease peristalsis and increase isotope retention within the diverticula (Brown & Azizkhan, 1999). Because the evidence is not conclusive that the pentagastrin or histamine$_2$ blockers clearly enhance accuracy, many institutions use the drugs only when the study result is not clearly positive or negative (Schropp, 2005). A limited Australian study reported an 87.5% enhanced sensitivity when they administered either oral or intravenous ranitidine for 24 hours before a repeated Meckel's scan after a previous false-negative result (Rerksuppaphol, Hutson, & Oliver, 2004). Meckel's diverticulum can occur anywhere in the abdomen but is most often found in the right lower quadrant (Jewett, Duszynski, & Allen, 1970).

The diagnostic Meckel's scan should be explained to the family. The excretion of isotope from the kidneys and bowel within 24 hours of administration should also be discussed. The nurse should explain why there are no long-term aftereffects from this small dosage to either the child or the family members.

If possible, the child should fast for 3 to 4 hours before the scan and optimally have had no barium studies, enemas, or laxatives within the previous 24 hours (Schropp, 2005). If the child is too young to be cooperative, it may be necessary to administer conscious sedation for the du-

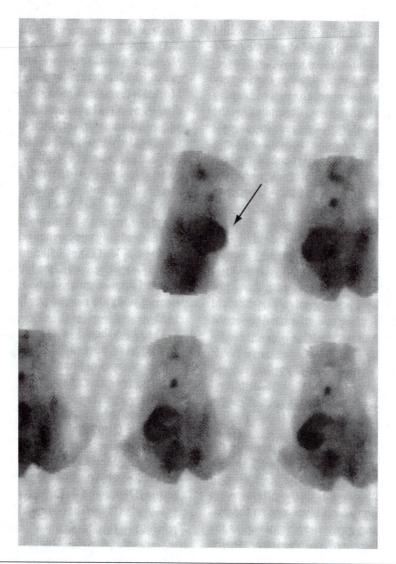

Figure 27-4 "Meckel's scan" or scintigraph showing the location of Meckel's diverticulum. (Courtesy of Dr. Cedric Priebe.)

ration of the scan. Rarely, the bleeding has been so great as to cause the child to be self-sedated throughout the procedure; the child becomes weak and lethargic from the blood loss. Close monitoring is necessary.

The Meckel's scan takes approximately 30 to 60 minutes to complete. As the isotope circulates, it quickly reaches the kidneys, bladder, stomach, and ectopic gastric mucosa. A positive study result is characterized by a focal tracer uptake that appears simultaneously with the stomach and increases over time (Schropp, 2005). Between 10% and 20% of it is absorbed into the soft tissues. Tc-pertechnetate has a half-life of 6 hours and is fully excreted from the body within 24 hours.

The differential diagnosis of the patient with a positive scan result includes ectopic gastric mucosa located elsewhere and a false-positive result (Sfakianakis &

Conway, 1981). Duplication cysts and Barrett's esophagus are two areas where gastric mucosa is found and that absorb a radiopharmaceutical. A duplication cyst, otherwise known as an *alimentary tract duplication*, can occur anywhere from the mouth to the anus and, in addition to being lined with normal gastrointestinal mucosa, has smooth muscle walls like those in the intestines. Barrett's esophagus is a disorder of the lower esophagus resulting from gastroesophageal reflux of acid from the stomach and causes a benign ulcer-like lesion in the area.

False-positive results can be caused by bleeding of the mucosa as in intussusception, bowel obstruction, ulcers, arteriovenous malformations, and urinary tract anomalies (Fries, Mortensson, & Robertson, 1984). An intestinal duplication is the second most common cause of a false-positive result. If the initial result is negative and there is a strong suspicion of a Meckel's diverticulum, the scan should be repeated. It is possible that the bladder, which rapidly fills with the isotope, may block the diverticulum from view. Bladder catheterization can enhance the sensitivity of the scan. Further, a patient with a bowel obstruction is not usually diagnosed before surgery with Meckel's diverticulum as the cause. Finally, if the intussusception containing a Meckel's diverticulum is reduced by a barium or air-contrast enema, the diagnosis may not be made at this time (Foglia, 1993). However, enema reduction of intussusception is seldom successful if the obstruction is due to the prolapse of the intestine through a patent omphalomesenteric fistula. In these cases, a characteristic "ram's horn" appearance may be seen. If the obstruction occurs because of a volvulus around a fibrous vitelline duct remnant that is not patent or because of an internal hernia beneath the vitelline artery, the diagnosis can be extremely difficult to make. The intestinal ischemia pain is sudden and severe, with few early signs of obstruction because of its location at the distal small bowel. Progression to lethal acidosis and shock can occur unless a high index of suspicion is maintained (Sawin, 2005).

Goyal and Bellah (1993) reported a 24-day-old male infant who presented with symptoms of bowel obstruction and was diagnosed before surgery by sonography. Because sonography is an excellent method of diagnosing many different disorders involving the bowel, it may be helpful in diagnosing Meckel's diverticulum, too. Sometimes, a combination of ultrasonography, computed tomography, and contrast enema can aid in the diagnosis of complicated case with a negative Meckel's scan result (Daneman, Lobo, Alton, & Shuckett, 1998). Other tests have been diagnostic but have rarely been used in children due to their more invasive nature, such as visceral angiography or isotope-labeled red blood cell scan (Sawin, 2005; Schropp, 2005). However, the new noninvasive diagnostic technique of swallowing a wireless capsule endoscopy may be able to pick up the Meckel's diverticulum as it takes pictures while passing through the intestinal tract (Schropp). Other sources of gastrointestinal bleeding can be identified with endoscopy, gastroduodenoscopy, or colonoscopy.

In cases in which there is a high index of suspicion of Meckel's diverticulum but the scan result is negative, the patient undergoes an exploratory laparotomy. It is at this time that the cause of the complete bowel obstruction is often found to be a Meckel's diverticulum (Foglia, 1993). The laparoscopic approach for diagnosis and excision of Meckel's diverticulum in children is described in the literature (Grosthwaite & Leather, 1997; Huang & Lin, 1993; Swaniker, Soldes, & Hirschi, 1999; Teitelbaum, Polley, & Obeid, 1994). This approach may be indicated instead of scintigraphic scanning in the assessment of the anemic pediatric patient with lower gastrointestinal bleeding and suspected Meckel's diverticulum (Swaniker et al.).

Treatment of Meckel's Diverticulum

Patients who have painless bleeding usually stop bleeding spontaneously, and the scan and surgery can be performed electively (Fig. 27-5). Patients who have active bleeding require fluid resuscitation provided as a blood transfusion and stabilization before going to the operating room. Patients with obstructive symptoms should be fluid resuscitated as rapidly as possible to expedite operative intervention to avoid ischemic bowel resection. Bleeding should not recur after excision of a Meckel's diverticulum (Foglia, 1993).

Considerable controversy exists over the value of performing a diverticulectomy if a Meckel's diverticulum is found incidentally at the time of laparotomy. Most surgeons believe that it is best to leave the Meckel's diverticulum alone and not excise it. Mackey and Dineen (1983) reported 32 cases of incidental Meckel's diverticula left in situ without subsequent complications. Leijonmarck, Bonman-Sandelin, Frisell, and Raf (1986) reported 28 additional cases of incidental Meckel's diverticula left in situ without complications during a mean follow-up of 7.8 years. They also reported a 6% reoperation rate for incidental Meckel's diverticula that were removed. However, if the Meckel's diverticulum is found in an infant or very young child, resection would be recommended because of the much higher incidence of symptomatic lesions under 2 years of age and lifelong potential for complications. It would also be indicated if it was found to be prone to develop symptoms, such as if it contained palpable ectopic mucosa, if there was any persistent omphalomesenteric remnants with abdominal wall attachments, if there was a prominent vitelline artery or fibrous vitelline artery remnant, if there was evidence of inflammation or a narrow base, or if there was a history of unexplained abdominal pain (Sawin, 2005). Whenever it is found in the older child or adult, the decision would be based on the clinical situation for the risks and benefits (Brown & Stevenson, 2002). If the lesion is not resected, it is imperative to inform the family and the primary care physician about the lesion and its possible associated symptoms (Sawin).

Operative Procedure

The patient must be hemodynamically stable at the time of surgery. If necessary, a blood transfusion should be administered. If this is an elective diverticulectomy, a rou-

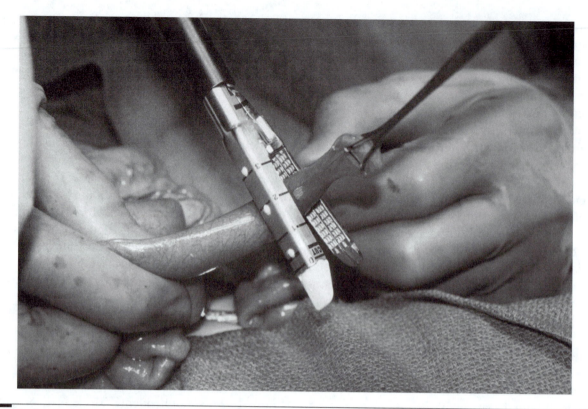

Figure 27-5 Endoscopic stapler used to resect a symptomatic Meckel's diverticulum.
(Courtesy of Tim Weiner, MD.)

tine bowel preparation may be given in some institutions, but is usually not necessary. The use of a laparoscopic approach has been described for this procedure in the past decade. Generally, the procedure uses an umbilical and two smaller ports. After insufflation, the cecum is located and the small bowel is inspected until the Meckel's diverticulum is located. Once resected and removed in an endoscopic bag, the diverticulum can be opened and evaluated for ulcers. If resection is determined to be necessary, the umbilical incision may be extended to allow for the procedure (Schropp, 2005).

The open procedure remains the traditional approach through a transverse right lower quadrant incision, or at the location noted on the Meckel's scan. An appendectomy should also be performed to avoid future diagnostic dilemmas (Brown & Stevenson, 2002). However, in some specific patients the appendix may be left for its potential use in future urologic drainage, Mitrofanoff, or other procedures, such as biliary drainage (Sawin, 2005). In patients with suspected intestinal obstruction, a generous transverse laparotomy incision should be used for rapid exposure and intestinal decompression with bowel resection as needed for any necrotic sections (Sawin). When located, the diverticulum is divided at the junction of the small intestine and closed with sutures or pos-

sibly staples if the child is older and larger. It is important not to narrow the lumen of the intestine when suturing or stapling because such narrowing may cause an intestinal obstruction after surgery (Cullen & Kelly, 1996).

If the patient has an intussusception, this should first be reduced and the diverticulum removed afterward. If a narrowing of the bowel and gangrene exist, it may be necessary to resect that portion of the bowel and anastomose or sew the ends of the bowel together. In the case of perforation with the absence of severe peritoneal soiling or hemodynamic instability, resection and primary anastomosis can be performed (Sawin, 2005). Occasionally, it may be necessary to give the patient a temporary stoma to allow for healing of the anastomosed bowel. If the obstruction has been caused by a volvulus or twisting of the bowel or by an internal hernia (caused by a remnant of the omphalomesenteric duct), the treatment consists of reduction of the volvulus or hernia and removal of the duct (Cullen & Kelly, 1996).

Major complications may occur as a result of the preceding presentations in conjunction with Meckel's diverticulum. Infection is the most common postoperative complication (Vane et al., 1987). As with any child who undergoes bowel surgery, the development of adhesions is a potential complication.

The risk of long-term complications, like strictures, adhesions, or subsequent bowel obstruction, developing 20 years after the surgery is between 2% and 6%. Men have a greater chance of suffering long-term complications than do women (Cullen & Kelly, 1996). Possible complications, such as postoperative bleeding and/or intestinal obstruction, should be discussed with the family.

Nursing Considerations

Nursing care for children undergoing diverticulectomy is similar to the care of children with splenectomy or cholecystectomy. Preoperative teaching focuses on the surgery, details about expected length of stay, and the recovery time. If the procedure has been performed laparoscopically with simple diverticulectomy, the patient can be offered fluids and have their diet advanced as tolerated shortly after surgery (Schropp, 2005). In the case of open procedures or ileal resection, the patient may remain NPO until bowel function returns. The diet is then advanced from clear liquids to regular as tolerated. Patients are usually discharged in 3 to 4 days if they meet the following criteria: no fever, ambulating, no infection, and tolerating a regular diet. School-age children are ready to return to school within 1 week and to full activities within 3 weeks. Information about signs of infection should be reinforced and information about pain medication provided. Follow-up should be planned with the surgical team in approximately 2 weeks.

■ Conclusion

Nurses caring for pediatric patients are frequently responsible for children who undergo splenectomy, cholecystectomy, and excision of a Meckel's diverticulum. The surgeries are generally well tolerated, requiring short hospital stays, ranging from 1 to 5 days and result in minimal morbidity. An understanding of the conditions necessitating these surgeries, the evaluation required, the operative procedure, and the nursing interventions is essential to providing quality care.

■ Educational Materials

APSNA invites you to download the following diagnosis-related teaching tools for Chapter 27, Splenectomy, Cholecystectomy, and Meckel's Diverticulum: 1) Splenectomy 2) Cholecystectomy. These teaching tools are available at the APSNA Web site (www.apsna.org) and the Jones and Bartlett Web site (www.jbpub.com). All teaching materials are available in English and Spanish and are free of charge. APSNA encourages their use for your patients and families.

References

American Academy of Pediatrics. (2000). Asplenic children. In L. K. Pickering (Ed.), *2000 red book*: *Report of the Committee on Infectious Diseases* (pp. 66–67). Elk Grove Village, IL: American Academy of Pediatrics.

Al-Salem, A. H., & Nourallah, H. (1997). Sequential endoscopic/laparoscopic management of cholelithiasis and choledocholithiasis in children who have sickle cell disease. *Journal of Pediatric Surgery, 21*, 1432–1435.

Arzoumanian, A., & Rosenthall, L. (1995). Splenosis. *Clinical Nuclear Medicine, 20*, 730–733.

Ashcraft, K. W. (1994). *Atlas of pediatric surgery*. Philadelphia: W.B. Saunders.

Baker, S., Barlow, S., Cochran, W., Fuchs, G., Klish, W., Krebs, N., et al. (2005). Overweight children and adolescents: A clinical report of the North American Society for Pediatric Gastroenterology, Hepatology and Nutrition. *Journal of Pediatric Gastroenterology and Nutrition, 40*(5), 533–543.

Balaguer, E. J., Price, M. R., & Burd, R. S. (2006). National trends in the utilization of cholecystectomy in children. *Journal of Surgical Research, 134*(1), 68–73.

Ben-Yehuda, D., Gillis, S., & Eldor, A. (1990). Clinical and therapeutic experience in 712 Israeli patients with idiopathic thrombocytopenic purpura. *Acta Hematologica, 91*, 1–6.

Brown, R. L., & Azizkhan, R. G. (1999). Gastrointestinal bleeding in infants and children: Meckel's diverticulum and intestinal duplication. *Seminars in Pediatric Surgery, 8*, 202.

Brown, R. L., & Stevenson, R. J. (2002). Meckel diverticulum. In C. D. Rudolph, A. M. Rudolph, M. K. Hostetter, G. Lister, & N. J. Siegel (Eds.), *Rudolph's pediatrics* (21st ed., pp. 1405–1407). New York: McGraw-Hill Medical Publishing Division.

Bussel, J. B. (1990). Autoimmune thrombocytopenic purpura. *Hematology Oncology Clinics of North America, 4*, 179–191.

Campbell, B. T., Narasimhan, N. P., Golladay, E. S., & Hirschl, R. B. (2004). Biliary dyskinesia: A potentially unrecognized cause of abdominal pain in children. *Pediatric Surgery International, 20*, 579–581.

Carney, D. E., Kokoska, E. R., Grosfeld, J. L., Engum, S. A., Rouse, T. M., West, K. M., et al. (2004). Predictors of successful outcome after cholecystectomy for biliary dyskinesia. *Journal of Pediatric Surgery, 39*, 813–816.

Caty, M. G., & Gibson, B. R. (2005). Gastrointestinal bleeding. In K. T. Oldham, P. M. Colombani, R. P. Foglia, & M. A. Skinner (Eds.), *Principles and practice of pediatric surgery* (Vol. 2, pp. 1141–1142). Philadelphia: Lippincott Williams & Wilkins.

Chirletti, P., Cardi, M., Bacillary, P., Vitale, A., Sammartino, P., Bolognese, A., et al. (1992). Surgical treatment of immune thrombocytopenic purpura. *World Journal of Surgery, 16*, 1001–1005.

Crawford, M. W., Speakman, M., Carver, E. D., & Kim, P. C. (2004). Acute chest syndrome shows a predilection for basal lung regions on the side of upper abdominal surgery. *Canadian Journal of Anaesthesia, 51*(7), 707–711.

Cullen, J. J., & Kelly, K. A. (1996). Current management of Meckel's diverticulum. *Advances in Surgery, 29*, 207–214.

Daneman, A., Lobo, E., Alton, D. J., & Shuckett, B. (1998). The value of sonography, CT and air enema for detection of complicated Meckel's diverticulum in children with nonspecific clinical presentation. *Pediatric Radiology, 28*, 928–932.

de Buys Roessingh, A. S., de Lagausie, P., Rohrlich, P., Berrebi, D., & Aigrain, Y. (2002). Follow-up of partial splenectomy in children with hereditary spherocytosis. *Journal of Pediatric Surgery, 37,* 1459–1463.

Digiacomo, J. C., & Cottone, F. J. (1993). Surgical treatment of Meckel's diverticulum. *Southern Medical Journal, 86,* 671–675.

Ein, S. H. (1993). Splenic lesions. In K. W. Ashcraft & T. M. Holder (Eds.), *Pediatric surgery* (pp. 535–545). Philadelphia: W.B. Saunders.

Esposito, C., Gonzalez Sabin, A., Corcione, F., Sacco, R., Esposito, G., & Settimi, A. (2001). Results and complications of laparoscopic cholecystectomy in childhood. *Surgical Endoscopy, 15,* 890–892.

Flake, A. W. (1997). Disorders of the gallbladder and biliary tract. In K. T. Oldham, P. M. Colombani, & R. P. Foglia (Eds.), *Surgery of infants and children: Scientific principles and practice* (pp. 1405–1414). Philadelphia: Lippincott-Raven.

Foglia, R. P. (1993). Meckel's diverticulum. In K. W. Ashcraft (Ed.), *Pediatric surgery* (2nd ed., pp. 435–439). Philadelphia: W.B. Saunders.

Fries, M., Mortensson, W., & Robertson, B. (1984). Technetium pertechnetate scintigraphy to detect ectopic gastric mucosa in Meckel's diverticulum. *Acta Radiologica, 25,* 417–422.

Friesen, C. A., & Roberts, C. C. (1989). Cholelithiasis: Clinical characteristics in children. *Clinical Pediatrics, 28,* 294–298.

George, C., Hammes, M., & Schwarz, D. (1995). Laparoscopic Swenson pull-through procedure for congenital megacolon. *ADRN Journal, 62,* 727–736.

Goyal, M. K., & Bellah, R. D. (1993). Neonatal small bowel obstruction due to Meckel diverticulitis: Diagnosis by ultrasonography. *Journal of Ultrasound Medicine, 12*(2), 119–122.

Grosthwaite, G. L., & Leather, A. J. M. (1997). Laparoscopy: The ultimate diagnostic tool for a bleeding Meckel's diverticulum. *Australia & New Zealand Journal of Surgery, 67,* 223–224.

Holcomb, G. W., & Greene, H. L. (1993). Fatal hemorrhage caused by disease progression after partial splenectomy for type III Gaucher's disease. *Journal of Pediatric Surgery, 28,* 1572–1574.

Holcomb, G. W., III, Olsen, D. O., & Sharp, K. W. (1991). Laparoscopic cholecystectomy in the pediatric patient. *Journal of Pediatric Surgery, 26,* 1186–1190.

Holcomb, G. W., III, & Pietsch, J. B. (1998). Gallbladder disease and hepatic infections. In J. A. O'Neill, Jr., M. I. Rowe, J. L. Grosfeld, E. W. Fonkalsrud, & A. G. Coran (Eds.), *Pediatric surgery* (5th ed., pp. 1495–1503). St. Louis, MO: Mosby.

Holcomb, G. W., III, Sharp, K. W., Neblett, W. W., III, Morgan, W. M., III, & Pietsch, J. B. (1994). Laparoscopic cholecystectomy in infants and children: Modifications and cost analysis. *Journal of Pediatric Surgery, 29,* 900–904.

Holcomb G. W., III, Morgan W. M., III, Neblett W. W., III, Peitsch, J. B., O'Neill, J. A., Jr., & Shyr, Y. (1999). Laparoscopic cholecystectomy in children: Lessons learned from the first 100 patients. *Journal of Pediatric Surgery, 34,* 1236–1240.

Holt, D., Brown, J., Terrill, K., Goldsby, R., Meyers, R. L., Heximer, J., et al. (2003). Response of intravenous immunoglobin predicts splenectomy response in children with immune thrombocytopenic purpura. *Pediatrics, 111*(1), 87–90.

Huang, C. S., & Lin, L. H. (1993). Laparoscopic Meckel's diverticulectomy in infants: Report of three cases. *Journal of Pediatric Surgery, 28*(11), 1486–1489.

Idowu, O., & Hayes-Jordan, A. (1998). Partial splenectomy in children under 4 years of age with hemoglobinopathy. *Journal of Pediatric Surgery, 33,* 1251–1253.

Jacir, N. N., Anderson, K. D., Eichelberger, M., & Guzzetta, P. C. (1986). Cholelithiasis in infancy: Resolution of gallstones in three of four infants. *Journal of Pediatric Surgery, 21,* 567–569.

Janu, P. G., Rogers, D. A., & Lobe, T. E. (1996). A comparison of laparoscopic and traditional open splenectomy in childhood. *Journal of Pediatric Surgery, 31,* 109–114.

Jewett, T. C., Jr., Duszynski, D. O., & Allen, J. E. (1970). The visualization of Meckel's diverticulum with 99mTc-pertechnetate. *Surgery, 68,* 567–570.

Jugenburg, M., Haddock, G., Freedman, M. H., Ford-Jones, L., & Ein, S. H. (1999). The morbidity and mortality of pediatric splenectomy: Does prophylaxis make a difference? *Journal of Pediatric Surgery, 34*(7), 1064–1067.

Kim, P. C. W., Wesson, D., Superina, R., & Filler, R. (1995). Laparoscopic cholecystectomy versus open cholecystectomy in children: Which is better? *Journal of Pediatric Surgery, 30,* 971–973.

King, D. E., Ginn-Pease, M. E., Lloyd, T. V., Hoffman, J., & Hohenbrink, K. (1987). Parenteral nutrition with associated cholelithiasis: Another iatrogenic disease of infants and children. *Journal of Pediatric Surgery, 22,* 593–596.

Krishnamurthy, G. T., Bobba, V. R., & Kingston, E. (1981). Radionuclide ejection fraction: A technique for quantitative analysis of motor function of the human gallbladder. *Gastroenterology, 80,* 482–490.

Krishnamurthy, S., & Krishnamurthy, G. T. (1997). Biliary dyskinesia: Role of sphincter of Oddi, gallbladder, and cholecystokinin. *Journal of Nuclear Medicine, 38,* 1824–1830.

Lachman, B. S., Lazerson, J., Starshak, R. J., Vaughters, F. M., & Werlin, S. L. (1979). The prevalence of cholelithiasis in sickle cell disease as diagnosed by ultrasound and cholecystography. *Pediatrics, 64,* 601–603.

Leijonmarck, C. E., Bonman-Sandelin, K., Frisell, J., & Raf, L. (1986). Meckel's diverticulum in the adult. *British Journal of Surgery, 73*(2), 146–149.

Loftus, W. K., & Metreweli, C. (1998). Ultrasound assessment of mild splenomegaly: Spleen/kidney ratio. *Pediatric Radiology, 28,* 98–100.

Lorberboym, M., Pastores, G. M., Kim, C. K., Herman, G., Glajchen, N., & Machac, J. (1997). Scintigraphic monitoring of reticuloendothelial system in patients with type I Gaucher disease on enzyme replacement therapy. *Journal of Nuclear Medicine, 38*(6), 890–895.

Mackey, W. C., & Dineen, P. A. (1983). A fifty-year experience with Meckel's diverticulum. *Surgery Gynecological Obstetrics, 156,* 56–64.

McCancre, K., & Huether, S. (1990). *Pathophysiology, the biological basis for disease in adults and children.* St. Louis, MO: Mosby.

Mehta, S. S., & Gittes, G. K. (2005). Lesions of the pancreas and spleen. In K. W. Ashcraft, G. W. Holcomb, III, & J. P. Murphy (Eds.), *Pediatric surgery* (4th ed., pp. 649–658). Philadelphia: Elsevier Saunders.

Minkes, R. K., Lagzdins, M., & Langer, J. C. (2000). Laparoscopic versus open splenectomy in children. *Journal of Pediatric Surgery, 35*(5), 699–701.

Monson, J. R. T. (1993). Advanced techniques in abdominal surgery. *British Medical Journal, 307,* 1346–1350.

Moore, K. L., & Persaud, T. V. N. (1993). *The developing human: Clinically oriented embryology.* Philadelphia: W.B. Saunders.

Pearson, H. A. (2002). The spleen. In C. D. Rudolph, A. M. Rudolph, M. K. Hostetter, G. Lister, & N. J. Siegel (Eds.), *Rudolph's pediatrics* (21st ed., pp. 1560–1562). New York: McGraw-Hill Medical Publishing Division.

Peter, G. (Ed.). (1994). *Red book: Report of the committee on infectious diseases* (23rd ed.). Elk Grove Village, IL: American Academy of Pediatrics.

Peter, G. (Ed.). (1997). *Red book: Report of the committee on infectious diseases* (24th ed.). Elk Grove Village, IL: American Academy of Pediatrics.

Reddy, V. S., Phen, H. H., O'Neill, J. A., Neblett, W. W., Pietsch, J. B., Morgan, W. M., et al. (2001). Laparoscopic versus open splenectomy in the pediatric population: A contemporary single-center experience. *American Surgeon, 67*(9), 859–863.

Rerksuppaphol, S., Hutson, J. M., & Oliver, M. R. (2004). Ranitidine-enhanced 99mtechnetium pertechnetate imaging in children improves the sensitivity of identifying heterotopic gastric mucosa in Meckel's diverticulum. *Pediatric Surgery International, 20*(5), 323–325.

Rescorla, F. J. (1997). Cholelithiasis, cholecystitis, and common bile duct stone. *Current Opinion in Pediatrics, 9*, 276–282.

Rescorla, F. J., Engum, S. A., West, K. W., Tres Schere, L. R. 3rd, Rouse, T. M., & Grosfeld, J. L. (2002). Laparoscopic splenectomy has become the gold standard in children. *American Journal of Surgery, 68*(3), 297–301.

Rice, H. E. (2005). Spleen: Pediatric spleen surgery. In K. T. Oldham, P. M. Colombani, R. P. Foglia, & M. A. Skinner (Eds.), *Principles and practice of pediatric surgery* (Vol. 2, pp. 1511–1522). Philadelphia: Lippincott Williams & Wilkins.

Rice, E. O., Miflin, T. E., Sakallah, S., Lee, R. E., Sansieri, C. A., & Barranger, J. A. (1996). Gaucher disease: Studies of phenotype, molecular diagnosis and treatment. *Clinical Genetics, 49*(3), 111–118.

Rice, H. E., Oldham, K. T., Hillery, C. A., Skinner, M. A., O'Hare, S. M., & Ware, R. E. (2003). Clinical and hematologic benefit of partial splenectomy for congenital hemolytic anemias in children. *Annals of Surgery, 237*(2), 281–288.

Rutherford, E. J., Livengood, J., Higginbotham, M., Miles, W. S., Koestner, J., Edwards, K. M., et al. (1995). Efficacy and safety of pneumococcal revaccination after splenectomy for trauma. *Journal of Trauma, 39*, 448–452.

Sawin, R. S. (2005). Appendix and Meckel's diverticulum. In K. T. Oldham, P. M. Colombani, R. P. Foglia, & M. A. Skinner (Eds.), *Principles and practice of pediatric surgery* (Vol. 2, pp. 1269–1282). Philadelphia: Lippincott Williams & Wilkins.

Schleef, J., Morcate, J. J., Steinau, G., Ott, B., & Willital, G. H. (1997). Technical aspects of laparoscopic splenectomy in children. *Journal of Pediatric Surgery, 32*, 615–617.

Schropp, K. P. (2005) Meckel's diverticulum. In K. W. Ashcraft, G. W. Holcomb, III, & J. P. Murphy (Eds.), *Pediatric surgery* (4th ed., pp. 553–556). Philadelphia: Elsevier Saunders.

Schutze, G. E., Mason, E. O. Jr., Barson, W. J., Kim, K. S., Wald, E. R., Givner, L. B., et al. (2002). Invasive pneumococcal infections in children with asplenia. *Pediatric Infectious Disease Journal, 21*(4), 278–282.

Sfakianakis, G. N., & Conway, J. J. (1981). Detection of ectopic gastric mucosa in Meckel's diverticulum and in other aberrations by scintigraphy: II. indications and methods—A 10-year experience. *Journal of Nuclear Medicine, 22*, 732–738.

Shaffer, E. A. (1996). Gallbladder disease. In W. A. Walker, P. R. Durie, J. R. Hamilton, J. A. Walker-Smith, & J. B. Watkins (Eds.), *Pediatric gastrointestinal disease: Pathophysiology, diagnosis, management* (5th ed., pp. 1399–1419). St. Louis, MO: Mosby.

Smith, B. M., Schropp, K. P., Lobe, T. E., Rogers, D. A., Presbury, G. J., Wilimas, J. A., et al. (1994). Laparoscopic splenectomy in childhood. *Journal of Pediatric Surgery, 28*, 975–977.

Soltero, M. J., & Bill, A. H. (1976). The natural history of Meckel's diverticulum and its relation to incidental removal. A study of 202 cases of diseased Meckel's diverticulum found in King County, Washington, over a fifteen year period. *American Journal of Surgery, 132*, 168–173.

Soutter, A. D., Ellenbogen, J., & Folkman, J. (1994). Splenosis is regulated by a circulating factor. *Journal of Pediatric Surgery, 29*, 1076–1079.

Swaniker, F., Soldes, O., & Hirschi, R. (1999). The utility of technetium 99m pertechnetate scintigraphy in the evaluation of patients with Meckel's diverticulum. *Journal of Pediatric Surgery, 34*(5), 760–764.

Svarch, E., Vilorio, P., Nordet, I., Chesney, A., Batista, J. F., Torres, L., et al. (1996). Partial splenectomy in children with sickle cell disease and repeated episodes of splenic sequestration. *Hemoglobin, 20*(4), 393–400.

Teitelbaum, D. H., Polley, T. Z., & Obeid, F. (1994). Laparoscopic diagnosis and excision of Meckel's diverticulum. *Journal of Pediatric Surgery, 29*(4), 495–497.

Tsakayannis, D. E., Kozakewich, H. P. W., & Lillehei, C. W. (1996). Acalculous cholecystitis in children. *Journal of Pediatric Surgery, 31*, 127–131.

Tulman, S., Holcomb, G. W., III, Karamanoukian, H. L., & Reynhout, J. (1993). Pediatric laparoscopic splenectomy. *Journal of Pediatric Surgery, 28*, 689–692.

Vane, D. W., West, K. W., & Grosfeld, J. L. (1987). Vitelline duct anomalies: Experience with 217 childhood cases. *Archives of Surgery, 122*, 542–547.

Wales, P. W., Carver, E., Crawford, M. W., & Kim, P. C. (2001). Acute chest syndrome after abdominal surgery in children with sickle cell disease: Is a laparoscopic approach better? *Journal of Pediatric Surgery, 36*(5), 718–721.

Zamir, O., Szold, A., Matzner, Y., Ben-Yehuda, D., Seror, D., Deutsch, I., et al. (1996). Laparoscopic splenectomy for immune thrombocytopenic purpura. *Journal of Laparoendoscopic Surgery, 6*(5), 301–304.

Nursing Care of Children with Complex Surgical Conditions

Biliary Atresia and Choledochal Cyst

By Laura M. Flanigan

The liver is the largest organ in the body and the site of varied and complex physiologic tasks. Included are vascular metabolic and storage functions as well as detoxification and excretion of drugs and chemical alteration and excretion of hormones. A vital excretory function of the liver is formation of bile, which then flows into the intestinal tract through a system of ducts. Bile salts are required for the digestion and absorption of fat. The extrahepatic biliary system is crucial as a means of excreting bilirubin, the end-product of hemoglobin degradation (Guyton, 1991).

Jaundice is a common presentation that implies an impairment of bile flow from internal biliary ducts to the duodenum. The causes of cholestasis in infants and children include anatomic abnormalities, metabolic disorders, hepatitis, and chromosomal anomalies. This chapter discusses the diagnosis and treatment of two anatomic abnormalities: biliary atresia and choledochal cyst.

■ Biliary Atresia

Description

Biliary atresia (BA) is an obstructive condition of the liver and bile ducts that presents in early infancy and results in obliteration of the extrahepatic biliary tree. Although the term *atresia* implies congenital absence of the biliary tree, this condition is a dynamic one. There is an ongoing, inflammatory process of bile duct epithelium that scleroses and obliterates the normal ductal system. The cause is unknown, but once fibrosis obliterates the bile ducts, bile can no longer be transported from the liver to the gastrointestinal tract. This results in profound cholestasis, jaundice, and progressive cirrhosis, ultimately leading to liver failure. Biliary atresia is the most common cause of chronic cholestasis in infants and children (Balistreri et al., 1996).

No causal relationship exists between the cholestatic jaundice of BA and the physiologic jaundice of the newborn that begins at 3 to 5 days of life and generally resolves by 2 weeks of age. The incidence of BA is approximately 1 in 15,000 live births. It is rarely seen in premature babies, and more females than males are affected. Polysplenia and intestinal malrotation are present in 15% to 20% of patients (Altman et al., 1997). Biliary atresia is the most common cause of death from liver disease in children (Ohi & Ibrahim, 1992). If untreated, BA results in progressive liver failure with a life expectancy of less than 2 years (Adelman, 1985).

Clinical Presentation

Most infants with BA have an uneventful perinatal course. Initially, the infant appears to be well and thrives in spite of the presence of jaundice that becomes apparent at 2 to 3 weeks of age (Wyllie & Hyams, 1993). Stools, which initially have a normal appearance, become acholic (pale or clay colored). Urine becomes dark in appearance, because the kidneys filter some excess bilirubin. In addition to being markedly icteric, the infant's liver is enlarged and firm. The gradual onset of the symptoms may go unnoticed by the parents and are often first appreciated by the primary health care provider at a regular visit at 4 to 8 weeks of life.

Differential Diagnosis and Work-Up

The presence of jaundice after 2 weeks of age is unlikely to be physiologic. Any jaundiced infant older than 2 weeks of age should be evaluated. Successful outcome in the treatment of BA is strongly influenced by the age at surgical intervention, which makes prompt diagnosis imperative. The likelihood of the surgical drainage procedure (Kasai procedure) being successful is markedly reduced in infants older than 10 weeks of age (Altman et al., 1997). No single test result is diagnostic of BA, but some may eliminate other conditions that present with jaundice in early infancy.

Laboratory Studies

Serum Bilirubin

An elevated bilirubin level may result from obstructive, metabolic, or infectious causes that result in cholestasis. The hyperbilirubinemia of physiologic jaundice is indirect (unconjugated), appearing at about 2 days of age and generally resolving by the second week of life. The jaundice of BA is characterized by direct (conjugated) hyperbilirubinemia, with the total bilirubin being elevated to 4 to 8 mg/dL or higher and the direct level being 15% to 20% of the total. This is indicative of obstructive process.

Liver Function

Liver enzymes are usually modestly elevated, indicative of hepatocellular injury. This is not specific to BA. At the onset, prothrombin time and partial thromboplastin time are usually normal because the synthetic functions of the liver are still intact (Altman, 1991).

Other

Hepatitis serology, TORCH (toxoplasmosis, other infections, rubella, cytomegalovirus infection, and herpes simplex) titers, and alpha1-antitrypsin studies are obtained to rule out some of the infectious and metabolic causes of jaundice. The hematocrit value, hemoglobin value, and white blood count are generally normal.

Radiologic Studies

Ultrasonography

An abdominal sonogram is a safe, noninvasive study that documents the presence and size of the gallbladder. In BA, the gallbladder is not visualized or is small (< 1.5 cm) and noncontractile. A fasting infant with a gallbladder greater than 1.5 cm that contracts with feeding is unlikely to have BA (Karrer, Lilly, & Hall, 1993).

Hepato-Iminodiacetic Acid (HIDA) Scan

The HIDA scan detects bile flow from the liver through the biliary tree and into the gastrointestinal tract. The isotope is quickly concentrated by the liver, and normally excretion begins immediately. It can be detected in the gallbladder within 5 minutes and in the small bowel by 30 minutes. If isotope activity is not detected in the small bowel within a few hours, a delayed scan is obtained in 24 hours. In infants with biliary obstruction, no excretion into the bowel is detectable. Infants with severe intrahepatic cholestasis, without extrahepatic biliary obstruction, may also demonstrate impaired excretion. Patients are prepared for the scan by receiving oral phenobarbital (5–10 mg/kg/day) for 3 to 5 days before the study. The choleretic effect of the phenobarbital may encourage bile flow in patients with cholestasis. This study helps to identify patients whose lack of bile excretion is due to parenchymal disease rather than extrahepatic ductal obstruction (Madj, Reba, & Altman, 1981).

Percutaneous Liver Biopsy

The percutaneous liver biopsy is performed with local anesthesia and sedation. Intramuscular vitamin K is administered before the biopsy to enhance clotting. The potential risk of bleeding following a percutaneous liver biopsy necessitates close observation and monitoring of the infant's hemodynamic status for 6 hours. The histologic findings consistent with a diagnosis of BA are bile duct proliferation, cholestasis (which may be mild, moderate, or severe), and portal tract fibrosis (Ohi & Ibrahim, 1992).

Exploratory Laparotomy and Intraoperative Cholangiogram

The work-up, to this point, cannot provide a secure diagnosis of BA. No test or combination of tests is absolutely diagnostic. Other causes of jaundice may be eliminated, and findings may provide evidence to support, but not make, the diagnosis. Diagnosis is confirmed with surgical exploration to identify the anatomy of the extrahepatic bile ducts.

With the patient under general anesthesia, a right upper quadrant incision is made. In BA, the liver is firm, and the surface appears greenish brown, coarse, and irregular. A generous liver specimen is obtained to confirm the findings of the previous percutaneous biopsy. If inspection of the extrahepatic biliary tree reveals complete fibrosis, the diagnosis of BA is confirmed. If the gallbladder has an obvious lumen, it is aspirated. If the contents are bilious, a cholangiogram is performed by instilling a small amount of radiopaque contrast. If the entire biliary tree, from the liver to the duodenum, can be visualized on the x-ray film, the diagnosis of BA is eliminated and the procedure terminated (Altman, 1991).

In BA, there are anatomic variations of the diseased extrahepatic ducts. In approximately 25% of patients, the distal common duct is patent to the duodenum. In 75%, the entire extrahepatic biliary tree is atretic. If the gallbladder is obviously fibrotic, a cholangiogram is deferred. Dissection in the portal area of the liver is then undertaken to identify the anatomy of the fibrotic biliary tree (Kasai, Kimura, & Asakura, 1968). If the diagnosis is confirmed by inability to visualize the complete biliary tree, the procedure converts from exploratory to therapeutic.

Surgery

Without surgical treatment to establish bile flow, BA is uniformly fatal. In 1968, after his earlier work in Japan, Kasai published the first report in the US literature on the hepatic portoenterostomy (Kasai et al., 1968). The results were extremely encouraging, and the procedure gained gradual acceptance as the definitive procedure for BA in the 1970s (Altman & Lilly, 1975).

The hepatoportoenterostomy, or Kasai procedure, involves excision of the fibrotic biliary tract and anastomosis of a 45 cm Roux-Y limb of the jejunum to the periductular tissue at the porta hepatis (Fig. 28-1) This newly created conduit provides a channel for bile flow from liver to intestine. Although there are three common variants of BA (Fig. 28-2), all require complete excision of the extrahepatic biliary tree and creation of the Kasai hepatoportoenterostomy. Many modifications of the conduit, including exteriorization of the jejunal limb, with cutaneous diversion of bile drainage and creation of an antireflux valve in the jejeunal limb (Karrer et al., 1993), have been proposed with the intent of reducing the incidence of ascending bacterial cholangitis. None of the modifications intended to reduce the incidence of cholangitis affects outcome (Altman et al., 1997).

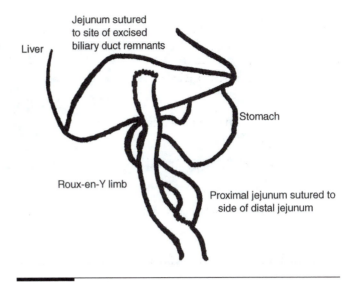

Figure 28-1 Kasai hepatoportoenterostomy.

The goal of the Kasai procedure is to establish bile flow from the liver. The first appearance of bile in the stool may be scant, streaky, and intermittent and usually occurs by the end of the first postoperative week. If adequate bile flow is achieved and maintained, the pigmented appearance of the stool gradually becomes normal.

Complications

The most common complication of the Kasai procedure is bacterial cholangitis. Initially, the bile flow from the liver may be sluggish. Infection results from the bile stasis and bacterial contamination from the intestinal conduit. All patients should receive intravenous antibiotics in the immediate postoperative period and continue oral prophylaxis for 12 to 24 months. Cholangitis is most likely within the first 2 years after surgery, although it may also occur later (McEvoy & Suchy, 1996). After a Kasai procedure, any patient with fever, leukocytosis, and a rising bilirubin level with no obvious other causes is presumed to have cholangitis and is treated with intravenous antibiotics and steroids. With each attack comes the risk of permanent liver damage with complete shutdown of bile flow. Institution of early treatment may prevent irreversible liver damage (Karrer et al., 1993).

Outcome

Kasai's hepatoportoenterostomy revolutionized the outlook for infants with BA. Early recognition, prompt, efficient work-up, and timely referral for surgical correction are critical to achieving the best outcome. Without biliary drainage, there is no possibility of altering the inexorable course of the disease. When surgery is carried out before the infant reaches 70 days, there is a significantly

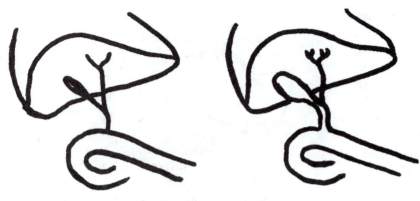

Type A Complete obliteration of bile ducts

Type B Patent distal biliary tree

Type C Minute intrahepatic ducts with patent proximal duct and gallbladder

Figure 28-2 Most common types of biliary atresia.

greater chance of achieving bile flow. Another factor influencing outcome is the diameter of microscopic biliary ductules at the porta hepatis where the fibrous biliary tree has been transected. Patients with larger ductal lumens have a significantly better chance of long term survival (Altman et al., 1997).

Bile drainage can be achieved in about 90% of patients who undergo a Kasai procedure at less than 10 weeks of age (Altman et al., 1997; Karrer et al., 1993). Approximately 30% to 40% of patients become jaundice-free, and liver functions return to normal, resulting in a very optimistic long-term outcome. Another 30% to 40% of patients have evidence of hepatic damage but with medical and nutritional support continue to grow and develop. The fibrotic liver may eventually decompensate, often precipitated by some physiologically stressful event. In nearly another 30% of patients, even with bile drainage having been achieved, the process causing BA continues uninterrupted with progressive biliary cirrhosis, leading to liver failure (Altman, 1991; Karrer et al.).

Portal hypertension is another potential problem after portoenterostomy, even with adequate bile flow. The portal vein carries blood and its newly acquired nutrients from the viscous into the liver. A scarred liver impedes this flow, increasing the portal venous pressure. Portal hypertension ultimately results in hypersplenism, ascites, and esophageal and gastric varices. Hemorrhagic bleeding from esophageal varices may be sudden, repeated, and life threatening. Varices are managed by endoscopic sclerosing or banding (Karrer et al., 1993).

At present, treatment for end-stage liver disease or severe portal hypertension is hepatic transplantation. Patients with BA make up the majority of the pediatric recipients undergoing liver transplantation (Whitington & Balistreri, 1991). It has been suggested that trans-plantation should replace the Kasai procedure as the treatment of choice (Azarow, Phillips, & Sandler, 1997). However, there is evidence from a large series that median survival is 15 years after biliary drainage is achieved with the Kasai. Some children may never need transplantation, whereas others survive with their native liver many years before needing transplantation. With the limited supply of organs available to infants, the decreased survival in infant recipients, and the problems associated with long-term immunosuppression, along with the likelihood that the portoenterostomy will extend pre-transplantation survival, the Kasai procedure and liver transplantation should be considered complementary therapies (Altman et al., 1997).

The advent of successful outcomes using living, related, and reduced-size orthotopic liver grafts has made it possible to plan liver transplantations for infants after a failed Kasai procedure. Transplantation may then take place before patients reach end-stage liver disease. For additional information on liver transplantation, refer to Chapter 30.

Developmental Considerations

When the Kasai procedure is successful in establishing biliary drainage and liver functions return to normal, there is a negligible impact on development. If the course of hepatic fibrosis is not interrupted by the portoenterostomy, delays in growth and development are inevitable. Fat, carbohydrate, and protein metabolism normally occur in the liver, and this process is increasingly impaired as hepatic fibrosis progresses. A critical indication of impaired hepatic function is an infant's failure to maintain his/her own curve on the growth chart for height, weight, and head circumference. As the child's nutritional status worsens, the ability to achieve expected developmental milestones becomes markedly impaired. Increasing abdominal girth secondary to hepatosplenomegaly and ascites make being placed in the prone position difficult, which interferes with development of head control. As nutrition worsens, the child develops muscle wasting and decreased strength and energy to perform normal, age-appropriate activities.

Susceptibility to infection may require isolating a child from his or her peer group and interferes with normal social development. Interventions designed to stimulate physical and social development should be encouraged. As children become sicker and require intermittent hospitalization, physical and occupational therapy and child life therapists can ensure that appropriate interventions and activities are available. Parents and the health care team should reinforce and participate in planned developmental activities.

Referrals

Several parent support groups may by helpful to parents as they struggle to cope with their child's diagnosis. For example the Biliary Atresia and Liver Transplant Network Inc. (BALT) and Children's Liver Association for Support Services (CLASS) are both organizations that can provide a support network for families of children with BA and chronic liver disease, both before and after transplantation. Refer to the Resource Chapter for additional information.

Referrals to home care agencies should be made as appropriate. If the biliary conduit is exteriorized, the family is referred to a home health agency for additional support and teaching until parents are comfortable caring for the ostomy. If the liver disease becomes progressive, parents may find themselves facing increasingly complex care issues at home. Equipment and home nursing support may be required for nasogastric feedings, total parenteral nutrition, central line care, and pain management.

■ Choledochal Cyst

Description

Choledochal cyst is a malformation of the biliary system, manifested by localized dilatation of all or some portion of the intra- and extrahepatic biliary tree. The first description appeared in the literature in the 17th Century (Douglas, 1852). In 1959, the entity was classified into three anatomic groups by Alonso-Lej, Rever, and Pessagano, and since then, two variants have been added (Caroli, 1968; Flanigan, 1975). The most common presentation is type I, cystic dilatation of the common bile duct, which represents more than 75% of cases. The other four classifications represent a spectrum of complex pathological anomalies in the biliary tree that together make up the remaining less than 25%. Type II represents a diverticulum of the common bile duct, and type III an intraduodenal dilatation of the common bile duct (also called *choledochocele*). In type IV, there is intrahepatic as well as extrahepatic cystic dilatation. If intrahepatic cysts are present with a normal extrahepatic biliary tree, it is classified as type V, also called Caroli's disease.

The origin of choledochal cyst formation is unclear, although many mechanisms have been proposed. It is likely that a number of factors lead to their formation and that the cysts actually represent a spectrum of anomalies in the pancreatobiliary system. The common features, in addition to cystic dilatation of the bile duct, include (1) anomalous junction of the pancreatic and common bile duct; (2) distal bile duct stenosis; (3) intrahepatic ductal dilatation; (4) abnormal histologic findings of the common bile duct; and (5) hepatic histology from normal to cirrhotic (Altman, 1992). The bile duct stenosis results in cholestasis, leading to cholangitis. The liver injury that results may range from mild, periportal infiltrates to marked biliary cirrhosis and subsequent portal hypertension (Lazar & Altman, 2000). Adenocarcinoma secondary to long-term inflammation of the bile ducts has also been reported (Howard, 1991). Surgical intervention is necessary to relieve the chronic obstruction that results.

Choledochal cyst is considered a rare entity with a worldwide incidence reported anywhere between 1:13,000 to 1:1,000,000 (Wyllie & Hyams, 1993). It is much more frequently seen in the Japanese, with an incidence of 1:1,000, but the incidence is only 1:15,000 in the United States (Howard, 1991). In all races, the female-to-male incidence is about 4:1.

Clinical Presentation

Choledochal cyst can be diagnosed at any age, but about 25% are diagnosed by a year and 60% by age 10. Clinical presentation in infants less than 6 months of age may include signs of complete extrahepatic biliary obstruction: jaundice, hepatomegaly, and acholic stools. These symptoms may initially make it indistinguishable from BA (Rowe, O'Neill, Grosfeld, Fonkalsrud, & Coran, 1995). Increased use of ultrasound as a screening technique has led to prenatal diagnosis in a number of cases (Holland & Lilly, 1992). Older infants or children are more likely to present with subtle, episodic, but recurrent, abdominal pain. The accompanying minimal jaundice may go unnoticed (Altman, 1992). Only about 15% of patients actually present with what is referred to as the classic triad: intermittent pain, jaundice, and abdominal mass. Pancreatitis and cholangitis may occur secondary to the bile stasis caused by the obstructive nature of the cyst (Lazar & Altman, 2000). Untreated choledochal cyst may result in chronic liver failure or biliary carcinoma (Karrer et al., 1993).

Diagnosis

The initial work-up depends on the nature, severity, and duration of the symptoms. Laboratory findings are nonspecific. The main finding is conjugated hyperbilirubinemia, which is generally more pronounced in the infant. There may also be increases in the alkaline phosphatase, transaminases, and gamma glutamyl transpeptidase. Abdominal ultrasonography and computed tomography establish the diagnosis. Both clearly define the dimensions of the cyst and the extent of involvement. In patients in whom symptoms are intermittent and marked cystic enlargement is not present, a DISIDA (technetium-99m) scan with follow-up scanning defines extrahepatic anatomy and pattern of bile excretion. Endoscopic retrograde cholangiopancreatography is also used, but the invasive nature risks precipitating cholangitis (Altman & Hicks, 1996). Recently, magnetic resonance cholangiopancreatography has begun to replace endoscopic retrograde cholangiopancreatography because it provides the same information noninvasively.

Recommended Therapy

The definitive treatment for choledochal cyst is surgical. Internal drainage by cystenterostomy is no longer the procedure of choice. Patients treated with this method suffered a high incidence of anastomotic obstruction, leading to bile stasis, cholangitis, biliary cirrhosis, and possible malignancy in the retained cyst wall (Flanigan, 1977).

Total cyst removal with reconstruction using a Roux-en-Y jejunostomy with anastomosis of the normal, proximal bile ducts to a limb of jejunum is now the preferred treatment in the majority of cases (Altman & Hicks, 1996). Anastomosis of the mucosa of the proximal bile duct to the mucosa of the jejunum is important to avoid postoperative stricture. If inflammation around the cyst makes resection hazardous, the entire mucosal lining may be removed, leaving the outer wall in place. In type V, where the cystic structure is inside the liver, a lobectomy may be indicated. If the disease affects both lobes, liver transplantation is the only treatment (Lazar & Altman, 2000).

Outcome

Early postoperative complications are generally minor. The most common late complications are cholangitis, obstructive jaundice, pancreatitis, and complications of portal hypertension, such as bleeding esophageal varices (Karrer et al., 1993). The long-term results after biliary reconstruction are favorable in patients who undergo surgery before the onset of advanced liver disease (Lazar & Altman, 2000).

Developmental Considerations

Early diagnosis and treatment alleviate the impact on a child's growth and development. Infants usually undergo surgery before chronic liver disease has any effect on growth and development. In older children, symptoms such as recurrent episodes of severe abdominal pain affect a child's ability to eat normally, go to school, and play.

Referrals

Most children recover with no long-term sequelae. Families with children who have chronic liver disease may find that contact with families in similar circumstances is helpful. The Children's Liver Association for Support Services (CLASS) is a support group for families of children with chronic liver disease.

■ Nursing Care of Infants and Children with Biliary Atresia and Choledochal Cyst

Preoperative Care

Families come with varied understanding about the diagnosis of BA or choledochal cyst, the treatment and possible outcomes. Most are overwhelmed and frightened by the news that their infant or child has a serious condition and needs an urgent, major surgical procedure. Some have limited knowledge about the diagnosis and its life-threatening implications, whereas others are well informed. With increasing frequency, parents come with information and lists of questions obtained from an Internet search.

If the patient with a presumptive diagnosis of BA is close to 70 days of age when referred to the pediatric surgeon, the situation must be treated with urgency to enhance the chances of a favorable income (Altman et al., 1997). On the contrary, when a prenatal diagnosis of choledochal cyst is made, an antenatal visit can allay parents' concerns that surgical excision is necessary immediately after birth.

Nursing assessment of the family's level of functioning makes it possible to provide the appropriate level of teaching and support. The nurse needs to repeat and reinforce the information about diagnosis, prognosis, and surgical procedure throughout the perioperative course.

Patients are admitted to the hospital the morning of surgery unless an inpatient bowel prep is required. If the synthetic functions of the liver are abnormal, intramuscular vitamin K should be administered to enhance clotting. If the possibility of transfusion is anticipated, parental concerns should be addressed when the urgency of the surgery negates the option of donor-designated blood. Nursing mothers should be assured that breastfeeding will be interrupted for only a few days. They should be provided with information and assistance with pumping and saving breast milk while their infant is unable to feed orally.

Parents often express concern about general anesthesia and need reassurance that anesthesia can be administered safely to infants and children. Specific concerns should be addressed by the anesthesiologist. Many centers allow parents to be present for anesthesia induction.

Because the diagnosis of BA cannot be absolutely confirmed before exploration, it is important to communicate with the family from the operating room. This may be achieved with a call or visit from a member of the surgical team.

Postoperative Care

Choledochal Cyst

Care after a Kasai procedure or choledochal cyst excision is similar to that as for any infant or child who undergoes major abdominal surgery and small-bowel anastomosis. It includes intravenous hydration, gastric/intestinal decompression, antibiotic coverage, and pain management.

Intravenous antibiotics are begun in the operating room. When the patient is tolerating feedings, this is changed to an oral antibiotic at a prophylactic dose. Adequate postoperative pain management requires narcotic infusion. This may be achieved quite safely, even in infants and small children with appropriate dosing and frequent assessment. The addition of rectal acetaminophen may potentiate the effect of the opioid, allowing reduction of the narcotic dose. This can result in fewer adverse effects (Tobias, 1996).

Either of the procedures requires a substantial right upper quadrant incision that should be covered with a small dressing to allow assessment of the wound. A drain is brought out through a stab wound several centimeters below the incision and dressed separately. This permits drainage of ascitic fluid or bile and is removed by the fifth postoperative day.

The patient remains NPO and has a nasogastric tube to low suction for decompression of the stomach and in-

testinal tract. Patency and position of the tube should be checked frequently. Presence of bowel sounds alone does not provide assurance that bowel function is sufficient to indicate removal of the tube. Reduced nasogastric drainage or passage of flatus or stool 3 to 5 days after surgery indicates return of bowel function. In infants, if small feedings of electrolyte solution or glucose water are tolerated, breast milk or formula can usually be successfully reintroduced. In toddlers and children, clear liquids are introduced, followed by an age-appropriate diet.

Biliary Atresia

In BA in which the native sclerosed, extrahepatic biliary tree has been resected, the appearance of bile in the stool indicates that the Kasai hepatoportoenterostomy has been successful in providing a conduit for bile flow from the liver to the gastrointestinal tract. The first stools may still be clay colored. The first appearance of bile is usually green plugs. Because of the severe intrahepatic cholestasis, bile flow is initially sporadic. Parents should be warned so that they are not alarmed by the passage of acholic stools. The flow of bile from the liver should increase gradually until the stools are normally pigmented. Within a few days of initiating feedings, patients begin ursodeoxycholic acid (Actigall), 12 to 20 mg/day in two divided doses. This is a choleretic agent that promotes bile flow and is continued for a minimum of 1 to 2 years if there is good return of liver function. Patients with continued evidence of cirrhosis may remain on it indefinitely.

In patients with BA, fat, carbohydrate, and protein metabolism that occur in the liver are usually impaired, and there is reduced presence of bile acids in the small intestine. This means that nutrition is an important consideration. After surgery, patients are fed breast milk or formula containing medium-chain triglycerides as the source of fat, such as Pregestimil and Alimentum. These formulas do not require the acids present in bile for digestion. Absorption of the fat-soluble vitamins A, D, E, and K is also compromised. These vitamins are available as a single preparation and should be started when the patient is tolerating oral feedings. Serum vitamin E levels can be monitored within 4 to 8 weeks. The dose can then be adjusted to maintain adequate levels (Hendricks & Walker, 1990).

Even with evidence of good biliary drainage, improvement in liver function parameters, including resolution of jaundice, cannot be expected for 4 to 6 weeks. Obtaining studies before that time creates unnecessary anxiety for the family and is not predictive of outcome. It will be several months before it can be established whether liver functions will return to normal, level off at some elevated level, or show continued deterioration.

Postoperative support for BA families is critical. If biliary drainage does not occur promptly, anxiety is heightened. Even in the face of successful biliary drainage, the likelihood of this being a chronic illness is dawning. Introduction of information on support groups for families of infants with BA is appropriate at this time. Families are discharged from the hospital not knowing whether the Kasai procedure will be successful in interrupting the course of the disease. It is still to be determined whether the child's liver will recover sufficiently or whether he or she will face the problems of chronic liver failure, ultimately requiring transplantation for survival.

Chronic Liver Disease

When the degree of hepatic fibrosis is significant or continues to worsen despite a portoenterostomy, the family must begin to deal with the sequelae of biliary cirrhosis. The patient and family benefit from continued nursing support, whether the child is managed at home or when hospitalization is required.

Maintaining the child's nutritional status at a level where growth and development continue to occur is critically important. Fat digestion and metabolism present the greatest problems, but initially, most babies gain weight on breast milk or MCT-oil formulas. Early introduction of solids that are higher in carbohydrates and have greater caloric density may be helpful. The addition of a carbohydrate supplement, such as Polycose, to both formula and solids boosts caloric intake. As the disease progresses, hepatosplenomegaly and ascites may compress the stomach so that small, frequent feedings become necessary. This is a difficult time for families as they begin to see their baby fail.

During the later stages of chronic liver disease, nasogastric feedings are needed either to supplement oral intake or as the primary source of nutrition. Admission to the hospital is usually required for parents to learn to pass the tube, secure it, and administer the feedings safely. Nighttime continuous feeding with oral feeding during the daytime allows maximum freedom. If enteral feeding is unsuccessful, total parenteral nutrition may be used but has the potential for further adverse affects on the liver. Optimizing the child's nutritional status improves chances of becoming a successful liver transplantation recipient. Failure to thrive with maximum nutritional support measures is an indication for transplantation in these babies (Whitington & Balistreri, 1991).

Many infants develop pruritus as a result of increased serum concentrations of bile salts. Bile salt deposits in the epidermis cause itching that can become severe. The child's nails should be kept short to prevent damage to the skin. Cloth mitts can be applied to prevent scratching so that hands need not be restrained. Cholestyramine may be administered to bind bile salts in the intestine and promote their excretion. However, this also reduces the bile salts available to aid in fat digestion. If bile is not present in the gastrointestinal tract, as evidenced by acholic stools, cholestyramine will not be effective (Wyllie & Hyams, 1993). Antihistamines may also be used. Severe, uncontrolled pruritus is considered an indication for transplantation.

Generalized edema and increasing ascites result from decreasing serum albumin levels and the presence of portal hypertension. Edema may become severe, resulting in discomfort and respiratory distress. Spironolactone (Aldactone) or furosemide (Lasix) may be used to control this problem (Wyllie & Hyams, 1993). Serum electrolyte levels should be monitored carefully after diuretics are initiated. Keeping the child's head elevated may also increase the his/her comfort level.

Research

Further research is required to identify the cause of BA. Genetic, ischemic, and infectious causes have been proposed as etiologies of the process that causes the sclerotic obliteration of the biliary tract. Most recently, an autoimmune basis has been proposed based on the presence of the inflammatory mediator ICAM-1, found in the ductal epithelium of six patients with BA (Dillon, Belchis, Minnick, & Tracey, 1997).

Conclusion

There are several causes of jaundice in early infancy. Only in the case of BA does early intervention have such a critical influence. Studies have shown that early diagnosis and surgical treatment are critical factors in achieving a successful outcome. Since the advent of the Kasai hepatoportoenterostomy, more than 30% of patients have liver function that returns to normal and remains stable. Another 30% gain enough improvement in liver function to be able to reach normal growth and developmental milestones for months or years before requiring transplantation. Less than one third of patients do not appear to gain any benefit from the procedure and require early liver transplantation to be rescued from liver failure.

Choledochal cysts can be diagnosed prenatally by ultrasound, but the child may not present with signs of extrahepatic biliary obstruction until later in infancy or early childhood. The preferred treatment for most types of choledochal cysts is total excision and a Roux-en-Y drainage procedure. Untreated cysts may result in liver failure or biliary carcinoma.

■ Acknowledgment

Thanks to Dr. R. Peter Altman, a recognized leader in the care of patients with biliary atresia and choledochal cyst, who has allowed me to share in their care. I am grateful that he listened when our teacher, mentor, and friend, Dr. Judson Randolph, said "Don't quit now."

In memory of Dr. John Lilly who never let us forget that we must always be striving to do better.

■ Educational Materials

APSNA invites you to download the following diagnosis-related teaching tool for Chapter 28, Biliary Atresia and Choledochal Cyst: 1) Biliary Atresia. This teaching tool is available at the APSNA Web site (www.apsna.org) and the Jones and Bartlett Web site (www.jbpub.com). All teaching materials are available in English and Spanish and are free of charge. APSNA encourages their use for your patients and families.

References

Adelman, S. (1985). Prognosis of uncorrected biliary atresia. *Journal of Pediatric Surgery, 20,* 529–534.

Alonso-Lej, F., Rever, W., & Pessagano, D. (1959). Congenital choledochal cyst with a report of 2 & an analysis of 94 cases. *International. Abstracts of Surgery, 108,* 1–30.

Altman, R. P. (1991). Infantile obstructive jaundice. In M. Schiller (Ed.), *Pediatric surgery of the liver, pancreas & spleen* (pp. 59–75).

Altman, R. P. (1992). Choledochal cyst. *Seminars in Pediatric Surgery, 1*(2), 130–133.

Altman, R. P., & Hicks, B. (1996). Choledochal cyst. In D. Carter, R. Russell, H. Pitt, & H. Bismuth (Eds.), *Hepatobiliary & pancreatic surgery* (pp. 362–368). London: Chapman & Hall Medical.

Altman, R. P., & Lilly, J. R. (1975). Technical details in the surgical correction of extrahepatic biliary atresia. *Surgery, Gynecology, & Obstetrics, 10,* 952.

Altman, R. P., Lilly, J. R., Greenfeld, J., Weinberg, A., vanLeeuwen, K., & Flanigan, L. (1997). A multivariate risk factor analysis of the portoenterostomy (Kasai) for biliary atresia: A twenty-five year experience from two centers. *Annals of Surgery, 226,* 348–355.

Azarow, K., Phillips, M., & Sandler, A. (1997). Should all patients undergo a portoenterostomy? *Journal of Pediatric Surgery, 32,* 168–174.

Balistreri, W., Grand, R., Hoofnagle, J., Suchy, F., Rykman, F., Perlmutter, D., et al. (1996). Biliary atresia: Current concepts & research directions. *Hepatology, 23,* 1682–1692.

Caroli, J. (1968). Disease of intrahepatic bile ducts. *Israeli Journal of Medical Science, 4,* 21–25.

Dillon, P., Belchis, D., Minnick, K., & Tracey, T. (1997). Differential expression of the major histocompatibility complex antigens & ICAM~1 on bile duct epithelial cells in biliary atresia. *Tohoku Journal of Experimental Medicine, 181,* 33–40.

Douglas, A. H. (1852). Case of dilatation of the hepatic bile duct. *Monthly Journal of Medical Science, 14,* 97.

Flanigan, D. P. (1975). Biliary cysts. *Annals of Surgery, 182,* 635–643.

Flanigan, D. P. (1977). Biliary carcinoma associated with biliary cysts. *Cancer, 40,* 880–883.

Guyton, A. C. (1991). *Textbook of medical physiology* (8th ed.) Philadelphia: W.B. Saunders.

Hendricks, K., & Walker, W. A. (1990). *Manual of pediatric nutrition* (2nd ed.). Toronto: B.C. Decker.

Holland, R., & Lilly, J. R. (1992). Surgical jaundice in infants: Other than biliary atresia. *Seminars in Pediatric Surgery, 2,* 126–129.

Howard, E. R. (1991). Choledochal cysts. In E. R. Howard (Ed.), *Surgery of liver disease in children.* Oxford: Butterworth-Heinemann.

Kasai, M., Kimura, S., & Asakura, Y. (1968). Surgical treatment of biliary atresia. *Journal of Pediatric Surgery, 3,* 665–675.

Karrer, F., Lilly, J. R., & Hall, R. J. (1993). Biliary tract disorders & portal hypertension. In K. W. Ashcraft & T. M. Holder (Eds.), *Pediatric surgery* (2nd ed., pp. 448–485). Philadelphia: W.B. Saunders.

Lazar, E., & Altman, R. P. (2000). Paediatric hepatobiliary surgery. In Morris & Woods (Eds.), *Oxford textbook of surgery* (2nd ed.). Oxford: Oxford University Press.

Madj, M., Reba, R., & Altman, R. P. (1981). Effect of phenobarbital on 99mTc-IDA scintigraphy in the evaluation of neonatal jaundice. *Seminars in Nuclear Medicine, 11,* 194–204.

McEvoy, C., & Suchy, F. (1996). Biliary tract disease in children. *Pediatric Clinics of North America, 43,* 75–98.

Ohi, R., & Ibrahim, M. (1992). Biliary atresia. *Seminars in Pediatric Surgery, 1,* 115–124.

Rowe, M., O'Neill, J., Jr., Grosfeld, J., Fonkalsrud, E., & Coran, A. (1995). Choledochal cyst. In *Essentials of pediatric surgery.* St. Louis, MO: Mosby.

Tobias, J. (1996). Postoperative pain management. In J. Deshpande & J. Tobias (Eds.), *Pediatric pain handbook* (p. 55). St. Louis, MO: Mosby.

Whitington, P. F., & Balistreri, W. F. (1991). Liver transplantation in pediatrics: Indications, contraindications, & pre-transplant management. *Journal of Pediatrics, 118,* 169–177.

Wyllie, R., & Hyams, J. (1993). Abnormalities of the bile duct. In R. Wyllie & J. Hyams (Eds.), *Pediatric gastrointestinal disease* (pp. 917–921). Philadelphia: W.B. Saunders.

Solid Tumors

By Laura E. San Miguel

The overall incidence of cancer in the pediatric population (children aged 0–19 years) has been essentially stable since the mid-1980s, and the mortality rates have steadily declined during this time (Smith & Ries, 2002). Still, cancer in childhood is the second leading cause of childhood mortality and the most common cause of death from disease in the United States in children aged 1 to 14 years (Smith & Ries). The incidence of cancer is greatest in the first year of life and again peaks at ages 2 to 3 years. This is followed by a steady decline in incidence until age 9, when the rate begins to increase again through adolescence (Gurney, Severson, Davis, & Robinson, 1995; Smith & Ries). There are approximately 2000 cancer-related deaths annually in the United States in children younger than 20 years (Ries, 2004; Smith & Ries). However, overall survival rates have improved dramatically. The 5-year survival rate after a cancer diagnosis in the 1960s was 28%. In the 1990s, that number rose to exceed 75% (Ries; Smith & Ries).

In the past, resection was the only treatment of solid tumors. It has now become an integral part of a combined program of treatment, along with chemotherapy, radiation therapy, and even immunotherapy. Each modality plays a specific role at a specific point, with each role being dependent on the one before and after it for success.

Leukemia accounts for approximately 30% of all childhood cancers, followed by central nervous system tumors (21%). The most common extracranial solid tumors are neuroblastoma, Wilms' tumor, Hodgkin's disease, non-Hodgkin's lymphoma, and rhabdomyosarcoma, in that order (Smith & Ries, 2002; American Cancer Society, Cancer Facts and Figures, 2005).

This chapter focuses on the cause, demographics, sites of origin, signs and symptoms, diagnostic testing, staging, and treatment of extracranial solid tumors, including neuroblastoma, Wilms' tumor, hepatoblastoma and hepatocellular carcinoma, and rhabdomyosarcoma.

■ Neuroblastoma

Each year in the United States, there are approximately 700 new cases of tumors of the sympathetic nervous system in children younger than age 20. Of these, about 650 are neuroblastomas (Goodman, Gurney, Smith, & Olshan, 2004). For incidence, see Table 29-1.

Neuroblastoma is one of the small, round, blue-cell tumors of childhood (which include Ewing's sarcoma, rhabdomyosarcoma, lymphoma, desmoplastic round-cell tumors, and primitive neuroectodermal tumors).

Table 29-1 **Incidence of Neuroblastoma, Wilms' Tumor, Hepatic Tumors, & Rhabdomyosarcoma**

Tumor Type	Incidence in Children < 20 Yr	Notes
Neuroblastoma	7.4% of malignancies 600–650 cases/yr M:F 1.1:1.0 W:B 1.2:1.0	Most common malignancy of infancy; 3rd most common malignancy 40.1% cases diagnosed < 1 yr; 89.4% cases diagnosed < 4 yr; 97.8% cases diagnosed ≤ 10 yr
Wilms' tumor	6% of malignancies 500 cases/yr M:F 0.92:1 unilateral disease M:F 0.60: 1 bilateral disease W:B 1.0:1.09	2nd most common extracranial tumor of childhood Occurs mainly in children < 5 yrs of age
Primary hepatic tumors	1.1% of malignancies 100–150 cases/yr M:F 1.5:1	**Hepatoblastomas:** Account for 2/3 of malignant liver tumors usually occurs in infancy with most cases < 4 yrs **Hepatocellular carcinoma:** mean age at diagnosis, 10 yrs Rare in children, most present in adolescence
Rhabdomyosarcoma	5.3% of malignancies 350 cases/yr M:F 1.4:1 W:B 0.9:1	Most common soft tissue sarcoma Two incidences of peak occurrence, with 2/3 of cases in children ≤ 6 yrs and second peak mid-adolescent years

M, male; F, female; W, white; B, black.

Neuroblastoma arises from neural crest cells, which normally give rise to the sympathetic nervous system (Brodeur & Maris, 2002; Weinstein, Katzenstein, & Cohn, 2003). There are three classic histopathologic patterns of neuroblastoma that correlate with the normal differentiation of the sympathetic nervous system. Neuroblastomas, ganglioneuroblastomas, and ganglioneuromas reflect a pattern of maturation and differentiation, with ganglioneuromas being the mature, benign counterpart to the highly malignant neuroblastoma (Brodeur & Maris).

The outcome for infants and children with neuroblastoma varies widely on the basis of age and stage of disease at diagnosis and tumor biology. In general, lower stages have better outcomes. Despite recent advances in treatment, however, advanced stage and older age at diagnosis are still poor prognostic indicators.

Etiology

The cause of neuroblastoma is unknown. There have been studies evaluating intrauterine exposures, parental occupations, and environmental impact, but none of these factors has been seen consistently or been confirmed in larger studies. No congenital anomaly or constitutional predisposition syndrome has been identified for neuroblastoma, and although a small percentage of patients report a family history, this percentage does not differentiate neuroblastoma from other embryonal cancers of childhood (Brodeur & Maris, 2002).

Sites of Origin

The location of the primary tumor in neuroblastoma can vary and change with age. Regardless of age, the most common primary site is the adrenal gland, which accounts for 40% of primary tumors in children and 25% in infants. Cervical and thoracic tumors are more commonly seen in infants, whereas pelvic tumors are more commonly seen in children. In about 1% of cases, no primary site is identified (Brodeur & Maris, 2002).

Clinical Presentation

The location of the primary tumor and the presence of metastatic disease dictate the presenting signs and symptoms for neuroblastoma (Brodeur & Maris, 2002; Kushner, 2004). Some tumors may be discovered incidentally when a child seeks medical attention for other reasons. However, most children with neuroblastoma are often not diagnosed until the disease has progressed, resulting in an ill appearance. Table 29-2 reviews the presenting signs and symptoms for neuroblastoma by anatomic site.

Table 29-2 **Presenting Signs and Symptoms for Neuroblastoma by Site**

Site	Signs and Symptoms
Generalized	Anorexia, irritability, fatigue, diarrhea, and hypertension
Orbital	Proptosis, periorbital ecchymosis
Superior stellate or cervical ganglion	Horner's syndrome, neurologic findings
Thoracic	Dysphagia, respiratory symptoms of infection, dyspnea, respiratory compromise, especially if tumor is displacing the trachea
Abdominal	Rapid increase in abdominal girth,[a] hard and fixed mass, complaints of fullness, vomiting, hepatomegaly
Adrenal	Difficult to palpate when small
Pelvic	Bladder and bowel compromise, a result of neuronal compression or mass effect
Paraspinal	Severe pain, weakness, or hypotonia of the extremities, scoliosis or paraplegia, depending on the location of the mass
Cortical bone	Pain, limping, refusal to ambulate
Bone marrow	Asymptomatic or anemia, thrombocytopenia, leukopenia, or pancytopenia
Skin nodules	Characteristic of stage IV-S disease and seen in children under age 1

[a]These tumors often occur with a rapid increase in abdominal girth, which is suggestive of malignancy compared with benign processes, which are more indicative of gradual abdominal distention.

Paraneoplastic Syndromes

A small percentage of patients (~2%) present with paraneoplastic syndromes, clinical findings not associated with the primary mass or the presence of metastatic disease (Kushner, 2004). In some patients, opsomyoclonus or cerebellar ataxia is observed. This consists of rapid involuntary chaotic conjugate eye movements and motor incoordination, which is manifested as frequent, irregular, jerking movements of muscles of the limbs and trunk (Lanzkowsky, 1995). This syndrome seems to be associated with a more favorable outcome, but often with long-term neurologic sequelae (Brodeur & Maris, 2002).

Tumors that produce vasoactive intestinal peptides cause a syndrome of intractable watery diarrhea. This is generally seen in patients with histologically mature tumors, and these patients generally have good outcomes. The diarrhea typically resolves after tumor resection (Kushner, 2004; Brodeur & Maris, 2002).

Diagnostic Work-Up

Screening for neuroblastoma can be divided into several study groupings: radiologic findings, urinary catecholamine metabolism, serum values; and pathological and histologic characteristics of the tumor (Fig. 29-1 and Table 29-3).

Histology

According to Brodeur et al. (1993), the definitive diagnosis of neuroblastoma is based on a pathological diagnosis from tumor tissue or the combination of tumor cells in the bone marrow *and* increased urine or serum catecholamines or metabolite levels. Obtaining tumor tissue to study for histopathology, *MYCN* gene copy number, tumor cell chromosome number, or expression of the *TRKA* gene is paramount to directing the choice of therapy (Brodeur & Maris, 2002).

Tumors are classified according to the International Neuroblastoma Pathology Classification System as either favorable or unfavorable. Classification depends on cell differentiation, schwannian stroma content, mitosis-karyorrhexis index, and age of the patient at diagnosis (Shimada et al., 1999; Weinstein et al., 2003). Favorable histology generally translates to better outcome.

Another predictor of outcome is the proto-oncogene *MYCN* (also known as N-myc). Multiple copies of *MYCN* are seen in aggressive tumors and are associated with advanced disease and poor prognosis (Kushner, 2004; Seeger et al, 1985). Tumor cell ploidy, chromosomal abnormalities, and expression of neurotrophin receptors are also studied to guide treatment and predict outcome (Kushner; Brodeur & Maris, 2002).

Spontaneous Regression

In selected patients with stage IV-S disease, neuroblastomas are able to regress or mature spontaneously. Actual overall incidence is probably 5% to 10%, and the tumor is seen almost exclusively in infants (Brodeur et al., 1992).

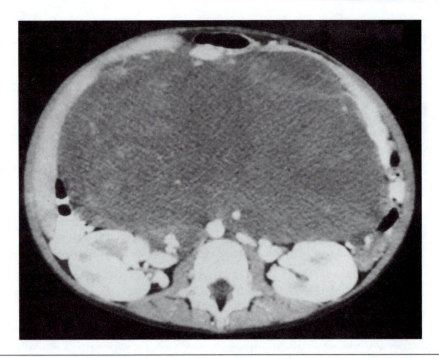

Figure 29-1 Computed tomographic scan of a huge, abdominal neuroblastoma.

Nickerson et al. (2000) found high survival rates in infants with IV-S disease whose tumors were not *MYCN* amplified. This study questioned minimizing or even eliminating treatment for these patients.

Staging

Patients with neuroblastoma are staged to predict survival and determine the intensity of treatment required. The International Neuroblastoma Staging System is used

Table 29-3	Diagnostic Evaluation for Suspected Neuroblastoma
Examination or Test	**Rationale**
History and physical examination	Assess general condition, underlying problems; size of primary tumor, areas of metastatic disease
Complete blood count	Anemia and/or thrombocytopenia may result from bone marrow replacement
Serum ferritin	Elevated levels indicative of advanced disease
Lactic dehydrogenase (LDH)	Elevated levels are indicative of malignancy
Neuron-specific enolase (NSE)	Tumor marker for neuroblastoma
Bone marrow aspirations (4 sites)	Single, positive site indicative for bone marrow involvement and metastatic disease
Bone marrow biopsies (2 sites)	
Chest radiograph	Assessment for metastatic disease
CT scan or MRI scan of the primary site	Evaluation of tumor size, invasiveness, enlargement of regional nodes
CT scan or MRI of possible metastatic sites	Head, neck, abdomen, liver, or chest
	Evaluate for presence, tumor size, and invasiveness
Meta-iodobenzylguanidine scintigraphy (MIBG)	Assesses primary tumor and metastasis not discovered with other diagnostic testing
Bone scan	Assesses cortical bone metastases, bone marrow involvement
Urinary catecholamines (homovanillic acid [HVA] and vanillylmandelic acid [VMA])	90% to 95% of tumors produce catecholamines; 24-hour urine levels measuring VMA and HVA are performed and elevation confirms the diagnosis

CT, computed tomography; MRI, magnetic resonance imaging.

to stage patients uniformly. This system is based on surgical and radiologic findings and bone marrow evaluation (Table 29-4) (Brodeur et al., 1993).

Treatment

The treatment of neuroblastoma is dictated by its classification as low, intermediate, or high risk. Low-risk tumors generally do not require chemotherapy or radiation therapy. Resection of the primary tumor is followed by close observation. Intermediate-risk tumors are treated with resection (stage 2) and resection followed by chemotherapy (stage 3) accordingly (Kushner et al., 1996; Matthay et al., 1998). High-risk tumors require a multimodality approach and still have overall survival rates of only 10% to 30% (LaQuaglia, 1997). Chemotherapy, radiation therapy, and surgery are all recommended treatments for high-risk disease.

Chemotherapy/Radiation Chemotherapy is the mainstay of treatment for intermediate- and high-risk neuroblastoma. Induction agents include cisplatin, doxorubicin, etoposide, cyclophosphamide, and vincristine (among others) and are generally used in combination (Brodeur & Maris, 2002; Kushner, 2004). The consolidation phase often includes myeloablative chemotherapy with bone marrow or stem cell rescue. Matthay et al. (1999) found that 13 cis-retinoic acid decreased relapse risk, and this agent has become part of the treatment for high-risk neuroblastoma.

Total-body irradiation is not commonly used because of toxicity concerns (Kushner, 2004). As part of a multimodality treatment plan, fractionated doses of radiation are used to control bulky tumors, for local control of surgical margins, for residual or disseminated disease, or for infants in respiratory distress due to significant hepatomegaly (Brodeur & Maris, 2002; Kushner et al., 2001; LaQuaglia et al., 2004). Radiation therapy should generally be administered after surgery because if it is given beforehand, excision of the tumor is more difficult.

Recurrent or refractory neuroblastoma is treated with novel cytotoxic agents, targeted radiation therapy, retinoids, and immune-mediated therapies. Unfortunately, the outcomes remain poor for this group of patients (Brodeur & Maris, 2002).

Surgical Management Although all aspects of the diagnostic work-up for neuroblastoma patients are important, the findings of the surgeon at the initial biopsy or primary resection define the stage, which in turn guides treatment (Brodeur & Maris, 2002). Most patients with suspected neuroblastoma have a central venous access device placed at the time of the initial biopsy or resection. This allows the administration of chemotherapy (if needed), antibiotics, blood products, total parenteral nutrition, and other intravenous needs. Perez et al. (2000) found that with surgery alone, patients with stage 1 and 2 neuroblastoma had a 98% survival rate, and Kushner

---

Table 29-4 **The International Neuroblastoma Staging System**

Stage	Definition
1	Localized tumor with complete gross excision, with or without microscopic residual disease, representative ipsilateral lymph nodes negative for tumor microscopically (nodes attached to and removed with the primary tumor may be positive).
2A	Localized tumor with incomplete gross excision; representative ipsilateral nonadherent lymph nodes negative for tumor microscopically.
2B	Localized tumor with or without complete gross excision, with ipsilateral nonadherent lymph nodes positive for tumor. Enlarged contralateral lymph nodes must be negative microscopically
3	Unresectable unilateral tumor infiltrating across the midline,[a] with or without regional lymph node involvement; or localized unilateral tumor with contralateral regional lymph node involvement; or midline tumor with bilateral extension by infiltration (unresectable) or by lymph node involvement.
4	Any primary tumor with dissemination to distant lymph nodes, bone, bone marrow, liver, skin and/or other organs (except as defined for stage 4S).
4S	Localized primary tumor (as defined for stage 1, 2A, or 2B), with dissemination limited to skin, liver, and/or bone marrow[b] (limited to infants <1 year of age).

NOTE. Multifocal primary tumors (e.g., bilateral adrenal primary tumors) should be staged according to the greatest extent of disease, as defined above, and followed by a subscript letter M (e.g., 3_M).

[a]The midline is defined as the vertebral column. Tumors originating on one side and crossing the midline must infiltrate to or beyond the opposite side of the vertebral column.

[b]Marrow involvement in stage 4S should be minimal, e.g., <10% of total nucleated cells identified as malignant on bone marrow biopsy or on marrow aspirate. More extensive marrow involvement would be considered to be stage 4. The meta-iodobenzylguanidine (MIBG) scan (if performed) should be negative in the marrow.

et al. (1996) reported that for non–stage 4 patients with no *MYCN* amplification, complete or partial resection without cytotoxic therapy is sufficient. However, high-risk neuroblastoma patients require a multimodality approach that includes biopsy for diagnostic testing, chemotherapy, tumor resection (usually after four or five cycles of chemotherapy), and possible radiotherapy and/or immunotherapy. Increased complication rates are reported when the resection is performed at the time of diagnosis *before* chemotherapy in high-risk neuroblastoma, and survival is not decreased with delayed surgery (DeCou et al., 1995; Shamberger, Allarde-Segundo, Kozakewich, & Grier, 1991). LaQuaglia et al. (2004) found that gross total resection of the primary tumor is correlated with local control, which is essential to long-term survival.

The general goal of the surgeon is initially to obtain tissue for study or to perform a primary resection for low-risk disease. Secondarily, for high-risk disease, the goal is resection after chemotherapy or removal of residual disease (Fig. 29-2). In all cases, care is taken to ensure that there is no injury or damage to vital structures during the surgery (Brodeur & Maris, 2002). Biopsy specimens need to be adequate both in size and in quality to appropriately stage the tumor. The surgical approach for primary resection of an abdominal tumor, especially one that involves the vena cava or major branches of the abdominal aorta, is a thoracoabdominal exposure, which is generally well tolerated. A complete vascular dissection and removal of all involved regional lymph nodes is the goal of resection (LaQuaglia, 2006). Surgical complications could include operative hemorrhage, nephrectomy, injury to surrounding vessels, or postoperative infection (LaQuaglia et al., 2004; Brodeur & Maris).

Prognosis

The most important variables in determining the prognosis for a child with neuroblastoma include the age of the patient at diagnosis, the stage of disease, the site of the primary tumor, and the histologic findings of the tumor (Brodeur & Maris, 2002). On the basis of the International Neuroblastoma Staging System criteria for neuroblastoma, the 3-year survival is as follows: stage 1 patients: 97%; stage 2A patients: 87%; stage 2B patients: 86%; stage 3 patients: 62%; stage 4 patients: < 40%; and stage 4S patients: 75%. The relapse rate is greater as the stage of the tumor increases. The exception is stage 4S tumors, which have a 75% relapse-free rate (LaQuaglia, 1997).

Future Directions

Length of survival for children diagnosed with neuroblastoma has improved over the years, and additional treatment modalities are under investigation. Already being studied are new drugs (e.g., topotecan and irinotecan), the use of radiolabeled metaiodobenzylguanidine (MIBG), antiangiogenesis therapies, and immunotherapy (Weinstein et al., 2003). Targeted immunotherapy (nonradiolabeled

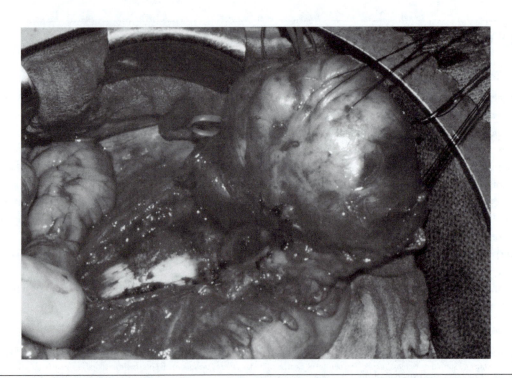

Figure 29-2 Intraoperative view of neuroblastoma.

monoclonal antibodies) does not overly suppress the immune system and has low toxicity, making it an attractive complement to already established treatments.

Future areas of research will focus on (1) identifying individuals who are genetically predisposed to neuroblastoma, (2) determining an ability to evaluate risk stratification based on a better understanding of biologic markers, which is key to predicting prognosis and hence guiding treatment, and (3) finding additional tumor markers that will allow researchers to study and follow the response to treatment (Brodeur & Maris, 2002; Brodeur & Brodeur, 1991).

■ Wilms' Tumor

Wilms' tumor, also known as nephroblastoma, is the most common primary malignant renal tumor of childhood, with approximately 500 new cases each year (Grundy et al., 2002; Bernstein, Linet, Smith, & Olshan, 2004). Wilms' tumor occurs most commonly in children younger than 5 years of age, and the incidence declines markedly with age, although it can be seen in adolescents and young adults (Table 29-1).

Wilms' tumor is a malignant embryoma of the kidney that arises from metanephric blastema. Individual tumors not only contain metanephric cells but may also have cartilage, skeletal muscle, and squamous epithelium. The classic tumor is an encapsulated or pseudoencapsulated intrarenal mass arising from the periphery of the renal cortex. Tumors are globular or spherical with a soft, gray-tan appearance. They appear to occupy an entire pole of the kidney, and calcification is not often present (Grundy et al., 2002). Although most tumors are solitary lesions, 7% involve both kidneys and 12% arise from multiple sites within the same kidney (Breslow, Beckwith, Ciol, & Sharples, 1988).

Wilms' tumor is considered a prototype for the success of cancer chemotherapy because the survival rates have improved from less than 30% to almost 90% since the advent of modern chemotherapy (Brodeur & Brodeur, 1991).

Etiology
Four genetic loci have been linked to the development of Wilms' tumor. Two are Wilms' tumor suppressor genes (*WT1* and *WT2*), and the other two are familial tumor loci (*FWT1* and *FWT2*) (Grundy et al., 2002). Inactivation of *WT1* may inhibit the protein contributing to normal kidney development. This gene was found when a link between a syndrome of aniridia, genitourinary malformation, and mental retardation and Wilms' tumor was made (a syndrome known as WAGR). Another association is with Beckwith-Wiedemann syndrome (macroglossia, omphalocele, and visceromegaly). Familial Wilms' tumor, hemihypertrophy, and genitourinary abnormalities have also been linked with Wilms' tumor (Grundy et al.; American Pediatric Surgical Association, 2005).

Clinical Presentation
An incidentally discovered abdominal mass in an otherwise healthy child is the most common presentation of Wilms' tumor. The mass is most often discovered by a family member or caregiver. The tumor may reach an enormous size before a diagnosis is made. The classic findings are abdominal pain, gross hematuria, and fever. The location and the size of the mass can help distinguish it from other causes. Notably, a Wilms' tumor tends to be a nontender, large, flank mass that does not move with respiration (Grundy et al., 2002).

A subset of patients have rapid abdominal enlargement associated with anemia, hypertension, gross hematuria, and sometimes fever, which is attributed to intratumoral hemorrhage and may be associated with spontaneous rupture (Grundy et al., 2002; LaQuaglia, 1997). Hypertension is noted in about 25% of cases as a result of an increase in renin activity (Steinbrecher & Malone, 1995).

On physical examination of the male, a varicocele may be evident as a result of obstruction of the spermatic vein, which may be associated with the presence of tumor thrombus in the renal vein or inferior vena cava. Persistence of the varicocele when the child lies supine is suggestive of venous obstruction (Grundy et al., 2002).

Diagnostic Work-Up
The chief differential diagnosis when a large abdominal mass is present is Wilms' tumor versus neuroblastoma, and to a lesser degree, hepatoblastoma. Differentiation is made easier with radiologic studies because most Wilms' tumors are intrarenal and most neuroblastomas arise from the adrenal gland. Imaging studies are restricted to those necessary to establish the presence of an intrarenal mass (Fig. 29-3). On ultrasound, a Wilms' tumor appears as a solid mass. Calcifications along the edge of the mass (rather than scattered throughout) also help differentiate the tumor from neuroblastoma. Additional important data include the presence and function of the opposite kidney, whether the opposite kidney has tumor involvement, and the presence and extent of intravascular tumor thrombus (Grundy et al., 2002) (Table 29-5).

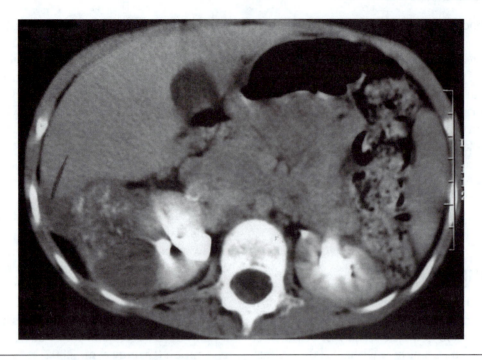

Figure 29-3 Computed tomographic scan of a right-sided intrarenal mass.

Staging

Staging depends on whether the primary tumor is confined to the renal capsule; whether the tumor ruptures before or during surgery; the presence or absence of abdominal lymph node involvement; hematogenous dissemination to distant sites, such as lung, liver, bone, or brain; and the presence of bilateral tumors (Grundy et al., 2002). Table 29-6 reviews staging.

Treatment

Once the stage of disease is determined by the surgeon and the pathologist, a treatment plan is initiated. In general, all patients receive postoperative chemotherapy. Until recently, the exceptions were children less than 24 months at diagnosis with stage I favorable histologic findings and with tumors weighing less than 250 g at resection. A recent study found local recurrence rates higher than ex-

Table 29-5	Diagnostic Evaluation for Suspected Wilms' Tumor
Examination or Test	**Rationale**
History and physical examination	Assess general condition and underlying problems
	Assesses size of primary tumor, areas of metastatic disease
Complete blood count	Bone marrow replacement is associated with anemia and thrombocytopenia, helps to differentiate from neuroblastoma because Wilms' tumor does not generally metastasize to the bone marrow
Liver function tests	Elevation indicates presence of malignancy and possible site of metastasis
Renal function tests	Assesses kidney function secondary to presence of disease; helps to determine ability to tolerate chemotherapy
Urinalysis	Assesses for presence of blood and renal function secondary to disease
Abdominal ultrasound/ Doppler ultrasound	Determines whether mass is cystic or solid, may identify organ of origin; Doppler study is done to identify intracaval extension, liver metastasis, or enlarged retroperitoneal lymph nodes; inferior vena cava thrombosis occurs with a 7% frequency
Computed tomography	Evaluates nature & extent of mass, liver & pulmonary metastasis, intra-abdominal tumor presence, & contralateral renal tumor presence
Chest radiograph	Assesses for pulmonary metastasis

Table 29-6	National Wilms' Tumor Study Group Staging System for Renal Tumors

Stage	Description
I	Tumor confined to the kidney and completely resected. No penetration of the renal capsule or involvement of renal sinus vessels.
II	Tumor extends beyond the kidney but is completely resected (negative margins and lymph nodes). At least one of the following has occurred: (a) penetration of the renal capsule (b) invasion of the renal sinus vessels (c) biopsy of tumor before removal (d) spillage of tumor locally during removal
III	Gross or microscopic residual tumor remains postoperatively, including inoperable tumor, positive surgical margins, tumor spillage involving peritoneal surfaces, regional lymph node metastases, or transected tumor thrombus.
IV	Hematogenous metastases or lymph node metastases outside the abdomen (e.g., lung, liver, bone, brain).
V	Bilateral renal Wilms' tumors at onset.

pected for this group, so the current recommendation is to give two-drug chemotherapy to these patients (Green et al., 2001).

Surgical Management Treatment strategies for Wilms' tumor are dependent on the histopathologic and surgical findings, making the role of the surgeon paramount (Grundy et al., 2002). The standard of care in the United States for Wilms' tumor is initial resection. "Exceptions to this rule include extensive intracaval tumors that require cardiopulmonary bypass for extraction, obviously unresectable tumors with documented invasion of contiguous structures, and possibly bilateral tumors, especially if it is unclear which side is more heavily involved" (LaQuaglia, 2006, p. 1964).

Resection usually requires a nephrectomy. A change in surgical practice involves eliminating the direct visualization and manual palpation of the contralateral kidney. Previously, this maneuver was the standard of care, but the renal committee of the Children's Oncology Group no longer recommends this approach (LaQuaglia, 2006). The resection of a Wilms' tumor begins with a thorough abdominal exploration using a wide transabdominal approach. Strict attention is paid to the local tumor extent or tumor rupture and status of the regional periaortic, interaortocaval, paracaval, and perirenal lymph nodes. The liver is carefully palpated for metastases, and both the peritoneal and diaphragmatic surfaces are inspected for metastatic disease (LaQuaglia, 1997).

Patients with extensive intracaval or unresectable tumors or with documented invasion of contiguous structures, and/or bilateral tumors with an unclear picture of which kidney is more heavily involved, benefit from preoperative chemotherapy and/or radiation therapy (Crombleholme, Jacir, Rosenfield, Lew, & Harris, 1994;

Lee, Saing, Leung, Mok, & Cheng, 1994; McLorie, Khoury, Weitzman, & Greenberg, 1996; Shaul, Srikanth, Ortega, & Mahour, 1992). After a thorough work-up, but before chemotherapy, these patients should still undergo exploration to obtain tissue for histopathologic study for proper staging and subsequent treatment.

Chemotherapy/Radiation Therapy Chemotherapy for Wilms' tumor involves several agents, including actinomycin-D, vincristine, doxorubicin, and cyclophosphamide. The doses, frequencies, and types of the drugs given are based on the stage of disease and histologic findings.

Radiation therapy, if applicable, is initiated when the patient is stable after surgery; is free of ileus, atelectasis, and/or diarrhea; has an absolute neutrophil count of greater than 100/mm³; and has a hemoglobin of at least 10 g/dL. Radiotherapy is not given after surgery to patients with stage 1 or 2 tumors with favorable histology who receive actinomycin-D and vincristine, and nominal doses are used in patients with stage 3 tumors with favorable histology if they receive vincristine, actinomycin-D, and doxorubicin after surgery (Grundy et al., 2002; Ritchey, Haase, & Shochat, 1993). For stage 4 patients, the tumor is staged as if the patient did not have metastatic disease, and radiation therapy is given concordantly. Radiotherapy is given in fractionated doses to the entire kidney bed and any other areas of gross residual disease. Unresectable liver metastases are irradiated, as are bulky nodal, brain, or skeletal sites of metastases. Patients with pulmonary metastases receive whole-lung fractionated radiation (Grundy et al., 2002; LaQuaglia, 2006).

Prognosis

Overall survival for children younger than 15 years of age with Wilms' tumor was 92% for the years 1985 to 1994, compared with 81% for 1975 to 1984 (Bernstein et al., 2004). Patients with favorable histology have better outcomes. Of those, patients with stage I tumors have a 94% 4-year relapse-free survival; stage II, 85%; stage III, 90%; and stage IV, 80.6%. For patients with unfavorable histology, those with stage I tumors have an 86% 4-year relapse-free survival; stage II, 70%; stage III, 56%; and stage IV, 47% (Grundy et al., 2002; LaQuaglia, 2006).

If a child with a favorable histology tumor has a recurrence, the prognosis is dependent on the site and the timing of the recurrence, the original tumor stage, and prior therapies. If the recurrence is more than 12 months after diagnosis, is in the subdiaphragmatic area (with no prior radiation), and no doxorubicin has been used for treatment, then aggressive therapies should be used. These children generally show a good response to further therapy. Approximately 50% of patients with anaplastic (unfavorable histology) tumors experience relapse or progression of their disease (Grundy et al., 2002).

The lungs are often a site of metastatic or recurrent disease, and biopsy and/or excision of these nodules can both confirm the diagnosis and reduce tumor burden before other therapies are used. Generally, doxorubicin (if not previously used) and the combination of etoposide and carboplatin are used for recurrent Wilms' tumor. The prognosis is poor if doxorubicin has already been used or if there is recurrence after abdominal radiation therapy (Grundy et al., 2002).

Future Directions

Similar to neuroblastoma, a goal of Wilms' tumor researchers is to better define genetic, biologic, and histologic factors that contribute to both the development and the aggressiveness of these tumors. Determining which patients require more intense therapy will not only improve survival for this group but will also minimize toxicities for those requiring less aggressive treatment (de Kraker & Jones, 2005; Grundy et al., 2002).

Additional and alternate therapies are also being evaluated. The National Wilms' Tumor Study Group (NWTSG), the International Society of Pediatric Oncology (SIOP), and the United Kingdom Children's Cancer Study Group (UKCCSG) are conducting trials evaluating predictive outcomes based on genetic findings, the use of pre-nephrectomy chemotherapy, and the role of doxorubicin and whole-lung radiation therapy in specific subsets of patients (de Kraker & Jones, 2005; Grundy et al., 2002).

■ Hepatic Tumors

Malignant liver tumors are rare in children, accounting for only 1.1% of all childhood tumors. There are ap-

proximately 100 to 150 new cases each year in the United States, and, of these, more than two thirds are hepatoblastomas. Hepatocellular carcinoma accounts for almost all other cases of primary malignant liver tumors (Bulterys, Goodman, Smith, & Buckley, 2004). For incidence, see Table 29-1. Most cases of hepatoblastoma occur in children younger than 5 years of age, in contrast to hepatocellular carcinoma, which is most common in the 15- to 19-year age group (Bulterys et al.; LaQuaglia, 1997).

Hepatoblastoma

Hepatoblastoma usually presents in the first 3 years of life and is slightly more common in males. Hepatoblastoma is an embryonal tumor, and there are several histologic subtypes ranging from undifferentiated to well differentiated (Tomlinson & Finegold, 2002). This tumor is most often unifocal, and the right lobe of the liver is more commonly affected (Weinberg & Finegold, 1983). Hepatoblastomas appear grossly as lobulated, bulging, tan masses. There are often areas of necrosis (Greenberg & Filler, 1997), and the tumor usually presents as a single pseudoencapsulated lesion (LaQuaglia, 2006).

Etiology

The exact cause of hepatoblastoma is not known, but hepatoblastoma is associated with some genetic syndromes. Children with Beckwith-Wiedemann syndrome and hemihypertrophy have a higher incidence of hepatoblastoma. It has also been reported in sibling pairs and in children with diaphragmatic or umbilical hernias, Meckel's diverticulum, and renal anomalies (Bowman & Riely, 1996).

Hepatoblastoma has also been associated with a variety of other genetic syndromes, including familial adenomatous polyposis, Li-Fraumeni syndrome, trisomy 18, and glycogen storage disease type I. There are some reports of environmental exposures and a link to hepatoblastoma. Paternal exposure to some metals and soldering fumes and maternal exposure to petroleum products and paints, oral contraceptives, and other hormones and alcohol have been noted in children who develop hepatoblastoma. This combined with an increasing incidence of the tumor in premature infants may indicate early organogenesis combined with a certain environmental exposure as a trigger for tumor development (Tomlinson & Finegold, 2002).

Clinical Presentation

Most children with hepatoblastoma present with an asymptomatic abdominal mass or abdominal swelling that is discovered by a parent or health care provider. Abdominal pain, irritability, fever, pallor, weight loss, nausea, and/or vomiting may be present but are usually associated with advanced disease. Jaundice is rare, and in almost all cases, there is normal hepatic function (Tomlinson & Finegold, 2002; LaQuaglia, 2006).

Diagnostic Work-Up
The work-up for hepatoblastoma involves physical assessment and laboratory and radiologic studies (Table 29-7 and Fig. 29-4). In more than 90% of patients with hepatoblastoma, the serum marker alpha fetoprotein (AFP) is elevated. In infants, who have a normally elevated AFP, distinguishing normal liver versus tumor may be difficult. By age 1, however, the AFP level is less than 10 ng/mL, and AFP is monitored in patients with hepatoblastoma to assess response to treatment and for recurrence (Tomlinson & Finegold, 2002; LaQuaglia, 2006).

Staging
Traditionally staging of hepatoblastoma has been based on operative findings. Stage I tumors are completely resectable, stage II are resectable with microscopic residual disease, stage III indicates gross residual disease with lymph node involvement (inability to resect the primary tumor), and stage IV disease indicates distant metastases regardless of the stage of the primary tumor (Tomlinson & Finegold, 2002). The International Society of Pediatric Oncology Group (SIOP) has developed an alternative staging system. This system (called PRETEXT—PRETreatment & EXTent of disease) looks at the site and number of involved liver segments. Studies in the United States still use the conventional staging system but also attempt to validate the PRETEXT system (Tomlinson & Finegold; LaQuaglia, 2006).

Treatment
The highest survival rates for patients with hepatoblastoma are when the tumor is resected initially. Approximately 60% of patients have resectable tumors, typically requiring a major anatomic resection (Tomlinson & Finegold, 2002; LaQuaglia, 2006).

Surgical Management Imaging studies cannot always correctly predict the resectability of liver tumors, making the surgeons role paramount in the staging and subsequent treatment of these tumors. A wide exposure is performed with a "generous bilateral subcostal incision" (LaQuaglia, 2006). Resection generally requires a hepatic lobectomy or trisegmentectomy, and technologic advances have added to the feasibility and safety of the procedure (Fig. 29-5). For patients with unresectable disease, surgical management should be directed toward obtaining diagnostic tissue, and once the tumor burden has been reduced with systemic therapy, resection can be performed. Pulmonary lesions that do not respond to chemotherapy or result from relapse are surgically resected as well (Tomlinson & Finegold, 2002; LaQuaglia).

Chemotherapy/Radiation Therapy For patients who present with unresectable disease, chemotherapy has been effective in reducing tumor burden, enabling resection, and treating metastatic disease. Unresectable tumors include those involving both lobes of the liver, cases with bulky lymphadenopathy, or those with involvement of

Table 29-7	**Diagnostic Evaluation for Hepatoblastoma/Hepatocellular Carcinoma**
Examination or Test	**Rationale**
Physical examination and history	Assess general condition and underlying problems
	Assess size of primary tumor, areas of metastatic disease
	Review neonatal history with focus on features suggesting Beckwith-Wiedemann syndrome
Complete blood count	Mild anemia and thrombocytosis are often seen
Liver function tests	Nonspecifically elevated
High serum cholesterol	High levels are associated with a poor prognosis
Alpha-fetoprotein (AFP)	Elevation occurs in >90% of cases and is often extreme; useful marker to monitor disease reduction
Abdominal radiograph[a]	Identifies presence of a right upper quadrant mass
Abdominal ultrasound	Distinguishes between space-occupying lesions and diffuse hepatomegaly
	Doppler ultrasound can assess tumor vascularity
Abdominal CT scan or MRI	Most sensitive for diagnostic discrimination and to assess operability; also identifies nodal disease
Chest CT scan	Assesses for pulmonary metastasis; evident in 10%–20% of patients

[a]The radiologic evaluation is the same for both diseases. Preoperative differentiation is difficult.

CT, computed tomography; MRI, magnetic resonance imaging.

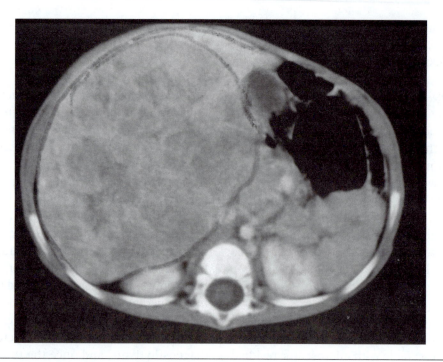

Figure 29-4 Computed tomographic scan of hepatoblastoma.

the porta hepatis. Patients receive vincristine, cisplatin, and 5-fluorouracil before surgery, converting some tumors to resectable status. Doxorubicin is used for refractory or recurrent tumors because of its high cardiotoxicity. All patients except those with initially resectable tumors with pure fetal histology receive either preoperative or postoperative chemotherapy to improve survival rates (Tomlinson & Finegold, 2002; LaQuaglia, 2006).

SIOP published a study in 2000 (Pritchard et al.) reporting survival rates of 75% in patients with both resectable and unresectable tumors treated with preoperative chemotherapy. The goal of the study was to minimize surgical complications, increase surgical resection rates, and treat any metastatic disease up front.

Radiation therapy is not currently part of hepatoblastoma treatment in the United States. It has been used

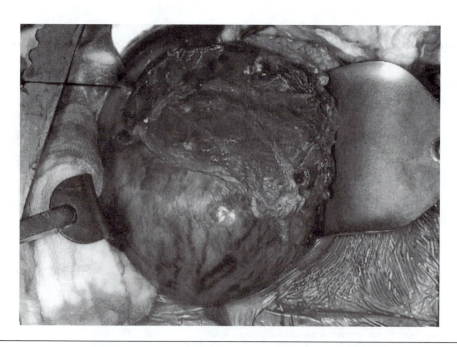

Figure 29-5 Intraoperative view of hepatoblastoma.

sparingly in tumors that are unresponsive to resection and aggressive chemotherapy but with minimal results (Tomlinson & Finegold, 2002).

Liver transplantation remains an option for patients with unifocal, intrahepatic tumors that remain unresectable after chemotherapy. A total hepatectomy is performed, followed by transplantation; 5-year survival rates approach 80% (Reyes et al., 2000).

Prognosis

Survival for children with hepatoblastoma has improved significantly. During the 1970s, only 20% to 30% of patients survived. The 2004 SEER data reported that the 5-year survival between 1975 and 1984 was 51% and rose to 59% between 1985 and 1994. For patients with resectable tumors, the combination of surgery and chemotherapy leads to a survival rate as high as 90%. For patients with unresectable primary tumors treated with chemotherapy and then complete resection, survival is still approximately 70%. Unfortunately, for children with unresectable tumors that do not respond well to chemotherapy, the prognosis remains poor (Tomlinson & Finegold, 2002).

Hepatocellular Carcinoma

Hepatocellular carcinoma (HCC) is the second most common liver malignancy in children, although far less common than hepatoblastoma. The usual age of presentation is after age 10. It usually occurs in the right lobe of the liver but, unlike hepatoblastoma, is usually multifocal. HCC is associated with hepatitis B and often occurs after the development of cirrhosis (Tomlinson & Finegold, 2002).

Clinical Presentation

Unlike hepatoblastoma, patients with hepatocellular carcinoma present with clinical symptoms. Abdominal pain is present with or without an accompanying abdominal mass. Fatigue, nausea, vomiting, anorexia, and weight loss frequently occur, and jaundice is slightly more common than with hepatoblastoma.

Diagnostic Work-Up

The diagnostic work-up for hepatocellular carcinoma and hepatoblastoma are the same (Table 29-7). A primary difference is that the AFP is less frequently elevated in HCC, and, when elevated, is less markedly so. On computed tomographic scan, the appearance of HCC is similar to that of hepatoblastoma, but HCC is more often multifocal, with local metastases and portal vein involvement. In 30% to 50% of patients, metastatic disease is present at diagnosis (LaQuaglia, 2006; Tomlinson & Finegold, 2002).

Staging

The staging system for hepatocellular carcinoma is the same as that for hepatoblastoma.

Treatment

Hepatocellular carcinoma is rare in children, inhibiting the ability to develop clinical trials in this age group. Children diagnosed with HCC are treated according to adult protocols. Cure is attainable if the tumor can be completely resected. Unfortunately, only about 10% to 20% of patients have resectable tumors. There is a subtype of HCC, called the *fibrolamellar variant*, which has higher survival rates (48%–60%). Unlike HCC, this variant typically occurs in the presence of an otherwise healthy liver. The fibrolamellar tumors tend to not have the bilateral involvement and extrahepatic extension that makes HCC so difficult to treat surgically (Tomlinson & Finegold, 2002; LaQuaglia, 2006). Chemotherapy is not effective for hepatocellular carcinoma, and there is a very limited role for radiotherapy.

Prognosis

Overall, survival rates for patients with hepatocellular carcinoma are only about 20%. Liver transplantation offers some hope to these children, but recurrence remains a significant obstacle and concern (Tomlinson & Finegold, 2002).

Future Directions

Liver transplantation, particularly in the setting of living related donors, offers a possibility for patients with primary malignant liver tumors. Similar to neuroblastoma and Wilms' tumor, early detection in light of known associated genetic syndromes or other potential triggering factors may help improve survival rates. The introduction of novel therapies, including new drugs and methods of delivery, will hopefully provide a better prognosis, particularly for those with hepatocellular carcinoma (LaQuaglia, 2006; Tomlinson & Finegold, 2002).

■ Rhabdomyosarcoma

Malignant tumors derived from primitive mesenchymal cells are called *sarcomas*. Mesenchymal cells mature into skeletal or smooth muscle, fat, fibrous tissue, bone, and/or cartilage. Sarcomas are divided into categories according to the mature cell type they resemble. For example, tumors that arise from the fat tissue are called liposarcomas. Sarcomas are highly aggressive tumors and tend to be locally invasive with a high propensity for local recurrence. Rhabdomyosarcoma is the most common soft tissue sarcoma in childhood, accounting for approximately 50% of all sarcomas (Wexler, Crist, & Helman, 2002; Gurney, Young, Roffers, Smith, & Bunin, 2004). It arises from tissue resembling striated muscle tissue, which contains rhabdomyoblasts or primitive muscle cells (Pack & Eberhart, 1985). Some sarcomas are called *undifferentiated* because they come from cells that are primitive and do not resemble any specific mature tissue type.

Soft tissue sarcomas rank fifth among all reported tumors, accounting for 7.4% of cancer cases.

There are four histopathologic subtypes of rhabdomyosarcoma: embryonal, alveolar, botryoid, and pleomorphic. Embryonal is the most common type in children, accounting for almost 75% of cases (Fig. 29-6). Usual primary sites of embryonal types are the head and neck, orbit, and genitourinary tract. Alveolar sites include extremities, trunk, and perineum. Botryoid sites include the bile ducts and submucosal locations, such as the bladder, vagina, and nasopharynx. The pleomorphic subtype is uncommon in infants and children, but when it occurs, the extremities and trunk are the usual locations (Lanzkowsky, 1995; Rowe, O'Neill, Grosfeld, Fonkalsrud, & Coran, 1995; Wexler et al., 2002).

Etiology

The cause of rhabdomyosarcoma is unknown, but there is some association with neurofibromatosis, Li-Fraumeni syndrome (LFS), and Beckwith-Wiedemann syndrome (Wexler et al., 2002).

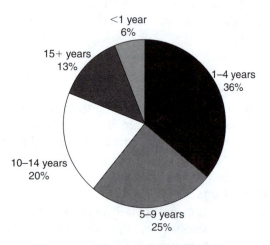

A. Age at Presentation

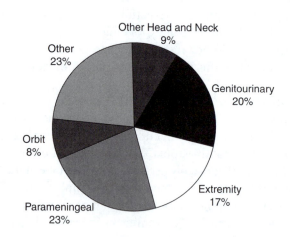

B. Site of Primary

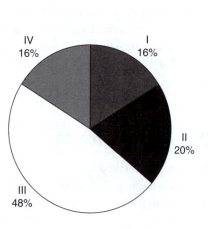

C. Clinical Group

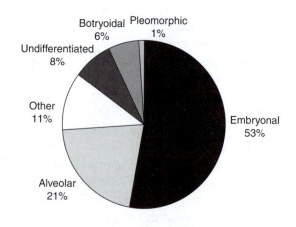

D. Histology

Figure 29-6 Clinical features of rhabdomyosarcoma.

Sites of Origin

Rhabdomyosarcoma can be found virtually everywhere in the body, and, like neuroblastoma, it is a small round blue cell tumor of childhood. The most common sites for rhabdomyosarcoma are the head and neck, accounting for 35% of cases, followed by genitourinary tract (22%), extremities (18%), and other sites (25%) (Wexler et al., 2002) (Fig. 29-6).

Clinical Presentation

Rhabdomyosarcoma is generally seen as a mass and/or a disturbance in bodily function resulting from the presence of the tumor. Presenting signs and symptoms depend on the tumor site and the presence of metastases. Table 29-8 details the signs and symptoms of rhabdomyosarcoma by anatomic locations.

Diagnostic Work-Up

Management of rhabdomyosarcoma depends on the tumor site and the extent of the disease. A thorough work-up to evaluate the primary tumor site and the presence and extent of metastases is necessary. A computed tomographic scan of the primary tumor site should be obtained to evaluate the tumor size and invasiveness, regional lymph node involvement, and other complicating features. Figure 29-7 demonstrates a computed tomographic scan of a large bladder rhabdomyosarcoma. Table 29-9 reviews the standard work-up. Additional examinations may be warranted for some tumor sites. For suspected rhabdomyosarcoma of the parameningeal and head and neck regions, ophthalmologic examination, cerebrospinal fluid cytologic studies, and an ear, nose, and throat examination with the patient under anesthesia provide further information (Lanzkowsky, 1995). After the initial work-up is complete, incisional biopsy of the primary tumor site and any metastatic regional lymph nodes is performed to provide tissue for pathological examination and biologic markers. Specific surgical management is discussed later, but if the tumor is small, noninvasive, and accessible, resection of the tumor with an attempt to obtain clear margins is performed after a complete work-up (Wexler et al., 2002; LaQuaglia, 2006).

Staging

Careful staging is important for both the treatment and the prognosis of rhabdomyosarcoma. The current Intergroup Rhabdomyosarcoma Study V (IRS-V) trial incorporates a tumor, node, metastases (TNM) classification system. It is a preoperative staging system that evaluates tumor size, invasiveness, lymph node involve-

Table 29-8	Presenting Signs and Symptoms of Rhabdomyosarcoma
Site	**Signs and Symptoms**
Vaginal	Discharge, bleeding from vaginal introitus, prolapse of polypoid mass with possible hemorrhage; urethral compression & constipation with advanced disease
Uterus	Prolapse of polyp through the cervix, abdominal pain, abdominal distention
Bladder	Urinary frequency or obstruction, frequent urinary tract infections, hematuria, dysuria, acute urinary retention, abdominal mass, hydrocephalus, urethral obstruction
Prostate	Pelvic mass, constipation, hematuria
Paratesticular	Unilateral, firm, mobile, painless mass palpable above and separate from the testes, sometimes associated with a hydrocele
Extremity	Presence of a mass, may be painless or painful, associated limp, overlying skin changes, pathological fracture (local bony invasion)
Nasopharyngeal	Local pain, sinusitis, epistaxis, dysphagia, airway obstruction
Middle ear	Pain, history of chronic otitis, aural discharge, polypoid mass in the external canal, Bell's palsy
Orbit	Eyelid swelling, proptosis, headache, decreased visual acuity, conjunctival mass, visual disturbances, extraocular muscle imbalance
Facial lesion	Painful swelling associated with trismus, skin discoloration or cellulitis over the mass
Laryngeal	Pertussis-like cough, hoarseness
Chest wall/paraspinal	Chest pain, mass, pleural effusion with occasional shortness of breath
Retroperitoneum	Abdominal pain, abdominal mass, compression of surrounding organs
Perianal/perineum	Subcutaneous mass, verrucous superficial tumor, constipation, dysuria
Bile duct tumors	Pain, fever, jaundice

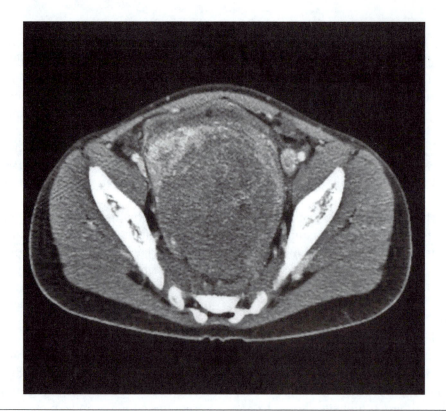

Figure 29-7 Computed tomographic scan of large bladder rhabdomyosarcoma.

ment, and primary site (Table 29-10). The combination of the clinical staging, TNM evaluation, and results of tissue pathological and histopathological studies provides the information needed to initiate treatment.

Treatment

A relatively new, but useful, method of determining treatment is risk-based assessment. Patients are considered low risk if they have embryonal rhabdomyosarcoma at a favorable site, embryonal type at an unfavorable site but with complete resection, or resection with positive microscopic margin. The intermediate-risk patients are those with embryonal rhabdomyosarcoma at an unfavorable site with gross residual disease after resection, those younger than 10 years of age with metastatic disease, and those with localized alveolar rhabdomyosarcoma. Any patients with metastatic disease over the age of 10 years at presentation are considered high risk. Risk-based assessment, combined with the staging information presented above, helps ensure treatment that is appropriate without exposing children to excess chemotherapy, thereby minimizing potential toxicity and long-term sequelae (LaQuaglia, 2006; Wexler et al., 2002).

Multimodality therapy, including surgery, chemotherapy, and radiation therapy, is paramount to achieving and maintaining remission for patients with rhabdomyosarcoma. The role of each modality depends on the stage and the classification of the tumor at presentation and the responsiveness to therapy. In 1972, the Intergroup Rhabdomyosarcoma Study group was organized to evaluate large numbers of patients being treated on or according to similar protocols. The results of these studies have been instrumental in "improving outcomes, identifying prognostic variables and developing risk-based therapies for patients with rhabdomyosarcoma" (Wexler et al., 2002, p. 953). The results of the IRS-V study indicate that therapy should be risk directed and based primarily on tumor site, tumor histology, and extent of disease (Crist et al., 2001).

Surgical Management Before the advent of chemotherapy and radiation therapy, surgery was the mainstay of treatment for patients with rhabdomyosarcoma. Survival rates have risen to 50% or greater with the addition of chemotherapy. At this point, the role of surgery became somewhat unclear. If tumors responded well to chemotherapy, was resection in fact indicated? And what is the impact of resection on survival? Given present-day survival rates, however, it would be unethical to randomly assign a patient to a nonsurgical arm of treatment (LaQuaglia, 1997).

Table 29-9 Diagnostic Evaluation for Suspected Rhabdomyosarcoma[a]

Examination or Test	Rationale
History and physical examination	Search for lymph nodes, size of primary mass, general condition, underlying conditions
Complete blood count	Bone marrow replacement associated with anemia or thrombocytopenia; bone marrow toxicity is the major side effect of chemotherapy
Electrolytes, renal and hepatic function tests, creatinine clearance	Renal toxicity associated with cisplatin and other alkylators; genitourinary tumors may obstruct ureters; hepatic toxicity with Dactinomycin
4-site bone marrow aspirations, 2-site bone biopsies	Bone marrow metastases: 6% of patients at diagnosis; 29% of stage 4 patients have marrow involvement; bone marrow assessment before chemotherapy
Bone scan	Possibility of bone and bone marrow metastases
CT of the primary site	Evaluation of tumor size, invasiveness, enlargement of regional nodes and complicating ureteral, biliary, bowel, or airway patency
CT of possible metastatic sites	CT scan lungs and liver: r/o parenchymal metastases. Superior to MRI for paraspinal, extremity, and head and neck (base of skull) lesions.
MR imaging	MR scan lungs and liver: r/o parenchymal metastases. More sensitive than CT to evaluate extent of viable tumor (T2-weighted imaging) and presence of hepatic metastases. Useful for evaluation of the epidural space in paraspinal or base of skull primaries.
Gallium scanning	Primary tumor & metastatic deposits may be identified by gallium scanning

[a]From Greenfield, *Surgery: Science principles and practice*, 2e, Reprinted with permission from Lippincott Williams & Wilkins.
CT, computed tomography; MRI, magnetic resonance imaging.

The goals of surgery are as follows:

1. Complete resection of the tumor without mutilating or debilitating consequences,
2. Procurement of tissue before the initiation of other therapies for tumor biology and histopathological study,
3. Debulking of the tumor before chemotherapy and radiation therapy,
4. Evaluation of response to therapy or excision of residual tumor, and
5. Placement of a central venous catheter for the administration of chemotherapy and other needs.

Surgical management varies with the site of disease (Table 29-11). Resection is the most rapid method to eradicate tumor and is the treatment of choice if it can be performed without significant cosmetic or functional deficit. Patients in whom tumors are resected at diagnosis fare better (Wexler et al., 2002). Re-excision is performed if surgical margins are positive for disease or if the existence of a neoplasm was unknown at the time of the initial excision. In the case of extremity tumors, if the tumor is deemed unresectable up front, it is of utmost importance that the surgeon plans the initial biopsy incision with regard for the future direction of resection. Some tumors are not amenable to surgical resection (e.g., parameningeal) but are responsive to chemotherapy. For these tumors, the role of surgery is biopsy to confirm the diagnosis and to obtain tissue for biologic studies. Incisional biopsy is generally performed, but computed tomography–guided needle biopsy is also an option (LaQuaglia, 2006; Wexler et al.).

If the tumor is large and gross total resection is not possible, debulking of the tumor may reduce tumor burden before the initiation of chemotherapy and/or radiation therapy. Second-look surgery is performed after other therapies have been initiated to evaluate responsiveness to therapy (and potentially limit further therapy) or for excision of residual tumor. Hays et al. (1990) found that for patients with selected tumor sites (clinical groups III and IV), excision of residual mass after intensive chemotherapy and radiotherapy may favorably influence outcome. Debilitating or disfiguring surgery is performed if residual disease is found after all other modes of therapy have been exhausted. LaQuaglia (2006, p. 1969) states that "amputation of extremity rhabdomyosarcoma does not enhance cure and should only be performed when lesions are bulky, invade neurovascular structures, or are recurrent."

Table 29-10	TNM Staging of Rhabdomyosarcoma: TNM Pretreatment Staging Classification for IRS-IV[a]				
Stage	**Sites**	**T Invasiveness**	**T Size**	**N**	**M**
1	Orbit	T1 or T2	a or b	N0, N1, or Nx	M0
	Head and neck[b]				
	Genitourinary[c]				
2	Bladder/prostate	T1 or T2	a	N0 or Nx	M0
	Extremity				
	Cranial parameningeal				
	Other[d]				
3	Bladder/prostate	T1 or T2	a	N1	M0
	Extremity		b	N0, N1, or Nx	M0
	Cranial parameningeal				
	Other[d]				
4	All	T1 or T2	a or b	N0 or N1	M1

[a]T (tumor): T1, confined to anatomic site of origin; T2, extension; a, ≤ 5 cm in diameter; b, > 5 cm in diameter. N (regional nodes): No, not clinically involved; N1, clinically involved; Nx, clinical status unknown. M (metastases): Mo, no distant metastases; Ml, distant metastasis present.
[b]Excluding parameningeal.
[c]Nonbladder/nonprostate.
[d]Includes trunk, retroperitoneal, and so on.

Chemotherapy

Multiagent chemotherapy is used for the treatment of rhabdomyosarcoma. Dosing, use of specific agents, and length of therapy depend on the stage and risk assessment at diagnosis. First-line effective agents for rhabdomyosarcoma include vincristine, actinomycin-D, and cyclophosphamide. Doxorubicin, etoposide, and ifosfamide have also been used. The drugs are used in combination for better response. Chemotherapy is used for the eradication of microscopic disease after resection, reduction of tumor size before resection of initially unresectable tumors, or cytoreduction before autologous bone marrow rescue. It is also used in the treatment of recurrent disease (Wexler et al., 2002).

Radiation Therapy Radiation therapy plays an essential role in the treatment of rhabdomyosarcoma. It is particularly useful for tumors in areas that are difficult to resect (e.g., head, neck, and pelvis). The use of radiation therapy is based on stage, and now, risk at diagnosis. Dose does not depend on age, although dose modifications have been made for young children to minimize long-term side effects. The IRS-V is using radiation therapy up front for high-risk advanced disease of the cranium and parameningeal areas, even when metastatic disease is not present. For low-risk disease, radiation therapy is initiated at 3 weeks of treatment; for intermediate risk, at 12 weeks; and for high risk, 15 weeks (Wexler et al., 2002).

Prognosis

The prognosis for patients diagnosed with rhabdomyosarcoma has greatly improved over the years. At present, predictors of outcome include primary tumor site, histologic findings, age at diagnosis, tumor invasion, metastases, and regional lymph node involvement (LaQuaglia et al., 1994). Favorable tumor sites include orbital, paratesticular, and vaginal primary tumors, and unfavorable sites include the parameningeal head and neck, extremities, urinary bladder and prostate, retroperitoneum, and trunk. Noninvasive, small, nonmetastatic tumors with no regional lymph node involvement have a more favorable outcome, as do those with the embryonal histology. There is a higher incidence of advanced disease and alveolar disease in children older than 7, making the prognosis better for children between 1 and 7 years of age (Lanzkowsky, 1995; Wexler et al., 2002).

Future Directions

Research efforts are now focused on patients with metastatic disease at presentation and on the use of risk-based assessment to guide treatment. Hyperfractionated versus conventional radiotherapy was evaluated in the IRS-IV study, and those results should be soon available. The use of autologous bone marrow transplantation or stem cell rescue after myeloablative chemotherapy and radiation therapy was evaluated but has not improved outcomes.

Table 29-11 The Role of Surgery for Primary Sites of Rhabdomyosarcoma in Children

Primary Site	Role of Surgery
Head and neck Superficial (scalp, temporal region, facial structures, neck)	Wide excision with normal margins of tissue provided no significant cosmetic and/or functional deficits occur.
Parameningeal (paranasal sinuses, nasopharynx, middle ear, pterygo-palatine fossa)	Rarely amenable to local excision; incisional biopsy for diagnosis; routine cervical lymph node sampling is unnecessary unless nodes are clinically suspicious.
Orbit and eyelid	Incisional biopsy only, orbital exenteration only for recurrent disease.
Genitourinary tract Paratesticular	Radical orchiectomy and resection of entire spermatic cord (inguinal approach to avoid scrotal contamination). For stage I, group I patients with no evidence of lymph node involvement, no retroperitoneal lymph node dissection is recommended; stages II–IV, groups II–IV, RPLN sampling is recommended to evaluate ipsilateral high infrarenal and low infrarenal nodes and bilateral iliac nodes.
Vulvar, vaginal	Respond well to chemotherapy; incisional biopsy for diagnosis, limited local excision after chemotherapy.
Uterine	Transvaginal biopsy for polypoid cases, D&C for intrauterine infiltrative tumors; radical resection is limited to patients with gross residual disease after initial resection, chemotherapy and radiation therapy or for those patients with progression despite therapy.
Bladder/prostate	Endoscopic, perineal, or suprapubic diagnostic biopsy; complete resection only if preservation of bladder and urethra assured.
Bladder dome	Partial cystectomy (ureteral reimplantation and bladder augmentation may be necessary), total cystectomy, anterior pelvic exenteration only if no local control is obtained after combination chemotherapy and radiation therapy.
Extremities	Complete surgical resection if limb function will not be greatly impaired (independent of whether or not microscopically clear margins can be obtained); biopsy of axillary, inguinal lymph nodes in upper and lower extremities; if immediate regional nodes are positive, more distal nodes should be explored; with an unplanned excision with positive margins, re-excision of the primary site to achieve tumor-free margins.
Trunk	Aggressive surgical management recommended with chest wall, diaphragmatic, and pulmonary resection; wide local resection of chest wall tumors includes removal of the entire soft tissue mass and a block of uninvolved tissue extending at least 1 rib above and below the lesion.
Retroperitoneum	Incisional biopsy for diagnosis, debulking before or after other therapies.

D&C, dilatation and curettage; RPLN, retroperitoneal lymph node.

Surgical approaches that combine interstitial brachytherapy and intraoperative radiation therapy at the time of the primary resection are being evaluated. Understanding more about cell lines and genetics will assist in tailoring treatment protocols to patient risk factors, which will potentially reduce toxicities of treatment. Maintaining or bettering current outcomes while minimizing short- and long-term side effects will remain a mainstay in the treatment of rhabdomyosarcoma (LaQuaglia, 2006; Wexler et al., 2002).

■ Conclusion

The care of the pediatric patient diagnosed with a solid tumor is complex. The role of surgery may be as simple as placement of a central line or as involved as a complicated tumor resection. Regardless of the complexity of the role, surgical nurses will find themselves caring for pediatric oncology patients. Understanding the disease process, expected outcomes, and potential complications prepares them to provide holistic and comprehensive care.

■ Acknowledgments

I would like to thank Barbara Ehrenreich, my original partner in crime for this project, for all the hard work she put into the first edition. I would also like to thank my colleagues at Memorial Sloan Kettering Cancer Center in New York City. In particular, I extend huge amounts of gratitude to Elsa Myers, Leonard Wexler, MD, Michael LaQuaglia, MD, and most especially Alex Chou, MD, without whom this would never have gotten off the ground!

■ Educational Materials

APSNA invites you to download the following diagnosis-related teaching tools for Chapter 29, Solid Tumors: (1) Thoracoabdominal neuroblastoma resection and (2) Extremity rhabdomyosarcoma resection. These teaching tools are available at the APSNA Web site (www.apsna.org) and the Jones and Bartlett Web site (www.jbpub.com). All teaching materials are available in English and Spanish and are free of charge. APSNA encourages their use for your patients and families.

References

American Cancer Society. (2005). *Cancer Facts and Figures, 2005.* Retrieved October 9, 2005, from http://www.cancer.org

American Pediatric Surgical Association. (2005). Retrieved October 9, 2005, from http://www.eapsa.org/parents/resources

Bernstein, L., Linet, M., Smith, M. A., & Olshan, A. F. (2004). Renal tumors. In L. A. G. Ries, M. P. Eisner, C. L. Kosary, B. F. Hankey, B. A. Miller, L. Clegg, et al. (Eds.), *SEER cancer statistics review, 1975–2002* (pp. 79– 90). Bethesda, MD: National Cancer Institute.

Bowman, L. C., & Riely, C. A. (1996). Management of pediatric liver tumors. *Surgical Oncology Clinics of North America, 5*(2), 451–459.

Breslow, N., Beckwith, J. B., Ciol, M., & Sharples, K. (1988). Age distribution of Wilms' tumor: Report from the National Wilms' Tumor Study. *Cancer Research, 48,* 1653–1657.

Brodeur, A. E., & Brodeur, G. M. (1991). Abdominal masses in children: Neuroblastoma, Wilms' Tumor, and other considerations. *Pediatrics in Review, 12*(7), 197–206.

Brodeur, G. M., Azar, C., Brother, M., Hiemstra, J., Kaufman, B., Marshall, H., et al. (1992). Neuroblastoma. *Cancer, 80*(6), 1685–1694.

Brodeur, G. M., & Maris, J. M. (2002). Neuroblastoma. In P. A. Pizzo & D. G. Poplack (Eds.), *Principles and practice of pediatric oncology* (4th ed., pp. 895–937). Philadelphia: Lippincott Williams & Wilkins.

Brodeur, G. M., Pritchard, J., Berthold, F., Carlsen, N., Castel, V., Castleberry, R. P., et al. (1993). Revisions of the international criteria for neuroblastoma diagnosis, staging, and response to treatment. *Journal of Clinical Oncology, 11*(8), 1466–1477.

Bulterys, M., Goodman, M. T., Smith, M. A., & Buckley, J. D. (2004). Hepatic tumors. In L. A. G. Ries, M. P. Eisner, C. L. Kosary, B. F. Hankey, B. A. Miller, L. Clegg, et al. (Eds.), *SEER cancer statistics review, 1975–2002* (pp. 91–97). Bethesda, MD: National Cancer Institute.

Crist, W. M., Anderson, J. R., Meza, J. L., Fryer, C., Raney, R. B., Ruymann, R. B., et al. (2001). Intergroup Rhabdomyosarcoma Study–IV: Results for patients with nonmetastatic disease. *Journal of Clinical Oncology, 19*(12), 3091–3102.

Crombleholme, T. M., Jacir, N. N., Rosenfield, C. G., Lew, S., & Harris, B. (1994). Preoperative chemotherapy in the management of intracaval extension of Wilms' tumor. *Journal of Pediatric Surgery, 29*(2), 229–231.

DeCou, J. M., Bowman, L. C., Rao, B. N., Santana, V. M., Furman, W. L., Luo, X., et al. (1995). Infants with metastatic neuroblastoma have improved survival with resection of the primary tumor. *Journal of Pediatric Surgery, 30*(7), 937–941.

de Kraker, J., & Jones, K. P. (2005). Treatment of Wilms' tumor: An international perspective. *Journal of Clinical Oncology, 23*(13), 3156–3157.

Goodman, M. T., Gurney, J. G., Smith, M. A., & Olshan, A. F. (2004). Sympathetic nervous system tumors. In L. A. G. Ries, M. P. Eisner, C. L. Kosary, B. F. Hankey, B. A. Miller, L. Clegg, et al. (Eds.), *SEER cancer statistics review, 1975– 2002* (pp. 65–72). Bethesda, MD: National Cancer Institute.

Green, D. M., Breslow, N. E., Beckwith, J. B., Ritchey, M. C., Shamberger, R. C., Haase, G. M., et al. (2001). Treatment with nephrectomy only for small, stage I/favorable histology Wilms' tumor: A report from the National Wilms' Tumor Study Group. *Journal of Clinical Oncology, 19,* 3719–3724.

Greenberg, M., & Filler, R. (1997). Hepatic tumors. In P. A. Pizzo & D. G. Poplack (Eds.), *Principles and practice of pediatric oncology* (3rd ed., pp. 717–732). Philadelphia: Lippincott-Raven.

Grundy, P. E., Green, D. M., Coppes, M. J., Breslow, N. E., Ritchey, M. L., Perlman, E. J., et al. (2002). Renal tumors. In P. A. Pizzo & D. G. Poplack (Eds.), *Principles and practice of pediatric oncology* (4th ed., pp. 865–893). Philadelphia: Lippincott Williams & Wilkins.

Gurney, J. G., Severson, R. K., Davis, S., & Robinson, L. L. (1995). Incidence of cancer in children in the United States. *Cancer, 76,* 2186–2195.

Gurney, J. G., Young, J. L. Jr., Roffers, S. D., Smith, M. A., & Bunin, G. R. (2004). Soft tissue sarcomas. In L. A. G. Ries, M. P. Eisner, C. L. Kosary, B. F. Hankey, B. A. Miller, L. Clegg, et al. (Eds.), *SEER cancer statistics review, 1975–2002* (pp. 111–123). Bethesda, MD: National Cancer Institute.

Hays, D. M., Raney, R. B., Crist, W. M., Lawrence, W. W. Jr., Ragab, A., Wharam, M. D., et al. (1990). Secondary surgical procedures to evaluate primary tumor status in patients with chemotherapy-responsive stage III and IV sarcomas: A report from the intergroup rhabdomyosarcoma study. *Journal of Pediatric Surgery, 25*(10), 1100–1105.

Kushner, B. H. (2004). Neuroblastoma: A disease requiring a multitude of imaging studies. *Journal of Nuclear Medicine, 45*(7), 1172–1188.

Kushner, B. H., Cheung, N. K., LaQuaglia, M. P., Ambros, P. F., Ambros, I. M., Bonilla, M. A., et al. (1996). Survival from locally invasive or widespread neuroblastoma without cytotoxic therapy. *Journal of Clinical Oncology, 14,* 373–381.

Kushner, B. H., Wolden, S., LaQuaglia, M. P., Kramer, K., Verbel, D., Heller, G., et al. (2001). Hyperfractionated low-dose radiotherapy for high-risk neuroblastoma after intensive chemotherapy and surgery. *Journal of Clinical Oncology, 19*(11), 2821–2828.

Lanzkowsky, P. (Ed.). (1995). *Manual of pediatric hematology and oncology* (pp. 419– 475). New York: Churchill Livingstone.

LaQuaglia, M. P. (1997). Childhood tumors. In L. J. Greenfield, M. W. Mulholland, K. T. Oldham, G. B. Zelenock, & K. D. Lillemore (Eds.), *Surgery: Scientific principles and practice* (pp. 2118–2140). Philadelphia: Lippincott-Raven.

LaQuaglia, M. P. (2006). Childhood tumors. In M. W. Mulholland, K. D. Lillemo, G. M. Doherty, R. V. Maier, & G. R. Upchurch, Jr. (Eds.), *Greenfields's surgery: Scientific principles and practice* (4th ed., pp. 1956–1981). Philadelphia: Lippincott Williams & Wilkins.

LaQuaglia, M. P., Heller, G., Ghavimi, F., Casper, E. S., Vlamis, V., & Hajdu, S. (1994). The effect of age at diagnosis on outcome in rhabdomyosarcoma. *Cancer, 73*(1), 109–117.

LaQuaglia, M. P., Kushner, B. H., Su, W., Heller, G., Kramer, K., Abramson, S., et al. (2004). The impact of gross total resection on local control and survival in high-risk neuroblastoma. *Journal of Pediatric Surgery, 39*(3), 412–417.

Lee, A. C. W., Saing, H., Leung, M. P., Mok, C. K., & Cheng, M. Y. (1994). Wilms' tumor with intracardiac extension: Chemotherapy before surgery. *Pediatric Hematology and Oncology, 11*, 535–540.

Matthay, K. K., Perez, C., Seeger, R. C., Brodeur, G. M., Shimada, H., Atkinson, J. B., et al. (1998). Successful treatment of stage III neuroblastoma based on prospective biologic staging: A children's cancer group study. *Journal of Clinical Oncology, 16*, 1256–1264.

Matthay, K. K., Villablanca, J. G., Seeger, R. C., Stram, D. O., Harris, R. E., Ramsay, N. K., et al. (1999). Treatment of high-risk neuroblastoma with intensive chemotherapy, radiotherapy, autologous bone marrow transplantation, and 13-cis-retinoic acid. *New England Journal of Medicine, 341*, 1165–1173.

McLorie, G. A., Khoury, A. E., Weitzman, S. S., & Greenberg, M. L. (1996). Preoperative chemotherapy in management of Wilms' tumor [editorial]. *Urology, 47*, 792–793.

Nickerson, H. J., Matthay, K. K., Seeger, R. C., Brodeur, G. M., Shimada, H., Perez, C., et al. (2000). Favorable biology and outcome of stage IV-S neuroblastoma with supportive care or minimal therapy: A children's cancer group study. *Journal of Clinical Oncology, 18*(3), 477–486.

Pack, G. T., & Eberhart, W. F. (1985). Rhabdomyosarcoma of skeletal muscle: Report of 100 cases. *Surgery, 32*, 1023.

Perez, C. A., Matthay, K. K., Atkinson, J. B., Seeger, R. C., Shimada, H., Haase, G. M., et al. (2000). Biologic variables in the outcome of stages I and II neuroblastoma treated with surgery as primary therapy: A children's cancer group study. *Journal of Clinical Oncology, 18*(1), 18–26.

Pritchard, J., Brown, J., Shafford, E., Perilongo, G., Brock, P., Dicks-Mireaux, C., et al. (2000). Cisplatin, doxorubicin and delayed surgery for childhood hepatoblastoma: A successful approach—results of the first prospective study of the International Society of Pediatric Oncology. *Journal of Clinical Oncology, 18*(22), 3819–3828.

Reyes, J. D., Carr, B., Kocoshis, S., Jaffe, R., Gerber, D., Mazariegos, G. V., et al. (2000). Liver transplantation and chemotherapy for hepatoblastoma and hepatocellular carcinoma in childhood and adolescence. *Journal of Pediatrics, 136*, 795–804.

Ries, L. A. (2004). Childhood cancer mortality. In L. A. G. Ries, M. P. Eisner, C. L. Kosary, B. F. Hankey, B. A. Miller, L. Clegg, et al. (Eds.), *SEER cancer statistics review, 1975–2002* (pp. 165–170). Bethesda, MD: National Cancer Institute.

Ritchey, M. L., Haase, G. M., & Shochat, S. (1993). Current management of Wilms' tumor. *Seminars in Surgical Oncology, 9*, 502–509.

Rowe, M. I., O'Neill, J. A., Grosfeld, J. L., Fonkalsrud, E. W., & Coran, A. G. (1995). *Essentials of pediatric surgery* (pp. 249–285). St. Louis, MO: Mosby.

Seeger, R. C., Brodeur, B. M., Sather, H., Dalton, A., Siegel, S. E., Wong, K. Y., et al. (1985). Association of multiple copies of the N-myc oncogene with rapid progression of neuroblastomas. *New England Journal of Medicine, 313*(18), 1111–1116.

Shamberger, R. C., Allarde-Segundo, A., Kozakewich, H. P., & Grier, H. E. (1991). Surgical management of stage III and IV neuroblastoma: Resection before or after chemotherapy? *Journal of Pediatric Surgery, 26*, 1113–1117.

Shaul, D. B., Srikanth, M. M., Ortega, J. A., & Mahour, G. H. (1992). Treatment of bilateral Wilms' tumor: Comparison of initial biopsy and chemotherapy to initial surgical resection in the preservation of renal mass and function. *Journal of Pediatric Oncology, 27*(8), 1009–1015.

Shimada, H., Ambros, I. M., Dehner, L. P., Hata, J., Joshi, V. V., Roald, B., et al. (1999). The international neuroblastoma pathology classification (The Shimada System). *Cancer, 86*, 364–372.

Smith, M. A., & Ries, L. A. (2002). Childhood cancer: Incidence, survival, and mortality. In P. A. Pizzo & D. G. Poplack (Eds.), *Principles and practice of pediatric oncology* (4th ed., pp. 1–12). Philadelphia: Lippincott Williams & Wilkins.

Steinbrecher, H. A., & Malone, P. S. J. (1995). Wilms' tumor and hypertension: Incidence and outcome. *British Journal of Urology, 76*, 241–243.

Tomlinson, G. E., & Finegold, M. J. (2002). Tumors of the liver. In P. A. Pizzo & D. G. Poplack (Eds.), *Principles and practice of pediatric oncology* (4th ed., pp. 847–864). Philadelphia: Lippincott Williams & Wilkins.

Weinberg, A. G., & Finegold, M. J. (1983). Primary hepatic tumors of childhood. *Human Pathology, 14*(6), 512–537.

Weinstein, J. L., Katzenstein, H. M., & Cohn, S. L. (2003). Advances in the diagnosis and treatment of neuroblastoma. *The Oncologist, 8*(3), 278–292.

Wexler, L. H., Crist, W. M., & Helman, L. J. (2002). Rhabdomyosarcoma and the undifferentiated sarcomas. In P. A. Pizzo & D. G. Poplack (Eds.), *Principles and practice of pediatric oncology* (4th ed., pp. 939–971). Philadelphia: Lippincott Williams & Wilkins.

CHAPTER

30

Pediatric Abdominal Organ Transplants

By Kathleen Falkenstein, Kurt Freer,
Michael J. Kinney, and Caroline Braas

The management of children with abdominal organ transplants challenges the entire transplant team before, during, and after this complex surgical procedure. For nurses, postoperative management of a child who receives an abdominal organ transplant (liver, small bowel, kidney) presents special problems in the intensive care unit (ICU) and on the transplant ward. To support a successful outcome, nurses must understand the unique physiologic changes that occur and be prepared to intervene appropriately. This chapter focuses on end-stage disease, surgical procedures, associated therapies, and possible complications that occur after transplantation.

Survival for solid-organ transplantation in the United States has improved dramatically over the past 2 decades. With the introduction of new immunosuppressive drugs, such as cyclosporine (1983) and tacrolimus (1994), along with more innovative surgical techniques, patient and graft survival continue to improve. Better long-term survival along with expansion of inclusion criteria for recipients has prompted an increase in referrals for transplantation. Today, more than 92,867 people are waiting for a solid-organ transplant, which has resulted in longer waiting times (UNOS Annual Report, 2004). In 2005, 6,443 liver transplantations were performed in the United States with 569 of the procedures in the pediatric

population (UNOS Annual Report, 2005). Eight hundred and ninety children younger than age 18 underwent kidney transplantation in 2005 (UNOS Annual Report).

■ Renal Transplantation

The first pediatric kidney transplant was performed in the early 1960s. The success of renal transplantation has improved within the past 3 decades, so transplantation is now the treatment of choice for children with end-stage renal disease (Mauer, Nevins, & Ascher, 1992). The transplantation process, including evaluation and the medical/surgical issues associated with these children, is reviewed here.

■ Preemptive Transplantation

According to data provided by the North American Pediatric Renal Transplant Cooperative Study (NAPRTCS) (Kohaut & Tejani, 1996), the most common diagnoses leading to chronic renal failure in children include congenital obstructive uropathy, aplastic/hypoplastic/dysplastic kidneys, focal segmental glomerulosclerosis, and reflux nephropathy (Warady, Herbert, Sullivan, Alexander, & Tejani, 1997).

Table 30-1   Indications for Organ Transplant

Renal	Liver	Intestinal
Renal dysplasia	Cholestatic	Intestinal atresia
Renal hyperplasia	Biliary atresia	Gastroschisis
Glomerulonephritis	Alagille's syndrome	Midgut volvulus
Prune belly syndrome	Neonatal hepatitis	Necrotizing enterocolitis
Wilms' tumor	Acute fulminant failure	Crohn's disease
Obstructive uropathy	Hepatitis A, B, or C	Gardner syndrome
Acquired disease	Neonatal hemochromatosis	TPN cholestasis
Alport's syndrome	Metabolic disease	Pseudo-obstruction
Juvenile nephrophthisis	Alpha-1 Antitrypsin deficiency	Congenital hepatic fibrosis
Hemolytic uremic syndrome	Wilson's disease	
Chronic pyelonephritis	Tyrosinemia	
Sickle cell nephropathy	Sclerosing cholangitis	
Polycystic kidney disease	Hepatoblastoma	
Oxalosis		
Congenital nephrotic syndrome		

TPN, total parenteral nutrition.

Tables 30-1 and 30-2 include indications for abdominal transplantation and clinical manifestations of end-stage organ disease. Various factors affect the decision regarding the best time to perform a transplantation. Preemptive transplantations are considered before renal replacement therapy with dialysis becomes necessary (Harada et al., 2001; Salvatierra et al., 1997). In some instances, preemptive transplantation is not an option because the child is initially seen with an acute episode of renal failure and dialysis has to begin immediately.

Transplantation Evaluation

The transplantation evaluation involves a thorough medical review to identify any contraindications to the patient receiving a kidney. An integral aspect of the evaluation involves identification of the potential recipient's ABO blood

Table 30-2   Clinical Manifestation of Kidney, Liver, and Intestinal Disease

Renal	Liver	Intestinal
Sodium retention	Jaundice	Jaundice
Metabolic acidosis (low CO_2)	Failure to thrive	Ascites
Hyperkalemia	Ascites	Malabsorption
Hypocalcemia	Hypoglycemia	Growth stunting
Hypokalemia	Hepatomegaly	
Anemia	Hypoalbuminemia	
Congestive heart failure	Prolonged clotting studies	
Hyperglycemia	Hyperammonemia	
Hyperlipidemia	Hypercholesterolemia or	
Peripheral neuropathy	hypocholesterolemia	
Renal osteodystrophy	Encephalopathy	
Growth stunting	Portal hypertension	
	Growth stunting	
	Hepatosplenomegaly	

type and human leukocyte antigen (HLA) tissue typing. These antigens are proteins that are present on the surface of kidney cells and other cells in the body (Bell, 1998). The antigens are divided into class I antigens, consisting of A, B, and C, and class II antigens, the DR category. The class I antigens present the major target for antibody and T-cell reactions to a transplanted organ. A perfect donor-recipient match is a six-antigen match based on these three sites. Parents always have at least a three-antigen match, an inherited haplotype. The human leukocyte antigen typing found in the transplanted kidney is the primary stimulus for the initiation of the immune response against the renal allograft (Suthanthiran & Strom, 1994). The more antigens that match, the less severe the rejection. Table 30-3 lists other testing performed in the transplantation evaluation. Children with congenital uropathies undergo a urologic evaluation in addition to the laboratory evaluation, physical examination, and radiologic studies. Ureterovesical reflux to the allograft ureter, native kidney, or ureteral stump increases susceptibility to urinary tract infection after renal transplantation (Zaontz, Hatch, & Firlit, 1988). Children with congenital reflux may require native ureteronephrectomies or ureteral reimplantation before transplantation to decrease the risk of urinary tract infection after transplantation.

Donor Selection

Selection of an optimal kidney donor involves numerous factors. When possible, a living donor should be considered because these recipients do significantly better than those receiving a cadaver organ (Salvatierra et al., 1997). The living donor may be a parent, sibling older than 18 years of age, or other relative. Many centers are now performing living related and living unrelated donor transplantations. This presents providers with an ethical dilemma of exposing a healthy donor to surgery with potential morbidity. Prospective living donors undergo a thorough medical and psychological evaluation before being accepted as donors. The donor evaluation includes the standard biochemical assessment with the addition of a glomerular filtrate rate; urine tests for protein, creatinine, and culture and sensitivity; and cancer screening for donors older than 40 years of age. Computed tomography (CT) is performed for prospective laparoscopic living related donors to identify the vascular anatomy. If a living donor is not identified or is found medically unacceptable, the child is placed on a waiting list for a cadaver graft. Although pediatric patients receive some priority according to their age, they may still wait several months to years for a medically suitable cadaveric organ. Whether receiving a living or cadaveric graft, the donor must be both ABO blood type and cross-match compatible. A positive T-cell cross-match indicates the possibility of hyperacute rejection, a contraindication to transplantation with that donor (Suthanthiran & Strom, 1994). A positive T-cell cross-match results in hyperacute rejection and graft loss within 24 hours.

Graft survival in pediatric renal transplant recipients is 96% and 76% at 1 and 5 years, respectively, for living donors. In contrast, cadaver graft survival is 94% and 59% at 1 and 5 years, respectively. Patient survival rates at 2 years are 96% for living donor recipients and 94% for cadaver donor recipients (Benfield, 2003).

Preoperative/Intraoperative Management

On admission for transplantation, the following studies should be performed: complete blood count, comprehensive metabolic panel, clotting studies, type and cross-match for two units of blood, and a final antibody cross-match. Patients receiving hemodialysis should be dialyzed the day before surgery, whereas those receiving peritoneal dialysis continue until 2 hours before surgery. Immunosuppression can be initiated preoperatively or intraoperatively according to the transplant center's protocol. Management during the operative procedure focuses on maintaining adequate central venous pressure and blood pressure, which are particularly vital during reperfusion of the allograft (Jones, Matas, & Najarian, 1994). The kidney is generally placed in the retroperitoneum unless the patient is an infant or small child, in which case it is placed in the peritoneal cavity. Two vascular anastomoses connect the donor's renal

---

Table 30-3 Renal Recipient Evaluation

- Physical examination
- Consultations (cardiology, social service, anesthesiology, nutrition)
- Renal ultrasound
- Chest radiographic film
- Electrocardiogram
- Comprehensive metabolic panel
- PPD
- ABO
- Complete blood cell count, clotting studies
- Urinalysis and urine cultures
- Voiding cystourethrogram
- Bone age
- Echocardiogram
- Viral titers: cytomegalovirus, Epstein-Barr virus, varicella, toxoplasmosis
- Immunization update
- Human leukocyte antigen

artery with the recipient's iliac artery and the donor's renal vein with the recipient's iliac vein (Jones et al.). After reperfusion of the kidney, the donor ureter is anastomosed to the bladder (ureteroneocystostomy).

Postoperative Management

Fluid and Electrolyte Therapy

Maintaining renal perfusion, adequate blood pressure, and intravascular fluid volume is extremely important in the immediate postoperative period to promote diuresis of the transplanted kidney. A combination of crystalloid and colloid solutions is administered to replace insensible water losses, urine output, gastrointestinal losses, and third-space distribution. During the initial 24 hours, milliliter per milliliter urine output replacement is delivered hourly with a 0.45% NaCl solution with sodium bicarbonate and potassium added as needed. Dextrose is avoided in urine replacement fluids to prevent the development of hyperglycemia. Insensible fluid losses are replaced with a dextrose solution.

Monitoring of the central venous pressure (CVP) is crucial during the early postoperative course to prevent hypovolemia, which may impair renal function, or hypervolemia with resultant pulmonary edema (Loertscher, Parfrey, & Guttmann, 1989). The CVP should be maintained in the range of 8 to 11 cm H_2O; 0.9% saline or 5% albumin should be administered at 5 to 10 mL/kg to support blood pressure and to maintain systolic measurements of at least 100 to 110 mm Hg (Alexander, 1990). Dopamine may be administered to maintain cardiac output and increase allograft perfusion (Alexander). Evaluation of the patient's clinical status, pulse oximetry, and chest radiography are important adjuncts to CVP measurements in differentiating fluid overload from hypovolemia. Biochemical imbalances are common during the early posttransplantation period. Close monitoring and correction of serum electrolytes, calcium, phosphorous, and glucose concentrations are necessary. In the immediate postoperative period, serum creatinine should be monitored every 6 hours to assess renal function. Initially, urine output is replaced milliliter per milliliter. Over the next 2 days, a fraction of the hourly urine output is replaced to promote a more manageable diuresis and to allow excretion of excess fluids (Mauer et al., 1992). Maintenance intravenous fluids are generally administered by the third postoperative day and adjusted according to oral intake.

Acute Renal Failure

Nonfunction of the allograft is caused by prerenal, renal, or postrenal factors. Prerenal graft nonfunction is caused by hypovolemia that is easily reversed by administering intravenous fluid resuscitation to maintain adequate CVP (Loertscher et al., 1989). A leading cause of postrenal allograft nonfunction is obstruction of the bladder outlet by a blood clot. The indwelling catheter should be irrigated or replaced if necessary (Keown & Stiller, 1986; Kirkman & Tilney, 1989). Once prerenal and postrenal factors have been eliminated, renal factors, such as acute tubular necrosis (ATN) must be considered. This condition is usually reversible and results from ischemia to the kidney either from prolonged donor hypotension or extended warm and/or cold ischemia time during the organ recovery and transplantation procedure (Shapiro & Simmons, 1991). Management of ATN includes avoidance of nephrotoxic drugs, such as cyclosporine and antibiotics, and conservative fluid replacement to prevent hypervolemia. Other causes of posttransplantation renal failure include acute allograft rejection, vascular complications, cyclosporine nephrotoxicity, recurrence of primary renal disease, or development of new disease (Singh, Stablein, & Tejani, 1997). A nuclear medicine renal scan and/or Doppler ultrasonography are obtained to evaluate graft function and abnormalities after surgery.

Surgical Complications

Bleeding after transplantation may occur from the site of the vascular anastomosis or from arterial branches that are not properly ligated during surgery (Kirkman & Tilney, 1989). Postoperative bleeding is manifested by tachycardia, hypotension, falling CVP, abdominal distention, pain, and oliguria that result from diminished perfusion of the allograft (Mauer et al., 1992). Restoration of the blood volume and surgical intervention to control the source of bleeding are required to stabilize the patient and avoid jeopardizing graft function.

Early graft loss caused by vascular thrombosis is a significant problem for pediatric renal transplant recipients (Kohaut & Tejani, 1996). This has been reported in 2.6% of all pediatric renal transplantations (Harmon, Stablein, Alexander, & Tejani, 1991; Singh et al., 1997). Children younger than 5 years of age are at highest risk for renal vascular thrombosis related to low-flow states. A young child's limited cardiac activity results in diminished renal blood flow and compromises the new graft. Renal artery thrombosis is seen as a sudden onset of anuria and is generally irreversible, requiring allograft nephrectomy. A related problem, renal artery stenosis, is caused by technical problems during organ procurement or the transplantation surgery. A stenosis is diagnosed by a Doppler ultrasonographic study that demonstrates decreased or turbulent flow through the renal artery

(Bunchman & So, 1994). Clinical symptoms include persistent and difficult to control hypertension, with or without erythrocytosis and deteriorating renal function (Tilney, Rocha, Strom, & Kirkman, 1984). Approximately one third of these cases are successfully treated with percutaneous transluminal angioplasty (Ingelfinger & Brewer, 1992).

In contrast, renal vein thrombosis (RVT) presents with persistent gross hematuria, graft swelling, and a gradual deterioration in renal graft function. RVT is more common in living related recipients younger than 6 years of age and recipients of young cadaver donor grafts, especially those with long cold storage times (Harmon et al., 1991). It may be possible to treat a partial RVT with heparin (Shapiro & Simmons, 1991).

Urologic Complications

Another source of complications after kidney transplantation is urologic problems related to technical difficulties in performing the ureteroneocystostomy (Mauer et al., 1992). Urinary extravasation occurs during the early postoperative period and develops at the ureterovesical anastomosis site. Clinical manifestations include unexplained fever, abdominal pain, decreased urine output, elevated serum creatinine, and wound drainage. Fluid from either the surgical drain or the incision may be analyzed for creatinine to determine whether the leakage is urine or lymph. Ultrasonography demonstrates a large fluid collection, and a nuclear medicine renal scan differentiates a urethral versus a bladder urinary leak (Salvatierra et al., 1997). Urine leaks are treated with prolonged indwelling catheter drainage for minor leakage (Shapiro & Simmons, 1991) or immediate surgical repair to avoid infection (Salvatierra et al.).

Obstruction at the ureterovesical anastomosis may occur at any time after transplantation, also causing oliguria, and usually requires surgical correction (Zaontz et al., 1988). After removal of the surgical drain, a lymphocele may develop because of the continued drainage of lymphatic fluid from the surface of the allograft or surrounding tissues. An ultrasound should be obtained to document the extraperitoneal collection. Needle aspirations and/or surgery may be required for large fluid collections, which compromise allograft function (Mauer et al., 1992).

The surgical incision should be monitored for signs of infection, including erythema, warmth, swelling, and drainage. The risk of wound infection after transplantation is increased for recipients with a history of chronic anemia, malnutrition, and current immunosuppressive therapy (Rubin, 1988). Three doses of prophylactic an-

tibiotics are administered at the time of surgery to prevent infection.

Medical Complications

According to NAPRTCS data, a high incidence of kidney allograft loss in children is due to rejection, both acute and chronic.

Acute Rejection

Acute rejection can occur as early as 2 weeks after transplantation. Table 30-4 lists clinical manifestations of acute organ rejection. In the first 2 years after transplantation as many as 72% of cadaver graft recipients and 56% of living donor recipients experience rejection (Kohaut & Tejani, 1996). Acute rejection is diagnosed clinically by progressive increases in creatinine levels, fever, allograft swelling and associated pain, proteinuria, hematuria, and hypertension and is confirmed by biopsy. The biopsy reveals glomeruli that are being invaded by lymphocytes. Induction drugs, such as antithymocyte globulin (ATG, thymoglobulin), OKT3, dacliximab (Zenapax), and basiliximab (Simulect) reduce early acute rejection to as low as 5% to 15% and prolong graft survival, thus increasing the supply of organs (Offner, Broyer, & Niaudel, 2002). Refer to Table 30-5 for immunosuppression regimens used in abdominal organ transplantations. A NAPRTCS report indicates that 50% of all kidney transplant recipients receive some form of induction therapy (Kohaut & Tejani).

Acute rejection can occur any time after the transplantation. Viral infection and medication noncompliance are two risk factors for late acute rejection. In the presence of acute rises in creatinine, with the suspicion of infection or noncompliance, a biopsy is obtained to diagnose acute rejection. Acute rejection is treated with steroid boluses at 10 mg/kg followed by a taper of steroids and maintenance of therapeutic drug levels of cyclosporine or tacrolimus. Acute rejection that is not responsive to steroid boluses requires treatment with OKT3. Some studies have suggested that there are clinically silent rejections, and, therefore, many centers have gone back to surveillance biopsies to better guide diagnosis and treatment of rejection (Rush, Nickerson, & Jeffery, 2000; Qureshi, Rabb, & Kasiske, 2002)

Chronic Rejection

Although effective strategies are being developed for treatment of acute rejection, chronic rejection remains a most troublesome problem. It is clinically characterized by slow and progressive increases in creatinine, often associated with hypertension and proteinuria, and is generally

Table 30-4 Clinical Manifestations of Acute Organ Rejection

Renal	Liver	Intestines
Fever	Fever	Fever
↑BUN	↑WBCs	Increased ostomy output
↑Creatinine	↑Liver enzymes	Diarrhea
Decreased urine output	Pain over graft	Abdominal pain
Weight gain	Dark urine	Metabolic acidosis
Abdominal pain	Jaundice	Vomiting
Irritability	Irritability	Abdominal distention

BUN, blood urea nitrogen; WBC, white blood cell.

unresponsive to present immunosuppressant agents. The cause of chronic rejection is probably multifactorial, but the most significant risk factor is a history of acute rejection (Paul, 1995). Chronic rejection is difficult to treat. The best approach is to prevent it by addressing identified risk factors, especially acute rejection (Tejani, Ho, Emment, & Stablein, 2002). An effective strategy is a change in immunosuppression and encouragement of medication compliance. When kidney function deteriorates, the child experiences symptoms of chronic renal failure that can be conservatively treated, such as by administration of phosphate binders, vitamin D therapy, recombinant erythropoietin to stimulate red blood cell production and decrease the severity of anemia, and, finally, retransplantation. Children are relisted for transplantation when they begin to show signs of renal failure, including growth stunting, fatigue, and poor school performance. Dialysis is reinstituted when biochemical parameters and physical findings indicate progressive renal failure. These include elevated BUN (> 100) and creatinine (> 6–8 mg/dL), hyperkalemia unresponsive to sodium polystyrene sulfonate (Kayexalate), hyperphosphatemia, and hypercalcemia. In general, there is an increased incidence of rejection of a subsequent transplant if the previous transplant was lost because of acute rejection as opposed to technical problems (Tejani, Cortes, & Stablein, 1996).

Hypertension

The cause of posttransplantation hypertension is also multifactorial, including the roles of renal factors (i.e., renin release in the face of decreased renal blood flow from ATN and cyclosporine toxicity) and hemodynamics (i.e., increased vascular volume in the presence of decreased urine output sometimes seen in rejection) (Mitsnefes, 2004). A frequent side effect of many immunosuppressants is hypertension (Ingelfinger & Brewer, 1992). Short-term effects of hypertension include head-

ache, vision problems, and light-headedness. Long-term hypertension contributes to the risk of kidney damage from glomerulosclerosis. Common treatment strategies include vasodilators, cardioselective agents, and diuretics. Frequently used antihypertensive agents are calcium-channel blockers that reduce blood pressure, treat ischemic heart disease, and reduce cyclosporine nephrotoxicity by antagonizing either the direct or indirect vasoconstrictive actions of the cyclosporine (Weir, 1990).

Maintenance Immunosuppression

Immunosuppression of children who have received an abdominal organ transplant is critically important to prevent rejection. Most centers use a combination of three immunosuppressant medications and/or induction therapy. Generally, these medications are continued throughout the patient's lifetime. Many centers reduce the dose of prednisone to alternate-day therapy or complete withdrawal. This strategy decreases the incidence of long-term side effects and promotes growth. Each of the medications acts on a different part of the cell cycle to block organ rejection. Immunosuppressive medications suppress humoral and cellular immunity. Cyclosporine and tacrolimus block the production of interleukin-2, thus interrupting events that lead to organ rejection. Corticosteroids decrease the number of activated lymphocytes. Both cyclosporine and tacrolimus require careful drug monitoring to adjust the dose in the early post transplantation period. A trough level is obtained during the hospitalization and follow-up of the patient (Lake & Kilkenny, 1992; Payne, 1992).

■ Liver Transplantation

The first human liver transplant was performed in Denver by Starzl in 1963. The patient survived only briefly, as did the next four recipients of liver transplants. Measurable

Table 30-5 Immunosuppression Therapy for Children with Abdominal Organ Transplant

Treatment	Dosage
Renal transplantation	
Cyclosporine microemulsion formula (Neoral)	6–12 mg/kg/day divided b.i.d.
	Trough levels (100–200 RIA or 150–300 TDX)
Antithymocytic globulin (ATG)	5–10 mg/kg/dose (until CYA level > 100)
Tacrolimus (Prograf)	0.1–0.15 mg/kg/day divided b.i.d.; trough levels, 5–10 ng
Azathioprine (Imuran)	1–1.5 mg/kg/day once a day
Mycophenolate mofetil (CellCept)	1,200 mg/kg/m²/day given b.i.d.
Solu-Medrol	5 mg/kg/day taper over 7 days to dose of 2 mg/kg/day (total not greater than 80 mg/day); days 8–14: 1.5 mg/kg/day (40 mg maximum)
Prednisolone	6–18 months 0.2 mg/kg/day
Liver transplantation	
Cyclosporine (Neoral)	12–20 mg/kg/day given b.i.d. or t.i.d.
	Trough levels, 1–3 months, 200–250; 6–12 months, 150–175; 1–2 years, 125
Tacrolimus (Prograf)	0.2–0.3 mg/kg/day p.o. b.i.d. to maintain trough levels of 15–20 ng/ml for first month; 2–12 months, 7–15 ng/mL; > 12 months, 5 ng/mL
Azathioprine	1–2 mg/kg/day given daily for 1 year
Mycophenolate mofetil	1,200 mg/kg/m²/day given b.i.d.
Prednisolone	10 mg/kg, day 1, and then wean to 2 mg/kg/day by day 5 and then 1 mg/kg/day daily or b.i.d. at discharge; wean at 0.2 mg/kg/every other month until total dose is 0.2 mg/kg dose, then q.o.d. times 2–3 months and discontinue
Small bowel transplantation	
Tacrolimus	0.15 mg/kg/day IV until tolerating oral. 0.30/mg/kg/day p.o. b.i.d. to maintain trough levels (15–30 ng/ml)
Methylprednisolone	10 mg/kg/day on day 1
	1 mg/kg/day with tapering doses over 5 days, to start on POD 2
Azathioprine	1 mg/kg/day IV or p.o.

Note: Each transplant center has individualized immunosuppressant regimens. This is just an example of management from the literature review.

success was not achieved until 1967, when a child with a hepatoma received a liver transplant and survived 13 months (Starzl, Swatsuki, & Van Thiel, 1982).

In the early 1980's, 20% to 50% of children who needed liver transplantation died before a child's donor liver became available; most of these patients weighed less than 10 kg (Broelsch, Edmond, & Thistlethwaite, 1988). To address the shortage of donor organs, investigators at the University of Chicago began using portions of young teen and adult livers for small children. This procedure is known as reduced size liver transplantation. Thereafter, the mortality rate for children on waiting lists for liver transplants decreased significantly to a reported national average of 7% to 10%. Living related liver transplantation (using a portion of a parent or relative liver for a small child) became a reality in 1989. This technique along with split liver techniques (one liver being used for two chil-

dren or a child and adult have continued to allow more children to be transplanted before they are in critical condition) (Hayashi et al., 1998).

Liver Structure and Function

See Table 30-6 for a review of the complex structure and physiology of the liver. The body's largest organ, the liver, rests in the right upper abdominal quadrant. The porta hepatis, located centrally behind the fourth segment of the liver, is the point of entry into the liver for the portal vein, hepatic artery, nerves, and lymph vessels and is the point where the bile duct emerges from the liver. The liver receives blood from two major sources: the hepatic artery and the portal vein. The hepatic artery conveys 20% of the blood supply as oxygenated blood; the portal vein supplies 80% as nutrient-filled blood from the stomach and intestines. The celiac axis carries oxygenated blood from the aorta to

Table 30-6	**Functions of the Liver**

A. Metabolism
  1. Carbohydrates: maintain normal glucose level (gluconeogenesis).
  2. Fats: oxidation of fatty acids for energy.
  3. Proteins: breaks down proteins, removes ammonia from blood.
B. Storage of vitamins: fat-soluble A, D, E, K, and B12.
C. Detoxification and removal of drugs from blood (alter doses with liver failure).
D. Secretion of bile: needed to break down fat globules and absorb fatty acids. Failure of bile flow results in malnutrition.
E. Synthesis of plasma protein: albumin, fibrinogen (blood coagulation).
F. Kupffer cell activity: destroys old and defective red blood cells and removes bacteria from blood.

the hepatic artery and to the spleen and stomach. The portal vein supplies 75% of the blood supply to the liver. When recipients have an occluded or small portal vein, the liver transplant is technically difficult. Both portal and hepatic blood flow are essential for the liver allograft to function normally (Starzl, Rutman, & Corman, 1987).

Bile is produced in the liver and secreted by parenchymal cells. Bile drains into cholangioles, small terminal bile ducts (canaliculi) that merge into the right and left hepatic ducts and form the common bile hepatic duct. The common hepatic duct joins the cystic duct from the gallbladder to form the common bile duct. The common bile duct exits the liver at the porta hepatis and empties into the duodenum to aid in digestion of fat. These ducts are not large, and any obstruction, whether mechanical or caused by disease, can cause liver decompensation.

The liver can function despite extensive damage; approximately 85% of the liver must be damaged before liver failure occurs. Fortunately, the liver has the unique ability to regenerate after injury; a damaged liver can regenerate within 3 weeks and resume normal function within about 4 months.

Indications for Liver Transplantation and Types of Liver Transplantations

The liver transplantation procedure can be performed as a whole-liver graft, reduced-size graft, split-liver procedure, or living donor operation. Reduced-size grafts can be obtained using a right-lobe, left-lobe, or left-lateral segment from either a cadaveric or a living donor. Left-lateral segment grafts are used in infants and small children. Older children may require a left-lobe graft to provide adequate liver tissue. Recently, living related transplantations have been performed on adult recipients who receive the right lobe. In a split-liver procedure, the liver is divided along the falciform ligament, producing two segments, a right-lobe graft that is used in an adolescent or a small adult and a left-lobe or left-lateral segment that can be used for an infant or small child.

Refer to Table 30-1 for indications for liver transplant (Otte, deVille, Goyet, & Reding, 2005).

Recipient Evaluation and Donor Selection

The evaluation of potential recipients for liver transplant includes a multidisciplinary approach and a thorough physical and laboratory evaluation (Table 30-7). Organs are allocated by blood group and body weight as well as the candidate's PELD score (see Table 30-8 for UNOS liver transplant status criteria).

Living related donor evaluations are performed on an outpatient basis. Initially, a family conference occurs to discuss risks and benefits of the procedure with the transplant team. Issues related to postoperative recov-

Table 30-7	**Liver Transplant Recipient Evaluation**

• Physical examination
• Laboratory tests: ABO
  Complete blood count
  Blood clotting studies
  Comprehensive metabolic panel
  Viral Titers
  –Hepatitis A, B, C
  –HIV
  –Epstein-Barr
  –Cytomegalovirus
  –Toxoplasmosis
  Quick Protein Reactive Antibody (PRA)
• Chest x-ray
• Ultrasound of liver
• Electrocardiogram
• PPD
• Liver biopsy
• Consultations:
  Cardiology
  Anesthesiology
  Social services
  Nutrition

Table 30-8	UNOS System for Liver Transplants	
UNOS Status	**Description of Status**	**Special Status Considerations**

MELD (Model for End-Stage Liver Disease)	• Numerical scale from 6 (less ill) to 40 (gravely ill)
	• Used with liver transplant candidates 12 years and older
	• Calculated using results of:
	  1. Bilirubin level
	  2. INR
	  3. Creatinine
		Exception: Status 1 (a patient with acute, sudden and severe onset liver failure with life expectancy of hours without a transplant (< 1% of candidates)

PELD (Pediatric End-Stage Liver Disease	• Used with a liver transplant candidate 11 years old or younger
	• Calculated using results of:
	  1. Bilirubin
	  2. INR
	  3. Albumin
	  4. Growth failure
	  5. Whether child < 1 year
		Exception: Status 1 (a patient with acute, sudden and severe onset liver failure with life expectancy of hours without a transplant (< 1% of candidates)

ery and return to work are discussed. The donor evaluation includes a history and physical examination with an adult hepatologist, laboratory evaluation (same as liver recipient), chest radiographic film, electrocardiogram, volumetric CT scan, liver biopsy (if necessary), and hepatic arteriogram to determine liver anatomy (Boone, Kelly, & Smith, 1992). Occasionally, unfavorable vascular anatomy is found. At this point, a different living donor is considered or the child continues to wait for an appropriate cadaver donor. The operation is scheduled after it has been determined that all study results are normal. In the case of acute liver failure, donors can be evaluated within approximately 6 to 8 hours and donate the same day. This has become a life-saving measure when children are in imminent danger of dying and no cadaveric organs are available (Casas, Falkenstein, Gallagher, & Dunn, 1999).

Pretransplantation Management and Complications

Because transplantation survival rates have continued to improve, liver transplantation is the modality of choice for children with end-stage liver disease. The most common reasons to initiate transplant in children with chronic liver disease are poor growth and development, portal hypertension, and mental changes (McDiarmid, 2003).

Nutritional and Developmental Concerns

Cognitive deficits are not unusual in children with liver disease because the children have organomegaly and mal-absorption, resulting in protein-calorie malnutrition and low energy levels (Stewart, Kennard, Waller, & Fixler, 1994). The brain is particularly vulnerable to the effects of protein energy malnutrition during early life. Malnutrition during the early months of life, independent of cause, has a deleterious effect on development (Stewart et al., 1989). Recognition and prevention of growth failure in a transplant candidate are necessary to assure maximal nutritional support (Balistreri, Bucuvalas, & Ryckman, 1995). The treatment of nutritionally depleted patients requires the administration of adequate calories to ensure optimal anabolic use of protein sources (Moukarzel et al., 1990).

Children who are in a better nutritional state before transplantation have better outcomes after transplantation (Moukarzel et al., 1990). When oral intake is not adequate to provide for calories and weight gain, nasogastric or gastrostomy tube feedings should be initiated (Kaufman, Murray, Wood, Shaw, & Vanderhoof, 1987).

Portal Hypertension

Children with chronic liver disease are at increased risk for esophageal varices that result from decreased blood flow to the liver and increased flow, by means of collateral circulation, to the spleen and stomach. These children require frequent evaluations because medical management is based on symptoms. Sclerotherapy is the temporizing treatment of choice for bleeding varices. Other therapies include propranolol (Inderal) or portal-venous surgical shunt procedure (Goh & Meyers, 1994).

Encephalopathy

Children with chronic liver disease may have obvious changes in mental status related to elevated ammonia levels. Changes in wake-sleep cycle, decreased concentration in school resulting in change in grades, frustration, and inability to perform simple fine motor skills are common. Evaluation and treatment with medications, such as neomycin and lactulose, and a decrease in dietary protein may help.

Infections

Children awaiting liver transplantation are at increased risk of infection because of chronic nutritional deficits and impaired liver function. Good hand washing and the avoidance of day care centers and large crowds while on the transplant list are recommended.

Surgical Procedure and Operative Management

When a liver becomes available, the recipient is brought to the hospital and preoperative blood work, including a comprehensive panel, complete blood count, prothrombin time/partial thromboplastin time, and type and crossmatch for blood products, is obtained. A chest radiographic film, urinalysis, and physical examination are part of the preoperative evaluation.

The surgical procedure is approximately 8 to 12 hours from induction of anesthesia and line placement to final skin closure. The procedure involves a bilateral subcostal incision to visualize and mobilize all major structures (portal vein, hepatic artery, and bile ducts) of the liver before the hepatectomy. Before removing the liver, the surgeon cross-clamps the suprahepatic and infrahepatic vena cavae, portal vein, and hepatic artery. Clamping of the vena cavae can lead to acidosis, hypotension, and bleeding. The donor liver is placed in an orthotopic position, and the vascular anastomoses are performed in the following order: suprahepatic vena cava, infrahepatic vena cava (which is flushed with 5% albumin to remove any leftover preservation solution), portal vein establishing blood flow to the graft, and, finally, the hepatic artery. Reperfusion of the graft occurs once portal venous blood flow is reestablished. During the reperfusion phase, the results of clamping can lead to swelling of the intestine, fluid shifts (third spacing), and renal failure. Children generally tolerate caval clamping well because of their collateral circulation (Falkenstein, 1993). Reconstruction of the biliary drainage involves a Roux-en-Y limb of the jejunum. Two to three Jackson-Pratt drains are also inserted. The child remains intubated and is transferred directly to the intensive care unit (Falkenstein).

The donor liver is stored in Wisconsin preservation solution and ice until it is prepared for implantation. Use of this solution has increased cold times from 8 to 24 hours. Extended preservation time permits careful inspection of the donor organ and reconstruction or back table surgery of the hepatic allograft. One of the advantages of living related donation is that the liver can be removed from the donor and almost immediately be placed in the recipient, thus decreasing cold ischemic time.

Postoperative Management

Postoperative care of the child after liver transplantation involves assessment and monitoring of the cardiovascular, pulmonary, neurologic, gastrointestinal, and immune systems; liver function; and fluid and electrolytes and nutrition (Falkenstein, 1993). Nursing care must also address the psychosocial and emotional needs of the child and family members.

Cardiovascular Monitoring

Adequate perfusion of body organs, especially the new liver, is important. Hypothermia may occur as a result of the large incision, the exposure of the bowel during surgery, and the transfusion therapy required. Hemorrhage is possible as a result of coagulopathy or bleeding from the anastomosis. To detect bleeding, one should observe for increased abdominal girth, oozing from suture lines, and large amounts of drainage from Jackson-Pratt drains. Children have an arterial line, two central lines, and peripheral lines in the upper extremities because of cross-clamping of the vena cava. Hypertension or hypotension may occur after surgery. Hypertension in the first 24 to 48 hours is usually related to the amount of colloids and blood products given in the operating room. It also may be due to altered function of the renin-angiotensin system from decreased renal flow caused by intravenous cyclosporine. Hypotension results from bleeding or depleted fluid volume.

Pulmonary Monitoring

Ventilatory support is usually required for the first 24 to 48 hours after liver transplantation. Children are less likely to breathe effectively on their own because of the large incision and large hepatic allograft. Gentle chest percussion and suctioning facilitated with adequate pain management should be provided.

Fluid and Electrolytes

CVP monitoring aids in evaluating the child's fluid status. A complicating factor of maintaining fluid and electrolyte balance is the shift of fluid into the vascular beds and abdomen that occurs after the portal vein and vena cava are unclamped in the operating room (Falkenstein, 1993). Children with this complication usually have a low CVP (l to 3 cm H_2O) and low urine output, suggesting hypovolemia, although they appear edematous and weigh more than their preoperative weight. Effective diuresis is accomplished with furosemide (Lasix) or ethacrynate sodium (Edecrin). Fluids are administered at 80% of maintenance. Electrolytes are monitored every 6 hours, and fluid and electrolyte correction is made accordingly (Falkenstein). Hypocalcemia, hypokalemia, and hypomagnesemia are common problems in the child immediately after liver transplantation. Intake and output (Jackson-Pratt drains, Foley catheter, nasogastric tube) should be accurately measured to monitor fluid balance. Decreased urine output (< 1 mL/kg/hr) may reflect early graft dysfunction or cyclosporine-induced nephrotoxicity. As liver function improves, urine volume and concentration improve, and urine changes from an orange to a straw color.

Neurologic Evaluation

Neurologic assessments should be performed using a modified Glasgow coma scale until the child is fully awake. Central nervous system status is a crucial indicator of allograft function. Seizure activity is uncommon and is usually limited to extremely ill children with multiple risk factors. Seizures may also occur if the tacrolimus level is elevated.

Gastrointestinal and Nutritional Management

A nasogastric tube is placed to keep the stomach decompressed and to prevent vomiting and aspiration postoperatively. Parenteral nutrition begins on day 2 or 3 and continues until the child is receiving adequate calories either orally or by nasogastric tube. Small children have an increased metabolic rate and require increased calories by mouth or nasogastric tube for at least 6 months after transplantation.

Care on the Transplant Unit

The average stay in the intensive care unit is 3 to 5 days, at which point children are moved to the transplant unit. The most common problems after transplantation are rejection and infection. Other complications include hepatic artery thrombosis, bile leaks, bowel perforation, hypertension, and fluid retention (Falkenstein, 1993). Nursing interventions include monitoring for signs and symptoms of rejection and infection, monitoring of blood pressure, and discharge teaching.

Surgical Complications

Hepatic Artery Thrombosis

Hepatic artery thrombosis (HAT) occurs 1 to 6 days after transplantation and is usually related to mechanical problems. HAT results in graft failure, necessitating prompt detection. Signs and symptoms include irritability, fever, increasing liver enzymes, and inability of clotting studies to normalize. Doppler ultrasonography is used to confirm the diagnosis. HAT requires thrombectomy and restoration of arterial blood flow (Heffron et al., 2005). Hyperbaric oxygen therapy has also been used for management of HAT (Mazariegos et al., 1999).

Late artery thrombosis may result from chronic rejection and is less damaging to the graft because of collateral circulation. Bile duct complications are common in all patients with hepatic artery thrombosis because the bile duct receives flow from the hepatic artery. Retransplantation may be required at a later time (Stevens et al., 1992).

Bile Duct Stricture

Bile duct stricture may occur at any time. Children who are at an increased risk for strictures are those with chronic rejection or cytomegalovirus infections or those who required placement of a stent for a small duct during anastomosis of the bile duct (Dunn et al., 1994). Serial bile duct dilatations or surgical repair may be necessary to treat this condition (Sung et al., 2004).

Bile Leaks

Bile leaks can develop at any time after transplantation. Leakage of bile is evidenced by a change in color of the drainage from the Jackson-Pratt drains. Diagnosis is confirmed by measuring bilirubin from the drain. If it is higher than the systemic bilirubin, a bile leak is suspected. Early diagnosis and treatment can prevent a major episode of infectious peritonitis. Surgical treatment may be warranted in some cases.

Bowel Perforation

Bowel perforation is relatively uncommon and usually occurs 5 to 7 days after surgery. This complication results from division of adhesions during surgery. Signs and symptoms are fever, abdominal pain, distention, and irritability. Diagnosis is confirmed by a lateral decubitus radiographic film of the abdomen, assessing for free air. Surgical repair is the only treatment and should be performed immediately (Oldham, Colombani, & Foglia, 1997).

Medical Complications

The first episode of acute rejection usually occurs 5 to 10 days after transplantation. Early signs of rejection include low-grade fever (38°C), increases in liver enzyme and bilirubin levels, abdominal pain over the liver graft, irritability, and ascites. Percutaneous liver biopsy confirms rejection. This procedure can safely be performed with the patient under local anesthesia with conscious sedation. Before the biopsy, prothrombin and partial thromboplastin time and a type and cross-match for 1 unit of blood should be available. After biopsy, the child should be placed on the right side for 2 to 4 hours in bed. The parent may hold a small infant. A hemoglobin level should be obtained 4 hours after the procedure as well as a chest x-ray to assess for pneumothorax. Any decrease should be reported to the transplant team, along with any change in vital signs or irritability. Signs and symptoms of rejection are similar to those of infection, but their treatment is different; therefore, careful evaluation and consideration of all differential diagnoses are vital. Bolus doses of corticosteroids used to treat rejection could enhance the process in a child with a viral infection. Initially, rejection is managed with methylprednisolone sodium succinate (Solu-Medrol). If liver enzymes continue to rise, a monoclonal antibody (OKT3) may be administered.

Chronic Rejection

Chronic rejection may be the most important cause of graft loss beyond the second year after transplantation and is not common in pediatric patients (Jain et al., 2003). Chronic rejection is defined as progressive loss of bile ducts, along with formation of fibrosis and cirrhosis. This process can begin in the first few months after transplantation, or it may occur many years later. The cause is still not well understood, but early chronic rejection is associated with several episodes of early acute rejection that led to tissue damage and scarring (Gupta, Hart, Millis, Cronin, Brady, 2001). Gupta et al. (2001) reported an increased incidence of chronic rejection in children who experience two or more episodes of acute rejection within 1 year after transplantation and in children with autoimmune hepatitis. They proposed that inconsistent immunosuppressive medication levels, secondary to malabsorption or noncompliance or related to chronic viral diseases, such as Epstein-Barr virus or cytomegalovirus, contributed to chronic rejection. Bile duct complications that result in strictures are also associated with chronic rejection after liver transplantation.

Hypertension

Hypertension in the immediate postoperative period is related to several factors: stress, pain, and administration of steroids. Hypertension is also a side effect of cyclosporin therapy. Antihypertensive agents are used to control high blood pressure. For many children, these episodes are transient and resolve within 3 to 6 months (Purath, 1995).

Renal Function

Renal impairment remains the most serious complication of continued reliance on calcineurin inhibitors (Alonso, 2004). Clinicians also realized that relying on serum creatinine as a serial measure of renal function underestimated the severity of the problem and that measuring glomerular filtration rate should be the standard of care (Berg, Ericzon, & Nemeth, 2001).

■ Intestinal Transplantation

Early attempts at human intestinal transplantation in the 1960s and 1970s, using prednisone and azathioprine as immunosuppression agents, resulted in survival rates of less than 2.5 weeks. It was not until the introduction of tacrolimus in the early 1990s that centers began to see better results (Kocoshis, 1994). There were 92 pediatric intestinal transplantations in 2004 in the United States (Mittal, Tzakis, Kato, & Thompson, 2003; UNOS Annual Report, 2004). From 1995 to 2002, UNOS reported at 1 year: 112 patients with a 58% to 78% survival rate and at 5 years, 61 patients with a 41% to 53.7% survival rate (UNOS Annual Report).

Although total parenteral nutrition (TPN) has significantly prolonged the lives of children with intestinal failure, it is often complicated by recurrent central venous line infections and sepsis, loss of venous access, and cholestatic liver disease (Bueno et al., 1999). Approximately 70% of pediatric recipients of intestinal transplants require a simultaneous liver transplant because of TPN-induced liver disease (Bueno et al.). Factors associated with high morbidity included bridging fibrosis, bilirubin > 3 mg/dL, platelet count < 100,000, prothrombin time > 15 seconds, and combined intestinal/liver transplantation. Early referral for intestinal transplantation should occur before the development of liver dysfunction, taking into consideration the preceding risk factors (Bueno et al.). Table 30-1 reviews the diseases leading to intestinal transplantation, and Table 30-2 reviews the signs and symptoms of intestinal failure.

Children who are dependent on TPN as the result of a variety of conditions causing short-bowel syndrome are considered for small-bowel transplantation. Exclusion criteria are incurable malignancy, severe cardiopulmonary insufficiency, and sepsis (Funovits, Staschak-Chicko, Kovalak, & Altieri, 1993).

Anatomy

The small intestine is a convoluted tube extending from the stomach to the large intestine. It measures approximately 7 m (23 feet) long and 4 cm (1.5 inches) in diameter in the adult. The small intestine is the site of digestion and absorption. It is divided into three sections: the first section (duodenum) measures 25 cm in length and is arranged in the shape of the letter C. The second (jejunum) makes up two fifths of the intestines and extends from the duodenum to the ileum. There is no structural line of distinction between the jejunum and the ileum. The ileum (third section) makes up the remainder of the intestine and terminates by joining the large intestine at the ileocecal valve. The villi that line the intestines are fingerlike projections of mucous membrane that enhance absorption of nutrients. The crypts of Lieberkühn are intestinal glands located in the epithelium of the mucosa that are responsible for enzymes that aid digestion (Warevich & Williams, 1980).

Recipient Evaluation

The preoperative evaluation for intestinal transplantation includes the standard biochemical assessment used for liver transplantation. Additional studies to ascertain the degree of malabsorption include mineral and trace elements, parenteral nutritional requirements, metabolic assessment, D-xylose tolerance test (carbohydrate absorption), fecal fat analysis (digestion), and nitrogen excretion studies. An endoscopic examination is obtained to document varices. Upper gastrointestinal radiography, Doppler ultrasonography, and an abdominal CT are used to assess hepatic, mesenteric, and venous vasculature. Magnetic resonance imaging may be performed if there is suspicion of subclavian vein occlusion (Reyes et al., 1998).

Donor Selection

The appropriate donor is ABO compatible, is of appropriate weight (no more than 20% greater than recipient), is free of infection, and has normal liver function. Donor preparation requires decontamination of the intestinal tract with a combination of GoLYTELY, colistin, gentamicin, and nystatin.

Transplantation Operation

The liver is included when there is TPN-induced end-stage liver disease. The intestinal graft is anastomosed on a vascular pedicle of superior mesenteric artery and superior mesenteric vein. The venous return is directed into the superior mesentery, splenic vein, inferior vena cava, or an interposition graft to the portal vein. In children who receive both liver and small-bowel grafts, the recipient vena cava is anastomosed and arterialized from the infrarenal aorta by means of conduit homograft. In the liver/small-bowel recipients, a permanent native portocaval shunt or a donor portal vein to native portal vein anastomosis is performed. Reconstruction of the gastrointestinal and biliary tracts uses a Roux-en-Y technique, and all children have an ileostomy performed as well as placement of a jejunostomy tube for feedings. The ostomy is reversed when the children consume all their nutrition through the enteral route (Reyes et al., 1998). Advances in surgical technique include reduction of graft size by removing the right lobe of the liver or part of the intestine. This has allowed timely transplantation in infants who would otherwise die (Misiakos et al., 2000).

Postoperative Phase

Care is similar to the postoperative care of liver transplant recipients, with the addition of ostomy output monitoring (Beath, Kelly, & Booth, 1994).

Surgical Complications

Complications after intestinal transplantation include stenosis or thrombosis of the arterial and/or vascular systems. Other complications include leaking at the intestinal anastomotic site and bowel perforation. Vascular problems can be assessed by observing the color and appearance of the stoma. Immediate surgical intervention is the treatment of choice.

Medical Complications

Rejection

Signs and symptoms of rejection are listed in Table 30-4. Diagnosis is confirmed by biopsy specimens from multiple small-bowel sites. Endoscopic changes, such as ulceration, bleeding, and decreased peristalsis, may be seen. Treatment depends on the severity of the rejection. Initially, the patient receives a bolus of steroids, and tacrolimus dosages are increased. If the child does not respond to this therapy, OKT3 or ATG is administered. Initially biopsy specimens of the intestines are obtained biweekly, then weekly for 4 weeks, then monthly or as indicated. There are no biochemical markers of rejection, although rejection may be accompanied by increased intestinal permeability. Biopsy is the only definitive method for the diagnosis of rejection (Atkison et al., 1997).

Graft-Versus-Host Disease (GVHD) GVHD may occur with other organ transplantations, but bowel transplantations have a greater incidence because of the abundance of lymphoid tissue in the intestines. GVHD results from donor T cells reacting against recipient tissue. The hypothesis is that donor lymphocytes settle in the recipient tissues as dormant cells that may reactivate with suboptimal immunosuppressant therapy (Abu-Elmagd, Fung, & Reyes, 1992). Pretreatment of the graft with radiation therapy, antilymphoid globulins, and OKT3 have been used to sterilize the donor graft before transplantation but have not successfully prevented GVHD (Funovits et al., 1993).

Infections/Translocation The child with short-bowel syndrome who is receiving parenteral nutrition and who undergoes isolated bowel or liver/bowel transplantation is at increased risk for opportunistic infections (Funovits et al., 1993). There is also an increased incidence of bacterial overgrowth in children requiring treatment with metronidazole and other agents to decontaminate the bowel. Surveillance stool cultures are obtained, and particular attention is given if rejection is suspected because bacteria may translocate from the bowel lumen through the damaged mucosa to the blood (Funovits et al.).

Gastrointestinal Motility Disorders These disorders, such as gastroesophageal reflux, gastric hypomotility, and pyloric spasm, are common and usually resolve 4 to 8 weeks after surgery. Diarrhea of unknown cause is managed with pectin, paregoric, octreotide (Sandostatin), and a low-fat diet. Surveillance stool cultures, endoscopy, and small-intestinal biopsy are strongly recommended at frequent intervals to rule out the possibility of graft rejection or enteric infection as a cause of diarrhea (Funovits et al., 1993).

■ Postoperative Care of the Pediatric Abdominal Transplant Recipient

Infections

The advent of newer, more powerful immunosuppressive agents has played a critical role in the improvement of the results in pediatric organ transplantation in the past decade. The reduction in rejection brings with it the consequences of oversuppression, which causes an increase in infections in this population. According to the annual report of the Studies of Pediatric Liver Transplantation, infection was the leading cause of mortality after transplantation (Renoult, Buteau, Lamarre, Turgeon, & Tapiero, 2005).

Bacterial Infection

Pediatric transplant recipients are at risk for bacterial infections. Common sites are intra-abdominal abscess, central lines, Jackson-Pratt drains, and urinary catheters. Children who are immunosuppressed may not respond to bacterial infections with a fever. The combination of ongoing immunosuppression and treatment with multiple antibiotics can lead to opportunistic infections.

Nursing assessment for signs and symptoms of infection in children with solid-organ transplantation includes assessing incisions for redness and drainage. A temperature of 38.5°C should be reported to the transplant team immediately.

Fungal Infection

Immunocompromised children are vulnerable to both common and rare pathogens, such as *Candida albicans*, *Aspergillus fumigatus*, and *Pneumocystis carinii* (Weil & Rovelli, 1990) because of prophylactic antibiotics administered with immunosuppressant agents in the early postoperative period. Prophylactic antifungal agents, such as clotrimazole (Mycelex) lozenges or nystatin swish and swallow are used for 4 to 6 weeks to prevent yeast infections. Amphotericin B is administered to treat systemic yeast infections, depending on the source of infection. In older children, oral or intravenous fluconazole can be used (American Academy of Pediatrics, 1997).

Viral Infection

Pediatric transplant recipients are immunologically naive compared with adults. Administration of immunosuppressant medications further increases the risk for primary viral infections with cytomegalovirus (CMV) and Epstein-Barr virus (EBV). Donor and recipient status for CMV should be identified, as demonstrated by the presence of a protective mismatch titer before transplantation. The least preferred match is a CMV positive donor organ in a CMV negative recipient. Serious problems occur when a CMV (+) donor organ is transplanted into a CMV (−) recipient. CMV-rich gamma globulin should be administered to provide passive immunity, or ganciclovir should be administered to treat early infection. Some centers have used both ganciclovir and acyclovir in differing protocols to reduce the effect of the CMV disease. A CMV (+) donor organ transplanted into a CMV (+) recipient raises the possibility of the recipient becoming infected with a different strain of CMV. CMV can be a pervasive disease, affecting the kidney, liver, lungs, and eyes (Dickens et al., 1991). Regardless of the cause, CMV infection, which presents with fever, decreased white blood cell count, and gastrointestinal symptoms, requires prompt treatment (Dunn et al., 1991). If a child develops a viral infection, immunosuppressive medications are tapered, and the appropriate antiviral agent is initiated (acyclovir, ganciclovir).

Epstein-Barr Virus

EBV is a serious complication for pediatric recipients if the child is seronegative and receives a seropositive organ. Undiagnosed EBV leads to posttransplantation lymphoproliferative disease (a malignancy) and death (Penn, 1998). The incidence of this disease is greatest in children who are younger than 5 years of age at the time of transplantation (Dharnidharka & Stevens, 2005; Green, 2002). Administration of potent immunosuppressive agents increases the incidence of this disease. Diagnosis is confirmed with biopsy of infected lymph nodes, polymerase chain reaction (PCR), DNA assay, and EBV titers. Treatment depends on the severity of infection. If a child has a positive PCR but is asymptomatic, decreasing immunosuppressive drugs may be the only treatment. If the child is symptomatic with lymphadenopathy, is febrile, and has a positive PCR titer, immunosuppression should be discontinued and treatment started with ganciclovir or acyclovir. A CT should be performed to identify any evidence of malignancy or tumors or dissemination to other organs. Early evaluation of signs and symptoms, such as fever, change in graft function, and lymphadenopathy, and prompt treatment may decrease mortality in this group of children. Evidence of lymphoma requires treatment with the appropriate chemotherapeutic agents (Martin, 1996).

Herpes Simplex

The herpes simplex virus can reactivate after transplantation but is rarely the source of a new infection. Children who have a prior history of herpes may be started on acyclovir after transplantation for 8 to 12 weeks or longer as a prophylaxis. The mouth should be examined routinely to detect whether the infection is present.

Pneumocystis carinii

This opportunistic pathogen may cause fatal infection after transplantation. Prophylaxis with sulfamethoxazole: trimethoprim (Bactrim) given daily three times a week has been effective in preventing *P. carinii* infections (Munoz, 1996).

Varicella

Varicella (chickenpox), a common childhood illness, can be life threatening to an immunocompromised child. The pretransplantation evaluation includes varicella titers. The varicella vaccine should be administered to children older than 1 year of age with negative titers. Siblings should receive the vaccine according to the American Academy of Pediatrics recommendations. Families and school nurses should be advised of children who are seronegative after transplantation and educated about the importance of notifying the transplant team of any exposure. If exposed, Acyclovir therapy must be started within 72 hours and given for 5 days. If disease does occur, intravenous or oral acyclovir is warranted. Varicella titers should be monitored 1 month after the disease presents. Protective immunity may not occur as a result of their immunocompromised condition, and these children are at risk for a subsequent infection. Pediatric transplantation patients are also at risk for the development of varicella zoster (shingles). Acyclovir should be administered for varicella zoster infections.

BK Virus

Polyoma virus (BK) has been emerging as an important cause of renal allograft dysfunction over the past decade. Most infections are asymptomatic, and the viruses remain latent in the kidney and in the lymphocytes after primary infection (Herman et al., 2004). BK virus may lead to graft failure in pediatric kidney transplant patients. Nurses should educate parents as to the importance of reporting fever or change in urine output or color in children after transplantation.

Pain Management

Pain management is an integral part of postoperative care of the transplant patient. Refer to Chapter 5 for specific strategies.

Immune Response

Immunosuppression

Immunosuppressive medications selectively prevent rejection. Double or triple immunotherapy is required initially to prevent humoral or cellular rejection. Perhaps the most challenging and the most dynamic aspect in caring for pediatric transplant recipients remains the selection of maintenance immunosuppression because there are now so many options from which to choose. The goal of maintenance immunosuppression is to maximize antirejection while minimizing potential side effects (Kahan & Ghobrial, 1994; Smith, Nemeth, & McDonald, 2003; Sollinger & Pirsch, 1995) (Table 30-5).

■ Living with a Transplant

Postoperative care of the pediatric transplant patient requires a collaborative relationship between the primary care physician and the transplant facility.

Growth

Current strategies to improve growth in the posttransplantation patient include low daily steroid dosing, alternate-day steroid dosing, steroid withdrawal, and steroid avoidance (Falkenstein & Dunn, 1998; Silverstein, Aviles, LeBlanc, Jung, & Vehaskari, 2005). In one study, discontinuation of corticosteroids was possible in 86% of children after liver transplantation, resulting in a significant increase in growth velocity and a low rate of acute rejection (Falkenstein & Dunn). The average follow-up period was 5 years, with no reported incidence of acute rejection. A small group of children became noncompliant with monotherapy immunosuppressant medication, which resulted in a 7% incidence of rejection. Recombinant human growth hormone prescribed in children with renal and liver disease offers a promising addition to the medical treatment of children who experience post-transplantation growth delay (Bartosh et al., 1992; Evans et al., 2005; Fine & Tejani, 2001).

Development

Children with chronic renal or liver disease may experience delays in sexual maturation. Adolescent girls note a delay in menarche, whereas males experience a delay in the development of secondary sex characteristics. Initial delays in menarche are ascribed to the hormonal imbalances caused by steroids (Armenti, Radmonski, Moritz, & Davidson, 2003).

Diet

A well-balanced diet should be encouraged. Children who are taking steroids are encouraged to consume a diet low in sugar and salt because of fluid retention and hyperglycemia (Pipes & Trahms, 1993).

Immunizations

As a result of illness, well-child immunizations are often neglected. All children awaiting organ transplantation should receive a full set of immunizations before transplantation on a regular or accelerated schedule. This decreases the risk of acquiring these infections after transplantation. After transplantation, live virus vaccines, such as varicella, and the measles, mumps, and rubella vaccine are being given only in a limited number of transplant centers (Campbell & Herold, 2005; Falkenstein, Stritzel, Kassman, & SPLIT Research Group, 2005; Neu, 2005).

Siblings can receive all immunizations. Smallpox vaccine recipients must not be in contact with the transplant recipient for four weeks after receiving the vaccine. This is especially important information for military families.

Yearly influenza vaccine is recommended for the recipient and family members. (Edvardsson et al., 1996).

Safety

Exercise restrictions should be advised for 6 weeks after surgery. Good hand washing is encouraged for the child and caregivers to decrease risk of infection. The use of sunblock, at least SPF 30, is recommended to prevent sunburn because these children are at increased risk for melanomas. Families should be provided with a Medic Alert application, and the importance of a bracelet in the event of an emergency should be discussed. Contact sports should be restricted for the first year. Encourage the use of bike helmets and car seat belts.

Screening

Children after transplantation require normal childhood hearing and vision screening because immunosuppressant medications and antibiotics make them more vulnerable to vision and hearing problems. Transplant recipients require a biannual vision test for the first year and then annually because of the risk of cataracts and pseudotumor cerebri (Lessell, 1992). An audiogram should be scheduled before discharge, 6 months after transplantation, and then yearly to assess for hearing loss related to the administration of ototoxic drugs.

Dental

Good dental habits with daily brushing and flossing and biannual check-ups should be encouraged. Children who receive cyclosporine or nifedipine (Procardia) are at increased risk for developing gingival hyperplasia. Prophylactic antibiotics should be prescribed for any dental procedure, including cleaning, to prevent a *Staphylococcus aureus* infection. The American Heart Association (AHA) guidelines for subacute bacterial endocarditis (SBE) prophylaxis with amoxicillin or penicillin 1 hour before procedure (50 mg/kg/dose; maximum, 3 g) should be followed.

Follow-Up Blood Work and Evaluation

Postoperative visits include physical examination and review of systems, including weight, height, and diet. Close follow-up is essential for the first several weeks. Visits are scheduled further apart as the child stabilizes. Monitoring includes a comprehensive blood panel, hepatic panel (liver and intestinal transplant recipients), complete blood count, magnesium, and drug level monitoring of immunosuppressive agents. Children who have undergone renal transplantation should have surveillance urinalysis, urine culture and sensitivity, renin, and 24-hour urine collection obtained every 6 months.

Behavioral Issues

Children who undergo transplantation must continue immunosuppressant therapy for the remainder of their lives. Often, this becomes a problem as children reach adolescence and try to "fit in" with their peers (Falkenstein, Flynn, Kirkpatrick, Casas, & Dunn, 2004; Jarzembowski et al., 2004; Meyers, Thomson, & Weiland, 1996; Nevins, 2002). Recipients suggest two reasons for missing medication: (1) forgetting to take their medicines or return for routine follow-up appointments and (2) avoidance of medication side effects. Several helpful strategies to improve noncompliance include simplifying the medication regimen, using weekly pill boxes to organize medications, or even investing in a watch with an alarm that gives a reminder so that medications are given on time.

Appearing different from one's peers can be a devastating experience. It should be recommended that adolescents use acne creams, nutritional counseling, depilatories for unwanted hair, and proper dental care to prevent the side effects of immunosuppressant medications.

In the posttransplantation phase when the children feel well, it is often difficult for the immediate and extended family to make the transition from illness to health (Jessop & Stein, 1988). In some of the pretransplantation and posttransplantation studies, parents have described the child with a transplant as dependent and irritable before the transplantation to defiant and aggressive afterwards (Stewart et al., 1994; Zitelli, Miller, Gartner, & Malatack, 1988). Shemesh and colleagues (2005) reported that children, unlike adults who have undergone a solid-organ transplant, have reported lower levels of depression and posttraumatic stress. It is critical for nurses and families to understand the psychosocial variables that contribute to psychological adjustment after transplantation (Shemesh et al.).

Schooling

Children with a transplant should be encouraged to attend school. Partnerships should be developed with the school nurse and the classroom teacher to promote the successful return of the child with a transplant to the classroom setting. Some successful strategies to build self-esteem include encouraging them to see themselves as "normal." They must be encouraged to develop new re-lationships at school, participate in sports and other extracurricular activities, and dream of a future.

■ Conclusion

Innovative surgical techniques and more specific immunosuppressive agents have improved the outcome and changed the goals of transplantation over the past decade. The multidisciplinary team approach is essential in order to manage this acquired chronic illness. Often, parents of children who undergo an organ transplantation live in constant fear of rejection and death (Hobbs & Sexton, 1995). Families may benefit from participation in support groups or chat lines. Nurses can support families to achieve a balance in normalizing their child's life and the complex management of their care.

■ Acknowledgments

The authors would like to acknowledge the work of Joanne Palmer in the development of this chapter in the first edition of this textbook. The Editors greatly appreciate the thoughtful review of this chapter by Kathy Iurlano, BSN, RN, CCTC. Ms. Iurlano currently practices as The Heart/Lung Transplant Coordinator at the Children's Hospital of Pittsburgh. Ms. Iurlano is the former Pediatric Liver and Intestine Transplant Coordinator at the same institution.

■ Educational Materials

APSNA invites you to download the following diagnosis-related teaching tools for Chapter 30, Pediatric Abdominal Organ Transplants: (1) Kidney Transplant and (2) Liver Transplant. These teaching tools are available at the APSNA Web site (www.apsna.org) and the Jones and Bartlett Web site (www.jbpub.com). All teaching materials are available in English and Spanish and are free of charge. APSNA encourages their use for your patients and families.

References

Abu-Elmagd, K., Fung, J. J., & Reyes, J. (1992). Management of intestinal transplantation in humans. *Transplant Proceedings, 24,* 1243–1244.

Alexander, S. R. (1990). Controversies in pediatric renal transplantation. *AKF Nephrology Letter, 7,* 5–21.

Alonso, E. (2004). Long term renal function in pediatric liver and heart recipients. *Pediatric Transplantation, 8*(4), 381–364.

American Academy of Pediatrics. (1997). *Red book: Report of the committee on infectious diseases.* Elk Grove Village, IL: Author.

Armenti, V., Radmonski, S., Mortiz, M., & Davidson, J. (2003). Pregnancy in female pediatric solid organ transplant recipients. *The Pediatric Clinics of North America, 50*(6), 1543–1560.

Atkison, P., Chatzipetrou, M., Tsaroucha, A., Lehmann, R., Tzakis, A., & Grant, D. (1997). Small bowel transplantation in children. *Pediatric Transplantation, 1,* 111–118.

Balistreri, W., Bucuvalas, J., & Ryckman, F. (1995). The effect of immunosuppression on growth and development. *Liver Transplantation and Surgery, 1*(5), 64–73.

Bartosh, S., Kaiser, B., Rervani, L., Plinsky, M., Palmer, J., & Dunn, S. (1992). Effects of growth hormone administration in pediatric allograft recipients. *Pediatric Nephrology, 6,* 68–73.

Beath, S., Kelly, D., & Booth, I. (1994). Post-operative care of children undergoing small bowel and liver transplantation. *British Journal of Intensive Care, 4,* 302–308.

Bell, J. (1998). Antigens and antibodies: The foreign language of transplantation. *Nephrology News & Issues, 12*(1), 12–13.

Benfield, M. (2003). Current status of kidney transplant: Update. *Pediatric Clinics of North America, 50*(6), 1301–1334.

Berg, U., Ericzon, B., & Nemeth, A. (2001). Renal function before and after liver transplantation in children. *Transplantation, 72*(4), 632–637.

Boone, P., Kelly, S., & Smith, C. D. (1992). Liver transplantation: Living related donations. *Critical Care Nursing Clinics of North America, 4*(2), 243.

Broelsch, C., Edmond, J., & Thistlethwaite, J. (1988). Liver transplantation with reduced size donor organs. *Transplantation, 45,* 519–524.

Bueno, J., Ohwada, S., Kocoshis, S., Mazariegos, G., Dvorchik, I., Sigurdsson, L., et al. (1999). Factors impacting the survival of children with intestinal failure referred for intestinal transplantation. *Journal of Pediatric Surgery, 34*(1), 27–33.

Bunchman, T. E., & So, S. K. (1994). Diagnosis and treatment of post operative allograft dysfunction. In A. Tejani & R. Fine (Eds.), *Pediatric renal transplantation* (pp. 257–268). New York: John Wiley & Sons.

Campbell, A. L., & Herold, B. C. (2005). Immunization of pediatric solid organ transplantation candidates: Immunization in transplant candidates. *Pediatric Transplantation, 9*(5), 652–661.

Casas, A., Falkenstein, K., Gallagher, M., & Dunn, S. P. (1999). Living related transplant for acute liver failure. *Pediatric Transplantation, 3,* 1–4.

Dharnidharka, V. R., & Stevens, G. (2005). Risk for post-transplant lymphoproliferative disorder after polyclonal antibody induction in kidney transplantation. *Pediatric Transplantation, 9*(5), 622–626.

Dickens, S., Luks, L., Braandt, M., Khazal, P., Weber, A., et al. (1991). Infectious complications of pediatric liver transplantation. *Transplantation, 57,* 544–547.

Dunn, S., Falkenstein, K., Lawrence, J., Meyers, R., Vinocur, C. D., Billmire, D. F., et al. (1994). Monotherapy with cyclosporin for chronic immunosuppression in pediatric liver transplant. *Transplantation, 57,* 512–515.

Dunn, S., Mayoral, J., Gilligham, K., Loeffler, C., Brayman, K., & Kramer, M. (1991). Treatment of invasive cytomegalovirus disease in solid organ transplant patients with Ganciclovir. *Transplantation, 51*(1), 98–106.

Edvardsson, V. O., Flynn, J. T., Deforest, A., Kaiser, B. A., Schulman, S. L., Bradley, A., et al. (1996). Effective immunization against influenza in pediatric renal transplant recipients. *Clinical Transplantation, 10,* 556–560.

Evans, I., Belle, S., Wei, Y., Penovich, C., Ruppert, K. & Detre, K. M. (2005). Post-transplant growth among pediatric recipients of liver transplantation. *Pediatric Transplant, 9*(4), 480–485.

Falkenstein, K., Stritzel, S., Kassman, K., & SPLIT Research Group. (2005). Immunization practices in pediatric liver transplant patients at studies of pediatric liver and transplant (SPLIT) centers. Abstract presentation. National Organization of Transplant Coordinators, July 26–30, 2005. Atlanta, GA.

Falkenstein, K., Flynn, L., Kirkpatrick, B., Casas, A., & Dunn, S. (2004). Noncompliance in children post-liver transplant. Who are the culprits? *Pediatric Transplantation, 6*(2), 150–158.

Falkenstein, K. (1993). Liver transplantation: Nursing care of pediatric recipients. *Med-Surg Nursing Quarterly, 1*(30), 51–86.

Falkenstein, K., & Dunn, S. (1998). Growth acceleration on cyclosporine monotherapy after transplantation in children. *Transplantation Proceedings, 30*(5), 1969–1972.

Fine, R., & Tejani, R. N. (2001). The contribution of renal transplantation to final adult height. *Pediatric Nephrology, 16,* 951–961.

Funovits, M., Staschak-Chicko, S., Kovalak, L., & Altieri, K. (1993). Transplantation of the small intestines. In M. T. Nolan & S. M. Augustine (Eds.), *Transplantation nursing* (pp. 319–345). Norwalk, CT: Appleton & Lange.

Goh, D., & Meyers, N. (1994). Portal hypertension in children. *Journal of Pediatric Surgery, 29*(5), 688–691.

Green, M. (2002). Viral infections and pediatric liver transplantation. *Pediatric Transplant, 6*(1), 20–24.

Gupta, P., Hart, J., Millis, J., Cronin, D., & Brady, L. (2001). De Novo hepatitis with autoimmune antibodies and atypical histology: A rare cause of late graft dysfunction after pediatric liver transplantation. *Transplantation, 71*(5), 664–668.

Harada, H., Seki, T., Nonomura, K., Chikaraishi, T., Takeuchi, I., Morita, K., et al. (2001). Pre-emptive kidney transplant in children. *International Journal of Urology, 8*(5), 205–211.

Harmon, W. E., Stablein, D., Alexander, S. R., & Tejani, A. (1991). Graft thrombosis in pediatric renal transplant recipients. *Transplantation, 51,* 406–412.

Hayashi, M., Cao, S., Concepcion, W., Monge, H., Ojogoho, O., So, S., et al. (1998). Current status of living related liver transplant. *Pediatric Transplantation, 2,* 16–25.

Heffron, T., Welsch, D., Pillen, T., Fasola, C., Red, D., Smallwood, G., et al. (2005). Low incidence of hepatic artery thrombosis after pediatric liver transplantation without use of intraoperative microscope. *Pediatric Transplantation, 9*(4), 486–490.

Herman, J., Van Ranst, M., Snocek, R., Beuselinck, K., Lerut, E., & Van Damme-Lombaerts, R. (2004). Polyomavirus infection in pediatric renal transplant recipients: Evaluation using a quantitative real time PCR technique. *Pediatric Transplantation, 8*(4), 485–492.

Hobbs, S., & Sexton, S. (1995). Cognitive development and learning in the pediatric organ transplant recipient. *Journal of Learning Disabilities, 26*(2), 28–32.

Ingelfinger, J. A., & Brewer, E. D. (1992). Pediatric post transplant hypertension: A review of current standards of care. *Child Nephrology and Urology, 12,* 139–146.

Jain, A., Mazariegos, G., Pokharna, R., Parizhskaya, M., Kashyap, R., Kosmach-Park, B., et al. (2003). The absence of chronic rejection in pediatric primary liver transplant patients who are maintained on tacrolimus-based immunosuppression: A long-term analysis. *Transplantation, 75*(7), 1020–1025.

Jarzembowski, T., Panaro, F., Heiliczer, J., Kraft, K., Bogettei, D., Sankary, H., et al. (2004). Impact of non-compliance on outcomes after kidney transplantation: An analysis in racial subgroups. *Pediatric Transplantation, 8*(4), 367–371.

Jessop, J. D., & Stein, R. (1988). Essential concepts in the care of children with chronic illness. *Pediatrics, 15,* 5–12.

Jones, J. W., Matas, A. J., & Najarian, J. S. (1994). Surgical technique. In A. Tejani & R. Fine (Eds.), *Pediatric renal transplantation* (pp. 187–200). New York: John Wiley & Sons.

Kahan, B. D., & Ghobrial, R. (1994). Immunosuppressive agents. *Surgical Clinics of North America, 74*(5), 1029–1053.

Kaufman, S., Murray, N., Wood, P., Shaw, B., & Vanderhoof, I. (1987). Nutritional support for the infant with extrahepatic biliary atresia. *The Journal of Pediatrics, 110*(5), 679–685.

Keown, P. A., & Stiller, C. R. (1986). Kidney transplantation. *Surgical Clinics of North America*, 66, 517–539.

Kirkman, R. L., & Tilney, N. L. (1989). Surgical complications in the transplant recipient. In E. Milford, B. Brenner, & J. Stein (Eds.), *Renal transplantation* (pp. 231–245). New York: Churchill Livingstone.

Kocoshis, S. (1994). Small bowel transplantation in infants and children. *Gastroenterology Clinics of North America*, 23(4), 727–742.

Kohaut, E. C., & Tejani, A. (1996). The 1994 Annual Report of the North American Pediatric Renal Transplant Cooperative Study. *Pediatric Nephrology*, 10, 422–434.

Lake, K. D., & Kilkenny, J. M. (1992). The pharmacokinetics and pharmacodynamics of immunosuppressive agents. *Critical Care Nursing Clinics of North America*, 4(2), 205–219.

Lessell, S. (1992). Pediatric pseudo tumor cerebri (idiopathic intracranial hypertension). *Survey of Ophthalmology*, 37(3), 155–166.

Loertscher, R., Parfrey, P. S., & Guttmann, R. D. (1989). Postoperative management of the renal transplant recipient and long term complications. In E. Milford, B. Brenner, & J. Stein (Eds.), *Renal transplantation* (pp. 197–230). New York: Churchill Livingstone.

Martin, S. (1996). Assessing and caring for the infant liver transplant recipient. *Critical Care Nursing*, 16(3), 734–743.

Mauer, S. M., Nevins, T. E., & Ascher, N. (1992). Renal transplantation in children. In C. Edelman (Ed.), *Pediatric kidney disease* (pp. 941–981). Boston: Little, Brown.

Mazariegos, G., O'Toole, K., Mieles, L. A., Dvorchik, I., Meza, M. P., Briassoulis, G., et al. (1999). Hyperbaric oxygen therapy for hepatic artery thrombosis after liver transplantation in children. *Liver Transplantation Surgery*, 5, 429–436.

McDiarmid, S. (2003). Current status of liver transplantation in children. *The Pediatric Clinics of North America*, 50, 1335–1374.

Meyers, K. E. C., Thomson, P. D., & Weiland, H. (1996). Noncompliance in children and adolescents after renal transplantation. *Transplantation*, 62(2), 186–189.

Misiakos, E. P., Kato, T., Levi, D., Ruiz, P., Cantwell, G. P., & Mittall, N. (2000). Pediatric small bowel transplantation. In A. H. Tejani, W. E. Harmon, & R. N. Fine (Eds.), *Pediatric solid organ transplantation* (1st ed., pp. 446–460). Copenhagen: Munksgaard.

Mitsnefes, M. (2004). Hypertension and end organ damage in pediatric renal transplantation. *Pediatric Transplantation*, 8(4), 394–399.

Mittal, M. D., Tzakis, M. D., Kato, T., & Thompson, J. (2003). Current status of small bowel transplantation in children. *The Pediatric Clinics of North America*, 50(6), 1419–1433.

Moukarzel, A., Najm, I., Vargas, J., McDiarmid, S., Busuttil, R., & Ament, M. (1990). Effect of nutritional status on outcome of orthotopic liver transplantation in pediatric patients. *Transplantation Proceedings*, 22(40), 1560–1563.

Munoz, S. (1996). Long-term management of the liver transplant recipient. *Medical Clinics of North America*, 80(5), 1103–1119.

Neu, A. (2005). Indications for varicella vaccine post-transplant. *Pediatric Transplantation*, 9(2), 141–144.

Nevins, T. E. (2002). Non-compliance and its management in teenagers. *Pediatric Transplantation*, 6, 475–479.

Offner, G., Broyer, M., & Niaudel, P. (2002). A multicenter, open label, pharmacokinetic safety, and tolerability study of basiliximab in pediatric De Novo renal transplant recipients. *Transplantation*, 74(7), 276–280.

Oldham, K., Colombani, P., & Foglia, R. (1997). *Surgery of infants and children*. Philadelphia: Lippincott-Raven.

Otte, J. B., deVille, J., Goyet, D., & Reding, R. (2005). Liver transplantation for hepatoblastoma. Indications and contraindications in the modern era. *Pediatric Transplantation*, 9(5), 557–566.

Paul, L. C. (1995). Chronic renal transplant loss. *Kidney International*, 47, 1491–1499.

Payne, J. L. (1992). Immune modification and complications of immunosuppression. *Critical Care Nursing Clinics of North America*, 4(1), 43–58.

Penn, I. (1998). De Novo malignancies in pediatric organ transplant recipients. *Pediatric Transplantation*, 2, 56–63.

Pipes, P., & Trahms, C. (1993). *Nutrition in infancy and childhood*. St. Louis, MO: Mosby.

Purath, J. (1995). Pediatric hypertension: Assessment and management. *Pediatric Nursing*, 21(2), 173–177.

Qureshi, F., Rabb, H., & Kasiske, B. L. (2002). Silent acute rejection during prolonged delayed graft function reduces kidney allograft survival. *Transplantation*, 74(100), 1400–1404.

Renoult, E., Buteau, C., Lamarre, V., Turgeon, N., & Tapiero, B. (2005). Infectious risk in pediatric organ transplant recipients: Is it increased with new immunosuppressive? *Pediatric Transplantation*, 9(4), 470–479.

Reyes, J., Bueno, J., Kocoshis, S., Green, M., Abu-Elmagd, K., Fuukawa, H., et al. (1998). Current status of intestinal transplantation in children. *Journal of Pediatric Surgery*, 33(2), 243–251.

Rubin, R. H. (1988). Infection in the renal and liver transplant patient. In R. Rubin & L. Young (Eds.), *Clinical approach to infection in the compromised host* (pp. 557–621). New York: Plenum.

Rush, D., Nickerson, P., & Jeffery, J. R. (2000). Protocol biopsies in the management of renal allograft recipients. *Current Opinions in Nephrology and Hypertension*, 9(6), 615–619.

Salvatierra, O., Tanney, D., Mak, R., Alfrey, E., Lemley, K., & Mackie, V. (1997). Pediatric renal transplantation and its challenges. *Transplantation Reviews*, II, 51–69.

Shapiro, R., & Simmons, R. L. (1991). Kidney transplantation. In L. Makowka (Ed.), *Handbook of transplantation management* (pp. 168–191). Austin, TX: R.G. Landes.

Shemesh, E., Annunziato, R. A., Shneider, B. L., Newcorn, J. H., Warshaw, J. K., Dugan, C., et al. (2005). Parents and clinicians underestimate distress and depression in children who had a transplant. *Pediatric Transplantation*, 9(5), 673–679.

Silverstein, D. M., Aviles, D. H., LeBlanc, P. M., Jung, F., & Vehaskari, V. M. (2005). Results of one-year follow-up of steroid-free immunosuppression in pediatric renal patients. *Pediatric Transplantation*, 9(5), 589–597.

Singh, A., Stablein, D., & Tejani, A. (1997). Risk factors for vascular thrombus in pediatric renal transplantation: A special report of the North American Pediatric Renal Transplant Cooperative Study. Transplantation, 63(9), 1263–1267.

Smith, J., Nemeth, T., & McDonald, R. (2003). Current immunosuppressive agents: Efficacy, side effects, and utilization. *The Pediatric Clinics of North America*, 50(6), 1233–1259.

Sollinger, H., & Pirsch, J. (1995). *Transplantation drug pocket reference guide*. Georgetown, TX: Landis.

Starzl, T., Rutman, C., & Corman, J. (1987). Transplantation of the liver. In E. Schiff (Ed.), *Diseases of the liver* (6th ed.). Philadelphia: Lippincott Raven.

Starzl, T., Swatsuki, S., & Van Thiel, T. (1982). Evaluation transplantation. *Hepatology*, 2(5), 261–265.

Stevens, L. H., Emond, J. C., Piper, J. B., Heffron, T. G., Thistlethwaite, J. R., Whitington, P. F., et al. (1992). Hepatic artery thrombosis in infants. *Transplantation*, 53, 396–399.

Stewart, S., Kennard, B., Waller, D., & Fixler, D. (1994). Cognitive function in children who receive organ transplantation. *Health Psychology*, 13(1), 3–13.

Stewart, S., Uauy, R., Waller, D., Kennard, B., Benser, M., & Andrews, W. (1989). Mental and motor development, social competence, and growth one year after successful pediatric liver transplantation. *The Journal of Pediatrics*, 114(4 Part 1), 574–581.

Sung, R. S., Campbell, D. A., Rudich, S. M., Punch, J. D., Shieck, V. L., Armstrong, J. M., et al. (2004). Long-term follow-up of percutaneous transhepatic balloon cholangioplasty in the management of biliary strictures after liver transplantation. *Transplantation, 77*(1), 110–115.

Suthanthiran, M., & Strom, T. B. (1994). Renal transplantation. *The New England Journal of Medicine, 331,* 365–376.

Tejani, A., Cortes, L., & Stablein, D. H. (1996). Clinical correlates of chronic rejection in pediatric renal transplantation: A report of the North American Renal Transplant Cooperative. *Transplantation, 61*(7), 1054–1058.

Tejani, A., Ho, P., Emment, L., & Stablein, D. (2002). Reduction in acute rejection decreases chronic rejection graft failure in children: A Report of the North American Pediatric Renal Transplantation in Children Cooperative. *American Journal of Transplant, 2,* 142–147.

Tilney, N. L., Rocha, A., Strom, T. B., & Kirkman, R. L. (1984). Renal artery stenosis in transplant patients. *Annals of Surgery, 199,* 454–460.

UNOS Annual Report. (2004). *The U.S. scientific registry of transplant recipients and the organ procurement and transplantation network, transplant data 1988–1994.* (International standard book number 1-88665113-2). Richmond, VA: United Network for Organ Sharing Printing Office.

U.S. Department of Health and Human Services. (2005). Annual report of the U.S. Organ Procurement and Transplantation Network and the Scientific Registry of Transplant Recipients: Transplant data 1995–2004. Rockville, MD: Health Resources and Services Administration, Healthcare Systems Bureau, Division of Transplantation.

Warady, B. A., Herbert, D., Sullivan, E. K., Alexander, S. R., & Tejani, A. (1997). Renal transplantation, chronic dialysis, and chronic renal insufficiency in children and adolescents. The 1995 Annual Report of the North American Pediatric Renal Transplant Cooperative Study. *Pediatric Nephrology, 11,* 49–64.

Warevich, R., & Williams, P. (1980). *Gray's anatomy.* Philadelphia: W.B. Saunders.

Weil, M., & Rovelli, M. (1990). Infectious disease and transplantation. In K. M. Sigardson-Poor & L. M. Haggerty (Eds.), *Nursing care of the transplant recipient* (pp. 89–113). Philadelphia: W.B. Saunders.

Weir, M. R. (1990). Calcium channel blockers in organ transplantation: Important new therapeutic modalities. *Journal of American Society of Nephrology, 1,* 528–538.

Zaontz, M. R., Hatch, D. A., & Firlit, C. F. (1988). Urologic complications in pediatric renal transplantation: Management and prevention. *Journal of Urology, 140,* 1123–1128.

Zitelli, B., Miller, J., Gartner, S., & Malatack, J. (1988). Changes in life style after transplantation. *Pediatrics, 82,* 173–178.

Further Readings

Bond, G. J., Mazariegos, G. V., Sindhi, R., Abu-Elmagd, K. M., & Reyes, J. (2005). Evolutionary experience with immunosuppression in pediatric intestinal transplantation. *Pediatric Surgery, 40*(1), 274–279.

Fine, R. N. (2002). Growth following solid-organ transplantation. *Pediatric Transplantation, 6*(1), 47–52.

First, M. R., & Schroeder, T. J. (1991). Solid-organ transplantation in the pediatric population. *Clinical Transplantation, 5*(2 part 2), 132–136.

Fuqua, J. S. (2006). Growth after organ transplantation. *Seminars in Pediatric Surgery, 15*(3), 162–169.

Hurwitz, M., Desai, D. M., Cox, K. L., Berquist, W. E., Esquivel, C. O., & Millan, M. T. (2004). Complete immunosuppressive withdrawal as a uniform approach to post-transplant lymphoproliferative disease in pediatric liver transplantation. *Pediatric Transplantation, 8*(3), 267–272.

Kosmach, B., Webber, S. A., & Reyes, J. (1998). Care of the pediatric solid organ transplant recipient. The primary care perspective. *Pediatric Clinics of North America, 45*(6), 1395–1418.

McDiarmid, S. V. (2003). Current status of liver transplantation in children. *Pediatric Clinics of North America, 50*(6), 1335–1374.

McDiarmid, S. V. (2000). Liver transplantation. The pediatric challenge. *Clinics in Liver Disease, 4*(4), 879–927.

Muehrer, R. J., & Becker, B. N. (2005). Life after transplantation: New transitions in quality of life and psychological distress. *Seminars in Dialysis, 18*(2), 124–131.

Salvatierra, O. Jr, Millan, M., & Concepcion, W. (2006). Pediatric renal transplantation with considerations for successful outcomes. *Seminars in Pediatric Surgery, 15*(3), 208–217.

An Adolescent Bariatric Weight Management Program

By Nancy Tkacz Browne and Beverly Bynum Haynes

The current epidemic of childhood and adolescent obesity represents a significant health problem to our nation's youth. This epidemic spans cultures, ethnicity, genders, socioeconomic levels and communities. Obesity threatens all children whether they are of normal weight or at the extreme end of the obesity spectrum. The primary goal of weight management policy is to prevent the development of obesity. However, if obesity is already present, the child needs a comprehensive approach to the management and resolution of obesity and its comorbidities.

Definition

Obesity is defined as an imbalance between caloric intake and energy expenditure. It is classified as either exogenous (taking in an excess of calories and/or decreased physical activity) or endogenous (inherent metabolic complications) (Hagarty, Schmidt, Bernaix, & Clement, 2004). The Centers for Disease Control and Prevention (CDC) recommend using the percentile body mass index-for-age and gender (BMI-for-age) charts to screen children who are at risk for becoming, or who actually are, obese (Ogden, Kuczmarski, et al., 2002). Children with BMI > 85th percentile are considered at risk for obesity and those with BMI > 95th percentile are considered obese.

Prevalence of Obesity in Adolescents

The CDC reports that the percentage of adolescents in the United States who are obese continues to increase. CDC data from the National Health and Nutrition Examination Survey: 1999–2000 reveal an overall obesity rate of 15.5% in 12- to 19-year-olds or almost 9 million adolescents (Ogden, Flegal, Carroll, & Johnson, 2002). This percentage has tripled since 1980 (CDC National Center for Health Statistics, 2005). Another 30% of adolescents are at risk for becoming obese. Adolescent obesity also differs among ethnic groups and gender, with the highest rates being found in Hispanic males (27.5%) and African-American females (26.6%). Increasing rates of obesity occur throughout the world, including developing countries in the Middle East, North Africa, and Latin America.

Etiology and Pathophysiology

Obesity is a chronic disease with multiple factors contributing to its etiology. Appetite, satiety, energy expenditure, and the regulation of subcutaneous and visceral fat stores are regulated by a complex interaction of the body's central nervous system, gastrointestinal tract, and fat cells. Hormones, proteins, and neuropeptides, such as ghrelin, leptin, glucagon, insulin, and adiponectin, affect body weight regulation (Greenway, Greenway, & Raum, 2004). Potential explanations of obesity include genetic, hormonal, physiologic, environmental, social, behavioral, and psychological theories (MacKenzie & Neinstein, 2002). Currently, a limited understanding of these interactions exists, and, therefore, the pathophysiology of obesity is poorly explained.

The relative contribution of an individual's genetics, culture, lifestyle, behaviors, psychology, environment, and metabolism in explaining the individual's obesity physiology is an ongoing debate (Baker et al., 2005). However, most experts agree that increased caloric intake from high-calorie food consumption, increased portion size, and decreased physical activity has contributed to the obesity epidemic in our youth over the past 3 decades. As the relationship between the physiologic mechanisms and environmental influences are better understood, better treatment options will be developed for the obese child and adolescent.

Comorbidities

Obesity is a significant health risk. As the incidence of childhood obesity grows, many chronic illnesses and risk factors for adult disease are now occurring in childhood.

Dietz (2004) estimates that 60% of obese adolescents have at least one risk factor for cardiovascular disease, with 25% having two or more risk factors. The cardiac risk factors of dyslipidemia and hypertension are highly correlated with high insulin levels in children (Freedman, Dietz, Srinivasan, & Berenson, 1999). Other comorbidities of obesity include insulin resistance and type 2 diabetes, sleep apnea, hypertension, hypercholesterolemia, dyslipidemia, polycystic ovary syndrome, dysmenorrhea, infertility, joint disease, pseudotumor cerebri, nonalcoholic fatty liver disease, asthma, renal focal nodular sclerosis, and skin disorders (Artz, Haqq, & Freemark, 2005; Daniels et al., 2005).

Obesity has a major impact on an individual's mental, psychosocial, and economic health (Dixon, Dixon, & O'Brien, 2001). Emotional comorbidities include low self-esteem, negative body image, and depression. Social comorbidities include social isolation, stigmatization, negative stereotyping, discrimination, teasing, and bullying (Koplan, Liverman, & Kraak, 2005). Obese children and adolescents have lower psychosocial quality of life scores than those diagnosed with cancer (Schwimmer,

Burwinkle, & Varni, 2003). Recently, researchers have validated for clinical use the Bariatric Quality of Life Index, which will provide more specific information to guide supportive treatment options (Weiner et al., 2005).

Obese individuals, including adolescents and children, are stigmatized in the specific areas of employment, education, and health care. Discriminatory practices and inconsistencies in the medical coverage of obesity-related comorbidities are also the norm (Puhl & Brownell, 2001). Weight-management programs are either poorly reimbursed or not compensated at all for any weight management care in 35% of children (Tershakovec, Watson, Wenner, & Marx, 1999).

Economic Impact

Obesity contributes to 300,000 US deaths annually. Health care costs associated with obesity-related illnesses are currently estimated at $90 to $117 billion dollars per year (Finkelstein, Fiebelkorn, & Wang, 2003). In addition to health care expenditures, economic productivity is compromised because of time lost at work due to illness. Safadi (2005) examines the history of obesity and bariatric surgery in the United States with the recent trend of third-party payers restricting and excluding coverage for bariatric medical and surgical treatment.

Prevention and Treatment for the Obese Adolescent

A partnership of family, community, schools, and health care professionals is necessary to address the complexities of the problem of childhood and adolescent obesity in our society. Models and guidelines exist for the prevention and treatment of childhood obesity (Baker et al., 2005; Speiser et al., 2005). Long-term results of obese children in a comprehensive, medically directed weight management program demonstrate a 20% reduction of excess weight after 10 years with 30% to 35% of children maintaining weight loss (Epstein, Paluch, Gordy, & Dorn, 2000; Epstein, Valoski, Wing, & McCurley, 1990). However, the remaining 70% of obese children were unsuccessful at achieving or maintaining weight loss. Guidelines for the combined use of behavioral therapy, restrictive diets, exercise, medications, and surgery currently exist for the treatment of adolescent obesity (Kirk, Scott, & Daniels, 2005). The remainder of this chapter focuses on a weight-management treatment plan for obese adolescents that includes bariatric surgery.

■ Bariatric Surgery and Adolescents

In 1991, The National Institutes of Health developed guidelines for patient selection for bariatric surgery. They recommended bariatric surgery be considered for individuals with a BMI > 40 or a BMI of 35 to 40 with at least one obesity related comorbidity (National Institutes of Health, 1991).

Bariatric surgery is a recognized subspecialty in the field of general surgery. Organizations such as the Association of Operating Room Nurses, the American Society for Bariatric Surgery, the Society of American Gastrointestinal Endoscopic Surgeons, the American Pediatric Surgical Association, and the American Academy of Pediatrics have developed practice guidelines for both open and minimally invasive bariatric surgery (AORN, 2004; Inge, Krebs, et al., 2004; Rogers, 2004; SAGES, 2003; Wittgrove, 2004). Although these guidelines differ slightly with respect to some parameters of the proposed criteria, all agree that these guidelines do not represent a rigid clinical algorithm. Adolescents must be evaluated individually to develop the best surgical treatment plan for their particular situation.

Studies in the United States and abroad suggest that bariatric surgery, when combined with a comprehensive weight-management program, is a safe and effective option for obese adolescents and improves their overall health (Barnett et al., 2005; Capella & Capella, 2003; Dolan, Creighton, Hopkins, & Fielding, 2003; Horgan et al., 2005; Inge, Krebs, et al.; Strauss, Bradley, & Brolin, 2001).

■ A Multidisciplinary Weight Management Program with Bariatric Component

The goals of a weight-management program are to achieve and maintain significant weight loss and to reverse or prevent obesity-induced comorbidities. The adolescent weight-management program with expertise in bariatric surgery should include at a minimum a pediatric/adolescent physician, pediatric surgeon (credentialed in bariatric surgery), nurse coordinator, registered dietitian, activity professional (exercise physiologist, physical therapist), child or adolescent psychologist, and bariatric anesthesiologist (Garcia, 2007; Speiser et al., 2005).

Team members are sensitive to the specific needs and challenges of obese adolescents and their families and share a philosophy that regards obesity as a chronic, life-long problem (Nadler & Kane, 2005). Education, equipment, policy, and procedure development, financing, and legal considerations are all part of the development of a comprehensive weight-management program for children and adolescents (Gallagher, 2005; Haynes, 2005).

■ Preoperative Evaluation

History

A complete health history of the obese adolescent by the multidisciplinary team is essential to rule out associated conditions and to ascertain current health status. Weight milestones, growth patterns, psychological issues, and activity and eating patterns are assessed. A review of systems approach screens for obesity related comorbidities.

Physical Examination

The physical examination ascertains the degree of obesity and determines any associated comorbidities. A review of systems approach is used. Results of this examination, along with the history, guide the diagnostic work-up.

Diagnostic Work-Up

The obese adolescent being prepared for bariatric surgery should undergo a complete diagnostic work-up to establish a preoperative baseline and to screen for obesity-related comorbidities. Selected studies are repeated periodically to assess for changes in nutritional status as well as existing comorbidities.

Nutrition

A complete 24-hour diet history includes an assessment of the adolescent's current eating patterns (frequency of meals, types of foods eaten, portion size, where meals eaten, who prepares meals, who buys food, and type of beverages and snacks consumed). The bariatric dietitian interviews the adolescent and the family member(s) responsible for meal planning and preparation and provides appropriate education.

Exercise

The exercise specialist develops a specific exercise program for the candidate before surgery and revises the regimen as necessary with postoperative needs in mind. Activities of daily living, sedentary time, and family activity are evaluated. Barriers to physical activity are determined. Barriers include physical, psychosocial, educational, environmental, and societal. The exercise professional prescribes an activity program that takes into consideration health related comorbidities. The adolescent is instructed to exercise three to seven times a week for 30 minutes, with walking being the exercise of choice for the first 2 weeks after surgery. Progress is closely monitored and is advanced as tolerated. Exercise routines favored by adolescents include treadmill, weights, walking, dancing, and swimming.

Behavior

The child psychologist screens the adolescent for stress at home or school, depression, abusive behavior (self-inflicted or maltreatment), and eating disorders. Readiness for change and family involvement are assessed using interview techniques. Psychological testing, such as the Beck Depression Index, can be helpful in identifying the individual's stresses. Most importantly, the psychologist can provide ongoing support for adolescents as they progress through the physical and psychological changes related to the weight loss experience.

Preoperative education is ongoing, and all members of the multidisciplinary team are involved. The nurse coordinator ensures that comprehensive education is provided at every phase of the perioperative process. A variety of mediums are used to ensure that the adolescent and his or her family are thoroughly prepared, not only for surgery, but also for the anticipated lifestyle changes after weight loss surgery.

■ Perioperative Considerations

Adolescents undergoing any bariatric surgical procedure are high-risk surgical candidates due to their large body size and associated comorbidities. In particular, the severely overweight adolescent has special needs in the areas of equipment, anesthesia, and positioning (Brenn, 2005; Ferraro, 2004b).

Facilities caring for the bariatric patient must have equipment that can accommodate a weight of 750 pounds or greater. This equipment includes, but is not limited to, hospital beds, operating room beds, commodes, scales, wheelchairs, and transport stretchers (Gianos, 2003). Appropriate-sized hospital gowns and blood pressure cuffs are essential. Operative equipment needs include high-flow insufflator, extra-long trocars, and an appropriate liver retractor to safely mobilize a potentially enlarged liver (Ferraro, 2004b).

Obese adolescents often are difficult to intubate because of excessive soft tissue and large neck circumference. Comorbidities, such as gastroesophageal reflux and sleep apnea, increase the intubation risk. Optimal medical management of these and other obesity related comorbidities reduces the risk of intubation and anesthesia (Brenn, 2005).

A well-organized surgical team that pays close attention to patient positioning in the operating room increases both patient and team member safety. Intermittent pneumatic sequential compression devices and subcutaneous heparin address this population's higher incidence of venous thromboembolic disease. After the procedure, the patient transfers directly to the bariatric bed.

■ Surgical Options

Bariatric surgical procedures are based on two mechanisms for inducing weight loss: intestinal malabsorption and gastric restriction (Hydock, 2005). Malabsorptive operations (jejunoileal bypass and biliopancreatic diversion with or without duodenal switch) shorten the functional length of the small-intestinal surface available for nutrient absorption. Restrictive procedures (adjustable gastric band [AGB] and the vertical banded gastroplasty) decrease the volume of food intake by creating a small upper gastric pouch. Some procedures (Roux-en-Y gastric bypass) combine both the malabsorptive and the restrictive components.

These operations can be performed by using either the open operative method or by the laparoscopic method (Schneider & Mun, 2005).

The nutritional consequences of the purely malabsorptive procedures make these operations less attractive for use in adolescents. Although this decision is made on a case-by-case basis, the two operations currently performed most frequently in the adolescent age group are the Roux-en-Y gastric bypass (RYGB) and the AGB (Inge, Zeller, Lawson, & Daniels, 2005).

Roux-en-Y Gastric Bypass

History of Gastric Bypass Surgery

Mason and Ito (1967) first described the gastric bypass technique. By 1977, the RYGB gastrojejunostomy was developed to alleviate problems associated with the original technique (Buchwald & Buchwald, 2002). Modifications of the RYGB procedure continued to evolve with technical revisions that addressed modifications of stomach division, pouch creation, and length of the Roux limb. By 1994, Wittgrove, Clark, and Tremblay had developed the laparoscopic technique for RYGB. Stanford et al. (2003) next applied the laparoscopic RYGB technique to adolescents and concluded that laparoscopic Roux-en-Y gastric bypass was safe in the adolescent population.

Description

The Roux-en-Y gastric bypass is both a restrictive and a malabsorptive procedure. It is restrictive in that the stomach is surgically decreased in size to limit the amount of food intake and also by creating a small outlet from the stomach to delay emptying. It is malabsorptive due to the bypassing of sections of the stomach and small intestine, which results in poor absorption of nutrients (Woodward, 2001).

Risks

Generic operative risks to the obese patient include development of pneumonia, development of venous thrombosis, difficulty with proper positioning on the operating table, and complications associated with obesity-related comorbidities. Risks associated specifically with RYGB include damage to internal organs, seroma/hematoma, diarrhea, internal hernia, gastritis, small bowel obstruction, potential micronutrient deficiencies, anastomotic stenosis, staple line disruption, incisional hernia, wound infection, gastrointestinal leakage, pulmonary embolism, bleeding, weight regain, and death (Inge et al., 2005).

Benefits

Although the risks seem formidable, the health benefits of weight loss surgery are many. They include improvement and/or resolution of obesity-related comorbidities, such as elevated blood sugar levels, hypertension, sleep apnea, pulmonary function, joint arthralgia, dyslipidemia, polycystic ovary syndrome, and improvement in psychosocial functioning. Weight loss of 33% of body weight 1 year after surgery has been demonstrated in adult series with similar results found in preliminary adolescent RYGB studies (Barrow, 2002; Inge et al., 2005).

Nutritional Education

The RYGB surgery candidate is introduced to the idea of lifetime changes, such as eating slowly and chewing thoroughly to break down food that will pass easily through the anastomosis and to aid in the digestive process. Patients learn that they will first be offered clear liquids after surgery and then will quickly advance to pureed food. Solids are allowed after 4 weeks if the patient is not expressing any difficulty swallowing. RYGB bariatric surgery patients are encouraged to consume 60% to 70% of their meals as protein and the rest as vegetables and some fruits (Elliot, 2003). Most RYGB diet plans call for a drastic reduction or elimination of carbohydrates. Carbohydrates, when eaten, should only make up 10% to 20% of the diet. RYGB patients are advised to drink at least 32 to 64 ounces of fluid a day but to avoid taking liquids with meals. Some patients complain of difficulty swallowing foods that are very dry, stringy, sticky, or gummy. These foods can cause vomiting and discomfort and should avoided (Marcason, 2004).

Malnutrition is a serious concern after a RYGB procedure. Adolescents are encouraged to report persistent nau-

sea and vomiting, edema, hair loss, and extreme fatigue (Shuster & Vazques, 2005). Prevention of protein-calorie malnutrition includes drinking protein shakes first during meals. Vegetable consumption is encouraged to maintain desirable levels of vitamins and minerals. A daily multivitamin is prescribed. Sweets should be avoided as excess intake can cause "dumping syndrome," a physiologic response to simple sugars causing a vasomotor response and gastrointestinal symptoms. The patient can experience heart palpitations, nausea, vomiting, abdominal pain, and diarrhea (Shuster & Vazques). Carbonated beverages are discouraged because they release gas that causes gastric pouch distention. Caffeine is limited because it stimulates appetite and has a diuretic effect (Elliot, 2003).

Regular laboratory blood and urine testing monitors metabolic changes. Ongoing counseling with a bariatric nutritionist reinforces preoperative teaching and counsels necessary dietary modifications.

Operative Technique

The stomach is divided to create a 20- to-30 mL proximal gastric pouch. The jejunum is then divided 60 to 80 cm from the ligament of Treitz. The proximal end of the jejunum is anastomosed to the side of the jejunum approximately 100 to 150 cm distally. The distal end of the jejunum is anastomosed to the upper gastric pouch. Sutures secure the bowel loop to the stomach and mesocolon to prevent slippage of the loop and possible internal herniation. A nasogastric tube is inserted into the upper gastric pouch and methylene blue injected to check for an anastomotic leak (Lujan, Hernandez, Frutos, Valero, & Parrilla, 2002). Figure 31-1 illustrates the completed Roux-en-Y procedure.

Postoperative Management

After surgery, the RYGB patient is transferred to the general pediatric unit or to the intensive care unit if the patient has been on continuous positive-airway pressure equipment at home. Aggressive pulmonary toilet is performed. Ambulation begins on the day of surgery with the patient out of bed twice before bedtime. Compression stockings placed on the patient in the operating room are required whenever the adolescent is not actually ambulating. Pain is treated presumptively with intravenous and oral medications, with patients transitioning to acetaminophen (Tylenol) within 1 to 3 days after surgery. All oral medications are given in liquid form.

The RYGB patient remains NPO until postoperative day 1 when an upper gastrointestinal x-ray study is completed to assess for anastomotic leaks. After a negative study, the patient is started on 30 mL of clear liquid, and

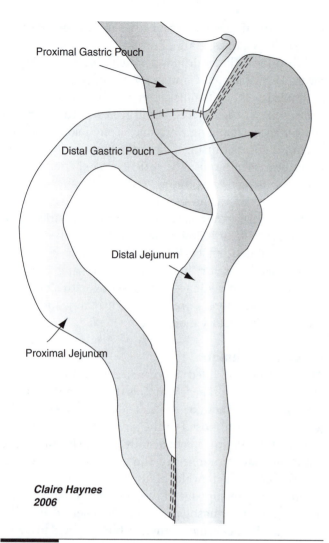

Proximal Gastric Pouch

Distal Gastric Pouch

Distal Jejunum

Proximal Jejunum

Claire Haynes
2006

Figure 31-1 Completed Roux-en-Y anatomy.
(Drawing by Claire Haynes.)

the volume is advanced as tolerated. The patient receives full liquids on the second postoperative day.

Medications

Ideally, humans take in all the nutrient requirements during the course of the day to maintain optimal health. This includes 13 vitamins. Due to anatomic changes and significant decreases in the amount of food the adolescent RYGB patient is able to ingest, there is a need for supplementation (Shuster & Vazques, 2005).

Supplementation medications are prescribed for adolescents after RYGB surgery. The rationale for these medications is based on adolescent growth and development principles as well as experience with adult RYGB surgery patients. After RYGB, adolescents are specifically at risk for iron-deficiency anemia, hypocalcemia (risk for decreased bone density), and vitamin B_{12} deficiency (pernicious anemia).

Supplementation medications include multivitamins, ursodiol, iron, calcium, and vitamin B_{12}. Vitamin B_{12} is supplemented orally on a daily basis or by intramuscular injection every 3 months (Alvarez-Leite, 2004; Shuster & Vazques, 2005).

Contraception

The female adolescent is counseled on the potential hazards of pregnancy during the rapid weight loss experienced with the RYGB procedure. Many female adolescents are taking oral contraceptives because of obesity-related menstrual irregularities or polycystic ovary syndrome. These medications are absorbed through the small bowel. Disruptions to the digestive system from RYGB surgery may interfere with absorption. With this in mind, oral contraceptives may not be the best form of pregnancy prevention (Inge et al., 2005).

Follow-Up

After RYGB surgery, the adolescent is monitored by visits to the multidisciplinary team, laboratory tests, biomeasurements (vital signs, weight, height, BMI, waist and hip circumferences), and other procedures as needed. The nutritionist, exercise specialist, psychologist, nurse, and surgeon counsel the adolescent at each visit. All patients are encouraged to participate in quality-of-life and other studies that track data over time in order to understand and predict changes that take place after RYGB in adolescents.

The Adjustable Gastric Band (AGB)

History

In 1986, Kuzmak introduced the first adjustable silicone gastric band, which featured an inflatable balloon connected by tubing to an implanted subcutaneous reservoir (Kuzmak, 1991). In the early 1990s, Belachew and colleagues (2001) modified the adjustable gastric band to allow its laparoscopic placement and implanted the first LAP-BAND® device (LAP-BAND®, Inamed Health, Santa Barbara, CA) (Belachew & Zimmermann, 2002). Modifications to the device and increased surgical experience over the past 20 years have significantly reduced the occurrence of complications (Fielding & Allen, 2002).

In 2001, after clinical trials, the US Food and Drug Administration approved a single device (LAP-BAND®) for implantation in the United States for individuals 18 years and older (Schneider & Mun, 2005). In 2005, the Food and Drug Administration authorized clinical trials at three US centers to evaluate the safety and efficacy of the AGB in adolescents (ages 14–17 years) involved in a multidisciplinary weight management program. Table 31-1 outlines a recommended protocol for assessment and testing of adolescents receiving the AGB.

Description

Adjustable gastric banding is a restrictive procedure. The AGB system has two components: the adjustable band and the access port (Fig. 31-2). The adjustable band component is a 13-mm-wide Silicone band that forms a circular ring around the proximal stomach. The band compresses the stomach to form a small opening for enteral contents to pass from the small, upper gastric pouch to the larger, lower gastric pouch. The inner lumen of the band is an inflatable balloon that allows the band to be either tightened (smaller opening between gastric pouches) or loosened (larger opening between gastric pouches).

Radiopaque, kink-resistant tubing connects the inflatable section to the subcutaneous access port.

Risks

Serious operative complications of laparoscopic gastric band surgery can theoretically include bleeding, damage to internal organs (liver, spleen), and gastric perforation. However, these complications are rare. Four recent AGB series (2,514 total adult patients) report one hemorrhage and one late death (Holloway, Forney, & Gould, 2004; Ponce, Paynter, & Fromm, 2005; Ren, Horgan, & Ponce, 2002; Spivak, Huewitt, Onn, & Half, 2005). The incidence of AGB complications has decreased (1.4%–10%) due to increased surgical experience and modifications of surgical technique (Ponce & Dixon, 2005). Minor postoperative complications include upper pouch enlargement,

Table 31-1 **Five-Year University of Illinois at Chicago Protocol for Adjustable Gastric Band in Adolescents Aged 14–17 Years of Age**

Evaluation	Preop	OR	1 wk	6 wk	3 mo	6 mo	9 mo	1 yr	Q 6 mo	Yearly
Medical	X	X	X	X	X	X	X	X	X	X
Psychological	X			X	X	X	X	X	X	X
Dietitian	X	X	X	X	X	X	X	X	X	X
Exercise specialist	X			X	X	X	X	X	X	X
Weight, height, body mass index	X	X	X	X	X	X	X	X	X	X
Blood pressure	X	X	X	X	X	X	X	X	X	X
Waist/neck circumference	X			X	X	X	X	X	X	X
Laboratory studies	X				X	X	X	X		X
Barium swallow	X							X		X
Bone age	X									
Bone density	X				X	X	X	X	X	X
Chest x-ray study	X							X		X
Electrocardiogram	X							X		
Echocardiogram	X							X		X
Esophageal manometry	X							X		X
Pulmonary function tests	X									
Sleep apnea consultation	X									
Gallbladder & liver ultrasound	X							X		X
Liver biopsy		X								
Visceral fat biopsy		X								

University of Illinois at Chicago, 2005.

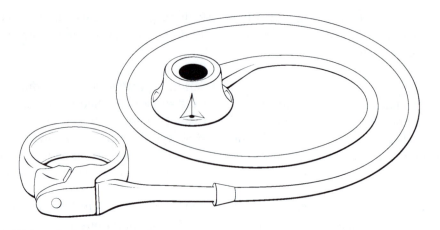

Figure 31-2 The adjustable gastric band and access port.
(Reprinted with permission by INAMED. LAP-BAND ® System.)

erosion of band through the stomach, band slippage, and food intolerance. Port-specific complications include infection, kinking, and tubing defects. Signs and symptoms of these complications can include vomiting, fever, sepsis, lack of satiety at previous volume of food intake, and failure to lose 1 to 2 pounds per week.

Benefits

The adjustable gastric band achieves weight loss comparable to that of other bariatric procedures while significantly reducing or eliminating obesity-related comorbidities (Parikh, Fielding, & Ren, 2005). Chapman et al. (2004) report an overall mortality of 0.05% and a morbidity rate of 11.3% with the adult AGB patients versus 0.5% and 23.6%, respectively, for the RYGB adults. Both procedures had comparable weight loss after 3 to 4 years of follow-up. These data suggest that AGB is among the least invasive of the bariatric procedures and is less morbid than the RYGB. It is reversible and adjustable and does not exclude any portion of the gastrointestinal tract from nutrient absorption. AGB patients have a slower and steadier weight loss over time, in contrast to RYGB patients. At 3 to 4 years after procedure, both sets of patients have comparable average excess weight loss (Jan, Hong, Pereira, & Patterson, 2005).

A potential advantage of the AGB in the adolescent age group is the necessity to return to the weight-management clinic for adjustments of the band system. This provides more opportunity for support and education by the weight-management team as well as allowing for earlier detection of complications.

Nutritional Education

Preoperative counseling of the AGB adolescent includes special attention to the perioperative diet regimen.

Preoperatively, a medically supervised calorie restricted liquid diet with sufficient protein is begun 2 to 4 weeks before the AGB surgery. This induced weight loss acutely decreases the size of the liver. Easier retraction of the liver and decreased overall intra-abdominal fat from the preoperative liquid diet improves the surgical exposure of the esophagogastric junction and increases the safety of the AGB placement. The bariatric dietitian also addresses healthy eating behaviors (eating slowly and chewing thoroughly), food selection (nutrient-dense, protein-dense foods vs. sweets), portion sizes (4 oz three times a day), menu planning, and separation of fluid intake from solid intake by at least 1 hour.

Operative Technique

The surgeon creates a small tract behind the upper stomach, passes an instrument through this tract to "grab" the end of the band, and brings the band around the stomach. The distal end of the tubing is threaded through an opening at the proximal end of the band and the device is then "locked" into a ring configuration. The surgeon then sutures stomach around a portion of the band to secure it anteriorly to the stomach. The distal end of the tubing is passed through an incision under the left ribs and attached to the band's reservoir port. The port is then securely sutured to the fascia, and the skin opening is closed. The balloon is left empty, allowing for maximal diameter of the band at the end of the operation (Fielding & Allen, 2002). Surgeons place the AGB laparoscopically with rare conversion to open technique.

Postoperative Management

As with the RYGB patient, pain management begins in the operating room and continues on a schedule for 24 hours. The patient converts to oral pain agents before discharge. Patients are instructed to either crush pills or use the liquid form of medications because whole pills may not pass through the banded area.

Within 6 to 18 hours of the AGB procedure, a limited barium swallow is performed to assess the placement of the band and the flow of liquid through the banded area.

Diet guidelines for the first 6 weeks after surgery are a gradual progression from full liquids to pureed foods to soft foods. Special attention is given to adequate protein intake. Equally important to what is eaten is the volume of intake at each setting. Patients are advised not to take more than 4 ounces at a time, separate liquids from solids, eat a balanced diet, avoid carbonated liquids, and chew thoroughly (Ferraro, 2004a).

The vast majority of AGBs are placed laparoscopically. Patients are mobilized quickly and often are out of bed within 4 hours after surgery. Ambulation is encouraged. Discharge is typically within 18–23 hours after surgery. Adolescents are instructed that they may have less stamina for the first 3 to 4 days after surgery, but that they have no activity restrictions. They may return to school within the first postoperative week.

AGB Adjustments

At the time of surgery, the balloon is left deflated to allow the maximum diameter of the band. With the larger 11-mm band, some surgeons prefer to leave 3 mL in the band's balloon at the time of surgery to provide a small level of restriction and satiety. At 6 weeks after surgery, the healing process of securing the band to the stomach has occurred, and the band's balloon is ready to be "adjusted" or filled.

Adjustments may be performed using fluoroscopy (barium swallow) or by patient feedback. Fluoroscopy is used to guide the adjustment by using real-time visualization of the upper gastric pouch and stoma size as the balloon is inflated or deflated (Horgan et al., 2005). Disadvantages of fluoroscopy include need of radiology equipment and radiation exposure to the patient. However, the visualization of the upper stomach pouch size and band placement during the adjustment can lead to early discovery of upper pouch enlargement. This potentially enables early successful management of this complication by band deflation in contrast to surgical revision.

The first adjustment is performed at 6 weeks after surgery. Subsequent adjustments are determined by assessing the patient for amount of food comfortably eaten at one setting, level of satiety, weight loss, and vomiting. Optimal rate of weight loss is 1 to 2 pounds per week, and portion size achieving satiety should be 4 to 5 ounces per meal (Ferraro, 2004b).

Follow-Up

Achieving and maintaining weight loss is a life-long process. At the present time, the AGB is placed with the intention to remain in use for the life of the patient. There is no evidence that the patient will be able to maintain their goal weight if the band is removed. Adolescent AGB programs collaborate with adult AGB programs to provide for a smooth transition from adolescence to adulthood.

Females who become pregnant after the placement of an AGB are followed closely to monitor the nutritional status of both mother and infant. The adjustability of the band allows the adaptation to the mother's or infant's needs during the pregnancy. Dixon, Dixon, & O'Brien (2005) prospectively studied the outcomes of 79 women in their first pregnancies after the placement of the AGB. They found that outcomes after AGB were consistent with the general community outcomes rather than outcomes of severely obese women. Careful monitoring and appropriate band adjustment seem to allow safe pregnancies for women after AGB placement.

■ Future Directions

As we learn more about the consequences of obesity in our youth, many unanswered questions remain. Current treatment options are an early attempt to reverse the co-morbidities of obesity. However, in order to continue to design effective treatment options, we need a better understanding of obesity's etiology, mechanisms, and environmental interactions. Long-term adolescent outcome data of the safety and efficacy of bariatric procedures and co-existing medical management options are a priority for ongoing research.

Exploration into the role and use of the implantable gastric stimulator (IGS) continues in adults and adolescents. The IGS system electrically stimulates the stomach with a pacemaker-like device. This device is implanted using a laparoscopic approach. The IGS appears to reduce appetite and increase satiety. Early results show significant excess weight loss but not as good as those achieved with RYGB or AGB (Favretti et al., 2004).

Another innovation, the intragastric balloon, is a saline-filled balloon that remains in the stomach for 6 months (Herve et al., 2005). This device is placed endoscopically and is used in conjunction with a weight-management program. Initial concerns with the device have been related to patient tolerance and failure to maintain weight loss (Vandenplas, Bollen, De Lange, Vandemaele, & De Schepper, 1999). However, because the intragastric balloon is reversible and placed endoscopically under conscious sedation, it may have a role in children and adolescents with less severe obesity or in the super obese as a bridge to a more definitive procedure.

Other areas of research that influence the future care of obese children and adolescents are the role of hormones (Park et al., 2006), genetics (Park et al., 2005), and medications (Wadden et al., 2005). As our understanding grows, it may be possible to combine less invasive therapies to achieve sustainable weight loss in children who are overweight with the ultimate goal of preventing obesity.

■ Conclusion

Obesity is the center of a "wheel" of comorbidities that affects every organ system, along with psychological, sociological, economic, and spiritual needs. Research will need to come from all avenues to combat a problem that reaches into all corners of our being. The Institute of Medicine of the National Academies calls for cooperation from family, schools, communities, federal and state government, media, and industry to address the prevention and treatment of childhood obesity (Koplan et al., 2005). No single group is responsible for this multifactorial problem, nor can one group acting alone bring it to resolution.

■ Acknowledgments

The authors express their appreciation to the following individuals for their thoughtful review and discussion of the material in this chapter: Allen F. Browne, Laura M. Flanigan, Carroll Harmon, Ai-Xuan L. Holterman, Mark J. Holterman, Marc Michalsky, Evan Nadler, Vern Vincent, Cynthia Yensel, & Jeffrey Zitsman. We also thank the weight management professionals at the Children's Hospital of Alabama and at the New Hope Pediatric & Adolescent Weight Management Project at the University of Illinois at Chicago.

■ Educational Materials

APSNA invites you to download the following diagnosis-related teaching tools for Chapter 31, An Adolescent Bariatric Weight Management Program: 1) Roux-en-Y gastric bypass and 2) Adjustable gastric band. These teaching tools are available at the APSNA Web site (www.apsna.org) and the Jones and Bartlett Web site (www.jbpub.com). All teaching materials are available in English and Spanish and are free of charge. APSNA encourages their use for your patients and families.

References

Alvarez-Leite, J. I. (2004). Nutrient deficiencies secondary to bariatric surgery. *Current Opinion Clinical Metabolic Care, 7*, 569–575.

AORN. (2004). AORN bariatric surgery guideline. *AORN, 79*, 1026–1052.

Artz, E., Haqq, A., & Freemark, M. (2005). Hormonal and metabolic consequences of childhood obesity. *Endocrinology & Metabolic Clinics of North America, 34*, 643–658.

Baker, S., Barlow, S., Cochran, W., Guchs, G., Klish, W., Krebs, N., et al. (2005). Overweight children and adolescents: A clinical report of the North American Society for Pediatric Gastroenterology, Hepatology and Nutrition. *Journal of Pediatric Gastroenterology and Nutrition, 40*, 533–543.

Barnett, S. J., Stanley, C., Hanlon, M., Acton, R., Saltzman, D. A., Ikramuddin, S., et al. (2005). Long-term follow-up and the role of surgery in adolescents with morbid obesity. *Surgery for Obesity and Related Diseases, 1*, 394–398.

Barrow, C. J. (2002). Roux-en-Y gastric bypass for morbid obesity. *AORN, 76*, 593–608.

Belachew, M., Legrand, M. J., & Vincent, V. (2001). History of Lap-Band®: From dream to reality. *Obesity Surgery, 11*, 297–302.

Belachew, M., & Zimmermann, J. M. (2002). Evolution of a paradigm for laparoscopic adjustable gastric banding. *The American Journal of Surgery, 184*, 21S–25S.

Brenn, B. R. (2005). Anesthesia for pediatric obesity. *Anesthesiology Clinics of North America, 23*, 745–764.

Buchwald, H., & Buchwald, J. N. (2002). Evolution of operative procedures for the management of morbid obesity 1950–2000. *Obesity Surgery, 12*, 705–717.

Capella, J. F., & Capella, R. F. (2003). Bariatric surgery in adolescence. Is this the best age to operate? *Obesity Surgery, 13*, 826–832.

CDC National Center for Health Statistics. (2005). Prevalence of overweight among children and adolescents: United States, 1999–2002. Retrieved February 2006, from www.cdc.gov/nchs/products/pubs/pubd/hestats/overwght99.htm

Chapman, A. E., Kiroff, G., Game, P., Foster, B., O'Brien, P., Ham, J., et al. (2004). Laparoscopic adjustable gastric banding in the treatment of obesity: A systematic literature review. *Surgery, 135*, 326–351.

Daniels, S. R., Arnett, D. K., Eckel, R. H., Gidding, S. S., Hayman, L. L., Kumanyika, S., et al. (2005). Overweight in children and adolescents: Pathophysiology, consequences, prevention, and treatment. AHA Scientific Statement. *Circulation, 111*, 1999–2012.

Dietz, W. H. (2004). Overweight in childhood and adolescence. *New England Journal of Medicine, 350*, 855–857.

Dixon, J. B., Dixon, M. E., & O'Brien, P. (2001). Quality of life after lap-band placement: Influence of time, weight loss, and comorbidities. *Obesity Research, 9*, 713–721.

Dixon, J. B., Dixon, M. E., & O'Brien, P. (2005). Birth outcomes in obese women after laparoscopic adjustable gastric banding. *Obstetrics & Gynecology, 106*, 965–971.

Dolan, K., Creighton, L., Hopkins, G., & Fielding, G. (2003). Laparoscopic gastric banding in morbidly obese adolescents. *Obesity Surgery, 13*, 101–104.

Elliot, K. (2003). Nutritional considerations after bariatric surgery (bariatric patients in the ICU). *Critical Care Nursing Quarterly, 26*, 133–138.

Epstein, L. H., Paluch, R. A., Gordy, C. C., & Dorn, J. (2000). Decreasing sedentary behaviors in treating pediatric obesity. *Archives of Pediatrics & Adolescent Medicine, 154*, 220–226.

Epstein, L. H., Valoski, A., Wing, R. R., & McCurley, J. (1990). Ten-year follow-up of behavioral, family-based treatment for obese children. *JAMA, 264*, 2519–2523.

Favretti, F., De Luca, M., Segato, G., Busetto, L., Ceoloni, A., Magon, A., et al. (2004). Treatment of morbid obesity with the transcend implantable gastric stimulator (IGS): A prospective survey. *Obesity Surgery, 14*, 666–670.

Ferraro, D. R. (2004a). Management of the bariatric surgery patient. *Clinician Reviews, 14*, 74–79.

Ferraro, D. R. (2004b). Preparing patients for bariatric surgery: The clinical considerations. *Clinician Reviews, 14*, 58–64.

Fielding, G. A., & Allen, J. W. (2002). A step-by-step guide to placement of the LAP-BAND adjustable gastric banding system. *The American Journal of Surgery, 184*, 26S–30S.

Finkelstein, E. A., Fiebelkorn, E. C., & Wang, G. (2003). National medical expenditures attributable to overweight and obesity: How much and who's paying? *Health Affairs, W3–219*, W213–W226.

Freedman, D. S., Dietz, W. H., Srinivasan, S. R., & Berenson, G. S. (1999). The regulation of overweight to cardiovascular risk factors among children and adolescents: The Bogalusa heart study. *Pediatrics, 103*, 1175–1182.

Gallagher, S. (2005). Caring for the child who is obese: Mobility, caregiver, safety, environmental accommodation, and legal concerns. *Pediatric Nursing, 31*, 17–20.

Garcia, V. F. (2007). Adolescent bariatric surgery. In H. Buchwald, G. Cowan, & W. J. Pories (Eds.), *Surgical managemenet of obesity.* (pp. 315–325). Philadelphia: Saunders.

Gianos, J. (2003). Special equipment for bariatric patients. *Critical Care Nursing Quarterly, 26*, 166.

Greenway, R. L., Greenway, S. E., & Raum, W. J. (2004). The physiology of the brain, the gut, and the fat cells in the morbidly obese. In L. E. Martin (Ed.), *Obesity surgery* (pp. 49–61). New York: McGraw.

Hagarty, M. A., Schmidt, C., Bernaix, L., & Clement, J. M. (2004). Adolescent obesity: Current trends in identification and management. *Journal of the American Academy of Nurse Practitioners, 16*, 481–489.

Haynes, B. (2005). Creation of a bariatric surgery program for adolescents at a major teaching hospital. *Pediatric Nursing, 31*, 21–22, 59.

Herve, J., Wahlen, C. H., Schaeken, A., Dallemagne, B., Dewandre, J. M., Markiewicz, S., et al. (2005). What becomes of patients one year after the intragastric balloon has been removed? *Obesity Surgery, 15*, 864–870.

Holloway, J. A., Forney, F. A., & Gould, D. E. (2004). The lap-band is an effective tool for weight loss even in the United States. *The American Journal of Surgery, 188*, 659–662.

Horgan, S., Holterman, M. J., Jacobsen, G. R., Browne, A. F., Berger, R. A., Moser, F., et al. (2005). Laparoscopic adjustable gastric banding for the treatment of adolescent morbid obesity in the United States: A safe alternative to gastric bypass. *Journal of Pediatric Surgery, 40*, 86–91.

Hydock, C. M. (2005). A brief overview of bariatric surgical procedures currently being used to treat the obese patient. *Critical Care Nursing Quarterly, 28*, 217–226.

Inge, T. H., Garcia, V. F., Daniels, S., Langford, L., Kirk, S., Roehrig, H., et al. (2004). A multidisciplinary approach to the adolescent bariatric surgical patient. *Journal of Pediatric Surgery, 39*, 442–447.

Inge, T. H., Krebs, N. F., Garcia, V. F., Skelton, J. A., Guide, K. S., Strauss, R. S., et al. (2004). Bariatric surgery for severely overweight adolescents: Concerns and recommendations. *Pediatrics, 114*, 217–223.

Inge, T. H., Zeller, M. H., Lawson, M. L., & Daniels, S. R. (2005). A critical appraisal of evidence supporting a bariatric surgical approach to weight management for adolescents. *Journal of Pediatrics, 147*, 10–19.

Jan, J. C., Hong, D., Pereira, N., & Patterson, E. J. (2005). Laparoscopic adjustable gastric banding versus laparoscopic gastric bypass for morbid obesity: A single-institution comparison study of early results. *Journal of Gastrointestinal Surgery, 9*, 30–41.

Kirk, S., Scott, B. J., & Daniels, S. R. (2005). Pediatric obesity epidemic: Treatment options. *Journal of the American Dietetic Association, 105*, S44–S51.

Koplan, J. P., Liverman, C. T., & Kraak, V. I. (2005). *Preventing childhood obesity: Health in the balance.* Washington, DC: National Academies Press.

Kuzmak, L. I. (1991). A review of seven years' experience with silicone gastric banding. *Obesity Surgery, 1*, 403–408.

Lujan, J. A., Hernandez, Q., Frutos, M. D., Valero, J. R., & Parrilla, P. (2002). Laparoscopic gastric bypass in the treatment of morbid obesity. *Surgical Endoscopy, 16*, 1658–1662.

MacKenzie, R. G., & Neinstein, L. S. (2002). Obesity. In L. S. Neinstein (Ed.), *Adolescent health care, a practical guide* (4th ed.). Philadelphia: Lippincott.

Marcason, W. (2004). What are the dietary guidelines following bariatric surgery? *Journal of the American Dietetic Association, 104*, 487–488.

Mason, E. E., & Ito, C. (1967). Gastric bypass in obesity. *Surgical Clinics of North America, 47*, 1845–1852.

Nadler, E. P., & Kane, T. D. (2005). Bariatric surgery. In R. P. Langer & C. T. Albanese (Eds.), *Pediatric minimal access surgery.* New York: Marcel Dekker.

National Institutes of Health. (1991). Gastrointestinal surgery for severe obesity, consensus development conference statement. Retrieved February 2006, from http://consensus.nih.gov/1991/1991GISurgeryObesity084html.htm

Ogden, C. L., Flegal, K. M., Carroll, M. D., & Johnson, C. L. (2002). Prevalence and trends in overweight among U.S. children and adolescents, 1999–2000. *JAMA, 288*, 1728–1732.

Ogden, C. L., Kuczmarski, R. J., Flegal, K. M., Mei, Z., Guo, S., Wei, R., et al. (2002). Centers for Disease Control and Prevention 2000 growth charts for the United States: Improvements to the 1977 national center for health statistics version. *Pediatrics, 109*, 45–60.

Parikh, M. S., Fielding, G., & Ren, C. J. (2005). U.S. experience with 749 laparoscopic adjustable gastric bands: Intermediate outcomes. *Surgical Endoscopy, 10*, 1631–1635.

Park, K. S., Shin, H. D., Park, B. L., Cheong, H. S., Choa, Y. M., Lee, H. K., et al. (2006). Polymorphisms in the leptin receptor (LERP)-putative association with obesity and T2DM. *Journal of Human Genetics, 51*(2), 85–91.

Park, K. S., Shin, H. D., Park, B. L., Cheong, H. S., Choa, Y. M., Lee, H. K., et al. (2005). Genetic polymorphisms in the transforming growth factor beta-induced gene associated with BMI. *Human Mutation, 25*, 322.

Ponce, J., & Dixon, J. B. (2005). Laparoscopic adjustable gastric banding. *Surgery for Obesity and Related Diseases, 1*, 310–316.

Ponce, J., Paynter, S., & Fromm, R. (2005). Laparoscopic adjustable gastric banding: 1,014 consecutive cases. *Journal of the American College of Surgeons, 201*, 529–535.

Puhl, R., & Brownell, K. D. (2001). Bias, discrimination, and obesity. *Obesity Research, 9*, 788–805.

Ren, C.J., Horgan, S., & Ponce, J. (2002). US experience with the LAPBAND system. *The American Journal of Surgery, 184*, 46S–50S.

Rogers, B. M. (2004). Bariatric surgery for adolescents: A view from the American Pediatric Surgical Association. *Pediatrics, 114*, 255–256.

Safadi, B. Y. (2005). Trends in insurance coverage for bariatric surgery and the impact of evidence-based reviews. *Surgical Clinics of North America, 85*, 665–680.

SAGES. (2003). Guidelines for the clinical application of laparoscopic bariatric surgery. Publication # 0030 Retrieved February 2006, from http://www.sages.org/sagespublication

Schneider, B. E., & Mun, E. C. (2005). Surgical management of morbid obesity. *Diabetes Care, 28*, 475–480.

Schwimmer, J. B., Burwinkle, T. M., & Varni, J. W. (2003). Health-related quality of life of severely obese children and adolescents. *JAMA, 289*, 1813–1819.

Shuster, M. H., & Vazques, J. A. (2005). Nutritional concerns related to Roux-en-Y gastric bypass: What every clinician needs to know. *Critical Care Nursing Quarterly, 28,* 227–260.

Speiser, P. W., Rudolf, M. C., Anhalt, H., Camacho-Hubner, C., Chiarelli, F., Eliakim, A., et al. (2005). Consensus statement: Childhood obesity. *Journal of Clinical Endocrinology & Metabolism, 90,* 1871–1887.

Spivak, H., Huewitt, M. F., Onn, A., & Half, E. E. (2005). Weight loss and improvement of obesity-related illness in 500 U.S. patients following laparoscopic adjustable gastric banding procedure. *The American Journal of Surgery, 189,* 27–32.

Stanford, A., Glascock, J. M., Eid, G. M., Kane, T. D., Ford, R. R., Ikramuddin, S., et al. (2003). Laparoscopic Roux-en-Y gastric bypass in morbidly obese adolescents. *Journal of Pediatric Surgery, 38,* 430–433.

Strauss, R. S., Bradley, L. J., & Brolin, R. E. (2001). Gastric bypass surgery in adolescents with morbid obesity. *Journal of Pediatrics, 138,* 499–504.

Tershakovec, A. M., Watson, M. H., Wenner, W. J., & Marx, A. L. (1999). Insurance reimbursement for the treatment of obesity in children. *Journal of Pediatrics, 134,* 573–578.

Vandenplas, Y., Bollen, P., De Lange, K., Vandemaele, K., & De Schepper, J. (1999). Intragastric balloons in adolescents with morbid obesity. *European Journal of Gastroenterology and Hepatology, 11,* 243–245.

Wadden, T. A., Berkowitz, R. I., Womble, L. G., Sarwer, D. B., Phelan, S., Cato, R. K., et al. (2005). Randomized trial of lifestyle modification and pharmacotherapy for obesity. *New England Journal of Medicine, 353,* 2111–2120.

Weiner, S., Sauerland, S., Fein, M., Bianco, R., Pomhoff, I., & Weiner, R. A. (2005). The bariatric quality of life (BQL) index: A measure of well-being in obesity surgery patients. *Obesity Surgery, 15,* 538–545.

Wittgrove, A. C. (2004). Surgery for severely obese adolescents: Further insight from the American Society for Bariatric Surgery. *Pediatrics, 114,* 253–254.

Wittgrove, A. C., Clark, G. W., & Tremblay, L. J. (1994). Laparoscopic gastric bypass, Roux-en-Y: Preliminary report of five cases. *Obesity Surgery, 4*(4), 353–357.

Woodward, B. G. (2001). *A complete guide to obesity surgery.* Victoria, British Columbia, Canada: Trafford.

VII

Nursing Care of the Injured Child

Pediatric Trauma

By Pam Pieper

Injuries, often preventable, occur in seconds and have the potential to kill or permanently change the life of a child. The goal of those involved in pediatric trauma is to prevent its occurrence and treat those affected so as to maximize their potential for recovery. This chapter presents an overview of the nursing care required by the pediatric trauma patient.

■ Epidemiology

Approximately 16 million injured children are seen in emergency departments (EDs) annually in the United States, with about 600,000 of them requiring hospitalization. Trauma is the number one killer of children over the age of 1 year, and 39% of the deaths in children under the age of 15 in 2002 (6,344 children) were caused by injuries (National Vital Statistics System, n.d.). The number of children estimated to have a permanent impairment secondary to trauma is greater than 50,000/year (Schafermeyer, 1993). Because the mechanisms of injury vary, review of local injury data is needed to develop prevention strategies that will be most effective in a particular area.

Host Factors

Common mechanisms of injury vary with the child's developmental level, usually correlating with the age of the child. Other host factors that affect injury rates are gender and race. Boys are more commonly injured than girls for every pediatric age group. According to 2002 data from the National Center for Injury Prevention and Control, 55% of homicide victims under the age of 15 were male, 56% were white, and 38% were black. In both males and females, 67% of the homicide victims were under the age of 5, with many of the deaths resulting from child abuse. Blacks and American Indian/Alaskan natives had homicide death rates of slightly more than 4 per 100,000, whereas the rate in whites was 1.28 per 100,000. Seventy-five percent of suicide deaths were males. However, more than three times as many girls as boys between the ages 10 and 14 injured themselves intentionally. The suicide rate for whites was nearly twice that of nonwhites.

Environmental Factors

The most significant environmental factor affecting injury patterns in children is their socioeconomic status. Nersesian, Petit, Shaper, Lemieux, and Naor reported in 1985 that children who live in poverty die 2.6 times more often than those who do not. Marcin, Schembri, He, and Romano (2003) performed a population-based analysis of injured children relative to socioeconomic and insurance status in Sacramento County, California, and determined that the gap continues to increase. The higher death rates from injury for poor children are not related to higher injury severity among hospitalized injured children, but rather because poor children sustain more injuries that require hospitalization. Risk factor exposure is higher in impoverished children; for example, they are less likely to be restrained in a motor vehicle or to wear a helmet when bicycle riding.

Intentional injuries include child abuse, interpersonal violence, and suicide. The actual rate of child abuse, which includes physical, emotional, and sexual abuse, is unknown. However, there were approximately 2.9 million referrals to child protective services in 2003 out of a total population of slightly more than 73 million children under the age of 18 in the United States. Of those, 26% were substantiated, with 167,900 cases of physical abuse and 87,600 cases of sexual abuse. Nearly half were boys (48%) and 10% of the victims were under the age of 1 year. There were 1,500 deaths from abuse or neglect; 35% of them were caused by neglect only, 28% by physical abuse only, and 29% by multiple maltreatment types (US Department of Health and Human Services, 2005). There were 1,082 homicide and 264 suicide deaths in children aged 0 to 14 years of age in 2002 (National Center for Injury Prevention and Control, n.d.).

Important indications that warrant further investigation into the mechanism of injury because of the possibility of nonaccidental trauma include a delay in seeking appropriate medical attention, seeking medical attention from multiple different providers for different injuries over time, histories that change with time or depending on who is providing the information, a history of behavior that is developmentally impossible, attributing the injury to a sibling, and a history that is inconsistent with the injury. Specific injuries are also suspicious for inflicted trauma, such as bite marks too large to have been inflicted by a child. Suspicions should also be raised when there is no history of severe trauma and certain injuries, such as rib fractures, are present. Mandelstam, Cook, Fitzgerald, and Ditchfield (2003) determined that both skeletal surveys and bone scintigraphies are needed in cases of suspected child abuse based on their review of 32 children, 30 of whom were under the age of 3, with a total of 124 fractures. Of these fractures, 77 were identified on the skeletal survey and 64 on the bone scintigraphy; six children had normal skeletal surveys with fractures visualized on bone scintigraphy and three children had fractures visible on bone scintigraphy not noted on their skeletal surveys. Rubin, Christian, Bilaniuk, Zazyczny, and Durbin (2003) recommend that either head computed tomography (CT)

or magnetic resonance imaging be included in the evaluation of abused children with normal neurologic status who meet any of the following criteria: younger than 6 months of age, multiple fractures, rib fractures, or facial injuries. Of the 51 infants in their study meeting these criteria who also underwent either CT or magnetic resonance imaging, 16 (31%) had either an intracranial injury or a skull fracture or both, none of which required operative intervention. Three other infants had only scalp hematomas that were not detected on physical examination. Funduscopic examinations were performed on 14 of this group of 19, all of which were normal.

Child abuse occurs in all socioeconomic classes. The importance of reporting any suspected or possible child abuse to the appropriate state authorities cannot be overstated. Removing a child from an abusive environment will prevent future injury, or even death, by that perpetrator.

■ Injury Prevention

Injury prevention is by far the most effective and cost-efficient method in which to address the issue of pediatric trauma. Primary care nurses have an important opportunity to provide developmentally appropriate anticipatory guidance at each well-child visit. Unfortunately, many nurses' first contact is only after a child has already been injured. In these cases, the child and family should be educated about injury prevention specifically related to the child's situation during the hospitalization and again shortly before discharge.

The most cost-effective, and therefore the highest-priority, injury prevention strategies involve automatic protection and elimination of environmental hazards. Airbags and automatic seat belts are two examples of design changes that provide automatic protection. Another strategy is legislative change that requires alteration in risk-taking behavior, such as bicycle helmet laws. The least effective strategy is education because it requires an audience motivated to change its behavior. Programs are most effective when there is significant local involvement and when they are aimed at a specific problem occurring within a defined high-risk population. Pressley, Barlow, Durkin, Jacko, Dominguez, and Johnson (2005) discuss program components of the injury prevention model used by the Robert Wood Johnson Foundation supported Injury Free Coalition for Kids. There are currently 40 Injury Free Coalition for Kids sites throughout the United States, with at least one in each of the 10 national trauma regions. Injury prevention strategies others have found to be successful include those published by Birkland (1993), Martin,

Langley, and Coffman (1995), and Stylianos and Eichelberger (1993).

Clinical Presentation

Prehospital Triage

Triage protocols are most important for those children with serious brain, internal, and skeletal injuries to avoid preventable death and disability. One method to determine which children should be treated at a trauma center is by using a scoring system, such as the Pediatric Trauma Score (see Table 32-1 for a modified version of the Pediatric Trauma Score) (Tepas, Mollitt, Talbert, & Bryant, 1987). The purpose of this scoring system is rapid assessment of the severity of a child's injury by prehospital providers in the midst of an often chaotic situation. A more detailed "Field Triage Decision Scheme" is presented in *Resources for Optimal Care of the Injured Patient: 1999* (Committee on Trauma, American College of Surgeons, 1998, p. 14).

Primary Survey

The three components of the Pediatric Assessment Triangle are appearance, work of breathing, and circulation to the skin. Use of the Pediatric Assessment Triangle gives experienced pediatric providers a general impression of a child's condition within 30 to 60 seconds simply by observing the child (Dieckmann, 2004). The primary survey includes evaluation of the child's airway with cervical spine immobilization, breathing and ventilation, circulation with hemorrhage control, disability in terms of neurologic status, and exposure with thorough examination for any obvious injuries. Although the assessment and treatment priorities are the same in children and adults, there are a number of anatomic and physiologic differences that must be taken into consideration.

Airway

The anatomy of the child's airway is different from that of an adult's (Table 32-2). One half to 1 inch of additional padding should be placed under the shoulders of infants and children who are placed on backboards or stretchers to prevent neck flexion from their relatively larger occiputs, which may occlude the airway. In a child without a possible neck injury, placing the child in the sniffing position easily opens the airway. If there is any possibility of a neck injury, the jaw thrust maneuver is used to open the airway while the cervical spine is maintained in

Table 32-1	**Color-Coded Pediatric Trauma Score**					
Component	**+2**		**+1**		**−1**	
Size	Orange, green[a] > 20 kg (≥ 44 lbs)	G	Yellow, white, blue[a] 10–20 kg (22–43 lbs)	G	Red, purple[a] < 10 kg (< 22 lbs)	B
Airway	Normal	G	Adjunct (e.g., O_2, mask, cannula, oral/nasal airway)	G	Assisted or intubated (BVM, ETT, EOA, Cric)	R
Consciousness	Awake	G	Amnesia or any reliable history of loss of consciousness	B	Altered mental status (drowsy/ lethargic/unresponsive) or paralysis or suspected spinal cord fracture	R
Circulation	Good peripheral pulses/ perfusion; SBP > 90 mm Hg	G	Carotid/femoral pulses palpable; SBP 50–90 mm Hg	B	Weak or no palpable pulses; SBP < 50 mm Hg	R
Fracture	None seen or suspected	G	Single closed fracture anywhere	B	Any open long bone fracture or multiple fractures	R
Cutaneous	No visible injury	G	Contusion, abrasion, or laceration ≤ 3 inches	G	Laceration > 3 inches or any penetrating injury to head, neck, or torso or amputation/tissue loss or 2°/3° burns to > 10% TBSA	R

R = any one (1): transport to trauma center
B = any two (2): transport to trauma center
G = follow local protocols
[a]Colors listed relate to those found on Broselow tape.
BVM, bag-valve-mask; Cric, cricothryrotomy; EOA, esophageal oral airway; ETT, endotracheal tube; TBSA, total body surface area.
From Tepas, J. J., III, Mollitt, D. L., Talbert, J. L., & Bryant, M. (1987). The pediatric trauma score as a predictor of injury severity in the injured child. *Journal of Pediatric Surgery, 22*, 15. Adapted with permission.

Table 32-2	**Airway and Breathing Differences in Children**
Airway	Pediatric airway more likely to become obstructed
	Diameter and length smaller
	Tongue relatively larger within oropharynx
	Head to body ratio larger → neck flexion
	Narrowest portion of airway at the cricoid cartilage (< 10 years old)
	Larynx funnel shaped (< 10 years old)
Breathing	Infants and young children are diaphragmatic breathers
	Compromised ventilation with impairment of diaphragmatic excursion
	Gastric distention most common reasons:
	Swallow air when crying
	Assisted ventilation with face mask
	Relieved with naso- or orogastric tube

From Hazinski, M. F., Zaritsky, A. L., Nadkarni, V. M., Hickey, R. W., Schexnayder, S. M., & Berg, R. A. (Eds.). (2002). *PALS provider manual* (pp. 82–83). Dallas: American Heart Association.

neutral position. Any obstructing material should be suctioned from the oropharynx; in addition, the nares of neonates should also be suctioned because they are obligate nasal breathers. If an oropharyngeal or nasopharyngeal airway is needed to maintain a patent airway, a nasopharyngeal airway should be used in conscious and semiconscious children to avoid eliciting the gag reflex and stimulating vomiting in these patients.

Oxygen should be provided at 100% by means of blow-by, mask, or nasal cannula in children with questionable airway reliability. Endotracheal intubation is indicated for children with a Glasgow Coma Score (GCS) of ≤ 8 (Table 32-3), those who are unable to maintain an adequate airway, or those who are hypovolemic to the extent that operative intervention is required. Orotracheal intubation is recommended either for all children who require resuscitation (Hazinski et al., 2002) or for those who are 8 years of age or younger (American College of Surgeons Committee on Trauma, 2004) because it is technically easier than nasotracheal intubation. The most accurate method for determining the appropriate-sized endotracheal tube (ETT) needed is a length-based measure such as the Broselow tape (Luten et al., 1992). If this tape is not available, an ETT with an outside diameter approximating the diameter of the child's little finger or external nares or the formula ETT mm internal diameter = (age in years/4) + 4 for children older than 2 years of age may be used. An uncuffed ETT should be used in children younger than 8 to 10 years of age. A natural seal is formed at the narrowest portion of their airway, the cricoid ring. Figure 32-1 shows a rapid-sequence intubation (RSI), or induction, protocol used for emergency intubation to decrease the possibility of regurgitation. An end-tidal carbon dioxide (CO_2) detector is used to confirm that the ETT is in the airway. The most frequent complication of endotracheal intubation in infants and children is right mainstem bronchial intubation because of the short length of their tracheas. Breath sounds and quality of chest rise should be assessed frequently after intubation. This is particularly important when the patient has been moved from one surface to another, such as when obtaining a computerized tomography (CT) scan.

Breathing

Infants and young children have compromised ventilation any time full diaphragmatic excursion is impaired because they are diaphragmatic breathers. The most common reason for this is gastric distention caused by swallowing air when the child is crying or receiving assisted ventilation with a face mask. Gastric distention is relieved by passing a nasogastric or orogastric tube and attaching the tube to suction.

Pulse oximetry is useful in assessing oxygenation as long as there is adequate peripheral perfusion. Carbon dioxide measurements may be followed in intubated patients with an end-tidal CO_2 monitor; the readings should be correlated with the partial pressure of arterial carbon dioxide ($PaCO_2$) from an arterial blood gas. A tension pneumothorax is suspected in an intubated child receiving positive-pressure ventilation whose respiratory status acutely deteriorates. Treatment of acidosis with sodium bicarbonate before the establishment of adequate ventilation and perfusion is contraindicated because it will lead to increased hypercarbia and acidosis.

Circulation

Reflex tachycardia and peripheral vasoconstriction in children allow them to present with normal blood pressures until they have lost approximately 30% (> 20 mL/kg) of their total blood volume (American College of Surgeons Committee on Trauma, 2004). However, tachycardia is caused not only by hypovolemia but also by pain and fear, both of which frequently occur in injured children. The use of capillary refill as an indicator of hypovolemia should be avoided because of the effect that ambient temperature has on capillary refill (Baraff, 1993; Gorelick, Shaw, & Baker, 1993). Systemic responses of children to hypovolemia are presented in Table 32-4. When a source of ongoing blood loss is visible, apply direct pressure and elevate the area.

Table 32-3	**Pediatric Coma Scale**		
Eye Opening			
< 1 Year		**> 1 Year**	**Score**
Spontaneously		Spontaneously	4
To shout		To verbal command	3
To pain		To pain	2
No response		No response	1
Best Verbal Response			
0–23 Months	**2–5 Years**	**> 5 Years**	
Smiles, coos appropriately	Appropriate words/phrases	Oriented and converses	5
Cries, consolable	Inappropriate words	Disoriented and converses	4
Persistent inappropriate crying and/or screaming	Persistent crying and screaming	Inappropriate words	3
Grunts, agitated, restless	Grunts	Incomprehensible sounds	2
No response	No response	No response	1
Best Motor Response			
< 1 Year		**> 1 Year**	
Spontaneous		Obeys	6
Localizes pain		Localizes pain	5
Flexion-withdrawal		Flexion-withdrawal	4
Flexion-abnormal (decorticate)		Flexion-abnormal (decorticate)	3
Extension (decerebrate)		Extension (decerebrate)	2
No response		No response	1

Source: Simon, J., & Goldberg, A. (1989). *Prehospital pediatric life support* (p. 11). St. Louis, MO: Mosby. Adapted with permission.

Vascular Access

Two large-bore peripheral intravenous (IV) lines are inserted, preferably in the upper extremities, to facilitate rapid infusion of fluids to restore circulating volume. Hazinski et al. (2002) suggest attempting an IV and intraosseous (IO) access at the same time in children who are receiving cardiopulmonary resuscitation or are in severe shock. IO access allows drugs, fluids, and blood products to be infused directly into the bone marrow. Placement of choice for an IO infusion is the proximal tibial plateau; it should not be placed in an injured extremity. Pressure infusion devices may be needed to maintain flow of the infusate. Central venous lines and peripheral venous cutdowns should be attempted only by those experienced in these procedures.

Any child who is suspected of being hypovolemic should receive an initial IV bolus of warmed normal saline or Ringer's lactate solution in addition to maintenance IV fluids. Approximately 3 mL of crystalloid is required to replace each milliliter of blood lost because all of the infused fluid does not remain in the intravas-

cular space, thus the "3 for 1 rule." The estimated blood volume in an infant is 80 mL/kg and in a child is 75 mL/kg. Children must lose approximately 25% to 30% of their blood volume before demonstrating a decrease in blood pressure; crystalloid boluses are therefore given in 20 mL/kg (25% of 80 mL/kg) increments. If there is no improvement after the second bolus, a third bolus or transfusion of 10 to 15 mL/kg O-negative or type-specific warmed packed red blood cells should be considered. Abnormal hemodynamic status after packed red blood cell transfusion indicates the need for operative intervention. Closely monitor the child's hemodynamic status until there is no longer any possibility of significant bleeding.

Disability

Brain injuries are the most frequent cause of death and morbidity in injured children. The AVPU (Alert, responds to Verbal stimuli, responds to Painful stimuli, or Unresponsive) is a simplified neurologic status evaluation tool that may be used initially. The gold standard for evaluation

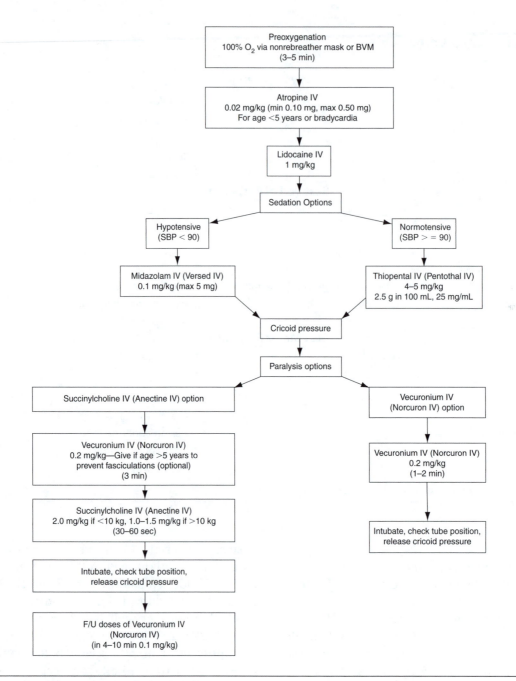

Figure 32-1 Rapid-sequence induction/intubation (RSI).
(Source: Jacksonville Pediatric Injury Control System.)

of neurologic status is the Glasgow Coma Scale (GCS, see Table 32-3). It is essential to record a baseline evaluation of the child's neurologic status with frequent re-evaluation and documentation of the GCS and pupillary size, responsiveness to light, and position.

Exposure

The final aspect of the primary survey requires complete exposure of the child, including rolling the child to one side to examine the back, to evaluate for any visible injuries while taking care to prevent hypothermia. Complications of hypothermia include metabolic acidosis and a shift in the oxygen hemoglobin dissociation curve to the left so that oxygen is bound more tightly to hemoglobin, leading to tissue hypoxia. Methods to prevent or treat hypothermia include using heated blankets; warming lights; and warmed IV fluids, blood, and inhaled gases. Temperatures should be periodically assessed and recorded during the resuscitation. Although rectal temperatures are generally considered to be the most accurate, Bernardo et al. (1996) found

Table 32-4	Systemic Responses to Blood Loss in the Pediatric Patient		
System	Mild (< 30%) Blood Volume Loss	Moderate (30%–45%) Blood Volume Loss	Severe (> 45%) Blood Volume Loss
Cardiovascular	Weak, thready peripheral pulses ↑ heart rate	Blood pressure low normal, narrowed pulse pressure Markedly ↑ heart rate Absent peripheral pulses; weak, thready central pulses	Hypotension Tachycardia then bradycardia
Central nervous system	Anxious, irritable, confused	Lethargic Dulled response to pain	Comatose
Skin	Cool, mottled Prolonged capillary refill	Cyanotic Markedly prolonged capillary refill	Pale, cold
Renal	Minimal ↓ in urinary output	Minimal urine output	No urinary output

From American College of Surgeons Committee on Trauma. (2004). *ATLS: Advanced trauma life support for doctors: Student course manual* (7th ed., p. 251). Chicago: American College of Surgeons. Adapted with permission.

that aural infrared temperatures were accurate enough for screening in children with moderate-to-severe injuries.

Secondary Survey

After the primary survey and initial stabilization, a secondary, systematic total body survey is performed. The child's vital signs and level of consciousness require frequent reassessment and recording during this time. All systems should be evaluated; however, the order in which the survey is performed varies depending on the child's suspected injuries.

History

Prehospital care providers provide valuable information regarding the injury mechanism and prehospital events. A simple mnemonic for this is AMPLE: Allergies, Medications, Past illnesses, Last meal, and Events related to the injury. In addition, the child's immunization status, particularly tetanus, should be obtained from the family.

■ Traumatic Brain Injuries (TBI)

Incidence

Ninety-seven percent of children under the age of 14 who die as a result of trauma have an intracranial injury; one third have an isolated brain injury (Lescohier & DiScala, 1993). Although minor brain injuries constitute the vast majority of brain injuries in children, they may also leave the child with permanent disabilities (Hawley, Ward, Magnay, & Long, 2004).

Primary and Secondary Injuries

Primary brain injuries occur at the time of the traumatic event and include scalp, skull, blood vessel, and intracranial injuries. Secondary injuries are precipitated by the damage caused by the traumatic event and include injuries from hypoxia, hypercarbia, increased intracranial pressure (ICP), and hypotension. These injuries are potentially avoidable and mandate that the ABCs (airway, breathing, and circulation) be adequately assessed and addressed in the brain-injured child. Hypotension within 24 hours of injury is the single most damaging secondary injury in terms of mortality, poor neurologic and functional outcomes, and length of hospital stay (Kokoska, Smith, Pittman, & Weber, 1998). Data from the Traumatic Coma Data Bank, that were prospectively collected, show that either prehospital hypotension (a single systolic blood pressure of < 90 mm Hg) or hypoxia (PaO_2 < 60 mm Hg on an arterial blood gas, cyanosis, or apnea) significantly increases the chance of poor outcome (as cited in Bullock et al., 2000).

Pathophysiology

The brain, cerebrospinal fluid (CSF), and blood fill the fixed intracranial vault. ICP is normally maintained at ≤ 10 mm Hg by minor volume variations in these three elements. When a child's brain is injured, it swells and displaces the CSF into the spinal subarachnoid space. If the swelling continues, eventually the ventricles become compressed or even obliterated. Hyperventilation causes cerebral vasoconstriction, thus decreasing cerebral blood flow and thereby decreasing ICP. However, prophylactic or prolonged hyperventilation ($PaCO_2 \leq 35$ mm Hg) during the first 24 hours after a brain injury is discouraged because cerebral blood flow is already reduced at that time. If the brain-injured child is hyperventilated to a $PaCO_2 < 25$ mm Hg, there is significant risk of causing cerebral ischemia. The potential for development of cerebral edema continues for 3 to 5 days post-injury. Prevention and early treatment of intracranial hypertension include normothermia, volume resuscitation, seizure prophylaxis, raising the head of the bed 30°, prevention of jugular venous drainage obstruction, sedation with possible pharmacologic paralysis, and maintaining a $PaO_2 > 60$ mm Hg. An algorithm for treatment of intracranial hypertension is found in Figure 32-2. ICP monitoring should

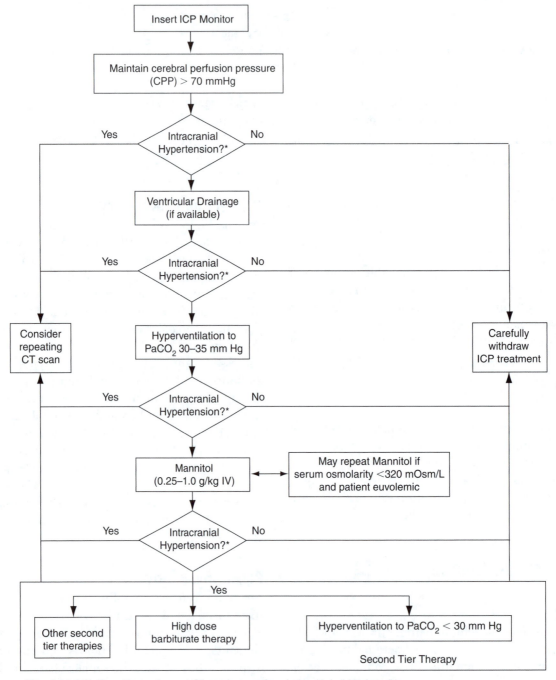

*Threshold of 20–25 mmHg may be used. Other values may be substitued in individual conditions.

Figure 32-2 Critical pathway for treatment of intracranial hypertension in the severe brain injury patient.
(Source: Bullock, M. R., Chestnut, R. M., Clifton, G. L., Gahjar, J., Marion, D. W., Naryan, R. K., et al (2000). *Management and prognosis of severe traumatic brain injury*. Brain Trauma Foundation and American Association of Neurological Surgeons. Adapted with permission.)

be initiated in children with a GCS of ≤ 8 after resuscitation who have evidence of compressed basilar cisterns or cerebral edema, hematomas, or contusions on the head CT. ICP relates directly to the cerebral perfusion pressure (CPP) by way of the equation: MAP (mean arterial pressure) − ICP = CPP. CPP is a more accurate predictor of outcome than the ICP. Hackbarth, Rzeszutko, Sturm, Donders, Kuldanek, and Sanfilippo (2002) analyzed predictive factors in brain-injured children and determined that survival was most strongly predicted by preservation of a CPP of at least 50 mm Hg.

Evaluation

Glasgow Coma Scale

GCS was developed to evaluate the level of consciousness in adults (Jennett & Teasdale, 1977). Modifications to this scale have been made so that it is applicable for use in infants and young children (see Table 32-3). Children whose GCS on admission is ≤ 8 are considered to have a major TBI. However, a very low GCS (3 to 5) is not always an accurate prognostic indicator in children.

Physical Examination

GCS evaluations and pupillary reflexes are serially documented to provide an ongoing record of the child's mental status. Results of inspection and gentle palpation of the head are also recorded. Any infant with a bulging fontanel should have a neurosurgical consultation, even if the baby is awake and alert, because sudden deterioration may occur (American College of Surgeons Committee on Trauma, 2004).

Radiologic Evaluation

The head CT is the standard method of evaluating for intracranial injuries. From their study of 98 children who presented with either brief loss of consciousness or amnesia, had a GCS of 13 to 15, and underwent a head CT, Halley, Silva, Foley, and Rodarte (2004) determined that physical examination was not predictive of a positive head CT. A neurosurgical consult is obtained for those children in whom the head CT demonstrates a neurosurgical lesion.

In this era of cost containment, the routine observation in the hospital of children with minor brain injuries is no longer standard. Discharge criteria from the ED for children with a minor brain injury include a normal head CT, a GCS of 15 (although they may have had a brief loss of consciousness or have amnesia), and a history of only minor trauma. In addition, there must be reliable parents, telephone and transportation access, and a home within a reasonable distance of medical care. Written and verbal recommendations need to be provided before discharge and a follow-up telephone call should be made within 48 hours. Caregivers need to have the child seen by health care personnel if the child becomes increasingly confused, sleepy, or cannot be awakened; has seizures or sudden, fixed staring; has several episodes of vomiting; complains of blurry or double vision or that neck stiffness or head pain becomes worse; has an unstable gait; or the caregiver notices that the child's pupils are not the same size.

Table 32-5 provides a list of specific brain injuries, their signs and symptoms, treatments, and complications.

Increased Intracranial Pressure

The most accurate, reliable, and cost-effective method currently available for monitoring ICP is a ventricular catheter attached to an external strain gauge. Ventricular catheters with either internal strain gauges or fiberoptic transduction impart analogous information, but they are more expensive. All of these catheters also allow for therapeutic CSF drainage. Other ICP monitors include those that are placed in the brain parenchyma. An ICP monitor is generally inserted by the neurosurgeon at the bedside or in the operating room. Elevated ICP is related to the potential for cerebral herniation. However, as the importance of the CPP has become better understood, it has become evident that there is no particular ICP for which treatment should be initiated. Present guidelines recommend treatment of ICP when it reaches 20 to 25 mm Hg. However, a portion of the brain may abnormally protrude, or herniate, through an opening in the skull at lower ICPs than that, depending on where the lesion is located. A higher ICP may be tolerated as long as the CPP is at least 70 mm Hg (Bullock et al., 2000).

An algorithm for the treatment of intracranial hypertension is seen in Figure 32-2. Steroids, including glucocorticoids, are not recommended for patients with severe TBI; they have been found to increase mortality (Alderson & Roberts, 2005). Because hyperthermia increases cerebral metabolism and therefore ICP, it needs to be controlled. If ventricular drainage is not available or does not decrease the ICP sufficiently, hyperventilation to a $PaCO_2$ of 30 to 35 mm Hg is initiated to attempt to control an elevated ICP. If this, too, is unsuccessful, the osmotic diuretic Mannitol may be used. Mannitol raises the serum osmolarity, thus pulling water into the bloodstream from the intracellular and interstitial spaces. However, once serum osmolarity reaches 320 mOsm/L, Mannitol should be stopped to prevent renal failure. If the ICP continues to remain elevated at this point, second-tier therapies, such as high-dose barbiturate-induced coma or craniectomy (removal of a portion of the skull), must be considered.

Table 32-5 — Specific Head Injuries

Injury	Diagnostics/Description	Treatment	Comments/Complications
Concussion	Brief loss of neurological function ± loss of consciousness or amnesia	Supportive care May need head computed tomography (CT)	If no persistent symptoms and reliable caregiver, may be observed at home
Scalp injuries			
Lacerations	Inspection	Irrigation and gentle débridement Sutures/staples as needed, remove in 5–7 days. May also use tissue adhesive; no removal necessary Thin layer of topical antibiotic ointment	If associated with open depressed skull fracture, laceration is a potential source of intracranial infection
Subgaleal hematomas	Inspection, palpation Injury to tissue external to the skull	None, reabsorb spontaneously Avoid aspiration (risk of infection)	
Skull Fractures	Head CT with bone windows		
Linear	Fine line visible on radiographs (CT or skull x-rays)	If not depressed or diastatic (traumatic separation through cranial suture lines), not treated	Most common skull fracture, usually insignificant
Depressed	Depression of bone visible on CT	If depressed ≥ thickness of skull, elevated in the operating room	Increased chance of post-injury seizures

Basilar	On inspection may have
	CSF rhinorrhea or otorrhea
	Battle's sign: posterior auricular ecchymosis
	Raccoon eyes: Periorbital ecchymosis
	Pneumocephalus on CT[a]
		Serial neurologic examinations
		Examinations of cranial nerves VII (facial) and VIII (acoustic)
			May not be visible radiographically
			Possible complications:
			  Seventh nerve palsy
			  Hearing deficit
			  Meningitis (if CSF leak)

Hematomas	Non–contrast enhanced head CT		
Epidural (extradural) hematoma (EDH)	Tearing of meningeal blood vessels May have brief loss of consciousness, a lucid interval, and then deterioration	Evacuation of large or rapidly expanding EDHs Surgical intervention also indicated for deteriorating LOC	Often rapid, marked recovery after evacuation w/minimal sequelae
Subdural hematoma (SDH)	Rupture of bridging cerebral veins	PICU observation with supportive care Craniotomy and evacuation of clot if symptomatic with significant lesion, decreasing LOC, or enlarging lesion on repeat CT Possible intracranial pressure monitor	Most common intracranial injury in infant victims of intentional trauma May have ipsilateral hemiparesis and oculomotor palsy[b]
Subarachnoid hemorrhages (SAH)	Bleeding of microvessels within the subarachnoid space (where the CSF circulates)	Observation for 24–48 hours	Possible complication: Hydrocephalus[b] May require shunt if hydrocephalus is severe[b]
Intracerebral hematoma/ cerebral contusion	Bleeding within the cerebral parenchyma Coup = at impact site Contrecoup = opposite impact site	Supportive care May rarely require operative intervention for large focal lesions	May cause increased ICP from edema and bleeding[b] May have significant morbidity, depending on where lesion located
Diffuse axonal injury (DAI)	Head CT MRI of brain provides better visualization of DAI than CT Diffuse shearing injury at gray/white matter boundary	See section on increased intracranial pressure in text	Most common cause of vegetative state and severe disability

[a]Graham, D. I. (1996). Neuropathy of head injury. In R. K. Narayan, J. E. Wilberger, & J. T. Povlishock (Eds.), *Neurotrauma* (pp. 44–52). New York: McGraw-Hill.
[b]Lowe, J. G., & Northrup, B. E. (1996). Traumatic intracranial hemorrhage. In R. W. Evans (Ed.), *Neurology and trauma* (pp. 140–147). Philadelphia: Saunders.
CSF, cerebrospinal fluid; CT, computed tomography; LOC, level of consciousness; MRI, magnetic resonance imaging; PICU, pediatric intensive care unit.

Strict urine output is monitored in children with TBI by means of an indwelling urinary catheter. Observation of the urine indicates whether two common complications of TBI, diabetes insipidus (DI) and the syndrome of inappropriate antidiuretic hormone secretion (SIADH), occur. The child's weight and urine sodium and osmolarity levels are monitored throughout treatment of both of these situations. In diabetes insipidus, antidiuretic hormone (ADH) is not released, which leads to free water loss and copious dilute urine output. Isotonic fluids are used as long as the child is hemodynamically unstable. Once the child is hemodynamically stable, treatment consists of administration of hypotonic replacement fluids. If this is not sufficient to increase the urine specific gravity to 1.010, antidiuretic hormone replacement is also required. SIADH is essentially the opposite problem: there is an excess reabsorption of water because of an overproduction of antidiuretic hormone. SIADH causes considerable free-water retention, which leads to electrolyte imbalances and decreased, concentrated urine output. Treatment of SIADH consists of significant fluid restriction until the urine sodium increases to at least 135 mmol/L. Severe cases may require IV boluses of 3% normal saline (Vernon-Levett, 2003).

Thoracic Injuries

Incidence and Pathophysiology

Serious intrathoracic trauma may be present in children without external or skeletal evidence of the significant energy that was transmitted causing the injury due to the increased flexibility of their highly cartilaginous chest walls. Thoracic trauma is the second most common cause of death from pediatric injury (Sartorelli & Vane, 2004), although only 6% of the 25,301 patients entered into the National Pediatric Trauma Registry (NPTR) between 1985 and 1991 had thoracic injuries. The vast majority, 86%, were caused by blunt mechanisms, with the automobile being involved in 74% of them. Gunshot wounds caused 60% of penetrating thoracic trauma. The most common intrathoracic injuries are pulmonary contusions and lacerations (48%), pneumothoraces and hemothoraces (41%), and rib fractures (30%) (Cooper, Barlow, DiScala, & String, 1994).

Evaluation

Evaluation for possible thoracic injuries includes inspection for external signs of trauma, such as contusions and abrasions from shoulder seat belts or penetrating injuries from gunshot wounds. The child's pulse oximetry and respiratory status should be continually re-evaluated. On percussion, the normally resonant sound heard over the lung changes to dullness when a hemothorax or atelectasis is present and is hyperresonant over a pneumothorax. Auscultation of breath sounds may demonstrate hemothoraces, pneumothoraces, or atelectasis by absent or decreased breath sounds over the affected area. The most common predictors for an abnormal chest radiograph or CT are abnormal auscultation of the chest, abnormal thoracic examination, increased respiratory rate, GCS of less than 15, fractured femur, and decreased systolic blood pressure, the latter three also being indicators of a significant transfer of energy during the injury (Holmes, Sokolove, Brant, & Kuppermann, 2002). Plain chest radiographs are frequently taken with a portable machine in the ED during resuscitation. They allow visualization of chest injuries in need of immediate attention as well as trauma to the thoracic skeleton. Thoracic CTs provide valuable additional data when further radiographic evaluation of the chest is needed. However, their significantly greater expense and radiation exposure prevents their use as the initial screening evaluation for chest injuries. Children who have received a significant impact to the chest should be screened with an electrocardiogram, which may be normal even when a cardiac contusion is present. The cardiac isoenzymes troponin I and creatine phosphokinase-MB, with the former being the more sensitive isoenzyme in the case of cardiac contusions, should also be drawn (Sartorelli & Vane, 2004).

Table 32-6 provides a list of specific thoracic injuries, their signs and symptoms, treatments, and complications.

Abdominal Injuries

Incidence and Pathophysiology

Blunt mechanisms cause 86% of abdominal injuries in children, most of which involve motor vehicles (Cooper et al., 1994). Although abdominal injuries occur slightly more frequently than thoracic injuries (8% vs. 6%), their mortality is approximately half that in children who have intrathoracic injuries. Factors contributing to abdominal trauma in young children include that they have less adipose tissue, less developed abdominal wall muscles, and that the solid organs are relatively larger. In addition, the liver and spleen are not as protected by the more pliable, shorter ribcage. Increased mobility and less fat provide the kidneys with less protection than in adolescents or adults.

Table 32-6	Specific Thoracic Injuries		
Injury	**Signs and Symptoms**	**Treatment**	**Complications**
Pulmonary contusion (bruise of lung)	Tachypnea, respiratory distress, may not appear for several hours	Pain management Respiratory support to maintain normal oxygen saturation Avoid fluid overloading Generally resolves in 7–10 days	Pneumonia Adult respiratory distress syndrome (ARDS)
Pneumothoraces (air in pleural space)	Visible on chest x-ray (CXR)	Respiratory support to maintain normal oxygen saturation	
Simple	Tachypnea Increased respiratory effort Decreased or absent breath sounds on affected side Hyperresonance on percussion	If comprises < 15% total lung volume and no respiratory distress, may just observe Chest tube	Respiratory distress
Tension (see Figure 32-3)	Sudden respiratory deterioration May have depressed diaphragm on ipsilateral side and mediastinal shift to contralateral side on CXR Most often related to mechanical ventilation	Immediate large-bore needle thoracostomy (rush of air out when needle reaches trapped air) One-way valve or underwater seal to needle until replaced with chest tube Chest tube	Decreased venous return to heart Decreased cardiac output
Open	Visible open sucking chest wound	Cover open wound and surrounding area with sterile occlusive dressing and tape securely on three sides Chest tube	Tension pneumothorax

Hemothorax (blood in pleural space)	Decreased breath sounds on affected side
	Dullness on percussion
	Elevation of hemidiaphragm or blunting of costophrenic angle on upright CXR
	Reevaluate on serial x-rays
		Chest tube if increasing hemothorax on serial CXRs
		Transfusion if hypovolemic shock
		Thoracotomy for:
		  Blood loss > 2–4 mL/kg/hr from chest tube[a]
		  Massive air leak[a]
			Shock
			Respiratory distress

Rib fractures	Tachypnea Shallow respirations Rib fractures on CXR	Pain management Prevention of atelectasis (forceful exhalation, e.g., blowing bubbles or a pinwheel) Evaluate infants/young children for nonaccidental trauma	Atelectasis and pneumonia Respiratory failure
Traumatic asphyxia	Visibly striking petechia and cyanosis on face, neck, and chest Retinal and subconjunctival hemorrhages	Supportive care Gradual spontaneous resolution	
Myocardial contusion (bruise of cardiac muscle)	Arrhythmias such as premature ventricular contractions (PVCs) and tachycardia	12-lead electrocardiogram (ECG) Cardiac isoenzymes troponin I and CPK-MB[b] Cardiac monitor and close observation for arrhythmias Most require no therapeutic intervention	Sudden dysrhythmias
Cardiac tamponade (blood in pericardial sac)	Hypotensive in spite of appropriate fluid resuscitation Positive ultrasound	Aspiration of nonclotting blood on pericardiocentesis is diagnostic and initial treatment Thoracotomy and repair of injury	Decreased cardiac output secondary to restriction of ventricular filling

[a]Cooper, A. (1995). Thoracic injuries. *Seminars in Pediatric Surgery, 4*, 109–115.
[b]Sartorelli, K. H., & Vane, D. W. (2004). The diagnosis and management of children with blunt injury of the chest. *Seminars in Pediatric Surgery, 13*, 98–105.

Evaluation

A detailed history of the mechanism of injury is very helpful in the initial evaluation of a child with abdominal trauma. Careful serial monitoring and recording of vital signs and repeated physical examinations are extremely important in determining hemodynamic stability in the child who may have ongoing blood loss from an intra-abdominal organ injury. Inspection of the abdomen may demonstrate such visible injuries as lap belt abrasions or contusions across the lower abdomen, the distinctive circular contusion from the end of a bicycle handlebar, or the site of a penetrating injury. These visible injuries provide clues to potential intra-abdominal organ injuries. Gastric distention occurs frequently in young children who have gulped air while crying, have had an esophageal intubation, or have received bag-valve-mask ventilation. Gastric distention caused by these mechanisms is relieved by placement of an orogastric tube connected to suction. Interpretation of a child's response to abdominal palpation is likely to be more difficult than that of an adult's in that they are often crying and frightened and state that it hurts anywhere they are touched.

The initial screening performed for peritoneal and pericardial fluid is often the focused abdominal sonography for trauma (FAST), performed by either radiologists or surgeons trained in this procedure. The results of these studies may demonstrate the presence of free fluid, which is indicative of a possible solid organ injury. However, ultrasound studies are operator dependent. If a FAST is performed immediately on arrival in the ED, sufficient blood may not have accumulated to be visible. If there is continuing suspicion of an abdominal organ injury, the FAST should be repeated or an abdominal/pelvic CT obtained to identify the presence of solid organ injury. The abdominal CT is the mode of choice for diagnosis of solid organ injuries because of its sensitivity, specificity, and accuracy (Alonso et al., 2003; Stylianos, 2005). Diagnostic peritoneal lavage (DPL) indicates the presence of blood or intestinal contents in the peritoneal fluid. It was frequently used before the wide availability of CTs but is used only rarely now, such as when a child is obtunded or requires immediate surgical intervention for other injuries and has a neurologic injury. Laparoscopy is also starting to be used for diagnosing and treating abdominal injuries in hemodynamically stable children (Feliz, Schultz, McKenna, & Gaines, 2006).

Hemodynamic stability after resuscitation is the most reliable determinant in the decision to manage a child with intra-abdominal solid organ injury nonoperatively (Alonzo et al., 2003). Serial hemoglobin and hematocrit levels correlate with solid and some hollow abdominal organ injuries. The decision to transfuse a child with decreasing hemoglobin and hematocrit levels is made on the basis of the presence of abnormal tissue perfusion and vital signs. Hemodynamically stable children with hemoglobin levels ≥ 7 g/dL do not require a blood transfusion (Umali, Andrews, & White, 1992); however, if hemorrhaging continues in a hemodynamically stable child, angiography and embolization should be considered.

Specific Injuries

Blunt abdominal trauma in children most commonly injures the spleen, liver, and kidney, with an occurrence rate of 28% to 30% in each category. In contrast, 70% of children with penetrating injuries have damage to the intestinal tract. The liver is the second most frequently injured intra-abdominal organ in penetrating trauma, occurring 27% of the time (Cooper et al., 1994).

Splenic Injuries

Children with splenic injuries have pain and guarding in the left upper abdomen. The pain may radiate to the left shoulder, a symptom known as Kehr's sign. King and Shumacker (1952) reported an "increased susceptibility to infection" in young infants in whom the spleen had been removed. Francke and Neu (1981) found that the complete removal of a child's spleen subjected the child to an 85 times greater risk of developing overwhelming post-splenectomy infection, the mortality rate of which is approximately 50% (Tepas, 2000). Therefore, children in whom a splenectomy is necessary should receive penicillin prophylaxis, Pneumovax, and the *Haemophilus influenzae* type B vaccine. Upadhyaya and Simpson (1968) were the first to advocate nonoperative management of hemodynamically stable children with splenic rupture. They found that children who had isolated splenic injuries often had almost stopped bleeding from the injury by the time a laparotomy was undertaken. Today, nonoperative management of children with most splenic injuries is the standard of care. The requirements for nonoperative management of a splenic injury include close monitoring of the child with the involvement of a surgical team able to operatively manage the injury should that become necessary, as well as immediate availability of both blood for transfusion and a fully staffed operating room. The presence of a brain injury should not affect the decision to conservatively manage a child's splenic injury. A protocol for care of children with blunt abdominal trauma is seen in Figure 32-3. The consensus guidelines for isolated spleen or liver injuries proposed by the American Pediatric Surgical Association Committee on

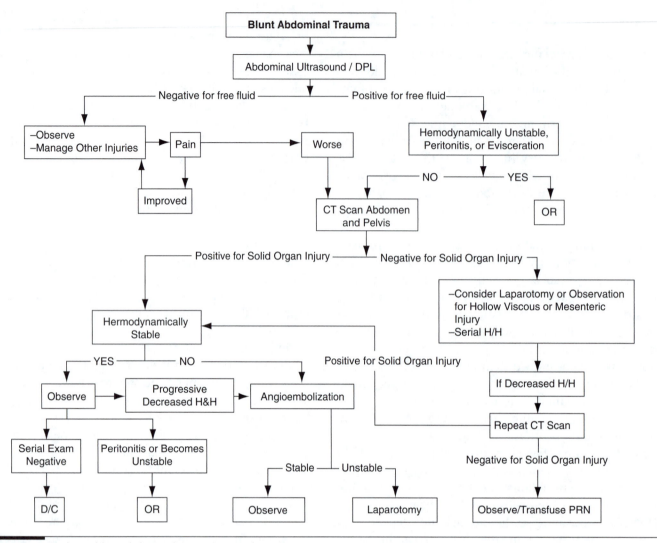

Figure 32-3 Pediatric blunt abdominal trauma protocol.
(Courtesy of J.J.Tepas, III, MD.)

Trauma are found in Table 32-7. Before discharge, the family should be instructed in the importance of restricting the child's activity, with guidelines for the length of time shown in the table. The length of time to radiographic evidence of a healed splenic injury is directly related to the significance of the injury.

Hepatic Injuries

Richie and Fonkalsrud first published the idea of nonoperative management of subcapsular liver hematomas in 1972. The same criteria used for surgical intervention for splenic injury (see Fig. 32-3) may also be applied for those hepatic injuries that do not involve damage to the hepatic veins, portal vein, or suprarenal inferior vena cava. Hemodynamically unstable children with liver injuries involving these major vessels or who have massive liver damage are at significant risk for exsanguination and re-

quire immediate operative intervention. Operative management is also indicated for children with a penetrating liver injury. A delayed, potentially disastrous, hemorrhage is more common in children who have hepatic rather than splenic injuries.

The most common long-term complication from liver injuries is bile leakage. As with splenic injuries, the length of time required for complete healing of a liver injury depends on the extent of the injury; consensus guidelines are presented in Table 32-7.

Pancreatic Injuries

The pancreas is relatively infrequently injured because of its retroperitoneal position. Motor vehicle crashes and bicycle handlebars, which compress the pancreas against the spine causing injury to the body or neck of the pancreas, are both common causes of pancreatic injuries.

Table 32-7	Proposed Guidelines for Resource Utilization in Children with Isolated Spleen or Liver Injury			
	CT Grade			
	I	**II**	**III**	**IV**
Intensive care unit days	None	None	None	1
Hospital days	2	3	4	5
Predischarge imaging	None	None	None	None
Postdischarge imaging	None	None	None	None
Activity restriction[a] (weeks)	3	4	5	6

Reprinted from *Current Opinion in Pediatrics*, 17, Stylianos, S. Outcomes from pediatric solid organ injury: Role of standardized care guidelines, p. 404, © (2005), with permission from Elsevier.

[a]Return to full-contact sports (i.e., football, wrestling, hockey, lacrosse, mountain climbing) should be at the discretion of the individual pediatric trauma surgeon. The proposed guidelines for return to unrestricted activity include "normal" age-appropriate activities.

Abdominal pain or tenderness and elevated levels of serum amylase and lipase are indications that an abdominal CT should be obtained to evaluate for a pancreatic injury. Treatment decisions are determined by the grade of the pancreatic injury on CT and the child's clinical status. Elevation of amylase levels may initially be delayed and may not correlate with the degree of injury to the pancreas. If there is no major ductal injury (grades I and II) and the child remains clinically stable, most pancreatic trauma may be managed nonoperatively. Nonoperative treatment for pancreatic injuries includes making the child NPO and initiating total parenteral nutrition until the elevated serum amylase levels approach normal and there is resolution of the abdominal pain. Shilyansky et al. (1998) reported that the average length of time to symptom resolution in children with nonoperatively managed pancreatic injuries was 15 days. The most common complication of pancreatic injuries is a pancreatic pseudocyst (40%), some of which require percutaneous drainage, whereas others resolve spontaneously.

Intestinal Injuries

Fourteen percent of children with intra-abdominal injuries from blunt mechanisms have damage to the gastrointestinal tract, involving the small bowel (64%) or the colon and rectum (21%) (Cooper et al., 1994). The most common of these mechanisms involves lap belts, where the child's torso is suddenly flexed at the hip and then thrown backward against the seat during rapid deceleration, compressing the abdominal contents between the lap belt and the child's spine. Careful evaluation for Chance fractures, burst fractures of lumbar vertebrae, should be made in any child with an intestinal injury caused by hyperflexion of the torso. Seventy percent of intra-abdominal injuries from penetrating trauma have damage to the gastrointestinal

tract involving the small bowel (40%) or the colon and rectum (39%) (Cooper et al.).

Prompt diagnosis of small bowel injuries remains problematic. Although extravasation of enteral contrast or pneumoperitoneum on CT indicates the presence of an intestinal injury, abdominal CT scans inconsistently demonstrate small bowel injuries. Other nonspecific findings on CT include bowel wall thickening, free intraperitoneal fluid without the presence of solid organ injury, and evidence of an ileus. Laboratory tests are nonspecific and do not aid in the diagnosis of small bowel injuries. Moss and Musemeche (1996) found that serial abdominal physical examinations in conscious patients were 100% diagnostic for small bowel injuries requiring operative intervention; all of them had abdominal tenderness on arrival. Jerby, Attorri, and Morton (1997) noted that children in their study who had diffuse abdominal tenderness were found to have major intestinal injuries at the time of surgery, in contradistinction to those with localized tenderness who had just minor intestinal injuries. Diagnostic laparoscopy is being used as an adjunct to CT to identify bowel injuries in some centers (Feliz et al., 2006).

Duodenal hematomas push the submucosa into the lumen of the duodenum, causing symptoms of a partial bowel obstruction. The diagnosis is made when a filling defect is seen on an upper gastrointestinal contrast study. Treatment includes gastric decompression, total parenteral nutrition, and resumption of enteral feeding as tolerated.

Renal Injuries

Renal injuries occur in 28% of children injured by blunt mechanisms and 10% by penetrating mechanisms. Ninety-five percent of renal injuries recorded in the NPTR-2 were blunt injuries (Cooper et al., 1994). Children are more likely to have renal injuries than adults because of the larger relative size of their kidneys and the general lack of protection of abdominal organs noted at the beginning of this section, in addition to children having less perirenal fat. The severity of a renal injury does not correlate to the degree of hematuria present. Children with clinical findings of abdominal or flank tenderness, blood at the urethral meatus, or pelvic instability should be further evaluated for genitourinary injuries regardless of the degree of hematuria.

Most children with renal injuries are hemodynamically stable and are managed nonoperatively. CT of the abdomen is the preferred diagnostic method for children with blunt trauma. It allows visualization of renal injuries while also evaluating for other intra-abdominal organ injuries. Before surgery, an intravenous pyelogram may be obtained even in children who are hemodynamically unstable secondary to gross renal pedicle disruption to demonstrate a functioning second kidney and for baseline renal perfusion. Children with penetrating injuries are evaluated with plain films and an intravenous pyelogram. Nonoperative management of renal injuries includes bed rest until gross hematuria clears and restricted activity until microscopic hematuria resolves. The potential for late-onset post-traumatic hypertension necessitates blood pressure evaluation every 6 months for at least 2 years after the injury.

■ Extremity Fractures

Incidence and Pathophysiology

Fifty-seven percent of the more than 31,000 pediatric trauma patients included in the NPTR-3 had at least one fracture, 21% of which were isolated extremity fractures. Of the 40% who had functional limitations at the time of discharge, 47% of those with 1 to 3 and 25% of those with ≥ 4 functional limitations had a fracture (DiScala, 1999). A significant impact is required to break a bone, and the most common mechanisms involve motor vehicles, with the patient being either inside the vehicle or struck by the vehicle, and falls. Nonaccidental trauma must also be considered in infants and young children who present with fractures if the stated mechanism is not consistent with the presenting injuries.

Evaluation

Evaluation of suspected extremity fractures includes the "five Ps": pain, pallor, pulses, paresthesias, and paralysis. Obvious or suspected fractures may be revealed by in-

spection. The bone may protrude through the skin, the extremity may have an abnormal bend or rotation when compared with the uninjured extremity, or there may be swelling or discoloration over suspected fracture sites. In addition, complaints of extremity pain should prompt further evaluation, including palpation of proximal and distal pulses and evaluation of sensation and movement distal to the area. A splint is applied to the extremity, including the joints above and below the injury. The splint stabilizes the fracture, prevents further neurovascular and soft tissue damage, decreases pain, and prevents a closed fracture from becoming an open one. There is the potential for significant blood loss into the dead space surrounding fracture sites. A sterile dressing is applied if there is an open wound present. In the ED, all extremities are evaluated, starting distally. Full gentle range of motion of joints in extremities without obvious fractures is performed. Injuries to soft tissues are recorded, as are the findings of the neurovascular examination of each limb. If open fractures are suspected, IV antibiotics are initiated. A tetanus shot is given if the child has not had one within the previous 5 years.

Anterior-posterior and lateral radiographs of any suspected fracture sites, including the joints above and below, are taken. Children have active growth plates and a significant amount of cartilaginous tissue in their skeletons, making the interpretation of their radiographs significantly more difficult than those of an adult. The growth plate is involved in up to one third of pediatric fractures, with possible long-term consequences of progressive angular deformity, limb length discrepancy, joint incongruity, and greater chance of refracture of the growth plate. Other fractures seen in children that are not found in adults include greenstick fractures, traumatic bowing or plastic deformation, and torus or buckle fractures.

Table 32-8 provides a list of specific extremity injuries, their signs and symptoms, treatments, and complications.

■ Psychosocial Issues

Care of the Child

Developmentally appropriate explanations of pending procedures should be provided to injured children, including those with a decreased level of consciousness. General pediatric nursing textbooks include information on developmental stages. Wong (1982) provides a concise review of developmentally appropriate nursing interventions specifically related to pediatric trauma patients. Child life therapists render a tremendous service by help-

Table 32-8 Specific Extremity Fractures

Bone Fractured	Common Injury Mechanisms	Treatment Modalities	Potential Complications

Humerus	If < 3 years old, often nonaccidental trauma[a,b]
	Backward fall onto outstretched hand
	Fall onto side of arm
	Direct force, high energy
		Proximal fractures[a]
		  Shoulder immobilizer if minimally displaced
		  May require OR or CR with PP
		Shaft fractures
		  Coaptation splint and sling[a,b]
		  Young children: sling and wrap around chest[c]
		Supracondylar fractures[b]
		  Nondisplaced: long-arm cast
		  Displaced
		    CR with cast, traction, or PP
		    OR usually followed by PP
			Supracondylar fractures[a]
			Brachial artery injuries
			Compartment syndrome
			Nerve damage
			Malunion

Radius and ulna	Forward fall onto outstretched hand	Immobilization with cast or splint
		Closed (almost all) or open reduction[b]
		May need Kirschner wires or IM fixation[c]
			Compartment syndrome, may be made worse by cast or splint. Split cast to prevent[b]
			  Malunion (most common)[a,b]
			  Peripheral nerve injury[a,b]
			  Refracture[a,b]
			  Growth arrest[b]

Femur	Nonaccidental trauma, especially if under age of 1[a,b] Hit by motor vehicle Bicycle crash High-speed motor vehicle crash	Traction splint in field Flexible IM rods[c] Immediate or early spica cast, especially in younger children with shortening < 3cm[d] Traction with delayed spica cast[c] Skin traction: generally if younger than 8 years old Skeletal traction: older children and subtrochanteric fractures needing 90°–90° position	Overgrowth causes longer than normal leg length when healed if not ~1 cm shortening in traction; best if side-to-side apposition of bones[c]

Tibia (~70% tibia with fibula[c])	Motor vehicle crash
	Hit by motor vehicle
	Falls
	Sports (older children)[d]
		Non- or minimally displaced fractures
		  CR, long-leg cast, non-weight bearing
		Unstable fractures
		  PP[d] or external or flexible IM fixation[a]
		Displaced fractures of tibia and fibula[d]
		  Knee and ankle immobilization in long-leg cast
		  Ice packs at fracture site
		  Leg elevation
		  Adolescents may need flexible IM fixation[c]
		Open fractures
		  External fixation or long-leg cast with window[d]
			Compartment syndrome[a,d]
			Vascular injuries[d]
			Leg length discrepancy[d]
			Delayed or nonunion[a,d]
			Angular deformity[d]
			Open fractures: high risk of infection[a,d]
			Valgus deformity worsens for 12 to 18 months after injury, then spontaneous improvement[a,d]

NOTE: All patients with open fractures need to have a tetanus booster (if none within past 5 years), IV antibiotics, and be taken urgently to the OR for débridement, irrigation, and fracture stabilization.[a-d]

[a]Price, C. T., Phillips, J. H., & Devito, D. P. (2001). In R. T. Morrissy & S. L. Weinstein (Eds.), *Lovell and Winter's pediatric orthopaedics* (Vol. 2, 5th ed., pp. 1319–1422). Philadelphia: Lippincott Williams & Wilkins.

[b]Herring, J. A. (2002b). Upper extremity injuries. In J. A. Herring (Ed.), *Tachdjian's pediatric orthopaedics* (pp. 2115–2250). Philadelphia: Saunders.

[c]Staheli, L. T. (2001). Trauma. In L. T. Staheli (Ed.), *Practice of pediatric orthopedics* (pp. 203–262). Philadelphia: Lippincott Williams & Wilkins.

[d]Herring, J. A. (2002a). Lower extremity injuries. In J. A. Herring (Ed.), *Tachdjian's pediatric orthopaedics* (pp. 2251–2438). Philadelphia: Saunders.

CR, closed reduction; IM, intramedullary; OR, open reduction; PP, percutaneous pinning.

ing to make the hospital a less threatening place and by decreasing the boredom. Regression and behaviors not usually exhibited at home are common among hospitalized children. Trauma or pediatric psychologists help the child and the family adapt to the stresses surrounding the child's injury, as well as providing significant support to the staff.

Post-traumatic stress disorder (PTSD) has been found at approximately the same rate in children exposed to violence and those involved in motor vehicle–related injuries. In addition, de Vries et al. (1999) found no correlation between the severity of injury and the emergence of PTSD. Presence of PTSD in parents was associated with younger children, children who had PTSD, and their having seen the injury occur. An elevated heart rate during ED triage and being female both independently were risk factors for development of PTSD (Kassam-Adams, Garcia-Espana, Fein, & Winston, 2005).

Care of the Family

Families of injured children are often initially distraught. One of the most precious things in their lives has been hurt and they frequently express feelings of guilt, "If only I had ____, this wouldn't have happened." It is important to encourage families to make use of pre-established support systems in addition to making them aware of services provided in the hospital, including pastoral care, social services, and the trauma psychologist. Particularly when a child is critically injured, they often cannot bring themselves to leave the premises for the first several days. They should be encouraged to have friends bring them food and clean clothes and to take care of responsibilities at home, such as other children or pets. The family needs to understand that the nursing staff will take care of their child, but only they can take care of their own personal needs, such as sleeping, eating, and showering. They need a great deal of energy to endure their child's hospital stay, even without any setbacks. The family may feel as if they are on an uncontrolled roller coaster ride, and tired parents are less capable of tolerating the situation. Parents should be encouraged to participate in their child's care and should be asked to share information about how their child has coped in the past. Families often want to share stories and pictures of their child before the injury, which helps the staff to better understand the dichotomy the family is attempting to reconcile.

Families often repeat the same questions. Let them know that their stress levels are so high that you do not expect them to remember all that they are told. They should be encouraged to ask if they do not understand something. The child's nurse should try to be present when physicians are talking to the family both to be sure that the family understands the explanation and so that the nursing staff is able to reinforce what the family has been told. Encourage families to write down the questions they have for a particular physician or service, to ensure that the questions are not forgotten when the appropriate person is available.

Families need to know about hospital and unit policies regarding visitors, including sibling visitation, food in the child's room, cellular phones, and to whom information regarding the child's status will be given over the telephone. Written information about the unit that includes these policies is helpful to families. It is important that policies are consistently enforced across all shifts.

■ Discharge Planning

Discharge planning for trauma patients ranges anywhere from making sure the child has a safe ride home in an appropriate car seat or restraint device to calling the organ procurement organization (OPO). Priorities for discharge planning must be set quickly because lengths of hospital stays continue to decrease. Before discharge, future problems that may occur as a result of the child's injuries should be discussed with the family. Many children who have survived brain injuries have difficulties transitioning back to school. Parents need to know that if their child starts having difficulties at home or school, the child may require a neuropsychological evaluation. The names and office telephone numbers of health care providers involved in their child's care should be provided to the parents. Managed care may complicate obtaining follow-up appointments with physicians who have provided care in the hospital. Insurance companies generally have a case manager who helps with discharge arrangements for home equipment, supplies, nursing, physical/occupational/speech therapies, and outpatient appointments. Arrangements for home tutoring should be made according to local guidelines.

Optimal rehabilitation for injured children allows them to reach their maximum post-injury potential. Unfortunately, not all children who could benefit from rehabilitation are given that option. A referral to an appropriate rehabilitation hospital should be made shortly after admission on any moderately to severely brain-injured child to prevent delay in transfer.

In some instances, children with severe brain injuries are candidates for organ donation. The OPO should be notified according to state and institutional guidelines. A perfusion scan that demonstrates absence of cerebral blood flow is presently considered the best brain death confirmatory study because the neurons cannot survive without oxygen carried by the blood. However, brain death determination must be made according to state regulations. The family should be told of that determination before the OPO discusses organ donation with the family unless the family requests to speak with them earlier. Many families are extremely grateful to have the opportunity to have something positive come from the death of their child.

■ Current and Potential Research

A tremendous amount of epidemiologic data have been collected regarding pediatric injuries, the largest repository of which is the NPTR. Movement toward a secure, HIPAA-compliant, web-based pediatric trauma registry will allow data entry and retrieval via the Internet from anywhere in the world, and that will allow researchers to write their own queries, is under way. These types of data are valuable in determining local and national directions for, and effectiveness of, injury prevention programs.

Research is currently being conducted on several aspects of brain injury, including more effective methods of intracranial hypertension control, the use of biomarkers to predict long-term outcomes of brain-injured patients, and long-term outcomes from minor brain injuries. Additionally, studies evaluating the connection between effective glycemic control and avoidable morbidity are under way. Other research involves the use of screening laboratory studies to assess for intra-abdominal injuries, with the potential for decreasing radiation exposure as compared with current screening methods.

■ Conclusion

Nurses who care for injured children need to be fully cognizant of pediatric anatomic and physiologic characteristics and to appreciate the differences in children of varying ages, developmental levels, and sizes. It is also necessary to anticipate what those differences will mean with respect to any given child's response to a traumatic injury and the treatments that follow. The most effective method to decrease the morbidity and mortality associated with pediatric trauma continues to be injury prevention.

■ Acknowledgments

I would like to thank Chris McKenna for reviewing this chapter and for her excellent suggestions, and Clara Lindley for all of her good-natured technical support.

References

Alderson, R., & Roberts, I. (2005). Corticosteroids for acute traumatic brain injury. Cochrane Library, retrieved September 23, 2005, from the Cochrane Database of Systematic Reviews.

Alonso, M., Brathwaite, C., Garcia, V., Patterson, L., Scherer, T., Stafford, P., et al. (2003). *Practice management guidelines for the nonoperative management of blunt injury to the liver and spleen.* Retrieved December 23, 2005, from the Eastern Association for the Surgery of Trauma Web site: http://www.east.org/tpg/livspleen.pdf

American College of Surgeons Committee on Trauma. (2004). *ATLS: Advanced trauma life support for doctors, student course manual* (7th ed.). Chicago: American College of Surgeons.

Baraff, L. J. (1993). Capillary refill: Is it a useful sign? [Commentary]. *Pediatrics, 92,* 723–724.

Bernardo, L. M., Clemence, B., Henker, R., Hogue, B., Schenkel, K., & Walters, P. (1996). A comparison of aural and rectal temperature measurements in children with moderate and severe injuries. *Journal of Emergency Nursing, 22,* 403–408.

Birkland, P. (1993). International update: Two successful Canadian programs teach teenagers trauma prevention. *Journal of Emergency Nursing, 19,* 35A–36A.

Bullock, M. R., Chestnut, R. M., Clifton, G. L., Ghajar, J., Marion, D. W., Narayan, R. K., et al. (2000). *Management and prognosis of severe traumatic brain injury.* Brain Trauma Foundation and American Association of Neurological Surgeons.

Committee on Trauma, American College of Surgeons. (1998). *Resources for optimal care of the injured patient: 1999.* Chicago: American College of Surgeons.

Cooper, A., Barlow, B., DiScala, C., & String, D. (1994). Mortality and truncal injury: The pediatric perspective. *Journal of Pediatric Surgery, 29,* 33–38.

de Vries, A. P. J., Kassam-Adams, N., Cnaan, A., Sherman-Slate, E., Gallagher, P. R., & Winston, F. K. (1999). Looking beyond the physical injury: Posttraumatic stress disorder in children and parents after pediatric traffic injury. *Pediatrics, 104,* 1293–1299.

Dieckmann, R. A. (2004). Pediatric assessment. In M. Gausche-Hill, S. Fuchs, & L. Yamamoto (Eds.), *APLS: The pediatric emergency medicine resource* (4th ed., pp. 20–49). Boston: Jones and Bartlett.

DiScala, C. (1999). *National pediatric trauma registry biannual report, October 1999.* Boston: Research and Training Center at Tufts University School of Medicine New England Medical Center and the American Pediatric Surgical Association.

Feliz, A., Shultz, B., McKenna, C., & Gaines, B. A. (2006). Diagnostic and therapeutic laparoscopy in pediatric abdominal trauma. *Journal of Pediatric Surgery, 41,* 72–77.

Francke, E. L., & Neu, H. C. (1981). Postsplenectomy infection. *Surgical Clinics of North America, 61,* 135–155.

Gorelick, M. H., Shaw, K. N., & Baker, M. D. (1993). Effect of ambient temperature on capillary refill in healthy children. *Pediatrics, 92,* 699–702.

Hackbarth, R. M., Rzeszutko, K. M., Sturm, G., Donders, J., Kuldanek, A. S., & Sanfilippo, D. J. (2002). Survival and functional outcome in pediatric traumatic brain injury: A retrospective review and analysis of predictive factors. *Critical Care Medicine, 30,* 1630–1635.

Halley, M. K., Silva, P. D., Foley, J., & Rodarte, A. (2004). Loss of consciousness: When to perform computed tomography? *Pediatric Critical Care Medicine, 5,* 230–233.

Hawley, C. A., Ward, A. B., Magnay, A. R., & Long, J. (2004). Outcomes following childhood head injury: A population study. *Journal of Neurology, Neurosurgery, and Psychiatry, 75,* 737–742.

Hazinski, M. F., Zaritsky, A. L., Nadkarni, V. M., Hickey, R. W., Schexnayder, S. M., & Berg, R. A. (Eds.). (2002). *PALS provider manual.* Dallas, TX: American Heart Association.

Holmes, J. F., Sokolove, P. E., Brant, W. E., & Kuppermann, N. (2002). A clinical decision rule for identifying children with thoracic injuries after blunt torso trauma. *Annals of Emergency Medicine, 39,* 537–540.

Jennett, B., & Teasdale, G. (1977). Aspects of coma after severe head injury. *The Lancet, 1*(8017), 878–881.

Jerby, B. L., Attorri, R. J., & Morton, D., Jr. (1997). Blunt intestinal injury in children: The role of the physical examination. *Journal of Pediatric Surgery, 32,* 580–584.

Kassam-Adams, N., Garcia-Espana, J. F., Fein, J. A., & Winston, F. K. (2005). Heart rate and posttraumatic stress in injured children. *Archives of General Psychiatry, 62,* 335–340.

King, H., & Shumacker, H. B. (1952). Splenic studies. *Annals of Surgery, 136,* 239–242.

Kokoska, E. R., Smith, G. S., Pittman, T., & Weber, T. R. (1998). Early hypotension worsens neurological outcome in pediatric patients with moderately severe head trauma. *Journal of Pediatric Surgery, 33,* 333–338.

Lescohier, I., & DiScala, C. (1993). Blunt trauma in children: Causes and outcomes of head versus extracranial injury. *Pediatrics, 91,* 721–725.

Luten, R. C., Wears, R. L., Broselow, J., Zaritsky, A., Barnett, T. M., Lee, T., et al. (1992). Length-based endotracheal tube and emergency equipment in pediatrics. *Annals of Emergency Medicine, 21,* 900–904.

Mandelstam, S. A., Cook, D., Fitzgerald, M., & Ditchfield, M. R. (2003). Complementary use of radiological skeletal survey and bone scintigraphy in detection of bony injuries in suspected child abuse. *Archives of Disease in Childhood, 88,* 387–390.

Marcin, J. P., Schembri, M. S., He, J., & Romano, P. S. (2003). A population-based analysis of socioeconomic status and insurance status and their relationship with pediatric trauma hospitalization and mortality rates. *American Journal of Public Health, 93,* 461–466.

Martin, V., Langley, B., & Coffman, S. (1995). Patterns of injury in pediatric patients in one Florida community and implications for prevention programs. *Journal of Emergency Nursing, 21,* 12–16.

Moss, R. L., & Musemeche, C. A. (1996). Clinical judgment is superior to diagnostic tests in the management of pediatric small bowel injury. *Journal of Pediatric Surgery, 31,* 1178–1182.

National Center for Injury Prevention and Control. (n.d.). *Overall: All Injury Causes: Nonfatal Injuries and Rates per 100,000—2004; Homicide Injury Deaths and Rates per 100,000—2002; Self-Harm: All Injury Causes: Nonfatal Injuries and Rates per 100,000—2002; Suicide Injury Deaths and Rates per 100,000—2002.* Retrieved December 23, 2005, from http://www.cdc.gov/ncipc/wisquars

National Vital Statistics System, National Center for Health Statistics, CDC. (n.d.). *10 Leading Causes of Death by Age Group—2002.* Retrieved September 23, 2005, from ftp://ftp.cdc.gov/pub/ncipc/10LC-2002/PDF/10lc-2002.pdf

Nersesian, W. S., Petit, W. R., Shaper, R., Lemieux, D., & Naor, E. (1985). Childhood death and poverty: A study of all childhood deaths in Maine, 1976 to 1980. *Pediatrics, 75,* 41–50.

Pressley, J. C., Barlow, B., Durkin, M., Jacko, S. A., Dominguez, D. R., & Johnson, L. (2005). A national program for injury prevention in children and adolescents: The Injury Free Coalition for Kids. *Journal of Urban Health: Bulletin of the New York Academy of Medicine, 82,* 389–402.

Richie, J. P., & Fonkalsrud, E. W. (1972). Subcapsular hematoma of the liver: Nonoperative management. *Archives of Surgery, 104,* 781–784.

Rubin, D. M., Christian, C. W., Bilaniuk, L. T., Zazyczny, K. A., & Durbin, D. R. (2003). Occult head injury in high-risk abused children. *Pediatrics, 111,* 1382–1386.

Sartorelli, K. H., & Vane, D. W. (2004). The diagnosis and management of children with blunt injury of the chest. *Seminars in Pediatric Surgery, 13,* 98–105.

Schafermeyer, R. (1993). Pediatric trauma. *Emergency Medicine Clinics of North America, 11,* 187–205.

Shilyansky, J., Sena, L. M., Kreller, M., Chait, P., Babyn, P. S., Filler, R. M., et al. (1998). Nonoperative management of pancreatic injuries in children. *Journal of Pediatric Surgery, 33,* 343–349.

Stylianos, S. (2005). Outcomes from pediatric solid organ injury: Role of standardized care guidelines. *Current Opinion in Pediatrics, 17,* 402–406.

Stylianos, S., & Eichelberger, M. R. (1993). Pediatric trauma: Prevention strategies. *Pediatric Clinics of North America, 40,* 1359–1368.

Tepas, J. J., III. (2000). Pediatric trauma. In K. L. Mattox, D. V. Feliciano, & E. E. Moore (Eds.), *Trauma* (4th ed., pp. 1075–1096). Stamford, CT: Appleton & Lange.

Tepas, J. J., III, Mollitt, D. L., Talbert, J. L., & Bryant, M. (1987). The pediatric trauma score as a predictor of injury severity in the injured child. *Journal of Pediatric Surgery, 22,* 14–18.

Umali, E., Andrews, H. G., & White, J. J. (1992). A critical analysis of blood transfusion requirements in children with blunt abdominal trauma. *The American Surgeon, 58,* 736–739.

Upadhyaya, P., & Simpson, J. S. (1968). Splenic trauma in children. *Surgery, Gynecology and Obstetrics, 126,* 781–790.

US Department of Health and Human Services, Administration on Children, Youth, and Families. (2005). *Child maltreatment 2003.* Retrieved October 14, 2005, from http://www.acf.hhs.gov/programs/cb/publications/cm03/cm2003.pdf

Vernon-Levett, P. (2003). Traumatic brain injury in children. In P. A. Moloney-Harmon & S. J. Czerwinski (Eds.), *Nursing care of the pediatric trauma patient* (pp. 171–188). Philadelphia: Saunders.

Wong, D. L. (1982). Childhood trauma: Its developmental aspects and nursing interventions. *Critical Care Quarterly, 5,* 47–60.

Burn Care of Children

By Robin Moushey, Lisa Meadows, and Jennifer Seigel

Almost half of the estimated 2 million burn injuries that occur each year involve children (Passaretti & Billmire, 2003). The burn insult is a devastating life event. The physical and psychological stability of the child is destroyed, disrupting the family and affecting caregivers. Improved management of burn patients, including such areas as fluid resuscitation, nutrition, and infection control, has resulted in a decline in burn mortality. A multidisciplinary approach is integral to the care of the burned child.

The skin is the largest organ in the body, making up 15% of total body weight (Sharp, 1993). The skin functions to protect from injury and infection, prevent loss of body fluids, regulate body temperature, and provide sensory contact with the environment, all of which are crucial to survival.

Younger children are at higher risk for a significant burn because they have a larger body surface area per pound of weight than adults. A child's epidermis is thinner, causing deeper injuries at shorter heat exposures. The type of agent and the length of time the child is exposed to the burning agent primarily determine the depth of the burn. Scald and contact burns occur most commonly in the birth to 2-year-old age range, and thermal burns occur most frequently in the 5- to 20-year-old group (Danks, 2003).

Children have a curious nature, an inability to protect themselves, and a thin epidermis, which makes them vulnerable to significant burn injuries. The stressors of the burn trauma to the child are numerous. Children suffer the painful and frightening occurrence of the trauma itself and are not able to integrate the experience to help them expand their coping mechanisms. Multiple family members may be involved in the actual trauma. Often, children feel guilty for the cause of the accident and for failure in saving the lives of others. Loss of siblings and/or parents compounds the grief that children experience. Burn injuries result from accidental or intentional events. The child should be carefully assessed and questions should be asked to determine the circumstances of the injury. Social work involvement is integral in the initial burn assessment. One should keep an open mind and provide support for the family throughout the child's hospitalization.

Many principles in this chapter can be used in caring for children with other devastating skin or tissue loss. This chapter discusses the following aspects of pediatric burn management: assessment of burn acuity and initial care, children's risk for airway obstruction, fluid requirements, assessment of body surface area and burn depth, pain management, burn wound management, nutrition, infection, and the multidisciplinary approach to care.

Assessing Burn Acuity

Prehospital care for burns includes all the components of trauma stabilization, including assessment and support of airway, breathing, and circulation. Prehospital interventions specific to burn care include the removal or extinguishing of the heat source followed by application of clean, dry materials to prevent hypothermia (Table 33-1). Moist coverings cause hypothermia and hypoperfusion to tissues and should be avoided. The body surface area burn (BSAB) should be estimated.

Assessing the burn wound percentage is a dynamic process. Various assessment methods exist. The rule of nines, which divides the body into areas of 9%, is used with adults but can result in dangerously high BSAB estimates in children because this method does not incorporate the increased body surface area of the head. The Lund and Browder chart, which divides each body part into a percentage, considers changes in body surface area that occur during childhood development (Fig. 33-1). A quick assessment is made by using the child's hand to equal 1% of his total body surface area. Field personnel without access to the Lund and Browder chart should use this palmar method or simply describe the injury to the receiving hospital (e.g., half of the arm).

Field personnel contact the burn center with the necessary information to prioritize care of the child in the acute management phase. These critical variables include age of the child, airway involvement, BSAB, location of the burn, burning agent, and time the burn occurred.

On admission to the hospital unit, the burn care team examines the child after removing all clothing, jewelry, and coverings used in transport. The burn is covered immediately with a warm, dry sheet or blanket. The child should not be exposed unnecessarily. Overhead warming lights or other exogenous heat sources should be used to maintain body temperature. The child's state of consciousness should be evaluated, and the presence of other injuries should be assessed. See Table 33-2 for a checklist of the initial assessment of the child with burns.

Children who fulfill one or more of the American Burn Association criteria adapted for the pediatric population are candidates for admission or transfer to a burn center (Table 33-3). One advantage of a pediatric burn center is its ability to provide intensive care monitoring. See Table 33-4 for suggested admission criteria to a burn intensive care unit.

Airway Management

All children with burn injuries should be immediately assessed for airway patency. Edema formation from fluid shifts (third spacing) and inflammation can compromise the airway of children with burns several hours after injury. These children should be reassessed continuously. Children with the following categories of burn injuries are at high risk for airway compromise: house fires; found in isolated confined area surrounded by flames (e.g., crib); burns covering the face, neck, or chest; electrical burns; and BSAB greater than 20%.

The child with a major burn is placed on a pulse oximeter with 100% oxygen administered. Blood gases and carboxyhemoglobin levels are obtained as indicated. The young child with a small airway diameter does not need circumferential burns around the neck or chest to have impaired ventilation. Early blood gases may have satisfactory results, but if airway edema progresses, hypercapnea results and respiratory acidosis develops.

The extent of smoke inhalation injury may be misleading in the young child. Children caught in a house fire often hide rather than escape. Flames may surround an isolated crib or playpen. Obvious signs of smoke inhalation are facial burns, soot in airways, singed hair, hoarseness, and dysphagia. History obtained from the scene includes altered level of consciousness and apnea.

Damage to the airway comes from varied factors. Direct thermal insult to the airway is usually limited to the upper airway (Smith, 2000). Toxins from combustion can be absorbed systemically or can cause direct injury to the tracheobronchial lining. Carbon monoxide and cyanide are absorbed systemically, whereas direct injury is caused by exposure to aldehydes, hydrochloride, chlorine, and ammonia (Sharp, 1993).

Carbon monoxide poisoning occurs when carbon monoxide has been inhaled and absorbed by the pul-

Table 33-1	**Tips to Transport the Burned Child**

1. Extinguish source of heat.
2. Remove clothes and jewelry.
3. Wrap in dry blanket or multiple sheets.
4. Do not soak burns in saline or water.
5. Keep child warm.
6. Cooling causes vasoconstriction, which decreases blood flow to both burned and unburned tissue. Soaking the burn in saline or water causes hypothermia and hypoperfusion. Keep the child warm!

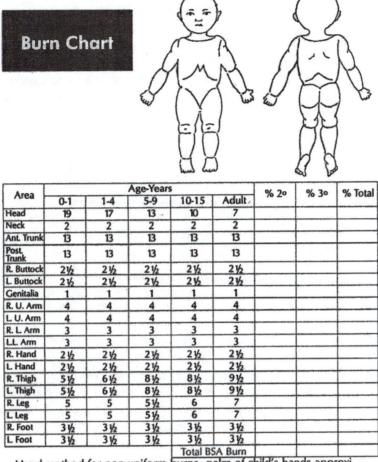

Burn Chart

Area	Age-Years					% 2°	% 3°	% Total
	0-1	1-4	5-9	10-15	Adult			
Head	19	17	13	10	7			
Neck	2	2	2	2	2			
Ant. Trunk	13	13	13	13	13			
Post. Trunk	13	13	13	13	13			
R. Buttock	2½	2½	2½	2½	2½			
L. Buttock	2½	2½	2½	2½	2½			
Genitalia	1	1	1	1	1			
R. U. Arm	4	4	4	4	4			
L. U. Arm	4	4	4	4	4			
R. L. Arm	3	3	3	3	3			
L.L. Arm	3	3	3	3	3			
R. Hand	2½	2½	2½	2½	2½			
L. Hand	2½	2½	2½	2½	2½			
R. Thigh	5½	6½	8½	8½	9½			
L. Thigh	5½	6½	8½	8½	9½			
R. Leg	5	5	5½	6	7			
L. Leg	5	5	5½	6	7			
R. Foot	3½	3½	3½	3½	3½			
L. Foot	3½	3½	3½	3½	3½			
					Total BSA Burn			

Hand method for non-uniform burns—palm of child's hands approximates 1 percent of child's total BSA burn.

Figure 33-1 Lund and Browder Chart (body surface area).

monary circulation, displacing oxygen from the red blood cells and decreasing the capacity of the blood to carry oxygen to the cells in the body. The carbon monoxide binds with the hemoglobin 250 times more readily than oxygen does and is then converted to carboxyhemoglobin. Oxygen levels decrease and hypoxemia develops.

Normal carboxyhemoglobin levels are 5% to 10%, with the half-life of carboxyhemoglobin being 5 hours on room air and 1 hour on 100% oxygen (Walker, 1996). Therefore, the carboxyhemoglobin level obtained in the emergency department may be lower than the level obtained in the field. Scherb (1990) states that "COHgb levels are not accurate indicators of the degree of poisoning. The signs and symptoms exhibited by the patient, especially the level of consciousness, are important when determining the severity of poisoning" (p. 144).

Symptoms of carbon monoxide poisoning include nausea and vomiting, headache, irritability, confusion, decreased consciousness, and respiratory failure. These symptoms may be confused with pain, hypoxia, head injury, electrolyte abnormalities, anxiety, or separation from parents. Cherry-red discoloration may be detected in mucous membranes but is difficult to assess because of irritation and inflammation from the injury itself. Once a child has been diagnosed with carbon monoxide poisoning, humidified oxygen should be supplied at 100% by means of a tight-fitting nonrebreather mask. The oxygen saturation may appear normal or falsely elevated in smoke inhalation because the hemoglobin molecule carrying carbon monoxide and/or oxygen is recognized by the pulse oximetry. Respiratory rate, depth, rhythm, and breath sounds should continue to be assessed, and arterial blood gases and carboxyhemoglobin levels should be followed.

A difficult decision is whether to intubate a child who initially is breathing on his own. When in doubt, the child should be intubated. Early intubation saves the child considerable airway trauma. The goal is to perform an

Table 33-2	Checklist for Initial Assessment of the Child with Burns
Airway	Facial/neck burns, perioral burns: (nose, lips, mouth, or throat); singed nasal hairs, eyebrows, facial soot, carbon particles in the mouth or sputum, circumferential burns of the chest. Observe for patency of airway: stridor/wheezing, difficulty swallowing, hoarseness, chest excursion, respiratory rate, depth, rhythm
Breathing	Place patient on 100% humidified O_2 + oximeter if at risk for compromised airway; evaluate respiratory rate, depth, rhythm, and breath sounds; obtain ABGs and carboxyhemoglobin as indicated. Assess for signs of CO poisoning; report of decreased respirations or apnea at scene; cherry red normal skin; confusion/coma; increased carboxyhemoglobin. Assist with intubation procedure if patient is not breathing effectively or obstruction is possible. Observe for circumferential full-thickness burns of the thorax that might decrease chest expansion. Assist with escharotomy, if necessary
Circulation	Cut clothing off and remove all watches, rings, other jewelry. Cover child with warm blankets. Cardio-respiratory monitor. Assess for signs of adequate cardiac output every 15 minutes: quality, rate, and rhythm of central and peripheral pulses; color; capillary refill; BP; level of consciousness; children with 10% but less than 15% BSA burn = maintenance IV fluid rate; children with 15%–20% BSAB = start 2 large-bore IVs
	Maintenance IV fluid rate + resuscitative fluid volume (4 mL lactated Ringer's × kg body weight × % BSAB); 1/2 total volume in first 8 hours (calculate based on time of initial burn injury), remainder 1/2 to be infused over 16 hr (hr 9–24); use fluid warmer to deliver IV fluids; maintain UO 1–2 mL/kg/hr
	Laboratory tests: CBC, comprehensive metabolic panel, type and cross-match
Secondary Survey	Weigh the patient; assist in assessment of BSAB; insert Foley catheter with > 20% BSAB
	Insert NG tube in children with > 20% BSAB. Monitor for nausea, vomiting, and presence of ileus
	Observe for circumferential full-thickness burns of the extremities; observe for any open wounds that might indicate open fractures related to the mechanism of injury or trauma; elevate injured extremities
	Make baseline assessment of all affected extremities and reassess every 15–30 minutes: Peripheral pulses (brachial, radial, popliteal, pedal), Doppler as needed
	Extremity temperature, color, and capillary refill, pain or paresthesia
	Prepare for possibility of escharotomy
	Obtain urinalysis

BSA, body surface area; BSAB, body surface area burn; O_2, oxygen; CO, carbon monoxide; ABG, arterial blood gas; BP, blood pressure; IV, intravenous; CBC, complete blood count; NG, nasogastric; UO, urine output.

intubation in a controlled setting with the child adequately sedated rather than as an emergency procedure. It is essential for physicians, nurses, and respiratory therapists to work together to maintain airway integrity. See Table 33-5 for suggestions for securing an endotracheal tube in a child with facial burns.

With a circumferential full-thickness chest burn, if blood gases are not satisfactory or chest excursion is lim-

Table 33-3	American Burn Association Referral Criteria for Transfer to a Burn Center

1. Partial-thickness burns greater than 10% total body surface area
2. Third-degree burns
3. Burns that involve the face, hands, feet, genitalia, perineum, or major joints
4. Inhalation injuries
5. Electrical burns, including lightning
6. Chemical burns
7. Children requiring special social, emotional, or long-term rehabilitation in burn centers with qualified personnel
8. Children with pre-existing medical disorders or concomitant trauma that may affect mortality

Table 33-4	**Admission Criteria to a Burn Intensive Care Unit**

Intensive care monitoring is required for:
- Children < 2 years of age with body surface area burns < 15%
- Children > 2 years of age with body surface area burns > 20%
- Electrical burns
- Inhalation injuries
- Burns covering face/neck with potential airway obstruction

ited after intubation, chest escharotomies may be warranted to allow sufficient pulmonary expansion and oxygenation (see "Wound Assessment" later in this chapter).

■ Intravenous Fluid Guidelines

The goals of burn fluid resuscitation are to restore vascular volume, perfuse the kidneys, and replace sodium losses. Loss of plasma and interstitial fluid from damaged skin and capillaries has an impact on the child's precarious water and electrolyte balance. Cytokines, histamines, and prostaglandins are some of the vasoactive mediators

Table 33-5	**Suggestions for Securing Endotracheal Tube on Child with Facial Burns**

Securing the endotracheal tube (ET) on children with burns on the face and neck is challenging. The following interventions are helpful:
- Use tracheostomy ties to secure the ET tube around the head. These ties are larger than umbilical tape and are less likely to cause pressure points on edematous tissue.
- Suture the ET tube. One suture is placed inside the mouth, and a second suture is inserted under the chin through the mandible. The ties are brought up and tied around the ET tube. Circum-mandibular stabilization causes less damage to nares; suture immediately after intubation.
- Wire ET tube to dental plate. Although this provides adequate security, it usually cannot be done immediately.
- Place isolation masks backward on the child, and use the ties to secure the ET tube. This is a short-term temporary intervention.
- Use protective skin barriers on unburned skin when possible to secure ties or tape.
- There are various commercial products to secure ET tubes, but these may prove to be less beneficial for the young child.

released in a stress response that effect edema formation (Demling, 2005). The lymphatic system is also disrupted. Sodium and protein molecules leave the capillaries and enter the interstitial space, raising oncotic pressure. This increase in oncotic pressure pulls water from the capillaries, causing a fluid shift from vascular to interstitial compartments, otherwise known as *third spacing*. This process is seen in both burned and unburned tissue. This process continues for approximately 24 hours after injury until capillary healing begins.

Other factors contribute to the complexity of fluid management in the patient with burns. Cardiac output is decreased in major burns by the release of a myocardial depressant factor. The release of antidiuretic hormone conserves water while aldosterone retains sodium with accompanying water retention. Both actions restrict urine output. Kidney perfusion and urine output can be severely disrupted 24 hours after burn injury unless fluid loss is replaced and hydration is maintained. Clinically, the child may have edematous interstitial tissue but a decreased vascular fluid volume.

Obtaining and maintaining adequate hydration of the child with burns require careful assessment and ongoing reevaluation. Overhydration can cause increasing tissue edema, compromising perfusion to body tissues. Insufficient fluid replacement decreases the flow of oxygen to the tissues, compromising kidney function. Adequate tissue perfusion enhances the oxygenation of both burned and unburned tissue, which is essential for optimal outcomes (Carvajal, 1994).

Composition of intravenous (IV) fluids and the most accurate assessment of satisfactory clinical outcomes for the child have been discussed in the burn community for decades. For simplicity, in this chapter, the pediatric resuscitative guidelines of the American Burn Life Support Manual (American Burn Association, 2005a) are used. Additional information can be found in the American Burn Association's publications that refer to burn assessment, management, thermal injuries and shock and fluid resuscitation (American Burn Association, 2005b, 2005c, 2005d).

Calculate fluid resuscitation from the time of initial burn injury, not from the time the child arrived at the emergency department. Appropriate fluid resuscitation depends on an accurate patient weight and BSAB after wound débridement (Cubison & Gilbert, 2005).

IV replacement fluids are calculated at 3 to 4 mL/kg/hr multiplied by the percent BSAB (American Burn Association, 2005a). One half of the total volume is given over the first 8 hours, and the remainder is given over the next 16 hours (Table 33-6). The maintenance fluid volume for

Table 33-6	General IV Guidelines According to BSA Burn (BSAB)		
	<10%	**10%–15%**	**>15%**
Location of IV line	Peripheral	Peripheral	Peripheral Difficult access: cutdown, central line, intraosseous infusion
Purpose	Hydration for child with limited PO intake Pain medication administration	Hydration for child with limited PO intake Pain medication administration	Resuscitation related to size of burn wound; hydration for child with limited PO intake or NPO status Pain medication administration
IVF rate	Maintenance	Maintenance	Maintenance fluid rate: + resuscitation: 3–4 ml LR × KGBW × BSAB 1/2 total volume over first 8 hr. Remainder given over next 16 hr.

IVF = Intravenous fluid

each child is added to the IV fluid replacement order (Fig. 33-2).

The composition of lactated Ringer's (LR) solution is close to normal body fluids and is a commonly used resuscitation IV fluid (275 mOsm/L; Na 130; K 4; Ca 3; Cl 109; lactate 28). Albumin is administered specific to each burn center's guidelines; however, it is usually not administered within the first 24 hours. Once initial fluid resuscitation orders are completed, IV fluids should be monitored and adjusted. Ongoing assessment of fluid status of the burn patient includes monitoring vital signs, physical examination, serial hematocrits, blood urea nitrogen, specific gravity, and adjusting for ongoing fluid losses. Urine output should be maintained at 1 to 2 mL/kg/hr.

As capillary and lymphatic function begins to return to the preburn state, kidney perfusion increases and diuresis occurs. Intravenous fluid composition and rates are adjusted to the child's response to therapy.

■ Wound Assessment

Skin exposure to a hot source can destroy the epidermis and the dermis-containing glands and hair follicles. Intense and prolonged heat exposure can damage subcutaneous and adipose tissue. The depth of tissue damage caused by fire and electrical sources may be evident immediately. However, burns occurring from grease, contact, and scalds can take 24 to 72 hours before the actual depth is mani-

Age	Kg	24° Maintenance IV Fluid	Hourly IV Rate* (for maintenance fluids)
1 mo	3	300 cc	13 cc/hr
3 mo	6	600 cc	25 cc/hr
6 mo	8	800 cc	33 cc/hr
1 yr	10	1000 cc	42 cc/hr
2 yr	12	1100 cc	46 cc/hr
4 yr	16	1300 cc	54 cc/hr
6 yr	20	1500 cc	63 cc/hr
8 yr	25	1600 cc	67 cc/hr
10 yr	30	1700 cc	71 cc/hr
12 yr	40	1900 cc	79 cc/hr
14 yr	50	2100 cc	88 cc/hr
*Add Burn IV Fluid Resuscitation if >15-20% BSA Burn (4cc/kg/%BSA burn)			

Figure 33-2 Pediatric intravenous maintenance rates.

fested. Overall goals for wound management include débriding, cleaning, and protecting the wound; minimizing infection; and maximizing function. Accurately describe the wound rather than labeling the depth of the burn (Table 33-7).

Full-thickness and partial-thickness injuries can occur simultaneously in a burn wound. Sensation and capillary refill should be assessed by gentle palpation only. Appearance of intact hair follicles during immediate wound assessment does not rule out the possibility of a full-thickness injury.

When edema is present in full-thickness injury, circumferential eschar prevents further expansion of tissues. Blood vessels become compressed, and ischemia develops. Although it is difficult to assess in a burned patient, the hallmark signs and symptoms of diminished circulation are cool, pale, painful, or tingling extremities, and/or pulselessness with immobile digits and poor capillary refill. Full-thickness circumferential burn injuries that result in vascular compromise require escharotomy. An escharotomy is indicated to allow blood flow to distal extremities or to enhance compliance of chest wall ventilation. By definition, a full-thickness burn has no sensation; however, the child's state of consciousness and level of anxiety require pharmacologic intervention before an escharotomy.

An escharotomy is performed with a scalpel or electrocautery and consists of making a longitudinal incision through both ends of the circumferential burn eschar. Minimal blood loss occurs. The incision should be deep enough to penetrate the eschar. As tissues release occurs, the subcutaneous fat bulges through the incision, tension is relieved, and effective blood flow returns. Once the initial incision is made, pulses should be reassessed. If they are nonpalpable, one should consider extending the incision to ensure that the incision extends through the entire eschar. Children with persistent signs of ischemia or those with fourth-degree injuries (e.g., involvement of muscle or bone, or electrical injury) may be at risk for compartment syndrome, necessitating fasciotomies.

■ Pain in Children with Burns

Children who are burned require appropriate pain management. Pain is a symptom of traumatic loss of body tissue and should be treated accordingly. Some burn dressing changes require general anesthesia for adequate pain management. A common mistake made in the pain management of a child with a burn is testing the child's tolerance to the initial procedure before increasing pain medication. Children enter a shocklike state after injury that can mask their expressive ability during the first burn dressing. Although it is difficult to predict the most effective pain management plan for a child with new burns, providing a dose that gives the maximum coverage for pain and anxiety is optimal. The initial experience of the child sets the stage for behavioral consequences for the rest of the hospitalization and after discharge.

Initial assessment criteria for appropriate pain management include the child's age and realistic behavioral expectations, BSAB, age of burn, burning agent, depth of burn, the child's previous experiences and coping mechanisms, and medical history. Additional issues are the response of the child and family, time necessary for débridement and whirlpool, nutritional concerns, and difficulty in maintaining IV access. During a dressing change, physical and occupational therapy can also increase the child's pain. This should be considered when the child's pain medication needs are assessed.

It is helpful to look at wound and pain management in three phases. The acute phase is usually 24 to 72 hours after injury. The goal during this period is aggressive pain control and wound débridement. Decisions are made regarding surgical débridement and/or skin grafting and application of alternative dressings. A combination of oxycodone and midazolam (Versed) decreases pain and anxiety in children before the dressing procedure. Nurses can administer dosages safely according to the institution's guidelines. Children may require supplemental IV medications (e.g., ketamine, morphine, propofol, fentanyl) or nitrous oxide to obtain adequate pain control. These agents should be given by trained personnel and monitored per hospital protocol.

The transition phase follows the acute phase when the switch is made from IV medications to oral pain medications or a combination of both. Children can participate more actively in wound care after their acute pain

Table 33-7	Classification of Depth of Burn Injury
Superficial (first degree)	Erythema; mild edema and pain; blanches with pressure
Partial thickness (second degree)	Pink to red; moist; moderate edema; extremely painful; vesicles
Full thickness (third degree)	Waxy-white to black; dry leathery; thrombosed vessels; edema; painless
(fourth degree)	Dry; leathery; black; painless; possible exposed bones, tendons, muscles

has been addressed. The exact timing of this phase depends on the treatment plan and the child's previous response to care. Antianxiety medication, such as midazolam, may still be required in addition to the narcotic analgesics. If the child displays uncontrollable irritability from the midazolam, the agent can be reversed with IV flumazenil (Romazicon), and the symptoms can be alleviated with IV morphine, acetaminophen with codeine, or diphenhydramine (Benadryl). Place the child in a nonstimulating environment.

Once most of the wound is epithelialized or grafted, the child enters the healing phase. Medications such as acetaminophen with codeine, combinations of acetaminophen and oxycodone, and/or diphenhydramine are used during the healing phase in the hospital and at home. Children with severe burns who have received narcotics for pain relief for an extended period require a plan to wean them carefully and methodically off the narcotics. Otherwise, signs and symptoms of withdrawal become evident.

Because there are tremendous variations in pain management methods, the side effects and the child's individual response to the medications should be continually assessed. Possible side effects of any sedative are respiratory depression, nausea, vomiting, and irritability. If the child with respiratory compromise responds quickly to oxygen and airway positioning, the medication should be resumed the following day. If the child does not respond quickly to the preceding measures, the daily medications should be changed, or taking the child to the operating room for future dressing changes and pain management should be considered.

To help alleviate the pain, the use of play, distraction, music and video therapy, toys, stories, and especially the child's participation with wound care is highly valued. A child as young as 18 months can press gauze between the toes or hold the tape to participate in wound care. Blowing bubbles is an optimal form of play and distraction for children. The pain service supports the acute phase with aggressive pain management during wound débridement. The transitional stage is a collaborative shift from pain management by the pain service to more psychological supportive efforts by child life service. These efforts are continued during the child's healing phase.

◼ Wound Care

The objective of wound care is to keep the burned area clean and moist. Epithelial cells thrive better in a moist environment. Epithelial cells are forced to exert more energy to burrow under the scar and lay down new cells

(David, 1987). Wound exudates consist of serum, colonizing bacteria, and dead leukocytes. Mechanical, chemical, or surgical débridement that decreases the accumulation of eschar is needed before healing takes place. This allows the effective use of topical ointments and/or the early use of alternative dressings.

Consistency is essential in burn care to assess the wound and evaluate the effectiveness of any treatment plan and dressing application. Wound care approaches are based on the stage of burn progression. Once-a-day dressing changes are adequate for débridement when a child is appropriately sedated. Wound treatment plans, although chosen for effectiveness and ease of use, should always consider patient comfort.

On initial débridement, all blisters should be removed, except those on the palms of the hands and the soles of the feet (Sharp, 1993). These blisters may require débridement if range of motion is restricted. Although intact blisters serve as a biologic dressing, clinical experience shows that they usually do not remain intact.

Historically, 1% silver sulfadiazine has been the most commonly used topical agent on burn wounds. It provides moisture and has an antimicrobial effect. Silver sulfadiazine cream, 1/16 to 1/8 inch thick, is applied to the wound before wrapping with gauze. A side effect of silver sulfadiazine is leukopenia, which may not be a true allergic reaction but rather the bone marrow's response to the stress of the burn. If a skin rash develops after reapplication of the silver sulfadiazine, the child may have an allergy to products with sulfa.

In the past several years, dressing impregnated with silver ions have become available and have been shown to be as effective as silver sulfadiazine. Many of these newer products do not require daily dressing changes, which decreases pain and anxiety for the child. The drainage from the burn wound activates the silver ions in the dressing, allowing a continuous release of silver into the wound. Biobrane-L (light adherence) is a synthetic substance that can be applied to a partial-thickness burn wound once it is cleaned and débrided. Biobrane consists of layers of collagen, silicone, and nylon and allows visibility of the wound. It is available in different sheet sizes or gloves. The Biobrane is stretched over a clean wound, and the edges are adhered onto nonburned areas with adhesive strips. This facilitates drainage to pass through the pores of the Biobrane instead of accumulating on the wound. A bulky dressing is wrapped over the Biobrane and then covered with an Ace wrap to provide additional pressure. To ensure Biobrane's adherence, movement and range of motion exercises are minimized 24 to 48 hours after application. Daily wound débridement is eliminated because Biobrane is left on the wound until it is healed.

Small burn injuries can be managed in the primary care setting. The same principles are used as in the inpatient management of burn wounds, including obtaining a history of the burn, evaluating the extent of the wound, and using pain management strategies. Families should be offered suggestions about burn wound management materials to avoid excessive costs. The list of options in wound management increases each year, and references to many of these are in the Wound Care Product Glossary in Appendix 33-A. Wounds can be wrapped with a white 100% cotton T-shirt, pillowcase, or sheet that has been cut up and rewashed for a cost-saving method. Tube socks can be cut and used over arms/legs. Panty liners without deodorant can be used for gauze.

Deep partial or full-thickness wounds that require an extended period of time to heal usually require excision and grafting in the operating room. Excisions may be tangential or fascial. In tangential excisions, thin layers of necrotic tissue are excised until bleeding tissue is reached. In deep excision, all necrotic burn and subcutaneous tissue is removed until the superficial fascia is visualized (Sadowski, 1992). The choice of excision method depends on the depth of burn and the surgeon's preference for the optimal graft bed.

Autografts are obtained from the child's own body and may be split thickness or full thickness. Split-thickness grafts consist of epithelium and part of dermis. These grafts are applied as either sheet grafts or mesh grafts, depending on the location of the burn and the surgeon's preference. A sheet graft is skin taken from a donor site and directly placed over the burn bed. A mesh graft is skin taken from a donor site and placed through a mesher that stretches the skin two to three times its size. If the child does not have adequate skin for autografting, donor skin is used. Allografts or homografts are tissue from same species (i.e., cadaver skin), whereas xenografts or heterografts are tissue from different species (e.g., pigskin).

Leaving the donor site open to air in children is not recommended. Children scratch the area, causing damage to budding tissue. Even when children are medicated for itching, protecting the donor site remains a problem in pediatric care.

Nutrition

The metabolic needs of children with burn injuries increase with tissue destruction, daily nitrogen losses, and postburn hypermetabolism (Sadowski, 1992; Sharp, 1993). The hypermetabolic state is 1.5 to 2 times the norm for the child and lasts until the wound is epithelialized or grafted (Sadowski). The patient should be assessed for an ileus and monitored for nausea and vomiting for 24 to 48 hours. A nasogastric tube is placed for decompression in any child with greater than 20% BSAB. Children with less than 15% BSAB should receive a high-calorie and high-protein diet with snacks or supplemental nutrition formulas. A feeding tube is placed in children with greater than 15% to 20% BSAB for continuous 12- to 24-hour enteral feedings with supplemental calorie intake to meet calorie needs. Caloric needs are adjusted based on the percentage of burn, activity level, and stress level (e.g., physical therapy, dressing changes, infection, fever, and operating room visits). Although they are able to consume an oral diet, few children are able to take in adequate calories. Often, nasogastric or nasojejunal feedings are needed to supplement oral intake. Early enteral feedings promote gut motility and prevent intestinal ischemia (Sadowski).

Translocation of the gastrointestinal flora, which is the release of gram-negative bacteria and endotoxins from the bowel lumen, contributes to the development of sepsis in the burned patient. Central venous total parenteral nutrition should only be used on those children who cannot tolerate enteral feedings. When enteral feedings are administered, the following are helpful hints for securing enteral tube position. Hydrocolloid wafers and transparent dressings are helpful when used on intact skin or the enteral tubing may be tied or secured to the endotracheal tube or around the head. The area under the ties should always be assessed for undue pressure caused by edema formation. Use arm cuffs when necessary to ensure that the tube stays properly placed.

Infection

One of the major risk factors for mortality in children with burn injuries is infection. The primary barrier to infection is lost when the body loses the skin's protective covering. The burn wound colonizes with organisms within 24 hours of exposure to the environment. The initial contaminant comes from the child's own skin flora. Additionally, many children admitted with burns may have a preexisting upper respiratory infection that is exacerbated with the trauma of the burn.

To heal the child, health care providers perform many procedural interventions that increase the risk of infection. Intubation, blood gas monitoring, IV access, Foley catheters, and nasogastric tubes are key risk factors. The use of systemic antibiotics has increased burn wound survival. However, the control of gram-negative/positive flora by broad-spectrum antibiotics may result in burn wounds becoming colonized by opportunistic yeast fungi. For this reason, antibiotics are used judiciously for the treatment of infections. Early surgical débridement and grafting allow for faster wound closure, establishing a new barrier to infection. Providing adequate nutrition stimulates the gastrointestinal tract, reduces the risk of translocation of organisms, and provides nutrients to heal (Periti & Donati, 1995).

Children who have been burned initially have difficulty maintaining body temperature. However, they soon enter a hypermetabolic state in which their hypothalamus "resets," and it is usual for them to run a low-grade temperature. Initial temperature spikes to 39 °C are common, but when they occur 48 hours after the burn, the child should be assessed for sepsis and other signs of common childhood infections (e.g., otitis media, influenza). White blood cell changes, the child's activity and appetite, and the appearance of the wound or grafts are all variables to be considered. The child should be assessed, not the temperature. Children who have an unusual fever, hypothermia, anorexia, and/or change in sensorium or vital signs should be evaluated for the development of sepsis. Blood cultures should be drawn after a careful patient assessment is made.

■ The Multidisciplinary Approach to Care

Burn treatment progresses through three major components of care and requires a multitude of team members. The physiologic impact of burn trauma is addressed throughout the acute management phase. Optimal wound care during this time is facilitated by aggressive treatment of pain and anxiety. Children may express thoughts concerning survival and death. Guilt feelings may be heightened if children have played with matches and caused harm to family members and/or belongings. The burn team should work closely together to maximize family and child support.

The transitional phase evolves when the plan of care is established. The focus is on wound care, nutrition, infection control, and therapy. It is normal that children and families initially reject the sight of the burn injury. Acceptance is accomplished over time with support and patience. In the hospital, mirrors can be covered with cards and greetings until facial swelling decreases. However, whenever children request to look, they should be accommodated. A mirror should be available during treatment. When grafts are explained to children and families,

it is important to focus on the value of covering the skin first and dealing with cosmesis later. Discuss how skin color returns and make a game for the child to find signs of new skin budding. Pain medications can be adjusted to allow children to participate in burn care routines. This gives the child and family some mastery and control of care in the hospital, which can continue at home.

The healing phase coordinates efforts for full functional recovery of both physiologic and psychological domains. Transition to home is optimized by minimizing contractions, providing as "near normal" an appearance as possible, maximizing the child's coping ability and personal strengths, and alleviating the anxiety and painful memories of burn treatment. Physical and occupational therapists are key members of the team during this phase. This process could continue for months or years.

The multidisciplinary team addresses all these patient needs from admission to postdischarge. Relationships formed from this collaborative process stimulate and support the team to foster successful patient outcomes.

■ Conclusion

Burns in children can result in devastating injuries to the child and significant emotional trauma to the child and family. Appropriate management of the child with a burn requires knowledgeable and skilled caregivers from the prehospital phase and initial resuscitation, throughout the hospitalization, to rehabilitation and return to the home, school, and community. In addition to management of the burn wound itself, airway and nutritional support, fluid and pain management, and prevention of infection are also particularly important. A multidisciplinary team aids in the provision of comprehensive medical, psychosocial, and rehabilitative care to the child and family.

References

American Burn Association. (2005a). Advanced burn life support manual. Chicago: American Burn Association.

American Burn Association. (2005b). Initial assessment and management. Chicago: American Burn Association.

American Burn Association. (2005c). Pediatric thermal injuries. Chicago: American Burn Association.

American Burn Association. (2005d). Shock and fluid resuscitation. Chicago: American Burn Association.

Carvajal, H. (1994). Fluid resuscitation of pediatric burn victims: A critical approach. Pediatric Nephrology, 8, 357–366.

Cubison, T., & Gilbert, P. (2005). So much for percentage, but what about weight? Emergency Medicine Journal, 22, 643–645.

David, I. (1987). Tissue damage and repair. In Smith & Martin (Eds.), Wound management (pp. 1–21). United Kingdom: Martin & Dunitz.

Danks, R. (2003). A comprehensive review of the epidemiology & treatment of burn victims. Journal of Emergency Medical Services, 28(5), 118–139.

Demling, R. (2005). The burn edema process: Current concepts. *Journal of Burn Care and Rehabilitation, 26*(3), 207–227.

Passaretti, D., & Billmire, D. (2003). Clinical experience: Management of pediatric burns. *Journal of Craniofacial Surgery, 14*(5), 713–718.

Periti, P., & Donati, L. (1995). Survival and therapy of burn patients at the threshold of the twenty-first century: A review. *Journal of Chemotherapy, 7*(6), 475–502.

Sadowski, D. (1992). Care of the child with burns. In M. F. Hazinski (Ed.), *Nursing care of the critically ill child* (pp. 875–927). St. Louis, MO: Mosby.

Scherb, B. J. (1990). Carbon monoxide poisoning: Hyperbaric oxygenation preparations. *Dimensions of Critical Care Nursing, 9*(3), 143–149.

Smith, M. (2000). Pediatric burns: Management of thermal, electrical, and chemical burns and burn-like dermatologic conditions. *Pediatric Annals, 29*(6), 367–378.

Sharp, R. (1993). Burns. In K. Ashcroft & T. Holder (Eds.), *Pediatric surgery burns* (pp. 89–102). Philadelphia: W.B. Saunders.

Walker, A. (1996). Emergency department management of house fire burns and carbon monoxide poisoning in children. *Current Opinion in Pediatrics, 8*(3), 239–242.

Suggested Readings

American Burn Association. (1988, March). Hospital and prehospital resources for optimal care of patients with burn injury: Guidelines for development and operation of burn centers. *Journal of Burn Care and Rehabilitation,11*(2), 98–104.

Benjamin, D., & Herndon, D. (2002). Special considerations of age: The pediatric burn patient. In D. Herndon (Ed.), *Total burn care* (2nd ed., pp. 427–438). Philadelphia: W.B. Saunders.

Dise-Lewis, J. (2000). A developmental perspective on psychological principles of burn care. *Journal of Burn Care and Rehabilitation, 21*(5), 255–260.

Foglia, R., Moushey, R., Meadows, L., Seigel, J., & Smith, M. (2004). Evolving treatment in a decade of pediatric burn care. *Journal of Pediatric Surgery, 39*(6), 957–960.

Foglia, R., & Moushey, R. (1994). *Burn care resource manual.* St. Louis, MO: St. Louis Children's Hospital.

Herndon, D., Rutan, R., Alison, W., & Cox, C. (1993). Management of burn injuries. In M. Eichelberger (Ed.), *Pediatric trauma: Prevention, acute care, rehabilitation* (pp. 568–590). St. Louis, MO: Mosby.

Merk, T. (2001). Beyond the burns: Managing the pain and consequences of pediatric burns. *Journal of Emergency Medical Services, 26*(9), 66–75.

Merz, J., Schrond, C., Mertens, D., Foote, C., Porter, K., & Regnold, L. (2003). Wound care of the pediatric burn patient. *AACN Clinical Issues, 14*(4), 429–441.

Monafo, W., & Bessey, P. (2002). Wound care. In D. Herndon (Ed.), *Total burn care* (2nd ed., pp.109–119). Philadelphia: W.B. Saunders.

Rose, J. K., & Herndon, D. N. (1997). Advances in the treatment of burn patients. *Burns, 23*(1), 519–526.

Sheridan, R. (2001). Comprehensive treatment of burns. *Current Problems in Surgery, 38*(9), 643–756.

Weed, R., & Berens, D. (2005). Basics of burn injury: Implications for case management and life care planning. *Lippincott's Case Management, 10*(1), 22–29.

Weisman, S., Bernstein, B., & Schlechter, N. (1998). Consequences of inadequate analgesia during painful procedures in children. *Archives of Pediatric and Adolescent Medicine, 152*, 147–149.

Appendix 33A		**Wound Care Product Glossary**

Product	Phase	Description/Use
Adaptic	Transitional Healing	Protective sterile dressing with a light petroleum coating. May be used to keep healing wound or donor site moist and clean; used in combination with Polysporin for small open areas and healed wounds that have been abraded.
Allevyn	Healing	Absorbent hydrophilic polyurethane dressing containing three layers: (1) nonadherent contact layer; (2) highly absorbent central layer (10 times more absorptive than 4 $\times$ 4s); and (3) waterproof outer layer. Placed on wound pink side up and generally used with IntraSite gel to calm granulation tissue.
Alloderm		Human dermal graft that can be applied to a debrided wound. It is then covered by an ultra-thin wide meshed skin graft.
Biobrane	Acute Transitional	An ultra-thin semipermeable silicone membrane mechanically bonded to a flexible knitted nylon fabric. Incorporates peptides and porcine collagen. Used over partial-thickness burns and sometimes over donor sites. Often used in conjunction with whirlpooling and occasionally with Silvadene. The large bore sheets are used to facilitate wound drainage. Comfortable dressing which protects nerve endings which are not irritated when the wound is cleaned. Decreases wound healing time. Not changed after first application.
Calcium Algonate	Transitional Healing	Generally used to control bleeding and absorb exudate. Promotes moist wound healing; may leave fibers in the wound.
Cultured Epithelial Autografts	Acute	Epithelial cells are harvested from the child's own skin to foster growth of epithelial cells and are used to cover large burned surface areas.
Elastogel	Healing	Gel-like substance used to soften scar areas and diminish keloid formation. May use under Jobst stocking.
Exudry	Acute Transitional	Permeable outer layer that allows wound to breathe; a cellulose layer used to promote a moist wound healing environment; a highly absorbent layer draws exudate and retains fluid; two nonadherent layers prevent shearing of grafts. Used for burns draining large amounts, or large burn surface area. Comes in sheets, pads, jackets, and gloves. Jacket application decreases endotracheal tube dislocation during dressing change.
Hyginet	Any	Elastic netting used to secure dressings, especially on scalp burns after wrapping with gauze.
Hypafix Tape	Any	Cloth-like tape that may be used to secure dressings. Works well on areas that are difficult to secure (areas with excessive sweating or moisture)
Integra		A bilayer skin replacement system. It contains a dermal replacement layer and an epidermal substitute layer (ESL). The ESL is eventually removed and covered with an autograft.
IntraSite Gel	Acute Transitional	Provides moist wound healing. Contains a starch substance that draws fluids out of the wound. Cleans and debrides the wound. Generally used on clean wounds with granulation tissue formation to help flatten tissue. Used on escharotomy/fasciotomy or avulsed wounds until closure can be performed.
Jobst Garment	Healing	Provides maximum pressure on a healed burn to minimize scar formation; fits tightly like a girdle. A positive pressure system measured to fit each area.
Mepiform	Healing	A silicone and polyurethane dressing that is used for the management of old and new hypertrophic and keloid scars. It is left on 24 hours. No supplemental adhesive needed.
Mepilex	Acute Transitional	A soft adhesive silicone foam pad that is non-adherent to moist wound beds. It is used on light to moderate draining wounds. It is left on the wound until strike-thru is seen on the outside of the dressing.
Mepitel	Acute Transitional	A silicone dressing bound to a porous net. Used for Epidermolysis Bullosa and low birth weight infants for skin protection, healing, and comfort (i.e., EKG leads). Change PRN. Topical antibiotic ointments are applied over the Mepitel.
N-Terface	Transitional Healing	Thin gossamerlike gauze dressing used in conjunction with Polysporin, Silvadene, or wet-to-dry dressing. Either surface may be placed next to the wound. It provides a protective covering and allows exudate to move away from the wound. Because it is protective, it allows some relief of discomfort. It may become adherent to the wound and may be left on for several days if wound is clean underneath. Use on wounds where no progression has been seen for several days, wounds with an angry red appearance, or in conjunction with Polysporin on open areas on healed wounds.
Scarlet Red	Transitional	Fine mesh, absorbent gauze impregnated with 5% scarlet red in a nonmedicinal blend of lanolin, olive oil, and petrolatum. Helps promote epithelial cell growth. Used to cover donor sites. Left in place under gauze dressing.
Transparent Dressing	Healing	Used over pink, clean burn wounds and to anchor Biobrane. Allows for easy visualization of wounds. Works better when wound is less weepy.
Tubigrip	Healing	Minimal support dressing used as an interim dressing pre-Jobst placement to help minimize keloid formation.
Xeroform	Transitional Healing	Petroleum-based antimicrobial dressing. Generally used as a moist protective dressing over skin grafts or as a donor site dressing.

Wound Management in Neonates, Infants, Children, and Adolescents

By Valerie E. Rogers

Caring for wounds is a fundamental part of the nursing care of children who have had surgery. Assessment, documentation, and communication regarding the condition of a wound are critical. Care and protection of the skin surrounding a wound are an essential part of wound care. Pain management is critical in postoperative wound care, both for the emotional well-being of the child and to expedite healing. Finally, wounds should be cared for as an integral part of the whole child and not as an entity that is somehow separate from the child.

Wounds in pediatric surgery patients are generally either the result of surgery, including closed and open incisions, or trauma. In addition, children occasionally develop nosocomial wounds, such as pressure ulcers. Nurses who care for children with wounds should develop an understanding of wound care in order to expedite wound healing, prevent infection, promote accurate communication both written and verbally, provide patient comfort, and prevent the development of institution-acquired wounds.

■ Wound Healing

Phases of Healing: An Orderly Progression

From the time of the initial injury, wounds follow an orderly and predictable progression through the wound healing process from injury to complete healing. This healing cascade is identical whether a wound is closed primarily or whether the wound is allowed to heal by secondary intention. Wound healing is an extraordinarily complex process. Many well-known cells in the body are involved in the healing process, including platelets, neutrophils, and lymphocytes, as well as many less well-known cells, such as keratinocytes, macrophages, and fibroblasts. Dozens of substances, including chemoattractants, hormones, and growth factors, are also recruited to the wound to take part in each phase of the intricate choreography of wound healing.

Wound healing progresses through four phases: hemostasis, inflammation, proliferation, and remodeling.

Although these phases overlap to some extent, each phase of healing occurs at a clearly identifiable time after sustaining a wound, and each has its own well-defined set of chemical and biochemical events that occur within that phase (Krummel & Blewett, 2003). Progression to a subsequent phase of wound healing depends on successful progression through the previous phase, so support of the healing process becomes imperative to closing a wound.

Immediately on sustaining a wound, the body senses disruption of the blood vessels in the wounded area and the phase of hemostasis begins. Platelets aggregate at the wound site and begin to form a fibrin clot to plug injured blood vessels. At the same time, vasoconstriction occurs to shunt blood away from the wound and prevent further blood loss. Vasoactive substances, chemoattractants, cytokines, and growth factors are released from the platelets as they break down, and these substances initiate and strengthen the inflammatory response, heralding the start of the second phase of wound healing.

Vasoactive substances cause local vasodilatation and increased permeability of the capillaries, leading to development of the common signs of the inflammatory phase, including erythema, edema, warmth, and exudate. Damage to the epidermis allows bacteria to penetrate one of the body's best defenses. In response, the body's cellular defenders are recruited to the wound within minutes to protect it from invading microorganisms. Early in the inflammatory phase, these cellular defenders are predominantly neutrophils. Within a day or so, monocytes are attracted to the wound from the circulatory system. Once in the wound, monocytes are renamed macrophages. The function of both neutrophils and macrophages is to engulf and destroy bacteria.

Necrotic tissue left in a wound continues to stimulate the inflammatory response and becomes detrimental to healing, so neutrophils and then macrophages act as a clean-up crew and cleanse the wound of dead cells and foreign matter. Macrophages produce chemoattractants that draw tissue-rebuilding cells to the wound, including fibroblasts and keratinocytes. The inflammatory phase peaks at about 3 days after injury and lasts for 4 to 6 days. Although critically important in cleaning and preparing a wound for closure, inflammation must be well regulated to allow the next phase of wound healing to proceed and to prevent engulfing the host in a systemic and life-threatening inflammatory response (Krummel & Blewett, 2003).

Once the clearing of bacteria and debris from a wound is well under way, the proliferation phase begins. During proliferation, which begins within hours of wounding, tissue is regenerated or replaced. Fibroblasts build a scaffolding or matrix of collagen, around which new granulation tissue is deposited. Granulation tissue forms as beefy red, puffy, vascular tissue that fills the defect created by the wound. Wounds closed by primary intention require little granulation tissue to fill the defect, and healing can proceed more quickly than in wounds healing by secondary intention, in which wound edges are not approximated.

Keratinocytes begin to resurface the wound with epithelial tissue. If hair follicles and other skin appendages are intact, as in partial-thickness wounds, keratinocytes harbored within these skin appendages spread out and around each appendage and regenerate the epidermis (Hunt, Hopf, & Hussain, 2000). In full-thickness wounds, however, the dermis is destroyed, and epithelialization, which is the process of replacing the epidermis, must proceed from the edges of the wound inward. At the same time, blood vessels are being formed in the new tissue, and the wound is contracting, or pulling inward. Contraction of the wound results in a smaller area to fill with granulation tissue and to cover with epidermis, thus speeding the process of healing. Although normally a useful component of wound healing, contraction of a wound over a joint can result in a contracture, limiting the mobility of the joint (Krummel & Blewett, 2003).

Once the wound is totally resurfaced with epithelium, proliferation slows down and finally ceases, and remodeling, the fourth stage of healing, begins. During the remodeling phase, the epidermis and underlying tissue mature and thicken. Tensile strength, or the ability of skin to withstand stretching without tearing, improves as collagen fibers reorganize along the skin's stress lines. However, tissue that heals by scar formation as a result of full-thickness tissue loss regains only 70% to 80% of the tensile strength of the skin prior to injury (Keswani & Crombleholme, 2005). Remodeling can last for a year or more. During this time, excess scar tissue is broken down, and the profile of a scar becomes less noticeable.

Factors Affecting Healing

Although wounds heal in an orderly and predictable way, there are a number of factors that can delay or inhibit healing. These factors can be local to the wound or systemic. Although not all factors that slow the healing process can be manipulated, understanding their effect on a wound allows the caregiver to anticipate problems and to create an environment that is most favorable to allowing a child's wounds to heal.

Local factors that impede wound healing include edema, pressure, desiccation or necrosis, maceration, and trauma. Edema is caused by leakage of serum from the capillaries during the inflammatory phase. During inflammation, capillaries become permeable in order to allow the escape of cells that are required at the wound site. Swelling is further exacerbated when the wound is in a dependent position. Fluid in the interstitial space squeezes closed the local capillaries supplying the wound, and blood flow is impeded. Therefore, circulation and the presence of edema around a wound should be assessed regularly, particularly in children with extremity wounds. As much as possible, wounded extremities should be positioned above the level of the heart to decrease venous congestion. Pressure also impedes blood flow to a wound. Capillaries are forced shut when they are squeezed between two hard objects, such as a mattress and a bony prominence. Children should be positioned to avoid pressure on their wound. If a child is not alert and mobile, and positioning is an issue because of a large wound or multiple wounds, pressure-relieving mattresses, and support devices should be employed.

Desiccation of a wound occurs when the wound is allowed to dry out. Fragile cells in the wound dehydrate and die, extending the area of tissue damage and destroying new tissue growth. Cell death creates necrotic tissue in a wound that prolongs inflammation and provides a medium for bacterial proliferation. A wound that has become desiccated becomes covered either with slough or with eschar. Both slough and eschar are dead tissue and are therefore undesirable. To prevent desiccation, the wound bed must be kept warm and moist. Maceration, on the other hand, occurs when too much fluid is allowed to sit in a wound. Surrounding skin becomes overhydrated and susceptible to irritation and breakdown. Both extremes should be avoided during wound healing, with the aim of maintaining a moist wound environment. Repeated trauma to a wound can also slow healing. Sources of trauma include dressings that damage new growth when removed, such as dry gauze that adheres to a wound; overly aggressive wound irrigation or cleansing, including the use of whirlpool; and use of harsh substances to cleanse a wound.

Systemic factors that delay wound healing include steroid use; connective tissue disorders, such as Ehlers-Danlos syndrome; diabetes; poor nutrition; pain; obesity; and infection. Steroids delay wound healing by inhibiting leukocyte and macrophage migration and by interrupting the inflammatory phase (Waldrop & Doughty, 2000). Elevated glucose levels in children with diabetes impair the ability of neutrophils to phagocytize bacteria and debris in a wound (West & Gimbel, 2000). Malnutrition is a major health problem in hospitalized patients (Stotts, 2000). It can occur in both acutely and chronically ill children and in premature infants born before their nutritional stores are fully developed. During wound healing, the body's metabolic demands are elevated. If, at the same time, a patient is malnourished, demands on the body for nutrients needed for tissue synthesis go unfulfilled, and healing can be delayed.

Obese children are often poorly nourished, but they have a number of other factors that impair wound healing as well. Compared with other tissues of the body, adipose tissue is poorly vascularized. As a result of poor perfusion, adipose tissue does not heal as well as other body tissues and is less able to combat infection. Tension on the suture line of an obese patient from the sheer weight of the tissue also impairs perfusion and predisposes to wound dehiscence. Obese individuals are prone to hematoma and seroma formation, and these pockets of fluid add to the pressure on the suture line and decrease tissue oxygenation. Finally, respiration can be impaired in obese individuals. Abdominal adipose tissue can impair excursion of the diaphragm during breathing and decrease tidal volume and vital capacity, reducing oxygenation (Wilson & Clark, 2004). Overall, obesity contributes to poor tissue oxygenation and delays healing.

Pain triggers a stress response that affects healing in two ways. Catecholamines are released during stress that cause vasoconstriction and diminished subcutaneous tissue oxygenation. Stress also causes secretion of adrenocorticotropic hormones that dampen the normal inflammatory response (Wilson & Clark, 2004). A comprehensive wound care plan must include measures to relieve stress and pain both pharmacologically, through appropriate pain medication and psychologically, using such measures as explaining procedures, involvement of a child life therapist during painful procedures, and use of distraction techniques.

Wound Infection and Surgical Site Infection

Infection can be both a local and a systemic cause of delayed healing of a wound. Infection disrupts the tensile strength of the developing tissue (Stotts, 2000) and often causes the wound to reopen. Local signs of wound infection include edema, induration, erythema and warmth of the periwound tissue, increasing or purulent drainage, change in wound or drainage odor, and increased wound pain. Systemic signs include fever, elevated leukocyte count with an increase in immature neutrophils (bands), and sudden elevation of blood glucose level (Stotts). Because of the increasing prevalence of antimicrobial-resistant bacteria, culturing infected wounds is recommended to identify infecting organisms and their antimicrobial susceptibility. Whenever possible, clean wound tissue rather than pus, slough, or eschar should be cultured.

Surgical site infection (SSI) or infection of a surgical wound, is a particular concern in children who have undergone surgery. An SSI is an incisional infection, or an infection that occurs in an organ or body cavity that has been entered or manipulated during surgery. Infection must occur within 30 days of the surgery to be classified as an SSI. Infection of implanted devices, such as central venous catheters with reservoirs or stainless steel bars placed for repair of pectus excavatum, can be considered an SSI for up to 1 year after surgery, if the infection can be attributable to the surgery. Stitch abscesses, infected newborn circumcisions, and infected burn wounds are not considered SSIs. Surgical site infections are the third most frequently reported nosocomial infection, making up 14% to 16% of nosocomial infections among hospitalized patients, and are the most common nosocomial infection among surgical patients. They are significant for increasing both the length and cost of hospitalization (Mangram, Horan, Pearson, Silver, & Jarvis, 1999). Although these statistics include all patients undergoing surgery and do not differentiate pediatric patients, pediatric surgery nurses are likely to care for children experiencing an SSI after surgery.

The most frequent organisms causing SSI are *Staphylococcus aureus*, coagulase-negative staphylococcus, *Enterococcus spp.* and *Escherichia coli*, with increasing frequency of *Candida albicans* and multiple antibiotic-resistant organisms, such as methicillin-resistant *S. aureus*, *Staphylococcus epidermidis*, and vancomycin-resistant enterococci (Mangram et al., 1999; Meakins & Masterson, 2003). Contributing patient factors are similar to those that delay wound healing, including diabetes, steroid use, obesity, and poor nutrition but also include infection at a remote site at the time of surgery, smoking, prolonged preoperative hospitalization, and extremes of age. Patients undergoing abdominal surgery or prolonged surgery are also at risk of developing SSI.

Although most SSIs are thought to be a result of endogenous contamination, nurses can help decrease their incidence in several ways. Before surgery, patients with remote sight infections, such as fungal diaper rashes or upper respiratory infections, can be identified and excluded from elective surgeries. Diabetic children should be maintained in tight glucose control during the perioperative period. If an adolescent is a known smoker, he or she should be encouraged to stop smoking before surgery. Although tobacco cessation is recommended for 30 days before surgery, even 1 week without smoking can help reduce the risk of SSI.

After surgery, the most important measure for preventing SSI is excellent hand-washing practices. Hands should be washed both before and after dressing changes and any contact with a surgical site. Even minimal contact with a colonized patient results in transfer of microorganisms. Meakins and Masterson (2003), for example, found that merely touching a patient's hand transferred 1,000 organisms. Postoperative incisions should be covered with a sterile dressing for 24 to 48 hours after surgery, sufficient time for epidermal resurfacing to occur and the barrier function of the skin to be restored (Cuzzell, 1990). At times, the initial postoperative dressing may require changing before 48 hours if it becomes saturated with blood or wound drainage, destroying the barrier function of the dressing. However, whenever possible, reinforcing a dressing during this period is preferable to environmental exposure of the surgical site during dressing change. Sterile technique should be maintained for all surgical dressing changes. Finally, families should be educated regarding proper incisional care and the signs of infection, because many SSIs occur after discharge (Mangram et al., 1999).

The Physiologic Wound Environment

Wounds heal best when a physiologic environment is maintained at the wound bed. A physiologic environment is one that mimics the environment of the body before wounding. Several factors are important in creating a physiologic environment, including moisture, temperature, perfusion, and bacterial burden. Maintaining moisture at the wound surface is probably the most important condition for healing. Moisture enhances removal of dead tissue and bacteria from the wound bed. It prevents desiccation of new tissue and sequesters growth factors and tissue building cells in the wound. Resurfacing of the epithelium occurs more rapidly with moisture. As a result, wounds that are kept moist heal faster, with less risk of infection and less scar formation than wounds that are allowed to desiccate.

Cells function best at normal body temperature. Allowing a wound to cool slows down wound repair. A decrease in temperature at the surface of the wound also causes vasoconstriction and diminishes blood flow to the wound. Cooling can occur through the use of dressings that permit evaporation of wound fluid, such as gauze; through frequent dressing changes that expose a wound to air; and through cleansing wounds with cold solutions. Warmth of a wound can be maintained through the use of moisture-retentive dressings and absorbent dressings that require minimal dressing changes, and by using room-temperature or warmed solutions for wound cleansing.

All wounds are contaminated by nature of their exposure to the external environment. However, they still heal along a normal trajectory if bacteria do not proliferate in the wound or invade healthy tissue. A high bacterial burden in a wound can slow healing. Maintenance of a moist and warm wound, proper wound cleansing to remove surface contamination, sterile technique during dressing changes, measures to prevent aerosolizing bacteria during dressing removal, and dressings that prevent bacteria from entering a wound all help control proliferation of microorganisms.

Communication in Wound Care

Understanding the Terminology of Wound Care

The use of common language in wound care is helpful in communicating with other health care providers. Familiarity with wound care terminology is also helpful in understanding the literature on wound care. Although there is no true standardization of terms and definitions, many terms have become established and accepted among people who research and provide wound care. Table 34-1 provides a list of terminology for wound care and descriptors of the terms. Many of these terms defy quantification or precise explanation, however, exemplifying the problem with standardization of a language to define wounds. Furthermore, these terms do not encompass the full range of descriptors needed for wound assessment. Nevertheless, they provide a starting point for communicating a patient's wound status for a nurse who is new to wound care.

Assessment and Documentation

Wound care involves much more than just changing a dressing. The healing status of a wound must be observed and communicated both verbally and in writing in the patient's record. This ensures that everyone involved in the care of a child with a wound is aware of the condition of that wound, of the care being performed on the wound, and of the progression of the wound toward closure. Not only are wound assessment and documentation legal obligations, they are essential for the development of team strategies to promote wound healing.

To assess the wound, the dressing must be removed. Old dressings should be manipulated and shaken as little as possible during removal, because microorganisms from the wound are aerosolized during dressing changes and can remain in the air for extended periods (Kerstein, 1995; Ovington, 2001), providing an exogenous source of wound contamination. The wound should be assessed and all pertinent information documented on the patient

record every time the wound is uncovered. Wounds closed by primary intention require fairly simple assessment, including approximation of the incision line; color of the surrounding skin; wound tenderness; presence of induration; presence, amount, and color of wound drainage; and presence of edema or any swelling at or near the incision. The integrity of sutures, staples, or adhesive strips should be noted. Any changes from the previous assessment should be documented and wounds showing signs of infection or deterioration should be reported. Finally, any wound care provided by the nurse should be recorded including type of dressing and its application, and actions taken when adverse wound outcomes are noted.

Documentation of wounds healing by secondary intention is more extensive than that of primarily closed wounds. Because most terms used in wound description are not quantifiable or standardized, assessments are judgmental and are greatly dependent on the wound care experience of the nurse. Assessment should include appearance of the wound and the periwound skin (the skin surrounding the wound); age of the wound (to determine the healing trajectory); size of the wound; presence of undermining (a cavity or empty space beneath the edge of the wound); type of tissue in the wound bed (e.g., granulation tissue, slough, eschar); amount and character of exudates; presence of an odor; and pain.

Wound status should always be compared with previous assessments so that progress can be noted. Consideration of the age of a wound gives some indication of the expected healing of the wound and whether healing is progressing as expected. For example, acute wound inflammation that extends beyond 4 days may indicate infection. The size of the wound should be measured with a measuring tape so that progression to closure can be assessed. The most reliable way to measure a wound is by measuring the longest length and the longest width of the wound (van Rijswijk, 2001). The axis along which these measurements are taken can be noted with the use of a clock face orientation, and a diagram can be drawn in the chart if needed for clarity. To measure the depth of a wound, place a cotton-tipped swab into the deepest part of a wound perpendicular to the skin. Mark the swab at skin level and compare the swab against a measuring tape. Occasionally, undermining is present in a wound. Undermining occurs as a result of tissue destruction and presents as an open pocket at the edge of a wound that extends beneath the intact periwound skin. A cotton-tipped applicator can gently be slipped into the area of undermining to measure its depth. Exposure of fascia, muscle, tendon, bone, or organ should be noted.

Table 34-1 Glossary of Wound Care Terms

Term	Definition
Adjuvant wound therapy	Therapeutic modalities used in wound care in addition to routine wound cleansing and use of advanced wound care dressings. Includes negative-pressure wound therapy, hyperbaric oxygen therapy, support (pressure reducing/relieving) surfaces, whirlpool, & physical therapy services.
Antiseptic	Substance that inhibits the growth and reproduction of microorganisms. Cytotoxic to healthy cells at full-strength dilutions. Includes povidone-iodine, hydrogen peroxide, silver, and sodium hypochlorite (Dakin solution).
Débridement	The process of removing dead or devitalized tissue and foreign matter from a wound. Four modalities include autolytic, chemical, mechanical, and surgical.
Autolytic débridement	The body's own enzymes and substances break down necrotic tissue.
Chemical débridement	Enzyme-containing agents applied to a wound to break down necrotic tissue without harming viable tissue. Include collagenase, papain/urea, and fibrinolysin, and deoxyribonuclease combination.
Mechanical débridement	Use of physical force to remove necrotic tissue. Can harm viable tissue. Includes wet-to-dry dressings, wound irrigation, whirlpool.
Surgical débridement	Removal of necrotic tissue with sharp instruments or laser.
Dehiscence	Separation of a surgical incision or closed wound. Caused by tension on the incision or fascia, infection, poor perfusion, connective tissue abnormalities, steroid use, immunosuppression.
Desiccation	Dehydration of living cells, leading to cell death.
Devitalized tissue	Dead or necrotic tissue. Includes eschar and slough.
Eschar	Thick, dry, black, leathery necrotic tissue in wound. Indicates full-thickness tissue destruction.
Slough	Stringy, loose, moist necrotic tissue in a wound, usually tan, yellow, or gray. Adheres to the underlying tissue.
Granulation tissue	Highly vascular tissue within a wound composed of cells and matrix (connective tissue). Supports the overlying epithelium in a healed, full-thickness wound.
Microbial wound status	Based on the presence, proliferation, and tissue invasion of microorganisms. Levels include contaminated, colonized, and infected.
Contaminated	Presence of microorganisms on a wound surface without proliferation. All wounds are contaminated.
Colonized	Presence and proliferation of infectious organisms within a wound. May or may not delay wound healing, but does not elicit signs of infection.
Infected	Proliferation of infectious organisms in a wound with invasion of healthy tissue. Host responds with signs of infection (erythema, edema, warmth, pain, change in exudate, odor).
Moist wound healing	Maintenance of moisture at the wound surface that is adequate to promote cellular activity and mobility, activate wound healing growth factors and enzymes, and prevent desiccation of tissue.
Surgical site infection (SSI)	Infection that occurs within an incision or a body cavity/organ that has been entered or manipulated during surgery. Occurs within 3 months of surgery, or in the case of an implant within 1 year of surgery, and can be attributed to the surgery.
Tissue rebuilding substances	Cells and substances involved in wound healing.
Chemoattractant	Substance that attracts cells and other necessary substances to a wound.
Collagen	Major structural proteins of the body. Gives skin its tensile strength.
Fibroblast	An immature connective tissue cell involved in the formation of granulation tissue and deposition of an extracellular matrix (framework for new tissue). Has a major role in protein synthesis and deposition of collagen in a wound.
Keratinocyte	Cell that differentiates into the layers of the epidermis.

(continues)

Macrophage	Type of leukocyte that migrates out of the circulatory system and into a wound during inflammation. Phagocytizes bacteria and secretes substances to clean the wound.
Wound closure	Methods of closing a wound. Includes primary, secondary, and delayed primary closure.
Primary wound closure	Skin edges are manually approximated, as with a surgical incision. Results in minimal scarring and low risk of infection.
Secondary wound closure	Skin edges are not approximated. The wound heals by granulation, epithelialization, and contraction.
Wound depth	Depth or layer of connective tissue involvement in a wound.
Partial-thickness wound	A wound that extends through the epidermis and into, but not through, the dermis. Dermal structures, such as hair follicles, sweat glands, sebaceous glands, nerves, and blood vessels, are preserved. Painful due to nerve exposure. Skin heals by regeneration.
Full-thickness wound	A wound that extends through both the epidermis and the dermis and may involve fascia, muscle, or bone. Pain may be limited due to nerve damage. Skin heals by scar formation.
Wound status	Healing trajectory of a wound as compared with the normal healing process.
Acute wound	Wound that proceeds through the repair process from injury to healing at a normal rate.
Chronic wound	Wound that fails to heal at a normal rate. Usually present for more than 30 days.

The type of tissue in a wound also gives a clue to its progression toward healing. One simple method of describing the type of tissue in a wound is the Red-Yellow-Black System of Wound Classification developed by Marion Laboratories Inc. in Europe (Cuzzell, 1988). Red denotes tissue that is clean, healthy, and granulating. Yellow denotes the presence in the wound of slough, a nonviable tissue created by the destruction of subcutaneous fat. Its presence indicates possible infection or the need for cleaning or débriding of a wound. Black denotes eschar, or dry, leathery necrotic tissue resulting from full-thickness tissue destruction (Cooper, 2000). When yellow or black tissue is present in a wound, the percent of the wound bed covered by that type of tissue should be recorded.

Exudate is either related to the leakage of blood or plasma into a wound and is *serous*, *sanguinous*, or *serosanguinous*, or is related to the phagocytic activity of leukocytes in the wound and the presence of infection and is *purulent*. Volume of exudate should be recorded. Guidelines for classifying the amount of exudate have been proposed by van Rijswijk (2001). However, the amount of exudate can be difficult to quantify when superabsorbent dressings are used. Wounds that are occluded often develop an odor. Some advanced wound care dressings, such as hydrocolloids, develop an odor as they react with wound fluid. Odor should be assessed after a wound is cleansed and should never be assessed by smelling the dressing.

The condition of periwound skin, or the skin adjacent to the wound, is predictive of healing (van Rijswijk, 2001) and should be documented. Periwound skin description should include color, temperature, presence of edema, and condition. Skin color is indicative of processes occurring beneath the skin, such as inflammation and infection. Periwound skin can be the same color as skin further from the wound, or any variation from pale pink, to bright pink, to red or erythematous. Darkly pigmented skin can be difficult to assess for color, but inflamed skin often becomes darker than the surrounding skin or appears bluish or purple. Skin reddened from pressure should be checked for the ability to blanch when pressed with a finger. Pressure-reddened skin that does not blanch indicates early tissue damage of a stage I pressure ulcer.

Skin temperature can be assessed with the back of the hand and compared with skin further from the wound. For more precise measurement, a liquid crystal skin thermometer, such as the type used to stick on children's foreheads, can be used. Be aware that in the early stages of healing, there is a normal zone of warmth around a wound. The area of warmth narrows as inflammation resolves and the wound heals. Skin that has decreased perfusion, such as edematous skin, may feel cool to the touch.

Early edema is a normal part of the inflammatory phase of healing. Prolonged edema decreases circulation to the wound and delays healing. Assessment should include the presence of edema around the wound. Skin with nonpitting edema may be taut or shiny. To assess for pitting edema, press the tissue firmly with a finger for 5 seconds. Pitting is graded on a scale of 0 to +3. If edema occurs on an extremity, both extremities should be measured at the same point and compared. Pulses should be assessed.

Condition of the periwound skin is judged against any changes from intact skin. Skin near a wound can be irritated, indicating redness and roughness without skin breakdown. Induration is a result of inflammation and is felt as hardness under the skin. Excessive moisture on the skin from exudate or incontinence can result in softening and weakening of the tissue, called *maceration*. Skin that is macerated appears either wrinkled—the way a child's fingers look when they get out of the bathtub—or pale, and possibly gray. Macerated skin is fragile and should be handled gently. Application of a skin sealant to periwound skin helps protect the skin from excessive moisture leaking from the wound. Trauma from tape or dressing removal, maceration, or skin infection such as *C. albicans* can damage the epidermis of the skin near the wound and result in denudement. Denuded skin lacks an epidermal covering, is moist and painful, and provides a portal of entry for microorganisms. The cause of skin denudement should be identified and corrected.

Wound and periwound pain should be noted. Pain that is out of proportion to the wound size and state of healing, or pain that is increasing is worrisome for infection and should be reported. Various pain measurement scales are available and the same scale should be used for interval comparisons. Children having painful procedures, such as wound cleansing and dressing changes, should be given appropriate pharmacologic and nonpharmacologic pain management before starting the procedure.

■ Caring for a Wound

Wound Cleansing

Cleansing a wound when changing the dressing helps to clean the wound of debris and to decrease the microbial count of the wound. The wound cleanser of choice is generally sterile normal saline. Saline is a physiologic solution. It does not add chemicals to the wound or change the pH and is safe to use on new tissue. Antiseptic solutions, including povidone-iodine, hydrogen peroxide, and sodium hypochlorite (Dakin solution), have been shown to be cytotoxic to new cells (Cooper, Laxer, & Hansbrough, 1991; Lineaweaver et al., 1985) and are no longer recommended for wound cleansing. Commercial wound cleansers are available that have been designed to be nontoxic to wound tissue and contain surfactants to help cleanse a wound, but their use probably has no benefit over saline in a wound that is clean and granulating. A 30- to 35-mL saline-filled syringe with an attached 18- or 19-gauge needle or blunt-end catheter can be used to irrigate a wound that has necrotic tissue, a significant amount of bacteria, or a large amount of exudate. This high-pressure irrigation helps cleanse a wound of bacteria and debris.

Wounds that are clean and granulating can be cleansed using low pressure, such as pouring saline directly from the bottle, using a bulb or piston syringe without a needle, or wiping gently with saline-soaked gauze (Barr, 1995; Hess, 2005). When a wound is cleansed with gauze-soaked saline, a separate piece of gauze is used for each swipe. The wound should be wiped in a circle or from top to bottom, working from the inside of the wound outward. The periwound skin should be cleansed at least 1 inch beyond the area that will be covered by the new dressing (Hess). Wiping must be carried out gently to avoid damaging fragile new tissue.

The process of cleaning dead tissue from a wound is called débridement. Wounds heal best when they are free of devitalized tissue. Wound débridement is achieved in one of four ways: surgical, chemical, mechanical, and autolytic. Devitalized tissue can be surgically removed using sharp instruments and can be removed either at the bedside or in surgery if a large amount of tissue must be removed. Nonviable tissue can also be removed from a wound by placing a chemical débriding agent into the wound. These chemicals break down devitalized tissue without harming healthy tissue. The use of wet-to-dry gauze dressings and whirlpool are types of mechanical débridement. Mechanical cleansing of a wound using wet-to-dry dressings involves placing wet woven gauze (do not use nonwoven gauze) into a wound and allowing it to dry. Devitalized tissue is mechanically removed with removal of the gauze. Wet-to-dry dressing changes are normally performed three or four times a day. They are painful and can damage healthy tissue, so they are not generally used on children. Several dressings promote autolytic débridement, or the body's ability to clean a wound. These dressings sequester enzymes and growth factors in wounds that are responsible for breaking down devitalized tissue. Dressings used for autolytic débridement in-clude hydrocolloids, hydrogels, alginates, hydrofibers, and transparent films and are discussed further in the next section. Autolytic débridement, although slow, is a gentle, effective, and safe method of débridement, provided that the wound is not infected.

Dressing a Wound

Advanced wound care dressings are dressings designed with technology that promotes a physiologic wound environment. There are several categories of advanced wound care dressings. These include hydrocolloid, hydrogel, alginate, hydrofiber, foam, and transparent film. Different dressing categories are used on different types of wounds depending on their size and depth, amount of exudate, amount of devitalized tissue, frequency of dressing removal for wound observation, availability, cost, and provider preference. Furthermore, each dressing category has an antimicrobial version that can be used on wounds at risk of infection. A description of dressing options, their indications, tips for use, and recommended changing frequency are found in Table 34-2.

In order for wounds to progress through the stages of healing and to promote unimpeded new tissue growth, a wound must be kept moist. Dressings should be chosen that manage exudate in a way that maintains a moist wound bed. Moisture retentive dressings, such as hydrocolloids, hydrogels, and transparent film dressings, should be used on wounds with scant-to-moderate drainage. Dressings that are moisture retentive either maintain the wound's own moisture through prevention of evaporation of wound fluid or they add moisture to the wound. Absorptive dressings, such as foams, alginates, and hydrofiber dressings, should be used on wounds with moderate-to-heavy drainage. These dressings absorb large amounts of drainage and keep the wound from becoming too wet.

Dead space is the space left in a wound where healthy tissue used to reside before injury. Eliminating dead space prevents the walls of a wound from healing closed prematurely and creating an abscess. A wound with depth should be filled with absorptive dressing material up to the level of the skin, including any areas of undermining. Dressings should be placed loosely in a wound, rather than being "packed" into it, so the microcirculation of the wound is not impeded by pressure and the wound is not prevented from contracting. A cotton-tipped applicator can be used to position the dressing into hard-to-reach places and into areas of undermining. Dressings placed in areas not easily seen during dressing changes, such as in areas of undermining, should extend out into the wound proper so that they are not forgotten at the

Table 34-2 The Well-Dressed Wound: Options in Dressings[a]

Dressing Type	Description	Indication	Tips	Change Frequency
Hydrocolloid				
DuoDERM CGF Dressing, ConvaTec, Princeton, NJ **Restore Wound Care Dressing,** Hollister, Inc., Libertyville, IL **Tegasorb Hydrocolloid Dressing,** 3M Health Care, St. Paul, MN	Occlusive or semi-occlusive dressing composed of carboxymethylcellulose, gelatin and pectin; Maintains a moist wound environment; Impermeable to bacteria	Primary or secondary dressing for dry to moist wounds; aids the body's ability to débride a wound; partial- and full-thickness wounds	May cause wound odor & residue sometimes mistaken for infection; Not for use with infected wounds; Smooth & press into place for best adhesion; comfortable; molds well to skin; does not adhere to wound; overlap periwound skin by at least 1 inch; don't stretch when applying; use under tape to protect fragile skin with tape removal	Up to 7 days, or before "melt-down" (saturation of dressing) When removing, gently lift dressing while pressing skin down and away from dressing
Hydrogel				
NU-GEL Collagen Wound Gel, Johnson & Johnson Wound Management, Somerville, NJ **SoloSite Wound Gel and Conformable Wound Dressing,** Smith & Nephew, Inc., Largo, FL	Water- or glycerin-based amorphous gel, impregnated gauze, or sheet dressing; Maintains moist wound environment	Primary dressing for dry or moist wounds; Aids the body's ability to débride a wound; Partial- and full-thickness wounds	Soothing, reduces pain; Does not adhere to wound; Minimal capacity for absorption unless also contains hydrocolloid; Rehydrates a wound bed; Requires secondary dressing to prevent dehydration; May macerate periwound skin; Gel may require rinsing from wound	Amorphous gel daily to t.i.d. Sheet and impregnated gauze up to 3 days if maintains moisture and doesn't become saturated with exudate
Alginate				
AlgiSite M Calcium, Smith & Nephew, Inc. **Kaltostat Wound Dressing,** ConvaTec **Sorbsan Topical Wound Dressing,** Bertek Pharmaceuticals, Research Triangle Park, NC	Absorbent dressing, derived from brown seaweed; contains calcium and sodium; Soft, nonwoven fibers shaped into pads, ropes; Maintains a moist wound environment	Primary dressing for moist or wet wounds; Aids the body's ability to débride a wound; Partial- and full-thickness wounds	Press into wound to contact all wound surfaces; absorbs 20 times its weight in wound fluid; forms a gel when in contact with wound fluid; gel may require rinsing from wound; requires cover dressing; theoretical risk of calcium absorption in large wound	Change dressing when totally gelled or signs of strikethrough on secondary dressing, up to 4 days

Type / Product	Description	Considerations	Wear Time
Hydrofiber			
Aquacel Hydrofiber Wound Dressing, ConvaTec	Made from sodium carboxymethylcellulose; Soft, nonwoven dressing shaped into pads, ribbons; Maintains a moist wound environment	Greater capacity for absorption than alginates; forms a gel when in contact with wound fluid to maintain moist wound bed; dressing maintains integrity when wet—can be lifted from wound; requires cover dressing	4 to 7 days, or until saturated
Similar in use to alginates; Primary dressing for moist or wet wounds; aids the body's ability to débride a wound; partial- and full-thickness wounds			
Foam			
Mepilex Soft Silicone Absorbent Foam, Mölnlycke Health Care, Newtown, PA; **3M Foam Dressing,** 3M Health Care; **PolyMem Dressing,** Ferris Manufacturing Corp., Burr Ridge, IL	Absorbent, nonlinting dressing; Nonadherent to wound; Maintains a moist wound environment	Some brands have top layer of transparent film to act as barrier to bacteria. Must apply non-film side toward wound; Provide thermal insulation; Some brands come with an adhesive border; Should overlap periwound skin	Up to 7 days, or until saturated
Primary or secondary dressing for moist or wet wounds; Partial- and full-thickness wounds; Can be placed around leaking gastrostomy tubes, tracheostomy tubes			
Gauze			
Curity Gauze Pads, Kerlix Rolls, Tyco Healthcare/Kendall, Mansfield, MA; **Medline Gauze Pads,** Medline Industries, Inc., Mundelein, IL	Cotton or synthetic, woven or nonwoven fabric; mildly to moderately absorptive; Not an advanced wound care dressing	Permeable to water, microorganisms; wet-to-dry dressing: moistened gauze placed in wound and allowed to dry over 4–6 hours; Removal pulls nonviable & sometimes viable tissue from wound; Removal can be painful. If not using for débridement can be moistened for easier removal; Can leave fibers in wound, stimulating inflammation	Daily or more frequently, depending on exudate amount; Limited absorptive capacity may necessitate several dressing changes per day; Not intended for extended wear
Cover dressing over a primarily closed surgical wound; wet-to-dry nonselective débridement of necrotic tissue; Inexpensive dressing filler in large, deep wounds; Inexpensive dressing for wounds requiring frequent inspection; primary or secondary dressing			
Transparent film			
Bioclusive Transparent Dressing, Johnson & Johnson Wound Management; **OpSite,** Smith & Nephew, Inc. **3M Tegaderm Transparent Dressing,** 3M Health Care	Adhesive, semipermeable, polyurethane membrane dressing; Waterproof, impermeable to bacteria; Maintains a moist wound environment	Do not stretch when applying or will blister skin; Not absorptive; Allows limited evaporation of wound moisture through the film; Not for use with infected wounds; Use cautiously on fragile skin; May be placed on skin to protect from abrasion; Must overlap periwound skin	Up to 7 days; Removal: grasp edge of dressing and pull it parallel with the skin surface, while supporting the skin under the dressing. This releases the adhesive without trauma
Primary or secondary dressing; Dry or slightly moist wound; Aids the body's ability to débride a wound			

(continues)

Table 34-2 *(continued)*

Dressing Type	Description	Indication	Tips	Change Frequency
Contact layer				
Conformant 2 Wound Veil, Smith & Nephew, Inc. **Mepitel Soft Silicone Wound Contact Layer,** Mölnlycke Health Care	Single layer "netting" placed on wound bed to prevent adhesion of overlying dressing to wound	Used as primary dressing on delicate wounds, painful wounds; Prevents pain and trauma to tissues with dressing changes	Allows exudate to pass through to secondary dressing; Not absorptive, requires secondary dressing; Secondary dressing can be changed without disturbing contact layer; Can be used under VAC; Can be used with topical medications	Up to 7 days
Antimicrobial				
Acticoat Antimicrobial Dressing, Smith & Nephew, Inc. **Aquacel AG Hydrofiber Dressing with Silver,** ConvaTec Contreet **Antimicrobial Dressing with Silver,** Coloplast Corp., Marietta, GA **SilvaSorb,** Medline Industries, Inc. **Silverlon,** Argentum Medical, LLC, Willowbrook, IL	Dressing impregnated with antimicrobial agent, such as silver or iodine; Releases active ingredient into wound slowly to preserve new tissue growth and provide continuous antimicrobial activity	Nonhealing wounds with high microbial burden; Wounds at risk of infection, such as burns, grafts, donor sites	Silver dressings available in every dressing category and many shapes; Broad range of antimicrobial activity; Reduces or prevents infection; May temporarily discolor wound or skin; Activated either by wound moisture or by dampening dressing with sterile water (not saline). Instructions are manufacturer-specific (read directions); Wound infection requires systemic antibiotic therapy; Silver cannot be used with debriding agents; Very costly dressings	3 to 7 days, depending on dressing type, manufacturer instructions, amount of exudate

aExamples are not inclusive of all products in the category.

next dressing change. Note should be made in the patient record of any concealed dressings. The presence of any concealed dressing can also be recorded on the cover dressing (the top dressing) to alert the next person who changes the dressing of their presence.

Occasionally, wounds drain so heavily that even the most absorbent dressing must be changed frequently. A strategy for managing copious wound drainage is to place an ostomy pouch or commercial wound pouch over the wound. By collecting drainage in a pouch, output can be measured and periwound skin is protected from maceration. Moreover, the child is spared repeated and possibly uncomfortable dressing changes.

Use of antimicrobial dressings is becoming increasingly common. Antimicrobial dressings are now available in every dressing category. In the antimicrobial dressing format, dressings are combined with a slow-release form of an antiseptic, such as silver or iodine. The antiseptic is slowly released from the dressing to maintain a constant level of antisepsis in the wound at a concentration low enough to prevent damage to newly developing tissue. Most antimicrobial dressings have an extended wear time, some exceeding 7 days. They are useful on wounds at risk of infection, such as burn wounds. They can also be used on infected wounds to decrease the surface bacteria. Antimicrobial dressings are only an adjunct treatment of wound infection, however, and should be used only in combination with systemic antimicrobial therapy. Most antimicrobial dressings are activated by moisture, either from the wound or from application of water to the dressing. Manufacturer instructions should be followed because directions vary with each type of dressing. Antimicrobial dressings, although efficacious, comfortable for the patient, and cost effective when used according to manufacturers' recommendations, are very expensive and are not suitable for wounds requiring daily dressing changes.

The use of sterile versus clean technique during wound care has become an area of controversy. A growing body of research supports the safety and cost-effectiveness of clean technique in the care of postoperative wounds (Stotts et al., 1997). However, most research has been carried out on chronic wounds and on adults (APIC, 2001; Gray & Doughty, 2001; Hollingsworth & Kingston, 1998). Until appropriate research is carried out in the pediatric population, sterile technique is still recommended for dressing changes involving surgical and other wounds in hospitalized children. However, sterile technique does not imply the same level of sterility as asepsis used in the operating room. Sterile dressing changes should include the use of a sterile field, sterile dressings, sterile irrigation solutions, and sterile gloves for placement of new dressings. Hands are one of the most significant transporters of bacteria and should be washed before and after handling a wound, and between removing an old dressing and replacing a new dressing, despite wearing gloves. Standard precautions should always be maintained.

Securing a dressing is the final step in completing a dressing change. This should be performed so that minimal damage to periwound skin is incurred with dressing removal, especially on children requiring frequent dressing changes. Several brands of adhesive tape are available that are gentle to the skin when removed. If skin is at risk of being denuded with tape removal, a hydrocolloid dressing can be placed on the skin and the tape placed over the hydrocolloid dressing. The hydrocolloid dressing can be left in place through repeated tape removals. Alternately, skin sealant can be applied to the skin beneath tape. Skin sealants should be allowed to dry completely before tape application, and should be reapplied each time tape is removed and replaced. Adhesive remover can be used to loosen tape without trauma to the skin. However, exposure to the chemicals present in adhesive remover is not benign. There have been reported cases of toxic epidermal necrolysis after exposure to adhesive remover (Ittmann & Bozynski, 1993), as well as allergic reactions. Adhesive removers contain petroleum distillates and are not water soluble, so they must be washed from the skin with soap and water before replacing the tape. Use of adhesive removers should be approached cautiously and only when necessary on infants, particularly premature infants. In lieu of tape, gauze rolls can be wrapped around a limb or torso to anchor a dressing. Other products that are useful in anchoring dressings without the use of tape include tubular stretch mesh and self-adhesive stretch wraps.

The child's attending provider should be kept informed of the wound status, and changes in the wound care routine should be made as needed. A wound is likely to require different treatment strategies and dressings as it cycles through the stages of wound healing. Nurses need to be aware that wound management carries with it significant liability, and orders for all wound care products and treatments should be documented on the patient record.

Negative-Pressure Wound Therapy

Negative-pressure wound therapy (NPWT) is an adjuvant wound care strategy being used increasingly in children. NPWT involves the application of controlled suction to the base of a wound to promote healing. Although suction has been used in heavily draining wounds for many years, the vacuum-assisted closure or VAC was introduced as an NPWT system in 1995 by KCI (Kinetic Concepts Inc., San Antonio, TX). The benefits of NPWT to wound healing are achieved through two mechanisms of action. First, the application of suction or subatmospheric pressure removes excess wound fluid, thereby preventing maceration, decreasing edema and third-space fluids, and decreasing bacterial count. Secondly, mechanical stretching of the cells in the wound creates stress and stimulates inflammation in the wound, enhances blood flow, and speeds cellular reproduction.

To apply the VAC to a wound, a prepackaged polyurethane foam sponge is cut to fit the shape of the wound. The sponge is placed into the wound and is covered with a transparent film dressing to occlude the wound. A suction catheter attached to a computer-controlled, vacuum-pressure pump is placed into the sponge, achieving an airtight seal. The pump is turned on and a uniform vacuum is created over the wound. Pump pressures can range from 50 to 200 mm Hg, but pressures used on children have generally been reported to be between 50 and 125 mm Hg, depending on the size of the child and the characteristics of the wound (Bookout, McCord, & McLane, 2004; Caniano, Ruth, & Teich, 2005). VAC dressing changes as well as pump setting changes should be performed by persons specially trained to do so. The pump must be turned on for at least 22 hours out of each 24 hours and may be run on either a continuous- or intermittent-suction mode. VAC dressing changes are recommended every 48 hours for most wounds. They can be painful and difficult for young children, so pain management should be addressed before the dressing is changed. Some institutions perform VAC dressing changes under brief anesthesia or with the use of conscious sedation.

NPWT has been used on virtually every type of wound and in all age groups over the past decade. Pediatric patients placed on NPWT have spanned the age range from neonate through adolescence. Indications for use of NPWT in children have included dehisced abdominal and sternal wounds, pilonidal cystectomy, soft tissue loss from intravenous extravasation, gunshot injuries, extensive tissue loss secondary to infectious complications, pressure ulcers, and compartment syndrome (Bookout et al., 2004; Caniano et al., 2005).

Contraindications to the use of NPWT include osteomyelitis, malignancy involving the wound site, nonenteric fistulas, bleeding, presence of necrotic wound tissue, and presence of exposed organs in the wound (although the use of NPWT over exposed organs is becoming more common). Although NPWT is a useful adjuvant wound therapy, it remains very costly, and its use must be weighed against other wound healing strategies.

■ Developmental Considerations in Wound Care

It comes as no surprise to anyone involved in the care of children that most wound research has been carried out on adults. However, it is thought that the physiology of wound healing in children is similar to that of adults. Children are generally treated according to the principles of adult wound care. However, there are physiologic and emotional differences in the pediatric population that should be taken into consideration when decisions are made regarding wound care for children (Garvin, 1990; Krummel & Blewett, 2003).

Differences between children and adults with wounds are varied. Children, in general, have less adipose tissue than adults, although there is currently an upward trend in body mass in the pediatric population. As pointed out previously, excess adipose tissue delays healing and increases the risk of wound infection. The generally lower body mass in children makes them less likely than their adult counterparts to develop obesity-related wound-healing complications. Children also generally have a healthier circulatory system, having had less time to develop circulatory impairment caused by diabetes and vascular disease (Krummel & Blewett, 2003). As a result, children usually have better perfusion of wounds and consequently heal better than do adults.

Newborns and premature infants present a special case in wound care. Many organ systems in infants are not fully mature, and this immaturity may affect wound healing. For example, the immune system is an integral part of the wound-healing cascade yet is not fully developed for several years after birth. Particularly during the first 6 months of life, infants are at increased risk of infection (Blackburn & Loper, 1992). However, the most conspicuously immature organ in the infant is the skin.

Premature infants have a poorly developed epidermis, as well as a tenuous connection between their dermis and epidermis. This predisposes them to stripping of the epidermis from the skin with adhesive removal. Breech of the epidermal barrier opens a portal for invasion of microorganisms and substantially increases fluid losses. Epidermal stripping is consequently an important source of morbidity and mortality in infants. The infant's thin epidermis and dermis allow absorption of substances through the skin that would not be absorbed by an adult. Their large skin surface area-to-body weight ratio, in relation to that of an adult, further increases transepidermal absorption and compounds the effects of absorbed substances.

In many ways, the most important differences between caring for wounded children and caring for adults are the developmental and psychological issues. Each stage of childhood development brings with it different interpretations by the child of illness, surgery, procedures, and pain. For example, infants can feel pain acutely but have no understanding of its cause. Toddlers and pre-schoolers have limited causal understanding. They often fill gaps in their understanding with fantasy and believe that their behavior is responsible for their condition. School-aged children begin to develop logical thinking and can understand cause and effect but fear losing control. Adolescents' understanding of a situation approaches that of adults, but they can be devastated by changes in body image (Garvin, 1990). Explanations of what is taking place should be offered and should be geared to the understanding of the child. Distraction techniques and security objects, as well as the presence of a supportive caregiver during procedures, are important nonpharmacologic interventions. Allowing participation and decision making in the process of wound care in older children imparts to them some control of the situation.

Pediatric Pressure Ulcers

A pressure ulcer (PU) is an area of localized tissue destruction that occurs when soft tissue is compressed between a bony prominence and an external surface for a prolonged period of time (National Pressure Ulcer Advisory Panel, 1989). The external surface is often a mattress but can be a wheelchair or any other firm surface. Although pressure ulcers are far more prevalent in adults, they do occur in children of all ages. Pressure ulcers are classified as stage I, stage II, stage III, or stage IV in increasing order of severity and based on the extent of tissue damage. The National Pressure Ulcer Advisory Panel (NPUAP), an independent not-for-profit professional organization dedicated to the prevention and management of pressure ulcers, established a PU classification system that is generally used (NPUAP). Although not all pressure ulcers are nosocomial wounds, critically ill children in hospitals are at risk of pressure ulcer development. A PU prevalence of 4.0% was reported in a survey of nine children's hospitals in 2004 (McLane, Bookout, McCord, McCain, & Jefferson, 2004). Nurses caring for pediatric surgery patients should be alert to the risk factors for the development of PUs and should be prepared to initiate preventive measures.

Multiple factors contribute to the development of PUs in children. Some of these factors are intrinsic to the patient and include poor nutrition, poor tissue perfusion, and poor oxygenation. Extrinsic factors contributing to PU development include skin moisture from incontinence or perspiration, friction against the skin from sources such as sheets, and shearing force created by the interaction of friction and gravity, as occurs when a patient placed in a sitting position slides down toward the foot of the bed. Certain children are at higher-than-average risk of developing PUs. Children who are immobile are at risk because they cannot turn themselves to shift their pressure points. Included in this group are children who are critically ill, those who are neurologically impaired, and those who undergo a prolonged operative procedure. Neurologically impaired children, including those with myelomeningocele, have decreased or absent sensation and lack the normal pain stimuli that reminds people to turn or move when pressure obstructs blood flow to the skin for a prolonged period. Malnourished children, including most hospitalized children, are at risk for PUs, as are children suffering from debilitating diseases. In the pediatric intensive care unit, mechanical ventilation and hypotension have been identified as additional risk factors (Quigley & Curley, 1996).

The primary sites for the development of PUs are age dependent. Infants and toddlers have heads that are disproportionately large for their body size and tend to develop PUs on the head, especially on the occiput. As children grow and become more similar in proportion to adults, their PU distribution more closely reflects that of the adult population, including development of PUs over the scapulae, elbows, arms, hands, and legs (McLane et al., 2004). Common locations for PUs in all pediatric age groups are the seat area, including the buttocks, sacrum/coccyx, ischium and trochanter, and feet.

Tools developed to determine risk of developing PUs in adults are not valid in the pediatric population because of differences in weight distribution and body proportions. A risk assessment tool, the Braden Q Scale, was developed as a modification of the adult Braden Scale (Bergstrom, Braden, Laguzza, & Holman, 1987) to predict the risk of PU development in children in the pediatric intensive care unit (Quigley & Curley, 1996). The tool measures seven subscales including sensory perception, skin moisture, activity, friction and sheer, mobility, nutritional status, and tissue oxygenation, with scores ranging from 7 to 28. A lower score indicates a higher risk of PU development. A modified Braden Q Scale, measuring three subscales (mobility, sensory perception, and tissue perfusion/oxygenation), was tested and validated in 2003, and the results were found to be consistent with the original seven-subscale Braden Q Scale (Curley, Razmus, Roberts, & Wypij, 2003). The Braden Q Scale has been difficult to apply to neonatal intensive care patients, however. The Neonatal Skin Risk Assessment Scale, or NSARS, is an instrument designed to measure PU risk in neonates (Huffines & Lodgson, 1997). This tool measures general physical condition based on gestational age, activity, and nutrition. No other PU risk assessment scales have been validated for the pediatric population.

Prevention strategies can be effective in reducing the incidence of PUs and include routine risk assessment and initiation of skin care measures. Measures to protect at-risk skin include routine turning schedules, suspending the patient's heels off the bed with pillows, occipital pressure relieving devices for immobile infants and toddlers, moisture barrier ointments for protection against incontinence, limiting elevation of the head of the bed to no more than 30 degrees (to prevent sliding) and for no more than 2 hours at a time, protecting areas of skin exposed to friction with the application of transparent film dressings, and initiation of pressure reducing and pressure relieving support surfaces for at-risk patients (Quigley & Curley, 1996).

■ Conclusion

This is an exciting time for nurses caring for children with surgical problems. Neonatal and pediatric wound care is an ever-evolving specialty with exciting advances on the forefront. Ongoing research improves our understanding of how to care for wounds. The development of better and more effective products improves physical outcomes and quality of life. As nurses caring for children with wounds, however, we need to step back and focus not just on the engrossing problem of the wound that will not heal, but also on the child.

Caring for children is an ever-changing adventure. Each age group presents its own challenges for nursing care, and each child brings his or her own individuality. We should never lose site of the beauty and joy in each and every one of "our" children. Their wounds are not just intriguing nursing challenges but are a small part of a very unique and wonderful person. Children with wounds, like all hospitalized children, deserve to be cared for as a whole and irreplaceable human being. They deserve the most tender, most age-appropriate, most passionate, most intelligent, and most evidence-based care that we can provide. Along with their families, they deserve the best we have to give them.

■ Acknowledgment

I would like to thank my daughter Carolyn R. Rogers, student at the University of Pittsburgh School of Medicine, for her support in the preparation of the chapter.

I would also like to acknowledge Gail Garvin, for her many contributions toward advancing the care of children with ostomies and wounds, including authorship of the chapter Caring for Children with Ostomies and Wounds in the first edition of this textbook.

References

Association for Professionals in Infection Control and Epidemiology, Inc. (APIC). (2001). Position statement: Clean vs sterile: Management of chronic wounds. *APIC News, 20*(1), 20–22, 31.

Barr, J. E. (1995). Principles of wound cleansing. *Ostomy Wound Management, 41*(7A Suppl.), 15S–22S.

Bergstrom, N., Braden, B. J., Laguzza, A., & Holman, V. (1987). The Braden scale for predicting pressure sore risk. *Nursing Research, 36*, 205–210.

Blackburn, S. T., & Loper, D. L. (1992). The immune system and host defense mechanism. In S. T. Blackburn & D. L. Loper (Eds.), *Maternal, fetal, and neonatal physiology: A clinical perspective* (pp. 439–490). Philadelphia: W.B. Saunders.

Bookout, K., McCord, S., & McLane, K. (2004). Case studies of an infant, a toddler, and an adolescent treated with a negative pressure wound treatment system. *JWOCN, 31*(4), 184–192.

Caniano, D. A., Ruth, B., & Teich, S. (2005). Wound management with vacuum-assisted closure: Experience in 51 pediatric patients. *Journal of Pediatric Surgery, 40*(1), 128–132.

Cooper, D. M. (2000). Assessment, measurement and evaluation: Their pivotal roles in wound healing. In R. A. Bryant (Ed.), *Acute and chronic wounds: Nursing management* (2nd ed., pp. 51–84). St. Louis, MO: Mosby.

Cooper, M. L., Laxer, J. A., & Hansbrough, J. F. (1991). The cytotoxic effects of commonly used topical antimicrobial agents on human fibroblasts and keratinocytes. *The Journal of Trauma, 31*(6), 775–784.

Curley, M. A., Razmus, I. S., Roberts, K. E., & Wypij, D. (2003). Predicting pressure ulcer risk in pediatric patients: The Braden Q scale. *Nursing Research, 52*(1), 22–33.

Cuzzell, J. Z. (1990). Choosing a wound dressing: A systematic approach. *AACN Clinical Issues in Critical Care Nursing, 1*(3), 566–577.

Cuzzell, J. Z. (1988). The new RYB color code. *American Journal of Nursing, 88*, 1342–1346.

Garvin, G. (1990). Wound healing in pediatrics. *Nursing Clinics of North America, 25*(1), 181–192.

Gray, M., & Doughty, D. (2001). Clean versus sterile technique when changing wound dressings. *JWOCN, 28*, 125–128.

Hess, C. T. (2005). *Clinical guide: Wound care* (5th ed.). Ambler, PA: Lippincott Williams & Wilkins.

Hollingsworth, H., & Kingston, J. E. (1998). Using a non-sterile technique in wound care. *Professional Nurse, 13*(4), 226–229.

Huffines, B., & Lodgson, M. C. (1997). The neonatal skin risk assessment scale for predicting skin breakdown in neonates. *Issues in Comprehensive Pediatric Nursing, 20*(2), 103–114.

Hunt, T. K., Hopf, H., & Hussain, Z. (2000). Physiology of wound healing. *Advances in Skin and Wound Care, 13*(Suppl. 2), 6–11.

Ittmann, P. I., & Bozynski, M. E. (1993). Toxic epidermal necrolysis in a newborn infant after exposure to adhesive remover. *Journal of Perinatology, 13*(6), 476–477.

Kerstein, M. D. (1995). Moist wound healing: The clinical perspective. *Ostomy Wound Management, 41*(7A Suppl.), 37S–44S.

Keswani, S. G., & Crombleholme, T. M. (2005). Wound healing: Cellular and molecular mechanisms. In K. T. Oldham, P. M. Colombani, R. P. Foglia, & M. A. Skinner (Eds.), *Principles and practice of pediatric surgery* (pp. 223–238). Philadelphia: Lippincott Williams & Wilkins.

Krummel, T. M., & Blewett, C. (2003). Wound healing. In M. M. Ziegler, R. G. Azizkhan, & T. R. Weber (Eds.), *Operative pediatric surgery* (pp. 179–189). New York: McGraw-Hill Professional.

Lineaweaver, W., Howard, R., Soucy, D., McMorris, S., Freeman, J., Crain, C., et al. (1985). Topical antimicrobial toxicity. *Archives of Surgery, 120*(3), 267–270.

Mangram, A. J., Horan, T. C., Pearson, M. L., Silver, L. C., & Jarvis, W. R. (1999). Guideline for prevention of surgical site infection, 1999. *Infection Control and Hospital Epidemiology, 20*(4), 247–278.

McLane, K. M., Bookout, K., McCord, S., McCain, J., & Jefferson, L. S. (2004). The 2003 national pediatric pressure ulcer and skin breakdown prevalence survey: A multisite study. *JWOCN, 31*(4), 168–178.

Meakins, J. L., & Masterson, B. J. (2003). Prevention of postoperative infection. In *ACS Surgery*. Retrieved August 5, 2005, from http://www.medscape.com/viewarticle/504449

National Pressure Ulcer Advisory Panel. (1989). Pressure ulcer cost, prevalence, and risk assessment: Consensus development conference statement. *Decubitus, 2*(2), 24–28.

Ovington, L. G. (2001). Hanging wet-to-dry dressings out to dry. *Home Healthcare Nurse, 19*(8), 477–483.

Quigley, S. M., & Curley, M. A. Q. (1996). Skin integrity in the pediatric population: Preventing and managing pressure ulcers. *Journal of the Society of Pediatric Nurses, 1*(1), 7–18.

Rijswijk, L. van. (2001). Wound assessment and documentation. In D. L. Krasner, G. T. Rodeheaver, & R. G. Sibbald (Eds.), *Chronic wound care: A clinical source book for healthcare professionals* (3rd ed., pp. 101–116). Wayne, PA: HMP Communications.

Stotts, N. A. (2000). Wound infection: Diagnosis and management. In R. A. Bryant (Ed.), *Acute and chronic wounds: Nursing management* (2nd ed., pp. 179–188). St. Louis, MO: Mosby.

Stotts, N. A., Barbour, S., Griggs, K., Bouvier, B., Buhlman, L., Wipke-Tevis, D., et al. (1997). Sterile versus clean technique in postoperative wound care of patients with open surgical wounds: A pilot study. *JWOCN, 24*(1), 10–18.

Waldrop, J., & Doughty, D. (2000). Wound-healing physiology. In R. A. Bryant (Ed.), *Acute and chronic wounds: Nursing management* (2nd ed., pp. 17–40). St. Louis, MO: Mosby.

West, J. M., & Gimbel, M. L. (2000). Acute surgical and traumatic wound healing. In R. A. Bryant (Ed.), *Acute and chronic wounds: Nursing management* (2nd ed., pp. 189–196). St. Louis, MO: Mosby.

Wilson, J. A., & Clark J. J. (2004). Obesity: Impediment to postsurgical wound healing. *Advances in Skin and Wound Care, 17*(8), 426–435.

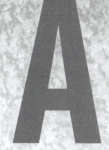

Resource Guide

Suzanne Borkowski, MS, PNP, ETN

The pediatric surgical nurse of 2007 faces the challenge of meeting the wide spectrum of needs for infants and children receiving modern pediatric surgical care.

A great deal of "technological care" has shifted from hospitals to home and community. Parents, families and caregivers are asked to assume more responsibility for their child's care than ever. Additionally, children may suffer from acute illnesses that require high-tech interventions such as intravenous antibiotics via indwelling lines.

Support groups are an integral part of this adjustment period and process. They are an important therapeutic intervention to create an opportunity to acquire information, new knowledge, coping strategies, and to share experiences. Appropriate resources and support groups of various types are available for many diseases, disabilities, conditions, and needs. These resources may be contacted via national organizations, government agencies, the internet, layperson email groups, parent-parent led and professionally led community groups.

On-going education and information regarding support groups and resources foster quality care. Be available and communicate with openness and honesty. Families will appreciate your support, concern, and trust.

■ Family Resources and Product Guides

Please note that references are correct as of publication date. Resources are updated on the APSNA Web site at www.apsna.org.

1. **American Burn Association**
   ABA Central Office—Chicago
   625 N. Michigan Ave., Ste 2550
   Chicago, Illinois 60611
   312-642-9260
   www.ameriburn.org

2. **Angel Flight North East Municipal Airport**
   492 Sutton Street, North Andover, MA 01845
   800-549-9980
   (Free transportation for those who cannot afford commercial transportation)

3. **American Cancer Society**
   National Headquarters
   1599 Clifton Rd. NE, Atlanta, GA 30329
   800-ACS-2345

4. **American Heart Association**
   7272 Greenville Ave., Dallas, TX 75231-4596
   800-AHA-USA1

5. **American Lung Association**
National Headquarter Office
61 Broadway, New York, NY 10006
212-315-8700   www.lungusa.org

6. **Biliary Atresia and Liver Transplant, Inc. (BALT)**
3835 Richmond Ave, Box 190
Staten Island, NY 10312
718-987-6200

7. **Biobrane biosynthetic wound dressing for burns**
UDL Laboratories, Inc.
1718 Northrock Court, Rockford, IL 61103

8. **Brain Injury Association**
105 North Alfred Street, Alexandria, VA 22314
800-444-6443   www.biausa.org

9. **Brave Kids**
800-568-1008 www.BRAVEKIDS.org

10. **Burnsurgery.org**
Education for Burn Care Professionals
www.burnsurgery.org

11. **Children's Liver Association for Support Services (C.L.A.S.S.)**
27023 McBean Parkway #126
Valencia, CA 91355
877-679-8256

12. **Children's Wish Foundation**
PO Box 28785 or 8615 Roswell Rd.
Atlanta, GA 30358
800-323-WISH; (fax) 770-393-0683

13. **Crohn's and Colitis Foundation of America (CCFA)**
386 Park Avenue South, 17th floor
New York, NY 10016-8804
800-932-2423   www.ccfa.org

14. **Cystic Fibrosis Foundation**
6931 Arlington Road, Bethesda, MD 20814
800-344-4823 www.cff.org

15. **Cystic Fibrosis**
www.cysticfibrosis.com
Email community (CF information and support)
Cystic-L or Cystic-l.org

16. **EA/TEF Child & Family Support Connection**
(National office)
111 West Jackson Boulevard, Suite 1145
Chicago, IL 60604-3502
312-987-9085 Phone   312-987-9086 Fax
www.eatef.org or info@eatef.org

17. **Gastrostomy Email Support Mailing List**
The family introduces the child and gives follow up, shares experiences, strategies, suggestions, and personal remedies for care of a GT.
Ward Scarff, Gtube List owner
http://www.gtube.org or GTUBE@LISTSERV.SYR.EDU

18. **MUMS**
Mother's United for Moral Support: National Parent Support Group
150 Custer St., Green Bay, WI 54301-1243
877-336-5333   www.netnet.net/mums/

19. **Pull-through Network**
2312 Savoy Street, Hoover, AL 35226-1528
205-978-2930   www.info@pullthrough.org

20. **National Dissemination Center for Children with Disabilities**
P.O. Box 1492, Washington, DC 20013
800-695-0285   www.nichcy.org

21. **National Kidney Foundation**
30 East 33rd St., New York, NY 10016
800-622-9010

22. **National Rehabilitation Information Center**
4200 Forbes Blvd Suite 202, Lanham, MD 20706
800-346-2742   www.naric.com

23. **National Spinal Cord Injury Association**
6701 Democracy Blvd. Suite 300-9, Bethesda, MD 20817
800-963-9629   info@spinalcord.org

24. **National Transplant Assistance Program**
150 North Radner Chester Rd. Suite F120, Radner, PA 19087
800-642-8399

25. **Pediatric Home Care Association of America**
228 Seventh St., SE, Washington, DC 20003
202-547-7424

26. **Phoenix Society for Burn Survivors, Inc.**
www.phoenix-society.org

27. **Ronald McDonald Houses Charities**
1 Croc Drive, Department 014, Oak Brook, Il 60523
630-623-7048 www.rmhc.com

28. **SIDS Alliance**
1314 Bedford Ave. Suite 210, Baltimore, MD 21208
800-221-7437 www.firstcandle.org

29. **Spina Bifida Association of America**
4590 McArthur Blvd. NW, #250
Washington, DC 20007-4226
800-621-3141

30. **TEF/Vater International Support Network**
15301 Greyfox Rd., Upper Marlboro, MD 20772
301-952-6837   www.tefvater.org

31. **Tracheo-Oesophageal Fistula Support (TOFS)**
International office
St. George's Centre, 91 Victoria Road, Netherfield
Nottingham, England NG4 2NN
T: +44 (0) 115-961-3092; F: +44 (0) 115-961-3097
www.tofs.org.uk

32. **United Ostomy Association of America, Inc. (UOAA)**
A new group is a national non-profit organization. The goal is to act as an umbrella organization for geographical focused support groups.
Ken Aukett, President of the Organizing Steer Committee
www.uoaa.org or kenaukett@uoaa.org

33. **Patient Teaching Material**
CR Bard Medical Division
8195 Industrial Blvd., Covington, GA 30014
800-526-4455 www.bardmedical.com

■ Product Guide

1. **3M Health Care. Steri-Drape ™**
St. Paul MN 55144-1000. 1-800-228-3957 www.3M.com.

2. **Cook Critical Care**
PO Box 4195, Bloomington, IN 47402-4195
1-800-457-4500 www.cookmedical.com

3. **Convatec**
100 Headquarter Park Dr. , Skillman, NJ 08558
800-422-8811 www.convatec.com

4. **Hollister**
2000 Hollister Dr., Libertyville, IL 60048
800-323-4060 www.hollister.com

5. **Kimberly Clark/Ballard Medical Products**
12050 Lone Peak Parkway, Draper, Utah 84020
800-528-5591 www.kchealthcare.com

6. **Mentor Corporation**
Self-Cath Coude Olive Tip with Guide Stripe (30/box)
8 Fr: order number 808; 10 Fr: order number 810
201 Mentor Drive, Santa Barbara, CA 93111
1-800-328-3863 www.mentorcorp.com

7. **Nutra/Balance Products**
Drink boxes: 27/case
Cookies: 12/12 count
7155 Wadsworth Way, Indianapolis, IN 46219
1-800-654-3691 www.nutra-balance-products.com (product information only)

8. **Specialty Surgical Products, Inc. Silicone Silo Bag-clear cast.**
Victor, MT 59875 1-406-951-0102 www.ssp-inc.com

Glossary

Leona L. Burnham

Abscess—A localized collection of pus in a tissue or body part resulting from the invasion of pyogenic bacteria.

Acholic—Absence of bile pigments in stool.

Adhesion—Fibrous band holding parts together that are normally separated.

Aganglionosis—The absence of ganglion cells (Hirschsprung's disease).

Anastomosis—Surgical joining of two segments of an organ, such as bowel, to allow flow from one segment to the other.

Anoplasty—One stage surgical repair utilized for low anorectal malformations.

Anorectal malformation—Congenital anomalies of the rectum, urinary and reproductive structures.

Antegrade Continent Enema (ACE)—Procedure where the appendix is brought up through the umbilicus to create a conduit for enema instillation.

Antiseptic—Substance that inhibits the growth and reproduction of microorganisms. Includes povidone iodine, hydrogen peroxide, silver and sodium hypochlorite (Dakins solution).

Aperture—An opening as in the skin barrier of an ostomy pouch.

Arteriovenous malformation—Tumor caused by abnormal collection of arteries and veins; characterized by a bruit or thrill.

Atresia—Congenital absence or closure of a normal body opening or tubular structure.

Balanitis—Inflammation of the skin covering the glans penis.

Barrett's esophagus—Inflammation and possible ulceration of the lower part of the esophagus.

Biliary dyskinesia—Impairment of the voluntary emptying of the gallbladder.

Branchial cleft cyst—Cyst or sinuses located around the ear and neck which result when branchial arches do not obliterate during fetal development.

Bronchogenic cyst—Mass of non-functioning pulmonary tissue containing cystic structures filled with fluid or mucus.

Bronchiolitis obliterans—Inflammation of the bronchioles from partial or complete obliteration of the bronchioles by nodular masses of granulation and fibrotic tissue.

Cecostomy—Procedure that secures access to the cecum and inserts a tube for enema instillation.

Celiotomy—Opening the abdominal cavity through an incision in the abdominal wall; see laparotomy.

Cholangiogram—A radiologic examination of the bile ducts using a radiopaque dye as contrast medium.

Cholangitis—Bile stasis with bacterial flora; usually presents with fever, leukocytosis, and elevated liver enzymes.

Cholecystectomy—Excision of the gallbladder.

Cholecystitis—Acute or chronic inflammation of the gallbladder.

Choledochal cyst—Malformation of the biliary system manifested by local dilation of all or some portion of the biliary tree.

Choledocholithiasis—Presence of stones in the common bile duct.

Cholelithiasis—Presence or formation of gallstones.

Cholestasis—A condition in which normal bile recirculation is defective and bile remains in the liver.

Cloaca—A complex malformation in females in which the rectum, vagina and urinary tract are fused together into a single common channel that communicates to the exterior through a single perineal orifice located at the normal urethra.

Cloacal Exstrophy—Complex anomaly including omphalocle, two exstrophied hemi-bladders with cecum, imperforate anus and abnormalities of the sexual structures.

Colonized—Presence and proliferation of infectious organisms within a wound without eliciting signs of infection.

Colostogram—Radiology study that pushes contrast material through the mucus fistula to identify the level of the fistula and examine distal bowel.

Colostomy—Surgical opening of the colon onto the abdomen.

Congenital Cystic Adenomatoid Malformation (CCAM)—Solid or cystic masses in the lung that communicate with the normal tracheobronchial tree and derive their vascular supply from the pulmonary circulation.

Contaminated—Presence of microorganisms on a wound surface, without proliferation.

Cryptorchidism—Failure of the testis to descend into the scrotum during gestation.

Cystic hygroma—A lymphangioma

Debridement—Process of removing devitalized tissue and foreign matter from a wound.

Defunctionalized—Disconnected organ, such as the bowel distal to a stoma.

Dehiscence—Separation of the edges of a previously approximated wound.

Denuded—Skin that has had the epidermis removed through trauma or exposure to caustic material.

Dissection—Separation of tissues.

Diverticulum— A blind pouch or structure leading from a larger canal.

Double barrel stoma—Two stomas, one created from the functional end and the other from the defunctionalized end of the GI or GU tract. The stomas are usually brought to the abdominal wall through the same fascial defect.

Duhamel procedure—Surgical treatment for Hirschsprung's Disease using a rectorectal pull-through technique.

Dumping syndrome— Syndrome of rapid emptying of stomach contents into small intestine; associated with symptoms of sweating and weakness after eating.

Dysmotility—A condition of the intestine in which normal peristalsis is disordered and does not move bowel contents in a coordinated, forward wave.

Effluent—Substance flowing through the GI or GU tract (stool or urine) and discharged out a stoma.

Effusion—A collection of fluid.

Empyema—An accumulation of thick infected fluid or pus in the lungs.

Enterocolitis—Inflammation of the small intestine and colon caused by an incomplete functional obstruction of the rectum with proximal dilation, stasis, and bacterial overgrowth.

Enteroplasty—A surgical procedure to improve the function of the bowel through lengthening or tapering.

ERCP (Endoscopic Retrograde Cholangiopancreatography)—Diagnostic or therapeutic procedure to obtain a radiograph of the pancreatic duct and the biliary tree and identify the caliber of the ducts, stones, or tumors with an endoscope.

Eschar—Thick, dry, leathery necrotic tissue in a wound, usually black.

Escharotomy—Removal of the eschar and underlying tissue of a severely burned patient.

Esophagostomy—Surgical opening of the esophagus onto the throat or chest to treat tracheoesophageal fistula.

Evisceration—Edges of the wound separate and the intestine protrude.

Exteriorization—A part of the body, such as a portion of the intestine, surgically exposed or brought outside the body.

Exudate—Discharge of fluid, cells and other substances from a wound.

Fasciotomy—Surgical incision and division of the fibrous membrane covering the muscle.

Fecalith—A stone or concretion of feces.

Fistula—An abnormal tube-like passage that connects two body tissues; may result from a congenital abnormality or injury.

Fundoplication—Surgical procedure for the treatment of gastroesophageal reflux involving wrapping the stomach fundus around the intraabdominal esophagus.

Gastric decompression—Removal of pressure in the stomach, usually by use of a nasogastric or gastrostomy tube connected to intermittent or constant suction.

Gastroschisis—A congenital abdominal wall defect involving herniation of intestine and other abdominal contents through an opening in the abdominal wall.

Gastrostomy—Surgical procedure to create an opening into the stomach, usually to insert a feeding tube, often called a "g-tube."

Granulation tissue—Highly vascular tissue within a wound composed of cells and connective tissue matrix.

Hamartoma—Tumor resulting from new growth of normal tissues.

Hartmann's pouch—Distal stump of a divided colon that is sutured closed and left in the abdomen.

Hemangioma—Benign tumor composed of dilated blood vessels.

Hernia—Protrusion of tissue through an abnormal opening.

HIDA Scan (hepato-iminodiacetic acid scan)—A nuclear medicine scan used to detect bile flow from the liver through the biliary tree and into the gastrointestinal tract. The addition of cholecystokinin injection (CCK-HIDA) can assess gallbladder contractility and function.

Hirschsprung's disease—A form of chronic intestinal obstruction caused by absence of ganglia in the bowel: also, known as aganglionic megacolon.

Hydrocele—Fluid-filled cyst in the scrotum formed by the tunica vaginalis.

Hypergranulation tissue—Beefy red, friable, inflamed epithelial tissue surrounding the gastrostomy progressing beyond the level of the stoma.

Ileostomy—Surgical opening of the ileum onto the abdomen

Ileus—An intestinal obstruction; the cause of an ileus may be a functional or mechanical obstruction.

Imbricated—The overlapping of the flat fibrous sheet of connecting tissue during abdominal surgery.

Imperforate anus—An anorectal malformation.

Incarceration—Condition in which an organ protrudes through an opening and can not be reduced.

Intussusception—The invagination or telescoping of one intestinal segment into another adjacent segment of bowel, creating an intestinal obstruction.

Jejunostomy—A surgical procedure for inserting a tube through the abdominal wall and into the jejunum to provide food or nutrients when gastrostomy feedings are not possible; often called a "j tube."

Kasai procedure—(Hepatoportoenterostomy) Surgical procedure to establish bile flow in biliary atresia.

Ladd's procedure—Surgical treatment of malrotation.

Laparotomy—Surgical opening of the abdomen.

Laparoscopy—Minimally invasive surgical procedure to explore the abdomen using a laparoscope.

Lithotripsy—The use of shock waves produced by a physical external source used to crush a calculus (stone) in the bladder or urethra.

Loop stoma—Loop of bowel brought to the abdominal wall, artficially divided and everted to create two openings in the same stoma—one opening to the proximal and the other to the distal bowel.

Lymphangioma—A tumor composed of lymph spaces and channels.

Maceration—Overhydration of skin caused by prolonged exposure to moisture. Skin becomes pale or gray, wrinkled, and susceptible to damage.

Malrotation—An asymptomatic anatomic variant that occurs as a result of failure to complete normal rotation and fixation of the bowel during fetal development.

Mucocutaneous junction—Suture line at the junction of the skin and the mucosa of a stoma.

Mucous fistula—Stoma created from the defunctionalized end of a completely divided bowel.

Myotomy—Surgical division or anatomical dissection of muscles.

Obturator sign—Pain on inward rotation of the hip caused by stretching of the obturator internus muscle. This sign may be present with acute appendicitis.

Omphalocele—An abdominal wall defect characterized by protruding intestines covered with a sac which is the amnion of the umbilical cord.

Orchidopexy/Orchiopexy—Surgical treatment of undescended testis.

Ostomy—A surgically created opening; another word for stoma.

Pectus—Chest deformity, including: carinatum— a protrusion of the chest wall and excavatum—a sunken chest wall.

PEG (percutaneous endoscopic gastrostomy)—A feeding gastrostomy tube inserted through a small abdominal incision using an endoscopic guidance.

PEG-J (percutaneous endoscopic gastro-jejunostomy)—A tube inserted with endoscopic guidance which allows simultaneous gastric decompression and jejunal feedings.

Peristomal plane—The area of skin adjacent to a stoma, including irregularities such as skin folds and scars.

Peritonitis—Inflammation of the peritoneum.

Pilonidal cyst or sinus—An abscess or chronic sinus located in the gluteal cleft.

Pneumatosis intestinalis—A condition in which gas-filled blebs are formed in the bowel wall.

Pneumoperitoneum—Air in the peritoneal cavity; indicates the position of the diaphragm.

Prolapse—Telescoping of the bowel out through an opening of a stoma or the anus.

Posterior Sagittal Anoplasty (PSAP)—A surgical procedure that is done for low anorectal malformations to relocate the rectum into the normal anatomic position.

Posterior Sagittal Anorectoplasty (PSARP or Pena Procedure)—Surgical procedure that is done for high anorectal malformations through a posterior approach to divide the rectum, urinary and reproductive structures and place the anus in the proper anatomic position.

Pseudocyst—An abnormal or dilated space resembling a cyst.

Psoas sign—Pain with passive hip flexion or extension.

Pull through—One of several operations to correct Hirschsprung's disease, including the Swenson, Duhamel, and Soave.

Pulmonary sequestration—An isolated lobe of lung tissue having no bronchial connection to the tracheobronchial system.

Pyelostomy—A surgically created opening or stoma into the renal pelvis.

Pyloromyotomy—Surgical treatment of pyloric stenosis.

Resection—Surgical removal of a portion of an organ or a mass of tissue.

Retention ring—Device, often a red rubber catheter, placed beneath the bowel of a loop stoma to hold the bowel above skin level until the suture line heals.

Rovsing's sign—Pain in the appendiceal area when pressure is applied to the opposite side of the abdomen.

Serosal layer—The outside layer of the gastrointestinal tract; extends from the stomach to the mesentery and contains nerves, lymphatics, and the blood vessels.

Short bowel syndrome—A condition in which there is inadequate bowel to provide full enteral nutrition. Also, known as Short gut syndrome.

Silo—Device used to contain bowel that is exterior to the body as in gastroschisis or abdominal compartment syndrome.

Slough—Stringy, loose, moist necrotic tissue in a wound, usually tan, yellow or gray.

Soave—Surgical treatment for Hirschsprung's disease using an endorectal pull-through.

Sternal cleft—A longitudinal opening or fissure of the sternum.

Stricturoplasty—The surgical opening of a stricture.

Stoma—Surgically created opening between the abdominal wall and the gastrointestinal or urinary tract to divert the flow of feces or urine.

Suppurative—Associated with the generation of or producing pus.

Swenson—Surgical treatment for Hirschsprung's disease performed through a combined abdominoperineal approach.

Thoracotomy—Surgical incision of the chest wall.

Thyroglossal duct cyst—Fluid-filled midline structure caused by abnormal development of the thyroid gland.

Tracheoesophageal fistula—Abnormal connection between the esophagus and trachea.

Twiddler's syndrome—Moving an implanted device by "twiddling" with the device.

Urachal sinus—a fistula from bladder to umbilicus. In fetal development, the urachus is a normal connection from bladder to umbilicus which usually obliterates after birth.

Urinary diversion—A surgical procedure that creates a route for urine to exit the body.

Urostomy—Surgically created opening between the abdominal wall and any part of the urinary tract.

VATS—Video assisted thoroscopic surgery.

Vesicostomy—Surgically created opening between the abdominal wall and the bladder.

Volvulus—Twisting or kinking of the midgut creating an intestinal obstruction.

Web—membrane.

Index

Page numbers followed by *t* and *f* indicate tables and figures, respectively.

A